Stahl's Essential Psychopharmacology

The Prescriber's Guide

THIRD EDITION

Stephen M. Stahl

University of California at San Diego,
San Diego, California

Editorial assistant
Meghan M. Grady

With illustrations by
Nancy Muntner

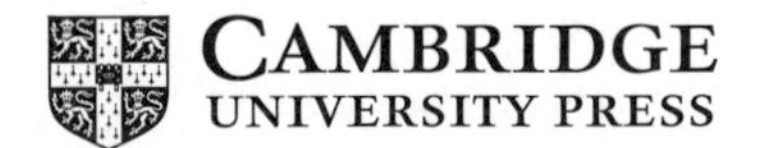

CAMBRIDGE UNIVERSITY PRESS
Cambridge, New York, Melbourne, Madrid, Cape Town, Singapore, San Paulo, Delhi

CAMBRIDGE UNIVERSITY PRESS
32 Avenue of the Americas, New York, NY 10013-2473, USA

www.cambridge.org
Information on this title: www.cambridge.org/9780521743990

First published 2005
Revised and updated edition published 2006
Third edition published 2009

Printed in the United States of America

A catalog record for this publication is available from the British Library.

Library of Congress Cataloging in Publication Data

ISBN 978-0-521-74399-0 paperback

Contents

Introduction

This *Guide* is intended to complement *Stahl's Essential Psychopharmacology*. *Stahl's Essential Psychopharmacology* emphasizes mechanisms of action and how psychotropic drugs work upon receptors and enzymes in the brain. This guide gives practical information on how to use these drugs in clinical practice.

It would be impossible to include all available information about any drug in a single work, and no attempt is made here to be comprehensive. The purpose of this guide is instead to integrate the art of clinical practice with the science of psychopharmacology. That means including only essential facts in order to keep things short. Unfortunately that also means excluding less critical facts as well as extraneous information, which may nevertheless be useful to the reader but would make the book too long and dilute the most important information. In deciding what to include and what to omit, the author has drawn upon common sense and 30 years of clinical experience with patients. He has also consulted with many experienced clinicians and analyzed the evidence from controlled clinical trials and regulatory filings with government agencies.

In order to meet the needs of the clinician and to facilitate future updates of this *Guide*, the opinions of readers are sincerely solicited. Feedback can be emailed to feedback@neiglobal.com. Specifically, are the best and most essential psychotropic drugs included here? Do you find any factual errors? Are there agreements or disagreements with any of the opinions expressed here? Are there suggestions for any additional tips or pearls for future editions? Any and all suggestions and comments are welcomed.

All of the selected drugs are presented in the same design format in order to facilitate rapid access to information. Specifically, each drug is broken down into five sections, each designated by a unique color background: ■ therapeutics, ■ side effects, ■ dosing and use, ■ special populations, and ■ the art of psychopharmacology, followed by key references.

Therapeutics covers the brand names in major countries; the class of drug; what it is commonly prescribed and approved for by the United States Food and Drug Administration (FDA); how the drug works; how long it takes to work; what to do if it works or if it doesn't work; the best augmenting combinations for partial response or treatment resistance; and the tests (if any) that are required.

Side effects explains how the drug causes side effects; gives a list of notable, life-threatening, or dangerous side effects; gives a specific rating for weight gain or sedation; and gives advice about how to handle side effects, including best augmenting agents for side effects.

Dosing and use gives the usual dosing range; dosage forms; how to dose and dosing tips; symptoms of overdose; long-term use; if habit forming, how to stop; pharmacokinetics; drug interactions; when not to use and other warnings or precautions.

Special populations gives specific information about any possible renal, hepatic, and cardiac impairments, and any precautions to be taken for treating the elderly, children, adolescents, and pregnant and breast-feeding women.

The art of psychopharmacology gives the author's opinions on issues such as the potential advantages and disadvantages of any one drug, the primary target symptoms, and clinical pearls to get the best out of a drug.

At the back of the guide are several indices. The first is an index by drug name, giving both generic names (uncapitalized) and trade names (capitalized and followed by the generic name in parentheses). The second is an index of common uses for the generic drugs included in the guide and is organized by disorder/symptom. Agents that are approved by the FDA for a particular use are shown in bold. The third index is organized by drug class, and lists all the agents that fall within each particular class. In addition to these indices there is a list of abbreviations; FDA definitions for the Pregnancy Categories A, B, C, D, and X, and, finally, an index of the icons used in the guide.

Readers are encouraged to consult standard references[1] and comprehensive psychiatry and pharmacology textbooks for more in-depth information. They are also reminded that the art of psychopharmacology section is the author's opinion.

It is strongly advised that readers familiarize themselves with the standard use of these drugs before attempting any of the more exotic uses discussed, such as unusual drug combinations and doses. Reading about both drugs before augmenting one with the other is also strongly recommended. Today's psychopharmacologist should also regularly track blood pressure, weight, and body mass index for most of his or her patients. The dutiful clinician will also check out the drug interactions of non-central-nervous-system (CNS) drugs with those that act in the CNS, including any prescribed by other clinicians.

Certain drugs may be for experts only and might include clozapine, thioridazine, pimozide, nefazodone, mesoridazine, and MAO inhibitors, among others. Off-label uses not approved by the FDA and inadequately studied doses or combinations of drugs may also be for the expert only, who can weigh risks and benefits in the presence of sometimes vague and conflicting evidence. Pregnant or nursing women, or people with two or more psychiatric illnesses, substance abuse, and/or a concomitant medical illness may be suitable patients for the expert only. Controlled substances also require expertise. Use your best judgment as to your level of expertise and realize that we are all learning in this rapidly advancing field. The practice of medicine is often not so much a science as it is an art. It is important to stay within the standards of medical care for the field, and also within your personal comfort zone, while trying to help extremely ill and often difficult patients with medicines than can sometimes transform their lives and relieve their suffering.

Finally, this book is intended to be genuinely helpful for practitioners of psychopharmacology by providing them with the mixture of facts and opinions selected by the author. Ultimately, prescribing choices are the reader's responsibility. Every effort has been made in preparing this book to provide accurate and up-to-date information in accord with accepted standards and practice at the time of publication. Nevertheless, the psychopharmacology field is evolving rapidly and the author and publisher make no warranties that the information contained herein is totally free from error, not least because clinical standards are constantly changing through research and regulation. Furthermore, the author and publisher disclaim any responsibility for the continued currency of this information and disclaim all liability for any and all damages, including direct or consequential damages, resulting from the use of information contained in this book. Doctors recommending and patients using these drugs are strongly advised to pay careful attention to, and consult information provided by, the manufacturer.

[1]For example, *Physician's Desk Reference* and *Martindale: The Complete Drug Reference.*

List of icons

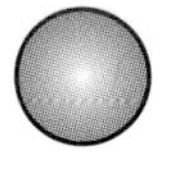
alcohol dependence treatment

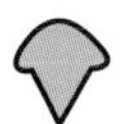
alpha 2 agonist

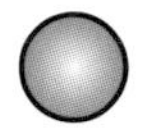
anticonvulsant

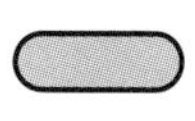
antihistamine

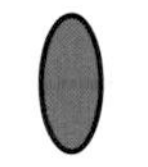
benzodiazepine

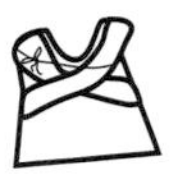
cholinesterase inhibitor

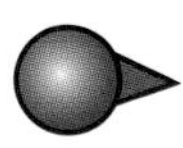
conventional antipsychotic

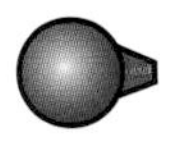
dopamine stabilizer

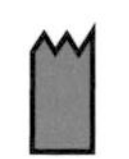
lithium

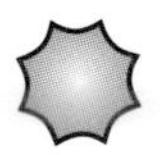
modafinil (wake-promoter)

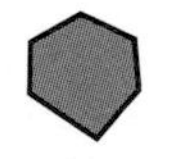
monoamine oxidase inhibitor

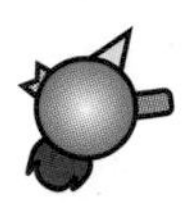
nefazodone (serotonin antagonist/reuptake inhibitor)

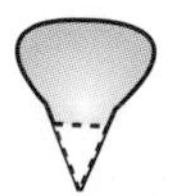
nicotinic partial agonist

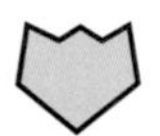

N-methyl-D-aspartate antagonist

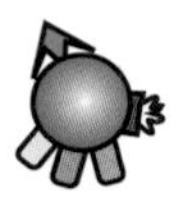

noradrenergic and specific serotonergic antidepressant

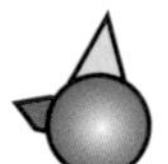

norepinephrine and dopamine reuptake inhibitor

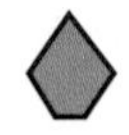

sedative-hypnotic

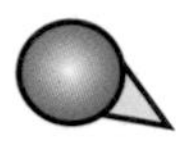

selective norepinephrine reuptake inhibitor

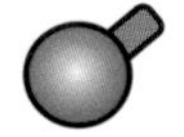

selective serotonin reuptake inhibitor

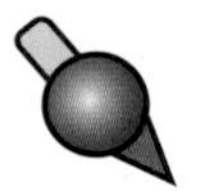

serotonin-dopamine antagonist

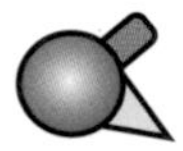

serotonin and norepinephrine reuptake inhibitor

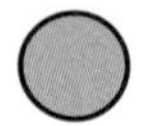

serotonin 1A partial agonist

stimulant

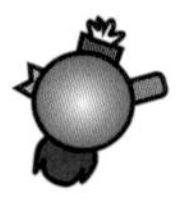

trazodone (serotonin antagonist/reuptake inhibitor)

tricyclic/tetracyclic antidepressant

How the drug works, mechanism of action

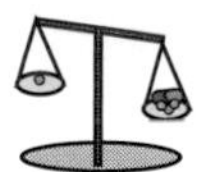

Best augmenting agents to add for partial response or treatment-resistance

Life-threatening or dangerous side effects

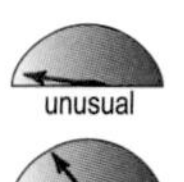

Weight Gain: Degrees of weight gain associated with the drug, with unusual signifying that weight gain has been reported but is not expected; not unusual signifying that weight gain occurs in a significant minority; common signifying that many experience weight gain and/or it can be significant in amount; and problematic signifying that weight gain occurs frequently, can be significant in amount, and may be a health problem in some patients

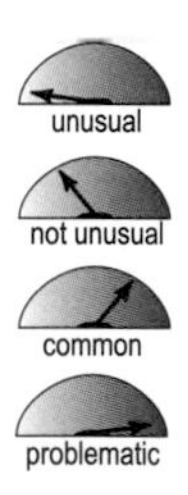

Sedation: Degrees of sedation associated with the drug, with unusual signifying that sedation has been reported but is not expected; not unusual signifying that sedation occurs in a significant minority; common signifying that many experience sedation and/or it can be significant in amount; and problematic signifying that sedation occurs frequently, can be significant in amount, and may be a health problem in some patients

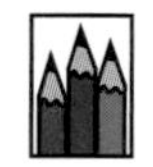

Tips for dosing based on the clinical expertise of the author

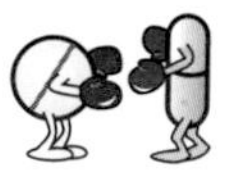

Drug interactions that may occur

Warnings and precautions regarding use of the drug

Dosing and other information specific to children and adolescents

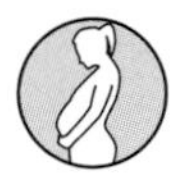

Information regarding use of the drug during pregnancy

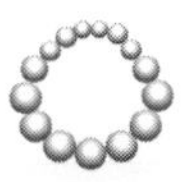

Clinical pearls of information based on the clinical expertise of the author

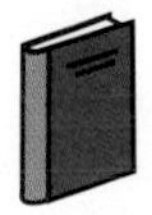

Suggested reading

THERAPEUTICS

Brands • Campral

see index for additional brand names

Generic? Not in U.S.

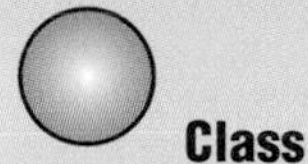

Class

- Alcohol dependence treatment

Commonly Prescribed for

(bold for FDA approved)

- **Maintenance of alcohol abstinence**

How the Drug Works

- Theoretically reduces excitatory glutamate neurotransmission and increases inhibitory gamma-aminobutyric acid (GABA) neurotransmission
- Binds to and blocks certain glutamate receptors, including metabotropic glutamate receptors
- Because withdrawal of alcohol following chronic administration can lead to excessive glutamate activity and deficient GABA activity, acamprosate can act as "artificial alcohol" to mitigate these effects

How Long Until It Works

- Has demonstrated efficacy in trials lasting between 13 and 52 weeks

If It Works

- Increases abstinence from alcohol

If It Doesn't Work

- Evaluate for and address contributing factors
- Consider switching to another agent
- Consider augmenting with naltrexone

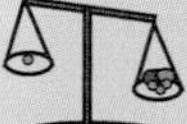

Best Augmenting Combos for Partial Response or Treatment Resistance

- Naltrexone
- Augmentation therapy may be more effective than monotherapy
- Augmentation with behavioral, educational, and/or supportive therapy in groups or as an individual is probably key to successful treatment

Tests

- None for healthy individuals

SIDE EFFECTS

How Drug Causes Side Effects

- Theoretically, behavioral side effects due to changes in neurotransmitter concentrations at receptors in parts of the brain and body other than those that cause therapeutic actions
- Gastrointestinal side effects may be related to large doses of a drug that is an amino acid derivative, increasing osmotic absorption in the GI tract

Notable Side Effects

- Diarrhea, nausea
- Anxiety, depression

Life-Threatening or Dangerous Side Effects

- Suicidal ideation and behavior (suicidality)

Weight Gain

- Reported but not expected

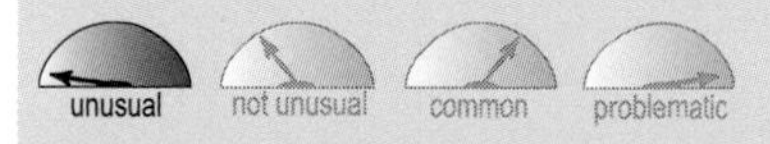

Sedation

- Reported but not expected

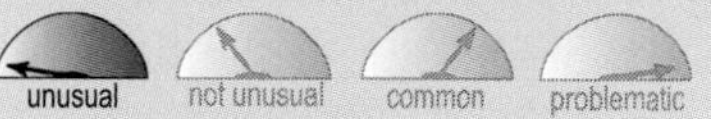

What to Do About Side Effects

- Wait
- Adjust dose
- If side effects persist, discontinue use

Best Augmenting Agents for Side Effects

- Dose reduction or switching to another agent may be more effective since most side effects cannot be improved with an augmenting agent

DOSING AND USE

Usual Dosage Range
- 666 mg three times daily

Dosage Forms
- Tablet 333 mg

How To Dose
- Patient should begin treatment as soon as possible after achieving abstinence
- Recommended dose is 666 mg three times daily; titration is not required

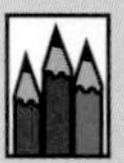

Dosing Tips
- Providing educational materials and counseling in combination with acamprosate treatment can increase the chances of success
- Patients should be advised to continue treatment even if relapse occurs and to disclose any renewed drinking
- Although absorption of acamprosate is not affected by food, it may aid adherence if patients who regularly eat three meals per day take each dose with a meal
- Adherence with three times daily dosing can be a problem; having patient focus on frequent oral dosing of drug rather than frequent drinking may be helpful in some patients

Overdose
- Limited available data; diarrhea

Long-Term Use
- Has been studied in trials up to one year

Habit Forming
- No

How to Stop
- Taper not necessary

Pharmacokinetics
- Terminal half-life 20–33 hours
- Excreted unchanged via the kidneys

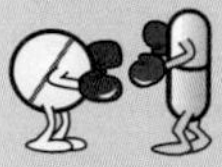

Drug Interactions
- Does not inhibit hepatic enzymes, and thus is unlikely to affect plasma concentrations of drugs metabolized by those enzymes
- Is not hepatically metabolized and thus is unlikely to be affected by drugs that induce or inhibit hepatic enzymes
- Concomitant administration with naltrexone may increase plasma levels of acamprosate, but this does not appear to be clinically significant and dose adjustment is not recommended

Other Warnings/Precautions
- Monitor patients for emergence of depressed mood or suicidal ideation and behavior (suicidality)
- Use cautiously in individuals with known psychiatric illness

Do Not Use
- If patient has severe renal impairment
- If there is a proven allergy to acamprosate

SPECIAL POPULATIONS

Renal Impairment
- For moderate impairment, recommended dose is 333 mg three times daily
- Contraindicated in severe impairment

Hepatic Impairment
- Dose adjustment not generally necessary

Cardiac Impairment
- Limited available data

Elderly
- Some patients may tolerate lower doses better
- Consider monitoring renal function

Children and Adolescents
- Safety and efficacy have not been established

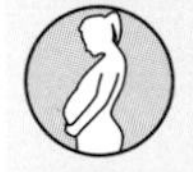

Pregnancy
- Risk Category C [some animal studies show adverse effects; no controlled studies in humans]
- Pregnant women needing to stop drinking may consider behavioral therapy before pharmacotherapy

- Not generally recommended for use during pregnancy, especially during first trimester

Breast Feeding

- Unknown if acamprosate is secreted in human breast milk, but all psychotropics assumed to be secreted in breast milk
- Recommended either to discontinue drug or bottle feed

THE ART OF PSYCHOPHARMACOLOGY

Potential Advantages

- Individuals who have recently abstained from alcohol
- For the chronic daily drinker

Potential Disadvantages

- Individuals who are not abstinent at time of treatment initiation
- For binge drinkers

Primary Target Symptoms

- Alcohol dependence

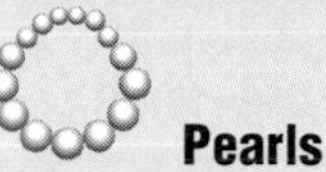

Pearls

- Because acamprosate serves as "artificial alcohol," it may be less effective in situations in which the individual has not yet abstained from alcohol or suffers a lapse
- Thus acamprosate may be a preferred treatment if the goal is complete abstinence, but may not be preferred if the goal is reduced-risk drinking

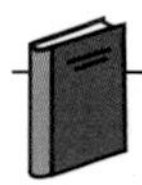

Suggested Reading

Anton RF, O'Malley SS, Ciraulo DA et al. Combined pharmacotherapies and behavioral interventions for alcohol dependence: the COMBINE study: a randomized controlled trial. JAMA 2006;295(17):2003–17.

Kranzler HR, Gage A. Acamprosate efficacy in alcohol-dependent patients: summary of results from three pivotal trials. Am J Addictions 2008;17:70–6.

Rosner S, Leucht S, Lehert P, Soyka M. Acamprosate supports abstinence, naltrexone prevents excessive drinking: evidence from a met-analysis with unreported outcomes. J Psychopharmacol 2008;22:11–23.

THERAPEUTICS

Brands • Xanax, Xanax XR

see index for additional brand names

Generic? Yes

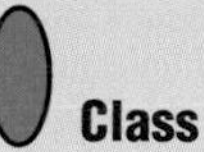

Class

- Benzodiazepine (anxiolytic)

Commonly Prescribed for

(bold for FDA approved)

- **Generalized anxiety disorder (IR)**
- **Panic disorder (IR and XR)**
- Other anxiety disorders
- Anxiety associated with depression
- Premenstrual dysphoric disorder
- Irritable bowel syndrome and other somatic symptoms associated with anxiety disorders
- Insomnia
- Acute mania (adjunctive)
- Acute psychosis (adjunctive)

How the Drug Works

- Binds to benzodiazepine receptors at the GABA-A ligand-gated chloride channel complex
- Enhances the inhibitory effects of GABA
- Boosts chloride conductance through GABA-regulated channels
- Inhibits neuronal activity presumably in amygdala-centered fear circuits to provide therapeutic benefits in anxiety disorders

How Long Until It Works

- Some immediate relief with first dosing is common; can take several weeks with daily dosing for maximal therapeutic benefit

If It Works

- For short-term symptoms of anxiety – after a few weeks, discontinue use or use on an "as-needed" basis
- For chronic anxiety disorders, the goal of treatment is complete remission of symptoms as well as prevention of future relapses
- For chronic anxiety disorders, treatment most often reduces or even eliminates symptoms, but not a cure since symptoms can recur after medicine stopped
- For long-term symptoms of anxiety, consider switching to an SSRI or SNRI for long-term maintenance
- If long-term maintenance with a benzodiazepine is necessary, continue treatment for 6 months after symptoms resolve, and then taper dose slowly
- If symptoms reemerge, consider treatment with an SSRI or SNRI, or consider restarting the benzodiazepine; sometimes benzodiazepines have to be used in combination with SSRIs or SNRIs for best results

If It Doesn't Work

- Consider switching to another agent or adding an appropriate augmenting agent
- Consider psychotherapy, especially cognitive behavioral psychotherapy
- Consider presence of concomitant substance abuse
- Consider presence of alprazolam abuse
- Consider another diagnosis, such as a comorbid medical condition

Best Augmenting Combos for Partial Response or Treatment Resistance

- Benzodiazepines are frequently used as augmenting agents for antipsychotics and mood stabilizers in the treatment of psychotic and bipolar disorders
- Benzodiazepines are frequently used as augmenting agents for SSRIs and SNRIs in the treatment of anxiety disorders
- Not generally rational to combine with other benzodiazepines
- Caution if using as an anxiolytic concomitantly with other sedative hypnotics for sleep

Tests

- In patients with seizure disorders, concomitant medical illness, and/or those with multiple concomitant long-term medications, periodic liver tests and blood counts may be prudent

SIDE EFFECTS

How Drug Causes Side Effects

- Same mechanism for side effects as for therapeutic effects – namely due to

excessive actions at benzodiazepine receptors
- Long-term adaptations in benzodiazepine receptors may explain the development of dependence, tolerance, and withdrawal
- Side effects are generally immediate, but immediate side effects often disappear in time

Notable Side Effects

* ✽ Sedation, fatigue, depression
* ✽ Dizziness, ataxia, slurred speech, weakness
* ✽ Forgetfulness, confusion
* ✽ Hyperexcitability, nervousness
- Rare hallucinations, mania
- Rare hypotension
- Hypersalivation, dry mouth

Life-Threatening or Dangerous Side Effects

- Respiratory depression, especially when taken with CNS depressants in overdose
- Rare hepatic dysfunction, renal dysfunction, blood dyscrasias

Weight Gain

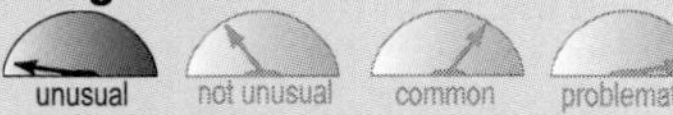

- Reported but not expected

Sedation

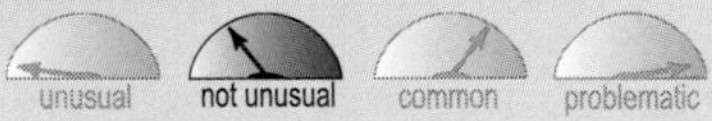

- Occurs in significant minority
- Especially at initiation of treatment or when dose increases
- Tolerance often develops over time

What to Do About Side Effects

- Wait
- Wait
- Wait
- Lower the dose
- Switch to alprazolam XR
- Take largest dose at bedtime to avoid sedative effects during the day
- Switch to another agent
- Administer flumazenil if side effects are severe or life-threatening

Best Augmenting Agents for Side Effects

- Many side effects cannot be improved with an augmenting agent

DOSING AND USE

Usual Dosage Range

- Anxiety: alprazolam IR: 1–4 mg/day
- Panic: alprazolam IR: 5–6 mg/day
- Panic: alprazolam XR: 3–6 mg/day

Dosage Forms

- Alprazolam IR tablet 0.25 mg scored, 0.4 mg (Japan), 0.5 mg scored, 0.8 mg (Japan), 1 mg scored, 2 mg multiscored
- Alprazolam IR orally disintegrating tablet 0.25 mg, 0.5 mg, 1 mg, 2 mg
- Alprazolam IR solution, concentrate 1 mg/mL
- Alprazolam XR (extended-release) tablet 0.5 mg, 1 mg, 2 mg, 3 mg

How To Dose

- For anxiety, alprazolam IR should be started at 0.75–1.5 mg/day divided into 3 doses; increase dose every 3–4 days until desired efficacy is reached; maximum dose generally 4 mg/day
- For panic, alprazolam IR should be started at 1.5 mg/day divided into 3 doses; increase 1 mg or less every 3–4 days until desired efficacy is reached, increasing by smaller amounts for dosage over 4 mg/day; may require as much as 10 mg/day for desired efficacy in difficult cases
- For panic, alprazolam XR should be started at 0.5–1 mg/day once daily in the morning; dose may be increased by 1 mg/day every 3–4 days until desired efficacy is reached; maximum dose generally 10 mg/day

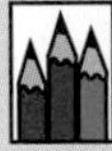

Dosing Tips

- Use lowest possible effective dose for the shortest possible period of time (a benzodiazepine-sparing strategy)
- Assess need for continued treatment regularly
- Risk of dependence may increase with dose and duration of treatment

- For interdose symptoms of anxiety, can either increase dose or maintain same total daily dose but divide into more frequent doses, or give as extended-release formulation
- Can also use an as-needed occasional "top up" dose for interdose anxiety
- Because panic disorder can require doses higher than 4 mg/day, the risk of dependence may be greater in these patients
- Some severely ill patients may require 8 mg/day or more
- Extended-release formulation needs to be taken only once or twice daily
- Do not break or chew XR tablets, as this will alter controlled-release properties
- Frequency of dosing in practice is often greater than predicted from half-life, as duration of biological activity is often shorter than pharmacokinetic terminal half-life
- Alprazolam and alprazolam XR generally dosed about one tenth the dosage of diazepam

❋ Alprazolam and alprazolam XR generally dosed about twice the dosage of clonazepam

Overdose

- Fatalities have been reported both in monotherapy and in conjunction with alcohol; sedation, confusion, poor coordination, diminished reflexes, coma

Long-Term Use

- Risk of dependence, particularly for treatment periods longer than 12 weeks and especially in patients with past or current polysubstance abuse

Habit Forming

- Alprazolam is a Schedule IV drug
- Patients may develop dependence and/or tolerance with long-term use

How to Stop

- Seizures may rarely occur on withdrawal, especially if withdrawal is abrupt; greater risk for doses above 4 mg and in those with additional risks for seizures, including those with a history of seizures
- Taper by 0.5 mg every 3 days to reduce chances of withdrawal effects
- For difficult to taper cases, consider reducing dose much more slowly after reaching 3 mg/day, perhaps by as little as 0.25 mg per week or less
- For other patients with severe problems discontinuing a benzodiazepine, dosing may need to be tapered over many months (i.e., reduce dose by 1% every 3 days by crushing tablet and suspending or dissolving in 100 mL of fruit juice and then disposing of 1 mL while drinking the rest; 3–7 days later, dispose of 2 mL, and so on). This is both a form of very slow biological tapering and a form of behavioral desensitization
- Be sure to differentiate reemergence of symptoms requiring reinstitution of treatment from withdrawal symptoms
- Benzodiazepine-dependent anxiety patients and insulin-dependent diabetics are not addicted to their medications. When benzodiazepine-dependent patients stop their medication, disease symptoms can reemerge or can worsen (rebound), and/or withdrawal symptoms can emerge

Pharmacokinetics

- Metabolized by CYP450 3A4
- Inactive metabolites
- Elimination half-life 12–15 hours

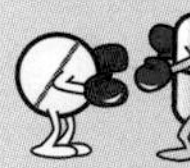

Drug Interactions

- Increased depressive effects when taken with other CNS depressants
- Inhibitors of CYP450 3A, such as nefazodone, fluvoxamine, fluoxetine, and even grapefruit juice, may decrease clearance of alprazolam and thereby raise alprazolam plasma levels and enhance sedative side effects; alprazolam dose may need to be lowered
- Thus, azole antifungal agents (such as ketoconazole and itraconazole), macrolide antibiotics, and protease inhibitors may also raise alprazolam plasma levels
- Inducers of CYP450 3A, such as carbamazepine, may increase clearance of alprazolam and lower alprazolam plasma levels and possibly reduce therapeutic effects

Other Warnings/ Precautions

- Dosage changes should be made in collaboration with prescriber
- Use with caution in patients with pulmonary disease; rare reports of death after initiation of benzodiazepines in patients with severe pulmonary impairment
- History of drug or alcohol abuse often creates greater risk for dependency
- Hypomania and mania have occurred in depressed patients taking alprazolam
- Use only with extreme caution if patient has obstructive sleep apnea
- Some depressed patients may experience a worsening of suicidal ideation
- Some patients may exhibit abnormal thinking or behavioral changes similar to those caused by other CNS depressants (i.e., either depressant actions or disinhibiting actions)

Do Not Use

- If patient has narrow angle-closure glaucoma
- If patient is taking ketoconazole or itraconazole (azole antifungal agents)
- If there is a proven allergy to alprazolam or any benzodiazepine

SPECIAL POPULATIONS

Renal Impairment

- Drug should be used with caution

Hepatic Impairment

- Should begin with lower starting dose (0.5–0.75 mg/day in 2 or 3 divided doses)

Cardiac Impairment

- Benzodiazepines have been used to treat anxiety associated with acute myocardial infarction

Elderly

- Should begin with lower starting dose (0.5–0.75 mg/day in 2 or 3 divided doses) and be monitored closely

Children and Adolescents

- Safety and efficacy not established but often used, especially short-term and at the lower end of the dosing scale
- Long-term effects of alprazolam in children/adolescents are unknown
- Should generally receive lower doses and be more closely monitored

Pregnancy

- Risk Category D [positive evidence of risk to human fetus; potential benefits may still justify its use during pregnancy]
- Possible increased risk of birth defects when benzodiazepines taken during pregnancy
- Because of the potential risks, alprazolam is not generally recommended as treatment for anxiety during pregnancy, especially during the first trimester
- Drug should be tapered if discontinued
- Infants whose mothers received a benzodiazepine late in pregnancy may experience withdrawal effects
- Neonatal flaccidity has been reported in infants whose mothers took a benzodiazepine during pregnancy
- Seizures, even mild seizures, may cause harm to the embryo/fetus

Breast Feeding

- Some drug is found in mother's breast milk
- ✽ Recommended either to discontinue drug or bottle feed
- Effects on infant have been observed and include feeding difficulties, sedation, and weight loss

THE ART OF PSYCHOPHARMACOLOGY

Potential Advantages

- Rapid onset of action
- Less sedation than some other benzodiazepines
- Availability of an XR formulation with longer duration of action

Potential Disadvantages

- Euphoria may lead to abuse
- Abuse especially risky in past or present substance abusers

Primary Target Symptoms

- Panic attacks
- Anxiety

Pearls

- * One of the most popular benzodiazepines for anxiety, especially among primary care physicians and psychiatrists
- Is a very useful adjunct to SSRIs and SNRIs in the treatment of numerous anxiety disorders
- Not effective for treating psychosis as a monotherapy, but can be used as an adjunct to antipsychotics
- Not effective for treating bipolar disorder as a monotherapy, but can be used as an adjunct to mood stabilizers and antipsychotics
- May both cause depression and treat depression in different patients
- Risk of seizure is greatest during the first 3 days after discontinuation of alprazolam, especially in those with prior seizures, head injuries, or withdrawal from drugs of abuse
- Clinical duration of action may be shorter than plasma half-life, leading to dosing more frequently than 2–3 times daily in some patients, especially for immediate-release alprazolam
- Adding fluvoxamine, fluoxetine, or nefazodone can increase alprazolam levels and make the patient very sleepy unless the alprazolam dose is lowered by half or more
- When using to treat insomnia, remember that insomnia may be a symptom of some other primary disorder itself, and thus warrant evaluation for comorbid psychiatric and/or medical conditions
- * Alprazolam XR may be less sedating than immediate-release alprazolam
- * Alprazolam XR may be dosed less frequently than immediate-release alprazolam, and lead to less interdose breakthrough symptoms and less "clock-watching" in anxious patients
- Slower rises in plasma drug levels for alprazolam XR have the potential to reduce euphoria/abuse liability, but this has not been proven
- Slower falls in plasma drug levels for alprazolam XR have the potential to facilitate drug discontinuation by reducing withdrawal symptoms, but this has not been proven
- * Alprozolam XR generally has longer biological duration of action than clonazepam
- * If clonazepam can be considered a "long-acting alprazolam-like anxiolytic," then alprazolam XR can be considered "an even longer-acting clonazepam-like anxiolytic" with the potential of improved tolerability features in terms of less euphoria, abuse, dependence, and withdrawal problems, but this has not been proven

Suggested Reading

DeVane CL, Ware MR, Lydiard RB. Pharmacokinetics, pharmacodynamics, and treatment issues of benzodiazepines: alprazolam, adinazolam, and clonazepam. Psychopharmacol Bull 1991;27:463–73.

Greenblatt DJ, Wright CE. Clinical pharmacokinetics of alprazolam. Therapeutic implications. Clin Pharmacokinet 1993; 24:453–71.

Jonas JM, Cohon MS. A comparison of the safety and efficacy of alprazolam versus other agents in the treatment of anxiety, panic, and depression: a review of the literature. J Clin Psychiatry 1993;54 (Suppl):25–45.

Klein E. The role of extended-release benzodiazepines in the treatment of anxiety: a risk-benefit evaluation with a focus on extended-release alprazolam. J Clin Psychiatry 2002;63 (Suppl 14):27–33.

Speigel DA. Efficacy studies of alprazolam in panic disorder. Psychopharmacol Bull 1998; 34:191–95.

THERAPEUTICS

Brands • Solian
see index for additional brand names

Generic? No

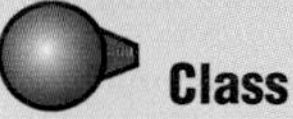

Class

- Atypical antipsychotic (benzamide; possibly a dopamine stabilizer and dopamine partial agonist)

Commonly Prescribed for

(bold for FDA approved)
- Schizophrenia, acute and chronic (outside of U.S., especially Europe)
- Dysthymia

How the Drug Works

- Theoretically blocks presynaptic dopamine 2 receptors at low doses
- Theoretically blocks postsynaptic dopamine 2 receptors at higher doses

✻ May be a partial agonist at dopamine 2 receptors, which would theoretically reduce dopamine output when dopamine concentrations are high and increase dopamine output when dopamine concentrations are low
- Blocks dopamine 3 receptors, which may contribute to its clinical actions

✻ Unlike other atypical antipsychotics, amisulpride does not have potent actions at serotonin receptors

How Long Until It Works

- Psychotic symptoms can improve within 1 week, but it may take several weeks for full effect on behavior as well as on cognition and affective stabilization
- Classically recommended to wait at least 4–6 weeks to determine efficacy of drug, but in practice some patients require up to 16–20 weeks to show a good response, especially on cognitive symptoms

If It Works

- Most often reduces positive symptoms in schizophrenia but does not eliminate them
- Can improve negative symptoms, as well as aggressive, cognitive, and affective symptoms in schizophrenia
- Most schizophrenic patients do not have a total remission of symptoms but rather a reduction of symptoms by about a third
- Perhaps 5–15% of schizophrenic patients can experience an overall improvement of greater than 50–60%, especially when receiving stable treatment for more than a year
- Such patients are considered super-responders or "awakeners" since they may be well enough to be employed, live independently, and sustain long-term relationships
- Continue treatment until reaching a plateau of improvement
- After reaching a satisfactory plateau, continue treatment for at least a year after first episode of psychosis
- For second and subsequent episodes of psychosis, treatment may need to be indefinite
- Even for first episodes of psychosis, it may be preferable to continue treatment indefinitely to avoid subsequent episodes

If It Doesn't Work

- Try one of the other first-line atypical antipsychotics (risperidone, olanzapine, quetiapine, ziprasidone, aripiprazole, paliperidone)
- If two or more antipsychotic monotherapies do not work, consider clozapine
- If no atypical antipsychotic is effective, consider higher doses or augmentation with valproate or lamotrigine
- Some patients may require treatment with a conventional antipsychotic
- Consider noncompliance and switch to another antipsychotic with fewer side effects or to an antipsychotic that can be given by depot injection
- Consider initiating rehabilitation and psychotherapy
- Consider presence of concomitant drug abuse

Best Augmenting Combos for Partial Response or Treatment Resistance

- Valproic acid (valproate, divalproex, divalproex ER)
- Augmentation of amisulpride has not been systematically studied

- Other mood-stabilizing anticonvulsants (carbamazepine, oxcarbazepine, lamotrigine)
- Lithium
- Benzodiazepines

Tests

✻ Although risk of diabetes and dyslipidemia with amisulpride has not been systematically studied, monitoring as for all other atypical antipsychotics is suggested

Before starting an atypical antipsychotic

✻ Weigh all patients and track BMI during treatment
- Get baseline personal and family history of diabetes, obesity, dyslipidemia, hypertension, and cardiovascular disease
- Get waistline circumference (at umbilicus), blood pressure, fasting plasma glucose, and fasting lipid profile
- Determine if patient is
  - overweight (BMI 25.0–29.9)
  - obese (BMI ≥30)
  - has pre-diabetes (fasting plasma glucose 100–25 mg/dL)
  - has diabetes (fasting plasma glucose >126 mg/dL)
  - has hypertension (BP >140/90 mm Hg)
  - has dyslipidemia (increased total cholesterol, LDL cholesterol, and triglycerides; decreased HDL cholesterol)
- Treat or refer such patients for treatment, including nutrition and weight management, physical activity counseling, smoking cessation, and medical management

Monitoring after starting an atypical antipsychotic

✻ BMI monthly for 3 months, then quarterly
- Consider monitoring fasting triglycerides monthly for several months in patients at high risk for metabolic complications and when initiating or switching antipsychotics
- Blood pressure, fasting plasma glucose, fasting lipids within 3 months and then annually, but earlier and more frequently for patients with diabetes or who have gained >5% initial weight
- Treat or refer for treatment and consider switching to another atypical antipsychotic for patients who become overweight, obese, pre-diabetic, diabetic, hypertensive, or dyslipidemic while receiving an atypical antipsychotic

✻ Even in patients without known diabetes, be vigilant for the rare but life-threatening onset of diabetic ketoacidosis, which always requires immediate treatment by monitoring for the rapid onset of polyuria, polydipsia, weight loss, nausea, vomiting, dehydration, rapid respiration, weakness and clouding of sensorium, even coma
- EKGs may be useful for selected patients (e.g., those with personal or family history of QTc prolongation; cardiac arrhythmia; recent myocardial infarction; uncompensated heart failure; or taking agents that prolong QTc interval such as pimozide, thioridazine, selected antiarrhythmics, moxifloxacin, sparfloxacin, etc.)
- Patients at risk for electrolyte disturbances (e.g., patients on diuretic therapy) should have baseline and periodic serum potassium and magnesium measurements

SIDE EFFECTS

How Drug Causes Side Effects

- By blocking dopamine 2 receptors in the striatum, it can cause motor side effects, especially at high doses
- By blocking dopamine 2 receptors in the pituitary, it can cause elevations in prolactin
- Mechanism of weight gain and possible increased incidence of diabetes and dyslipidemia with atypical antipsychotics is unknown

Notable Side Effects

✻ Extrapyramidal symptoms

✻ Galactorrhea, amenorrhea

✻ Atypical antipsychotics may increase the risk for diabetes and dyslipidemia, although the specific risks associated with amisulpride are unknown
- Insomnia, sedation, agitation, anxiety
- Constipation, weight gain
- Rare tardive dyskinesia

Life-Threatening or Dangerous Side Effects

- Rare neuroleptic malignant syndrome
- Rare seizures
- Dose-dependent QTc prolongation

- Increased risk of death and cerebrovascular events in elderly patients with dementia-related psychosis

Weight Gain

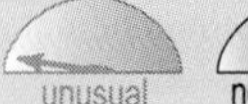
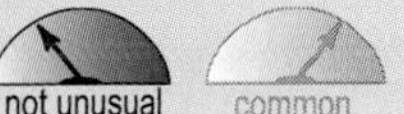

- Occurs in significant minority

Sedation

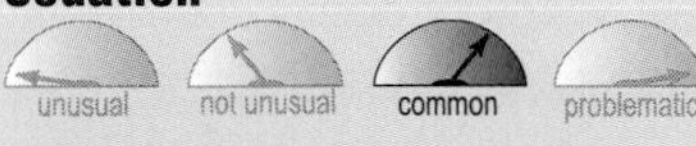

- Many experience and/or can be significant in amount, especially at high doses

What to Do About Side Effects

- Wait
- Wait
- Wait
- Lower the dose
- For motor symptoms, add an anticholinergic agent
- Take more of the dose at bedtime to help reduce daytime sedation
- Weight loss, exercise programs, and medical management for high BMIs, diabetes, dyslipidemia
- Switch to another atypical antipsychotic

Best Augmenting Agents for Side Effects

- Benztropine or trihexyphenidyl for motor side effects
- Many side effects cannot be improved with an augmenting agent

DOSING AND USE

Usual Dosage Range

- Schizophrenia: 400–800 mg/day in 2 doses
- Negative symptoms only: 50–300 mg/day
- Dysthymia: 50 mg/day

Dosage Forms

- Different formulations may be available in different markets
- Tablet 50 mg, 100 mg, 200 mg, 400 mg
- Oral solution 100 mg/mL

How To Dose

- Initial 400–800 mg/day in 2 doses; daily doses above 400 mg should be divided in 2; maximum generally 1,200 mg/day

Dosing Tips

- * Efficacy for negative symptoms in schizophrenia may be achieved at lower doses, while efficacy for positive symptoms may require higher doses
- Patients receiving low doses may need to take the drug only once daily
- * For dysthymia and depression, use only low doses
- * Dose-dependent QTc prolongation, so use with caution, especially at higher doses (>800 mg/day)
- * Amisulpride may accumulate in patients with renal insufficiency, requiring lower dosing or switching to another antipsychotic to avoid QTc prolongation in these patients

Overdose

- Sedation, coma, hypotension, extrapyramidal symptoms

Long-Term Use

- Amisulpride is used for both acute and chronic schizophrenia treatment

Habit Forming

- No

How to Stop

- Slow down-titration (over 6–8 weeks), especially when simultaneously beginning a new antipsychotic while switching (i.e., cross-titration)
- Rapid discontinuation may lead to rebound psychosis and worsening of symptoms

Pharmacokinetics

- Elimination half-life approximately 12 hours
- Excreted largely unchanged

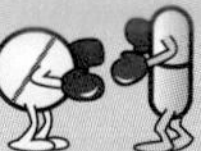

Drug Interactions

- Can decrease the effects of levodopa, dopamine agonists
- Can increase the effects of antihypertensive drugs
- CNS effects may be increased if used with a CNS depressant
- May enhance QTc prolongation of other drugs capable of prolonging QTc interval
- Since amisulpride is only weakly metabolized, few drug interactions that could raise amisulpride plasma levels are expected

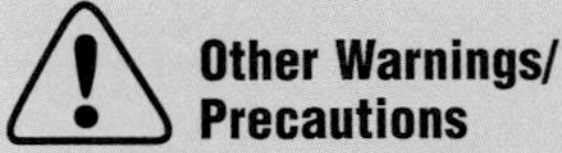

Other Warnings/ Precautions

- Use cautiously in patients with alcohol withdrawal or convulsive disorders because of possible lowering of seizure threshold
- If signs of neuroleptic malignant syndrome develop, treatment should be immediately discontinued
- Because amisulpride may dose-dependently prolong QTc interval, use with caution in patients who have bradycardia or who are taking drugs that can induce bradycardia (e.g., beta blockers, calcium channel blockers, clonidine, digitalis)
- Because amisulpride may dose-dependently prolong QTc interval, use with caution in patients who have hypokalemia and/or hypomagnesemia or who are taking drugs that can induce hypokalemia and/or magnesemia (e.g., diuretics, stimulant laxatives, intravenous amphotericin B, glucocorticoids, tetracosactide)
- Use only with caution if at all in Parkinson's disease or Lewy body dementia, especially at high doses

Do Not Use

- If patient has pheochromocytoma
- If patient has prolactin-dependent tumor
- If patient is pregnant or nursing
- If patient is taking agents capable of significantly prolonging QTc interval (e.g., pimozide; thioridazine; selected antiarrhythmics such as quinidine, disopyramide, amiodarone, and sotalol; selected antibiotics such as moxifloxacin and sparfloxacin)
- If there is a history of QTc prolongation or cardiac arrhythmia, recent acute myocardial infarction, uncompensated heart failure
- If patient is taking cisapride, intravenous erythromycin, or pentamidine
- In children
- If there is a proven allergy to amisulpride

SPECIAL POPULATIONS

Renal Impairment

- Use with caution; drug may accumulate
- Amisulpride is eliminated by the renal route; in cases of severe renal insufficiency, the dose should be decreased and intermittent treatment or switching to another antipsychotic should be considered

Hepatic Impairment

- Use with caution, but dose adjustment not generally necessary

Cardiac Impairment

- Amisulpride produces a dose-dependent prolongation of QTc interval, which may be enhanced by the existence of bradycardia, hypokalemia, congenital or acquired long QTc interval, which should be evaluated prior to administering amisulpride
- Use with caution if treating concomitantly with a medication likely to produce prolonged bradycardia, hypokalemia, slowing of intracardiac conduction, or prolongation of the QTc interval
- Avoid amisulpride in patients with a known history of QTc prolongation, recent acute myocardial infarction, and uncompensated heart failure

Elderly

- Some patients may be more susceptible to sedative and hypotensive effects
- Although atypical antipsychotics are commonly used for behavioral disturbances in dementia, no agent has been approved for treatment of elderly patients with dementia-related psychosis
- Elderly patients with dementia-related psychosis treated with atypical antipsychotics are at an increased risk of death compared to placebo, and also have an increased risk of cerebrovascular events

Children and Adolescents

- Efficacy and safety not established under age 18

Pregnancy

- Although animal studies have not shown teratogenic effect, amisulpride is not recommended for use during pregnancy

- Psychotic symptoms may worsen during pregnancy and some form of treatment may be necessary
- Amisulpride may be preferable to anticonvulsant mood stabilizers if treatment is required during pregnancy

Breast Feeding

- Unknown if amisulpride is secreted in human breast milk, but all psychotropics assumed to be secreted in breast milk
- ✻ Recommended either to discontinue drug or bottle feed

THE ART OF PSYCHOPHARMACOLOGY

Potential Advantages

- Not as clearly associated with weight gain as some other atypical antipsychotics
- For patients who are responsive to low-dose activation effects that reduce negative symptoms and depression

Potential Disadvantages

- Patients who have difficulty being compliant with twice daily dosing
- Patients for whom elevated prolactin may not be desired (e.g., possibly pregnant patients; pubescent girls with amenorrhea; postmenopausal women with low estrogen who do not take estrogen replacement therapy)
- Patients with severe renal impairment

Primary Target Symptoms

- Positive symptoms of psychosis
- Negative symptoms of psychosis
- Depressive symptoms

Pearls

- ✻ Efficacy has been particularly well demonstrated in patients with predominantly negative symptoms
- ✻ The increase in prolactin caused by amisulpride may cause menstruation to stop
- Some treatment-resistant patients with inadequate responses to clozapine may benefit from amisulpride augmentation of clozapine
- Risks of diabetes and dyslipidemia not well studied, but does not seem to cause as much weight gain as some other atypical antipsychotics
- Has atypical antipsychotic properties (i.e., antipsychotic action without a high incidence of extrapyramidal symptoms), especially at low doses, but not a serotonin dopamine antagonist
- Mediates its atypical antipsychotic properties via novel actions on dopamine receptors, perhaps dopamine stabilizing partial agonist actions on dopamine 2 receptors
- May be more of a dopamine 2 antagonist than aripiprazole, but less of a dopamine 2 antagonist than other atypical or conventional antipsychotics
- Low-dose activating actions may be beneficial for negative symptoms in schizophrenia
- Very low doses may be useful in dysthymia
- Compared to sulpiride, amisulpride has better oral bioavailability and more potency, thus allowing lower dosing, less weight gain, and fewer extrapyramidal symptoms
- Compared to other atypical antipsychotics with potent serotonin 2A antagonism, amisulpride may have more extrapyramidal symptoms and prolactin elevation, but may still be classified as an atypical antipsychotic, particularly at low doses
- Patients have very similar antipsychotic responses to any conventional antipsychotic, which is different from atypical antipsychotics where antipsychotic responses of individual patients can occasionally vary greatly from one atypical antipsychotic to another
- Patients with inadequate responses to atypical antipsychotics may benefit from a trial of augmentation with a conventional antipsychotic or switching to a conventional antipsychotic
- However, long-term polypharmacy with a combination of a conventional antipsychotic with an atypical antipsychotic may combine their side effects without clearly augmenting the efficacy of either
- Although a frequent practice by some prescribers, adding two conventional antipsychotics together has little rationale and may reduce tolerability without clearly enhancing efficacy

Suggested Reading

Burns T, Bale R. Clinical advantages of amisulpride in the treatment of acute schizophrenia. J Int Med Res 2001; 29 (6): 451–66.

Curran MP, Perry CM. Spotlight on amisulpride in schizophrenia. CNS Drugs 2002; 16 (3): 207–11.

Leucht S, Pitschel-Walz G, Engel RR, Kissling W. Amisulpride, an unusual "atypical" antipsychotic: a meta-analysis of randomized controlled trials. Am J Psychiatry 2002; 159 (2): 180–90.

THERAPEUTICS

Brands
• Elavil

see index for additional brand names

Generic?
Yes

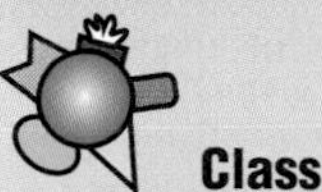

Class
- Tricyclic antidepressant (TCA)
- Serotonin and norepinephrine/noradrenaline reuptake inhibitor

Commonly Prescribed for
(bold for FDA approved)
- **Depression**
- **Endogenous depression**
- * Neuropathic pain/chronic pain
- * Fibromyalgia
- * Headache
- * Low back pain/neck pain
- Anxiety
- Insomnia
- Treatment-resistant depression

How the Drug Works
- Boosts neurotransmitters serotonin and norepinephrine/noradrenaline
- Blocks serotonin reuptake pump (serotonin transporter), presumably increasing serotonergic neurotransmission
- Blocks norepinephrine reuptake pump (norepinephrine transporter), presumably increasing noradrenergic neurotransmission
- Presumably desensitizes both serotonin 1A receptors and beta adrenergic receptors
- Since dopamine is inactivated by norepinephrine reuptake in frontal cortex, which largely lacks dopamine transporters, amitriptyline can increase dopamine neurotransmission in this part of the brain

How Long Until It Works
- May have immediate effects in treating insomnia or anxiety
- Onset of therapeutic actions usually not immediate, but often delayed 2–4 weeks
- If it is not working within 6–8 weeks for depression, it may require a dosage increase or it may not work at all
- May continue to work for many years to prevent relapse of symptoms

If It Works
- The goal of treatment of depression is complete remission of current symptoms as well as prevention of future relapses
- The goal of treatment of chronic pain conditions such as neuropathic pain, fibromyalgia, headaches, low back pain, and neck pain is to reduce symptoms as much as possible, especially in combination with other treatments
- Treatment of depression most often reduces or even eliminates symptoms, but not a cure since symptoms can recur after medicine stopped
- Treatment of chronic pain conditions such as neuropathic pain, fibromyalgia, headache, low back pain, and neck pain may reduce symptoms, but rarely eliminates them completely, and is not a cure since symptoms can recur after medicine is stopped
- Continue treatment of depression until all symptoms are gone (remission)
- Once symptoms of depression are gone, continue treating for 1 year for the first episode of depression
- For second and subsequent episodes of depression, treatment may need to be indefinite
- Use in anxiety disorders and chronic pain conditions such as neuropathic pain, fibromyalgia, headache, low back pain, and neck pain may also need to be indefinite, but long-term treatment is not well studied in these conditions

If It Doesn't Work
- Many depressed patients have only a partial response where some symptoms are improved but others persist (especially insomnia, fatigue, and problems concentrating)
- Other depressed patients may be nonresponders, sometimes called treatment-resistant or treatment-refractory
- Consider increasing dose, switching to another agent, or adding an appropriate augmenting agent
- Consider psychotherapy
- Consider evaluation for another diagnosis or for a comorbid condition (e.g., medical illness, substance abuse, etc.)
- Some patients may experience apparent lack of consistent efficacy due to activation of latent or underlying bipolar disorder, and

require antidepressant discontinuation and a switch to a mood stabilizer

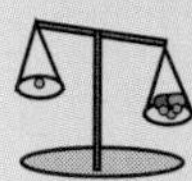

Best Augmenting Combos for Partial Response or Treatment Resistance

- Lithium, buspirone, thyroid hormone (for depression)
- Gabapentin, tiagabine, other anticonvulsants, even opiates if done by experts while monitoring carefully in difficult cases (for chronic pain)

Tests

- None for healthy individuals

✻ Since tricyclic and tetracyclic antidepressants are frequently associated with weight gain, before starting treatment, weigh all patients and determine if the patient is already overweight (BMI 25.0–29.9) or obese (BMI ≥30)

- Before giving a drug that can cause weight gain to an overweight or obese patient, consider determining whether the patient already has pre-diabetes (fasting plasma glucose 100–25 mg/dL), diabetes (fasting plasma glucose >126 mg/dL), or dyslipidemia (increased total cholesterol, LDL cholesterol and triglycerides; decreased HDL cholesterol), and treat or refer such patients for treatment, including nutrition and weight management, physical activity counseling, smoking cessation, and medical management

✻ Monitor weight and BMI during treatment

✻ While giving a drug to a patient who has gained >5% of initial weight, consider evaluating for the presence of pre-diabetes, diabetes, or dyslipidemia, or consider switching to a different antidepressant

- EKGs may be useful for selected patients (e.g., those with personal or family history of QTc prolongation; cardiac arrhythmia; recent myocardial infarction; uncompensated heart failure; or taking agents that prolong QTc interval such as pimozide, thioridazine, selected antiarrhythmics, moxifloxacin, sparfloxacin, etc.)
- Patients at risk for electrolyte disturbances (e.g., patients on diuretic therapy) should have baseline and periodic serum potassium and magnesium measurements

SIDE EFFECTS

How Drug Causes Side Effects

- Anticholinergic activity may explain sedative effects, dry mouth, constipation, and blurred vision
- Sedative effects and weight gain may be due to antihistamine properties
- Blockade of alpha adrenergic 1 receptors may explain dizziness, sedation, and hypotension
- Cardiac arrhythmias and seizures, especially in overdose, may be caused by blockade of ion channels

Notable Side Effects

- Blurred vision, constipation, urinary retention, increased appetite, dry mouth, nausea, diarrhea, heartburn, unusual taste in mouth, weight gain
- Fatigue, weakness, dizziness, sedation, headache, anxiety, nervousness, restlessness
- Sexual dysfunction (impotence, change in libido)
- Sweating, rash, itching

Life-Threatening or Dangerous Side Effects

- Paralytic ileus, hyperthermia (TCAs + anticholinergic agents)
- Lowered seizure threshold and rare seizures
- Orthostatic hypotension, sudden death, arrhythmias, tachycardia
- QTc prolongation
- Hepatic failure, extrapyramidal symptoms
- Increased intraocular pressure
- Rare induction of mania
- Rare activation of suicidal ideation and behavior (suicidality) (short-term studies did not show an increase in the risk of suicidality with antidepressants compared to placebo beyond age 24)

Weight Gain

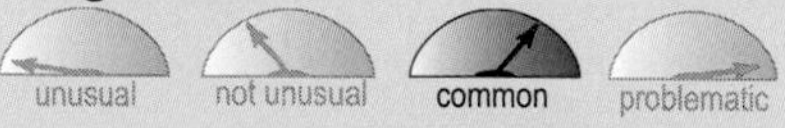

- Many experience and/or can be significant in amount

- Can increase appetite and carbohydrate craving

Sedation

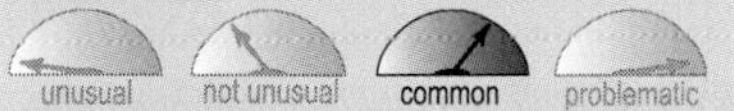

- Many experience and/or can be significant in amount
- Tolerance to sedative effects may develop with long-term use

What to Do About Side Effects

- Wait
- Wait
- Wait
- Lower the dose
- Switch to an SSRI or newer antidepressant

Best Augmenting Agents for Side Effects

- Many side effects cannot be improved with an augmenting agent

DOSING AND USE

Usual Dosage Range

- 50–150 mg/day

Dosage Forms

- Capsule 25 mg, 50 mg, 100 mg

How To Dose

- Initial 25 mg/day at bedtime; increase by 25 mg every 3–7 days
- 75 mg/day in divided doses; increase to 150 mg/day; maximum 300 mg/day

Dosing Tips

- If given in a single dose, should generally be administered at bedtime because of its sedative properties
- If given in split doses, largest dose should generally be given at bedtime because of its sedative properties
- If patients experience nightmares, split dose and do not give large dose at bedtime
- Patients treated for chronic pain may require only lower doses
- If intolerable anxiety, insomnia, agitation, akathisia, or activation occur either upon dosing initiation or discontinuation, consider the possibility of activated bipolar disorder, and switch to a mood stabilizer or an atypical antipsychotic

Overdose

- Death may occur; CNS depression, convulsions, cardiac dysrhythmias, severe hypotension, EKG changes, coma

Long-Term Use

- Safe

Habit Forming

- No

How to Stop

- Taper to avoid withdrawal effects
- Even with gradual dose reduction, some withdrawal symptoms may appear within the first 2 weeks
- Many patients tolerate 50% dose reduction for 3 days, then another 50% reduction for 3 days, then discontinuation
- If withdrawal symptoms emerge during discontinuation, raise dose to stop symptoms and then restart withdrawal much more slowly

Pharmacokinetics

- Substrate for CYP450 2D6 and 1A2
- Plasma half-life 10–28 hours
- Metabolized to an active metabolite, nortriptyline, which is predominantly a norepinephrine reuptake inhibitor, by demethylation via CYP450 1A2

Drug Interactions

- Tramadol increases the risk of seizures in patients taking TCAs
- Use of TCAs with anticholinergic drugs may result in paralytic ileus or hyperthermia
- Fluoxetine, paroxetine, bupropion, duloxetine, and other CYP450 2D6 inhibitors may increase TCA concentrations
- Fluvoxamine, a CYP450 1A2 inhibitor, can decrease the conversion of amitriptyline to nortriptyline and increase amitriptyline plasma concentrations
- Cimetidine may increase plasma concentrations of TCAs and cause anticholinergic symptoms
- Phenothiazines or haloperidol may raise TCA blood concentrations

- May alter effects of antihypertensive drugs; may inhibit hypotensive effects of clonidine
- Use of TCAs with sympathomimetic agents may increase sympathetic activity
- Methylphenidate may inhibit metabolism of TCAs
- Activation and agitation, especially following switching or adding antidepressants, may represent the induction of a bipolar state, especially a mixed dysphoric bipolar II condition sometimes associated with suicidal ideation, and require the addition of lithium, a mood stabilizer or an atypical antipsychotic, and/or discontinuation of amitriptyline

Other Warnings/ Precautions

- Add or initiate other antidepressants with caution for up to 2 weeks after discontinuing amitriptyline
- Generally, do not use with MAO inhibitors, including 14 days after MAOIs are stopped; do not start an MAOI until 2 weeks after discontinuing amitriptyline, but see Pearls
- Use with caution in patients with history of seizures, urinary retention, narrow angle-closure glaucoma, hyperthyroidism
- TCAs can increase QTc interval, especially at toxic doses, which can be attained not only by overdose but also by combining with drugs that inhibit TCA metabolism via CYP450 2D6, potentially causing torsade de pointes-type arrhythmia or sudden death
- Because TCAs can prolong QTc interval, use with caution in patients who have bradycardia or who are taking drugs that can induce bradycardia (e.g., beta blockers, calcium channel blockers, clonidine, digitalis)
- Because TCAs can prolong QTc interval, use with caution in patients who have hypokalemia and/or hypomagnesemia, or who are taking drugs that can induce hypokalemia and/or magnesemia (e.g., diuretics, stimulant laxatives, intravenous amphotericin B, glucocorticoids, tetracosactide)
- When treating children, carefully weigh the risks and benefits of pharmacological treatment against the risks and benefits of nontreatment with antidepressants and make sure to document this in the patient's chart
- Distribute the brochures provided by the FDA and the drug companies
- Warn patients and their caregivers about the possibility of activating side effects and advise them to report such symptoms immediately
- Monitor patients for activation of suicidal ideation, especially children and adolescents

Do Not Use

- If patient is recovering from myocardial infarction
- If patient is taking agents capable of significantly prolonging QTc interval (e.g., pimozide, thioridazine, selected antiarrhythmics, moxifloxacin, sparfloxacin)
- If there is a history of QTc prolongation or cardiac arrhythmia, recent acute myocardial infarction, uncompensated heart failure
- If patient is taking drugs that inhibit TCA metabolism, including CYP450 2D6 inhibitors, except by an expert
- If there is reduced CYP450 2D6 function, such as patients who are poor 2D6 metabolizers, except by an expert and at low doses
- If there is a proven allergy to amitriptyline or nortriptyline

SPECIAL POPULATIONS

Renal Impairment

- Use with caution; may need to lower dose

Hepatic Impairment

- Use with caution; may need to lower dose

Cardiac Impairment

- TCAs have been reported to cause arrhythmias, prolongation of conduction time, orthostatic hypotension, sinus tachycardia, and heart failure, especially in the diseased heart
- Myocardial infarction and stroke have been reported with TCAs
- TCAs produce QTc prolongation, which may be enhanced by the existence of bradycardia, hypokalemia, congenital or acquired long QTc interval, which should

be evaluated prior to administering amitriptyline
- Use with caution if treating concomitantly with a medication likely to produce prolonged bradycardia, hypokalemia, slowing of intracardiac conduction, or prolongation of the QTc interval
- Avoid TCAs in patients with a known history of QTc prolongation, recent acute myocardial infarction, and uncompensated heart failure
- TCAs may cause a sustained increase in heart rate in patients with ischemic heart disease and may worsen (decrease) heart rate variability, an independent risk of mortality in cardiac populations
- Since SSRIs may improve (increase) heart rate variability in patients following a myocardial infarct and may improve survival as well as mood in patients with acute angina or following a myocardial infarction, these are more appropriate agents for cardiac population than tricyclic/tetracyclic antidepressants

✻ Risk/benefit ratio may not justify use of TCAs in cardiac impairment

Elderly

- May be more sensitive to anticholinergic, cardiovascular, hypotensive, and sedative effects
- Initial dose 50 mg/day; increase gradually up to 100 mg/day
- Reduction in risk of suicidality with antidepressants compared to placebo in adults age 65 and older

Children and Adolescents

- Carefully weigh the risks and benefits of pharmacological treatment against the risks and benefits of nontreatment with antidepressants and make sure to document this in the patient's chart
- Use with caution, observing for activation of known or unknown bipolar disorder and/or suicidal ideation, and inform parents or guardians of this risk so they can help observe child or adolescent patients
- Monitor patients face-to-face regularly, particularly during the first several weeks of treatment
- Not generally recommended for use in children under age 12
- Several studies show lack of efficacy of TCAs for depression
- May be used to treat enuresis or hyperactive/impulsive behaviors
- Some cases of sudden death have occurred in children taking TCAs
- Adolescents: initial dose 50 mg/day; increase gradually up to 100 mg/day

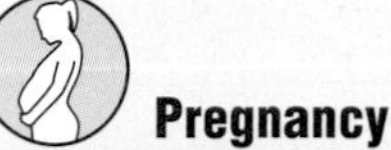

Pregnancy

- Risk Category C [some animal studies show adverse effects; no controlled studies in humans]
- Crosses the placenta
- Adverse effects have been reported in infants whose mothers took a TCA (lethargy, withdrawal symptoms, fetal malformations)
- Must weigh the risk of treatment (first trimester fetal development, third trimester newborn delivery) to the child against the risk of no treatment (recurrence of depression, maternal health, infant bonding) to the mother and child
- For many patients this may mean continuing treatment during pregnancy

Breast Feeding

- Some drug is found in mother's breast milk

✻ Recommended either to discontinue drug or bottle feed

- Immediate postpartum period is a high-risk time for depression, especially in women who have had prior depressive episodes, so drug may need to be reinstituted late in the third trimester or shortly after childbirth to prevent a recurrence during the postpartum period
- Must weigh benefits of breast feeding with risks and benefits of antidepressant treatment versus nontreatment to both the infant and the mother
- For many patients this may mean continuing treatment during breast feeding

THE ART OF PSYCHOPHARMACOLOGY

Potential Advantages

- Patients with insomnia
- Severe or treatment-resistant depression
- Patients with a wide variety of chronic pain syndromes

Potential Disadvantages
- Pediatric and geriatric patients
- Patients concerned with weight gain
- Cardiac patients

Primary Target Symptoms
- Depressed mood
- Symptoms of anxiety
- Somatic symptoms
- Chronic pain
- Insomnia

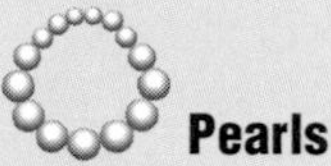

Pearls
- Was once one of the most widely prescribed agents for depression
- Remains one of the most favored TCAs for treating headache and a wide variety of chronic pain syndromes, including neuropathic pain, fibromyalgia, migraine, neck pain, and low back pain

✻ Preference of some prescribers for amitriptyline over other tricyclic/tetracyclic antidepressants for the treatment of chronic pain syndromes is based more upon art and anecdote rather than controlled clinical trials, since many TCAs/tetracylics may be effective for chronic pain syndromes

- Tricyclic antidepressants are no longer generally considered a first-line treatment option for depression because of their side effect profile

✻ Amitriptyline has been shown to be effective in primary insomnia

- TCAs may aggravate psychotic symptoms
- Alcohol should be avoided because of additive CNS effects
- Underweight patients may be more susceptible to adverse cardiovascular effects
- Children, patients with inadequate hydration, and patients with cardiac disease may be more susceptible to TCA-induced cardiotoxicity than healthy adults
- For the expert only: although generally prohibited, a heroic but potentially dangerous treatment for severely treatment-resistant patients is to give a tricyclic/tetracyclic antidepressant other than clomipramine simultaneously with an MAO inhibitor for patients who fail to respond to numerous other antidepressants
- If this option is elected, start the MAOI with the tricyclic/tetracyclic antidepressant simultaneously at low doses after appropriate drug washout, then alternately increase doses of these agents every few days to a week as tolerated
- Although very strict dietary and concomitant drug restrictions must be observed to prevent hypertensive crises and serotonin syndrome, the most common side effects of MAOI/tricyclic or tetracyclic combinations may be weight gain and orthostatic hypotension
- Patients on TCAs should be aware that they may experience symptoms such as photosensitivity or blue-green urine
- SSRIs may be more effective than TCAs in women, and TCAs may be more effective than SSRIs in men
- Since tricyclic/tetracyclic antidepressants are substrates for CYP450 2D6, and 7% of the population (especially Caucasians) may have a genetic variant leading to reduced activity of 2D6, such patients may not safely tolerate normal doses of tricyclic/tetracyclic antidepressants and may require dose reduction
- Phenotypic testing may be necessary to detect this genetic variant prior to dosing with a tricyclic/tetracyclic antidepressant, especially in vulnerable populations such as children, elderly, cardiac populations, and those on concomitant medications
- Patients who seem to have extraordinarily severe side effects at normal or low doses may have this phenotypic CYP450 2D6 variant and require low doses or switching to another antidepressant not metabolized by 2D6

Suggested Reading

Anderson IM. Meta-analytical studies on new antidepressants. Br Med Bull 2001; 57:161–78.

Anderson IM. Selective serotonin reuptake inhibitors versus tricyclic antidepressants: a meta-analysis of efficacy and tolerability. J Aff Disorders 2000;58:19–36.

Barbui C, Hotopf M. Amitriptyline v. the rest: still the leading antidepressant after 40 years of randomised controlled trials. Br J Psychiatry 2001;178:129–44.

Bryson HM, Wilde MI. Amitriptyline. A review of its pharmacological properties and therapeutic use in chronic pain states. Drugs Aging 1996;8:459–76.

THERAPEUTICS

Brands • Asendin
see index for additional brand names

Generic? Yes

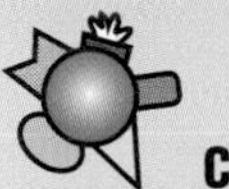

Class

- Tricyclic antidepressant (TCA), sometimes classified as a tetracyclic antidepressant
- Norepinephrine/noradrenaline reuptake inhibitor
- Serotonin 2A antagonist
- Parent drug and especially an active metabolite are dopamine 2 antagonists

Commonly Prescribed for

(bold for FDA approved)

- **Neurotic or reactive depressive disorder**
- **Endogenous and psychotic depressions**
- **Depression accompanied by anxiety or agitation**
- Depressive phase of bipolar disorder
- Anxiety
- Insomnia
- Neuropathic pain/chronic pain
- Treatment-resistant depression

How the Drug Works

- Boosts neurotransmitter norepinephrine/noradrenaline
- Blocks norepinephrine reuptake pump (norepinephrine transporter), presumably increasing noradrenergic neurotransmission
- Since dopamine is inactivated by norepinephrine reuptake in frontal cortex, which largely lacks dopamine transporters, amoxapine can thus increase dopamine neurotransmission in this part of the brain
- A more potent inhibitor of norepinephrine reuptake pump than serotonin reuptake pump (serotonin transporter)
- At high doses may also boost neurotransmitter serotonin and presumably increase serotonergic neurotransmission
- Blocks dopamine 2 receptors, reducing positive symptoms of psychosis

How Long Until It Works

- Onset of therapeutic actions usually not immediate, but often delayed 2–4 weeks
- If it is not working within 6–8 weeks for depression, it may require a dosage increase or it may not work at all
- May continue to work for many years to prevent relapse of symptoms

If It Works

- The goal of treatment is complete remission of current symptoms as well as prevention of future relapses
- Treatment most often reduces or even eliminates symptoms, but not a cure since symptoms can recur after medicine stopped
- Continue treatment until all symptoms are gone (remission)
- Once symptoms gone, continue treating for 1 year for the first episode of depression
- For second and subsequent episodes of depression, treatment may need to be indefinite
- Use in anxiety disorders may also need to be indefinite

If It Doesn't Work

- Many patients have only a partial response where some symptoms are improved but others persist (especially insomnia, fatigue, and problems concentrating)
- Other patients may be nonresponders, sometimes called treatment-resistant or treatment-refractory
- Consider increasing dose, switching to another agent, or adding an appropriate augmenting agent
- Consider psychotherapy
- Consider evaluation for another diagnosis or for a comorbid condition (e.g., medical illness, substance abuse, etc.)
- Some patients may experience apparent lack of consistent efficacy due to activation of latent or underlying bipolar disorder, and require antidepressant discontinuation and a switch to a mood stabilizer

Best Augmenting Combos for Partial Response or Treatment Resistance

- Lithium, buspirone, thyroid hormone

Tests

- None for healthy individuals

❋ Since tricyclic and tetracyclic antidepressants are frequently associated with weight gain, before starting treatment,

weigh all patients and determine if the patient is already overweight (BMI 25.0–29.9) or obese (BMI ≥30)
- Before giving a drug that can cause weight gain to an overweight or obese patient, consider determining whether the patient already has pre-diabetes (fasting plasma glucose 100–25 mg/dL), diabetes (fasting plasma glucose >126 mg/dL), or dyslipidemia (increased total cholesterol, LDL cholesterol and triglycerides; decreased HDL cholesterol), and treat or refer such patients for treatment, including nutrition and weight management, physical activity counseling, smoking cessation, and medical management
- ✻ Monitor weight and BMI during treatment
- ✻ While giving a drug to a patient who has gained >5% of initial weight, consider evaluating for the presence of pre-diabetes, diabetes, or dyslipidemia, or consider switching to a different antidepressant
- EKGs may be useful for selected patients (e.g., those with personal or family history of QTc prolongation; cardiac arrhythmia; recent myocardial infarction; uncompensated heart failure; or taking agents that prolong QTc interval such as pimozide, thioridazine, selected antiarrhythmics, moxifloxacin, sparfloxacin, etc.)
- Patients at risk for electrolyte disturbances (e.g., patients on diuretic therapy) should have baseline and periodic serum potassium and magnesium measurements

SIDE EFFECTS

How Drug Causes Side Effects
- Anticholinergic activity may explain sedative effects, dry mouth, constipation, and blurred vision
- Sedative effects and weight gain may be due to antihistamine properties
- Blockade of alpha adrenergic 1 receptors may explain dizziness, sedation, and hypotension
- Cardiac arrhythmias and seizures, especially in overdose, may be caused by blockade of ion channels

Notable Side Effects
- Blurred vision, constipation, urinary retention, increased appetite, dry mouth, nausea, diarrhea, heartburn, unusual taste in mouth, weight gain
- Fatigue, weakness, dizziness, sedation, headache, anxiety, nervousness, restlessness
- Sexual dysfunction, sweating
- ✻ Can cause extrapyramidal symptoms, akathisia, and theoretically, tardive dyskinesia

Life-Threatening or Dangerous Side Effects
- Paralytic ileus, hyperthermia (TCAs/tetracyclics + anticholinergic agents)
- Lowered seizure threshold and rare seizures
- Orthostatic hypotension, sudden death, arrhythmias, tachycardia
- QTc prolongation
- Hepatic failure, extrapyramidal symptoms
- Increased intraocular pressure
- Rare induction of mania
- Rare activation of suicidal ideation and behavior (suicidality) (short-term studies did not show an increase in the risk of suicidality with antidepressants compared to placebo beyond age 24)

Weight Gain

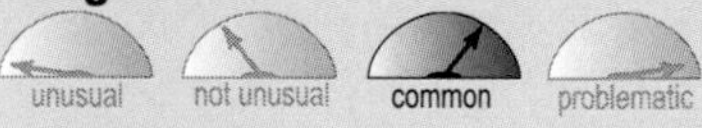

- Many experience and/or can be significant in amount
- Can increase appetite and carbohydrate craving

Sedation

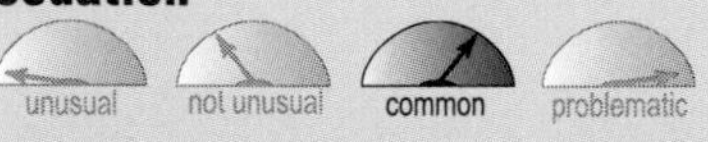

- Many experience and/or can be significant in amount
- Tolerance to sedative effect may develop with long-term use

What to Do About Side Effects
- Wait
- Wait
- Wait
- Lower the dose
- Switch to an SSRI or newer antidepressant

Best Augmenting Agents for Side Effects

- Many side effects cannot be improved with an augmenting agent
- May use anticholinergics for extrapyramidal symptoms, or switch to another antidepressant

DOSING AND USE

Usual Dosage Range

- 200–300 mg/day

Dosage Forms

- Tablets 25 mg, 50 mg, 100 mg, 150 mg

How To Dose

- Initial 25 mg 2–3 times/day; increase gradually to 100 mg 2–3 times/day or a single dose at bedtime; maximum 400 mg/day (may dose up to 600 mg/day in inpatients)

Dosing Tips

- If given in a single dose, should generally be administered at bedtime because of its sedative properties
- If given in split doses, largest dose should generally be given at bedtime because of its sedative properties
- If patients experience nightmares, split dose and do not give large dose at bedtime
- If intolerable anxiety, insomnia, agitation, akathisia, or activation occur either upon dosing initiation or discontinuation, consider the possibility of activated bipolar disorder, and switch to a mood stabilizer or an atypical antipsychotic

Overdose

- Death may occur; convulsions, cardiac dysrhythmias, severe hypotension, CNS depression, coma, changes in EKG

Long-Term Use

- Generally safe
- Some patients may develop withdrawal dyskinesias when discontinuing amoxapine after long-term use

Habit Forming

- Some patients may develop tolerance

How to Stop

- Taper to avoid withdrawal effects
- Even with gradual dose reduction some withdrawal symptoms may appear within the first 2 weeks
- Many patients tolerate 50% dose reduction for 3 days, then another 50% reduction for 3 days, then discontinuation
- If withdrawal symptoms emerge during discontinuation, raise dose to stop symptoms and then restart withdrawal much more slowly

Pharmacokinetics

- Substrate for CYP450 2D6
- Half-life of parent drug approximately 8 hours

✻ 7- and 8-hydroxymetabolites are active and possess serotonin 2A and dopamine 2 antagonist properties, similar to atypical antipsychotics

✻ Amoxapine is the *N*-desmethyl metabolite of the conventional antipsychotic loxapine

- Half-life of the active metabolites approximately 24 hours

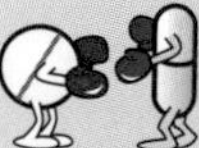

Drug Interactions

- Tramadol increases the risk of seizures in patients taking TCAs
- Use of TCAs/tetracyclics with anticholinergic drugs may result in paralytic ileus or hyperthermia
- Fluoxetine, paroxetine, bupropion, duloxetine, and other CYP450 2D6 inhibitors may increase TCA/tetracyclic concentrations
- Cimetidine may increase plasma concentrations of TCAs/tetracyclics and cause anticholinergic symptoms
- Phenothiazines or haloperidol may raise TCA/tetracyclic blood concentrations
- May alter effects of antihypertensive drugs; may inhibit hypotensive effects of clonidine
- Use of TCAs/tetracyclics with sympathomimetic agents may increase sympathetic activity
- Methylphenidate may inhibit metabolism of TCAs/tetracyclics
- Activation and agitation, especially following switching or adding antidepressants, may represent the induction of a bipolar state, especially a mixed dysphoric bipolar II condition

sometimes associated with suicidal ideation, and require the addition of lithium, a mood stabilizer or an atypical antipsychotic, and/or discontinuation of amoxapine

Other Warnings/ Precautions

- Add or initiate other antidepressants with caution for up to 2 weeks after discontinuing amoxapine
- Generally, do not use with MAO inhibitors, including 14 days after MAOIs are stopped; do not start an MAOI until 2 weeks after discontinuing amoxapine, but see Pearls
- Use with caution in patients with history of seizure, urinary retention, narrow angle-closure glaucoma, hyperthyroidism
- TCAs/tetracyclics can increase QTc interval, especially at toxic doses, which can be attained not only by overdose but also by combining with drugs that inhibit its metabolism via CYP450 2D6, potentially causing torsade de pointes-type arrhythmia or sudden death
- Because TCAs/tetracyclics can prolong QTc interval, use with caution in patients who have bradycardia or who are taking drugs that can induce bradycardia (e.g., beta blockers, calcium channel blockers, clonidine, digitalis)
- Because TCAs/tetracyclics can prolong QTc interval, use with caution in patients who have hypokalemia and/or hypomagnesemia, or who are taking drugs that can induce hypokalemia and/or magnesemia (e.g., diuretics, stimulant laxatives, intravenous amphotericin B, glucocorticoids, tetracosactide)
- When treating children, carefully weigh the risks and benefits of pharmacological treatment against the risks and benefits of nontreatment with antidepressants and make sure to document this in the patient's chart
- Distribute the brochures provided by the FDA and the drug companies
- Warn patients and their caregivers about the possibility of activating side effects and advise them to report such symptoms immediately
- Monitor patients for activation of suicidal ideation, especially children and adolescents

Do Not Use

- If patient is recovering from myocardial infarction
- If patient is taking agents capable of significantly prolonging QTc interval (e.g., pimozide, thioridazine, selected antiarrhythmics, moxifloxacin, sparfloxacin)
- If there is a history of QTc prolongation or cardiac arrhythmia, recent acute myocardial infarction, uncompensated heart failure
- If patient is taking drugs that inhibit TCA/tetracyclic metabolism, including CYP450 2D6 inhibitors, except by an expert
- If there is reduced CYP450 2D6 function, such as patients who are poor 2D6 metabolizers, except by an expert and at low doses
- If there is a proven allergy to amoxapine or loxapine

SPECIAL POPULATIONS

Renal Impairment

- Use with caution – may require lower than usual adult dose

Hepatic Impairment

- Use with caution – may require lower than usual adult dose

Cardiac Impairment

- TCAs/tetracyclics have been reported to cause arrhythmias, prolongation of conduction time, orthostatic hypotension, sinus tachycardia, and heart failure, especially in the diseased heart
- Myocardial infarction and stroke have been reported with TCAs/tetracyclics
- TCAs/tetracyclics produce QTc prolongation, which may be enhanced by the existence of bradycardia, hypokalemia, congenital or acquired long QTc interval, which should be evaluated prior to administering amoxapine
- Use with caution if treating concomitantly with a medication likely to produce prolonged bradycardia, hypokalemia, slowing of intracardiac conduction, or prolongation of the QTc interval
- Avoid TCAs/tetracyclics in patients with a known history of QTc prolongation, recent

acute myocardial infarction, and uncompensated heart failure
- TCAs/tetracyclics may cause a sustained increase in heart rate in patients with ischemic heart disease and may worsen (decrease) heart rate variability, an independent risk of mortality in cardiac populations
- Since SSRIs may improve (increase) heart rate variability in patients following a myocardial infarct and may improve survival as well as mood in patients with acute angina or following a myocardial infarction, these are more appropriate agents for cardiac population than tricyclic/tetracyclic antidepressants

✻ Risk/benefit ratio may not justify use of TCAs/tetracyclics in cardiac impairment

Elderly
- May be more sensitive to anticholinergic, cardiovascular, hypotensive, and sedative effects
- Initial dose 25 mg/day at bedtime; increase by 25 mg/day each week; maximum dose 300 mg/day
- Reduction in risk of suicidality with antidepressants compared to placebo in adults age 65 and older

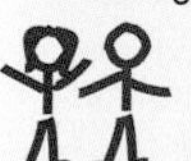

Children and Adolescents
- Carefully weigh the risks and benefits of pharmacological treatment against the risks and benefits of nontreatment with antidepressants and make sure to document this in the patient's chart
- Use with caution, observing for activation of known or unknown bipolar disorder and/or suicidal ideation, and inform parents or guardian of this risk so they can help observe child or adolescent patients
- Monitor patients face-to-face regularly, particularly during the first several weeks of treatment
- Not generally recommended for use in children under age 16
- Several studies show lack of efficacy of TCAs/tetracyclics for depression
- May be used to treat enuresis or hyperactive/impulsive behaviors
- Some cases of sudden death have occurred in children taking TCAs/tetracyclics
- Adolescents: initial 25–50 mg/day; increase gradually to 100 mg/day in divided doses or single dose at bedtime

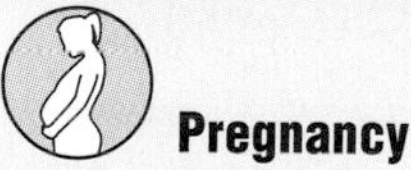

Pregnancy
- Risk Category C [some animal studies show adverse effects; no controlled studies in humans]
- Amoxapine crosses the placenta
- Adverse effects have been reported in infants whose mothers took a TCA (lethargy, withdrawal symptoms, fetal malformations)
- Evaluate for treatment with an antidepressant with a better risk/benefit ratio

Breast Feeding
- Some drug is found in mother's breast milk

✻ Recommended either to discontinue drug or bottle feed

- Immediate postpartum period is a high-risk time for depression, especially in women who have had prior depressive episodes, so drug may need to be reinstituted late in the third trimester or shortly after childbirth to prevent a recurrence during the postpartum period
- Evaluate for treatment with an antidepressant with a better risk/benefit ratio

THE ART OF PSYCHOPHARMACOLOGY

Potential Advantages
- Severe or treatment-resistant depression
- Treatment-resistant psychotic depression

Potential Disadvantages
- Pediatric and geriatric patients
- Patients concerned with weight gain
- Cardiac patients
- Patients with Parkinson's disease or tardive dyskinesia

Primary Target Symptoms
- Depressed mood

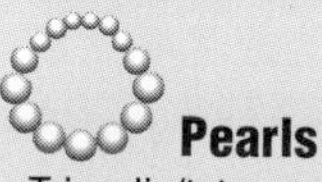

Pearls
- Tricyclic/tetracyclic antidepressants are no longer generally considered a first-line

treatment option for depression because of their side effect profile

- Tricyclic/tetracyclic antidepressants continue to be useful for severe or treatment-resistant depression
- ❋ Because of potential extrapyramidal symptoms, akathisia, and theoretical risk of tardive dyskinesia, first consider other TCAs/tetracyclics for long-term use in general and for treatment of chronic patients
- TCAs may aggravate psychotic symptoms
- Alcohol should be avoided because of additive CNS effects
- Underweight patients may be more susceptible to adverse cardiovascular effects
- Children, patients with inadequate hydration, and patients with cardiac disease may be more susceptible to TCA-induced cardiotoxicity than healthy adults
- For the expert only: although generally prohibited, a heroic but potentially dangerous treatment for severely treatment-resistant patients is to give a tricyclic/tetracyclic antidepressant other than clomipramine simultaneously with an MAO inhibitor for patients who fail to respond to numerous other antidepressants
- Use of MAOIs with clomipramine is always prohibited because of the risk of serotonin syndrome and death
- Amoxapine may be the preferred trycyclic/tetracyclic antidepressant to combine with an MAOI in heroic cases due to its theoretically protective 5HT2A antagonist properties
- If this option is elected, start the MAOI with the tricyclic/tetracyclic antidepressant simultaneously at low doses after appropriate drug washout, then alternately increase doses of these agents every few days to a week as tolerated
- Although very strict dietary and concomitant drug restrictions must be observed to prevent hypertensive crises and serotonin syndrome, the most common side effects of MAOI/tricyclic or tetracyclic combinations may be weight gain and orthostatic hypotention
- Patients on TCAs/tetracyclics should be aware that they may experience symptoms such as photosensitivity or blue-green urine
- SSRIs may be more effective than TCAs/tetracyclics in women, and TCAs/tetracyclics may be more effective than SSRIs in men
- ❋ May cause some motor effects, possibly due to effects on dopamine receptors
- ❋ Amoxapine may have a faster onset of action than some other antidepressants
- ❋ May be pharmacologically similar to an atypical antipsychotic in some patients
- ❋ At high doses, patients who form high concentrations of active metabolites may have akathisia, extrapyramidal symptoms, and possibly develop tardive dyskinesia
- ❋ Structurally and pharmacologically related to the antipsychotic loxapine
- Since tricyclic/tetracyclic antidepressants are substrates for CYP450 2D6, and 7% of the population (especially Caucasians) may have a genetic variant leading to reduced activity of 2D6, such patients may not safely tolerate normal doses of tricyclic/tetracyclic antidepressants and may require dose reduction
- Phenotypic testing may be necessary to detect this genetic variant prior to dosing with a tricyclic/tetracyclic antidepressant, especially in vulnerable populations such as children, elderly, cardiac populations, and those on concomitant medications
- Patients who seem to have extraordinarily severe side effects at normal or low doses may have this phenotypic CYP450 2D6 variant and require low doses or switching to another antidepressant not metabolized by 2D6

Suggested Reading

Anderson IM. Meta-analytical studies on new antidepressants. Br Med Bull 2001; 57:161–78.

Anderson IM. Selective serotonin reuptake inhibitors versus tricyclic antidepressants: a meta-analysis of efficacy and tolerability. J Aff Disorders 2000;58:19–36.

Hayes PE, Kristoff CA. Adverse reactions to five new antidepressants. Clin Pharm 1986; 5:471–80.

Jue SG, Dawson GW, Brogden RN. Amoxapine: a review of its pharmacology and efficacy in depressed states. Drugs 1982; 24:1–23.

THERAPEUTICS

Brands
- Dexedrine
- Dexedrine Spansules
- Dextro Stat

see index for additional brand names

Generic? Yes

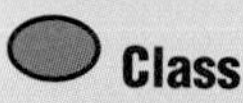

Class
- Stimulant

Commonly Prescribed for
(bold for FDA approved)
- **Attention deficit hyperactivity disorder (ADHD) (ages 3–16)**
- **Narcolepsy**
- Treatment-resistant depression

How the Drug Works
✻ Increases norepinephrine and especially dopamine actions by blocking their reuptake and facilitating their release
- Enhancement of dopamine and norepinephrine actions in certain brain regions may improve attention, concentration, executive function, and wakefulness (e.g., dorsolateral prefrontal cortex)
- Enhancement of dopamine actions in other brain regions (e.g., basal ganglia) may improve hyperactivity
- Enhancement of dopamine and norepinephrine in yet other brain regions (e.g., medial prefrontal cortex, hypothalamus) may improve depression, fatigue, and sleepiness

How Long Until It Works
- Some immediate effects can be seen with first dosing
- Can take several weeks to attain maximum therapeutic benefit

If It Works (for ADHD)
- The goal of treatment of ADHD is reduction of symptoms of inattentiveness, motor hyperactivity, and/or impulsiveness that disrupt social, school, and/or occupational functioning
- Continue treatment until all symptoms are under control or improvement is stable and then continue treatment indefinitely as long as improvement persists
- Reevaluate the need for treatment periodically
- Treatment for ADHD begun in childhood may need to be continued into adolescence and adulthood if continued benefit is documented

If It Doesn't Work (for ADHD)
- Consider adjusting dose or switching to another formulation of d-amphetamine or to another agent
- Consider behavioral therapy
- Consider the presence of noncompliance and counsel patient and parents
- Consider evaluation for another diagnosis or for a comorbid condition (e.g., bipolar disorder, substance abuse, medical illness, etc.)

✻ Some ADHD patients and some depressed patients may experience lack of consistent efficacy due to activation of latent or underlying bipolar disorder, and require either augmenting with a mood stabilizer or switching to a mood stabilizer

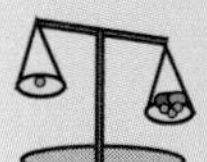

Best Augmenting Combos for Partial Response or Treatment Resistance
✻ Best to attempt other monotherapies prior to augmenting
- For the expert, can combine immediate-release formulation with a sustained-release formulation of d-amphetamine for ADHD
- For the expert, can combine with modafinil or atomoxetine for ADHD
- For the expert, can occasionally combine with atypical antipsychotics in highly treatment-resistant cases of bipolar disorder or ADHD
- For the expert, can combine with antidepressants to boost antidepressant efficacy in highly treatment-resistant cases of depression while carefully monitoring patient

Tests
- Blood pressure should be monitored regularly
- In children, monitor weight and height

SIDE EFFECTS

How Drug Causes Side Effects

- Increases in norepinephrine peripherally can cause autonomic side effects, including tremor, tachycardia, hypertension, and cardiac arrhythmias
- Increases in norepinephrine and dopamine centrally can cause CNS side effects such as insomnia, agitation, psychosis, and substance abuse

Notable Side Effects

✻ Insomnia, headache, exacerbation of tics, nervousness, irritability, overstimulation, tremor, dizziness
- Anorexia, nausea, dry mouth, constipation, diarrhea, weight loss
- Can temporarily slow normal growth in children (controversial)
- Sexual dysfunction long-term (impotence, libido changes) but can also improve sexual dysfunction short-term

Life-Threatening or Dangerous Side Effects

- Psychotic episodes, especially with parenteral abuse
- Seizures
- Palpitations, tachycardia, hypertension
- Rare activation of hypomania, mania, or suicidal ideation (controversial)
- Cardiovascular adverse effects, sudden death in patients with preexisting cardiac structural abnormalities

Weight Gain

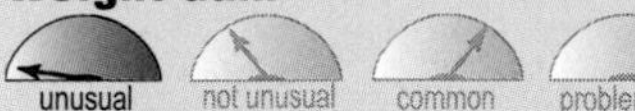

- Reported but not expected
- Some patients may experience weight loss

Sedation

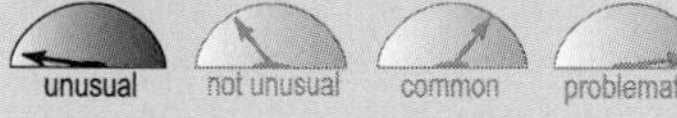

- Reported but not expected
- Activation much more common than sedation

What to Do About Side Effects

- Wait
- Adjust dose
- Switch to a long-acting stimulant
- Switch to another agent
- For insomnia, avoid dosing in afternoon/evening

Best Augmenting Agents for Side Effects

- Beta blockers for peripheral autonomic side effects
- Dose reduction or switching to another agent may be more effective since most side effects cannot be improved with an augmenting agent

DOSING AND USE

Usual Dosage Range

- Narcolepsy: 5–60 mg/day (divided doses for tablet, once-daily morning dose for Spansule capsule)
- ADHD: 5–40 mg/day (divided doses for tablet, once-daily morning dose for Spansule capsule)

Dosage Forms

- Spansule capsule 5 mg, 10 mg, 15 mg
- Tablet 5 mg scored, 10 mg

How To Dose

- Narcolepsy (ages 12 and older): initial 10 mg/day; increase by 10 mg each week; give first dose on waking
- ADHD (ages 6 and older): initial 5–10 mg/day in 1–2 doses; increase by 5 mg each week; give first dose on waking
- Can give once-daily dosing with Spansule capsule or divided dosing with tablet (every 4–6 hours)

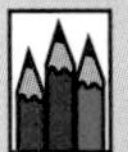

Dosing Tips

- Clinical duration of action often differs from pharmacokinetic half-life

✻ Immediate-release dextroamphetamine has 3–6 hour duration of clinical action

✻ Sustained-release dextroamphetamine (Dexedrine spansule) has up to 8-hour duration of clinical action
- Tablets contain tartrazine, which may cause allergic reactions, particularly in patients allergic to aspirin
- Dexedrine spansules are controlled-release and should therefore not be chewed but rather should only be swallowed whole

* Controlled-release delivery of dextroamphetamine may be sufficiently long in duration to allow elimination of lunchtime dosing in many but not all patients
* This innovation can be an important practical element in stimulant utilization, eliminating the hassle and pragmatic difficulties of lunchtime dosing at school, including storage problems, potential diversion, and the need for a medical professional to supervise dosing away from home
- Avoid dosing late in the day because of the risk of insomnia
* May be possible to dose only during the school week for some ADHD patients
- Off-label uses are dosed the same as for ADHD
* May be able to give drug holidays over the summer in order to reassess therapeutic utility and effects on growth and to allow catch-up from any growth suppression as well as to assess any other side effects and the need to reinstitute stimulant treatment for the next school term
- Side effects are generally dose-related
- Taking with food may delay peak actions for 2–3 hours

Overdose
- Rarely fatal; panic, hyperreflexia, rhabdomyolysis, rapid respiration, confusion, coma, hallucination, convulsion, arrhythmia, change in blood pressure, circulatory collapse

Long-Term Use
- Often used long-term for ADHD when ongoing monitoring documents continued efficacy
- Dependence and/or abuse may develop
- Tolerance to therapeutic effects may develop in some patients
- Long-term stimulant use may be associated with growth suppression in children (controversial)
- Periodic monitoring of weight, blood pressure, CBC, platelet counts, and liver function may be prudent

Habit Forming
- High abuse potential, Schedule II drug
- Patients may develop tolerance, psychological dependence

How to Stop
- Taper to avoid withdrawal effects
- Withdrawal following chronic therapeutic use may unmask symptoms of the underlying disorder and may require follow-up and reinstitution of treatment
- Careful supervision is required during withdrawal from abusive use since severe depression may occur

Pharmacokinetics
- Half-life approximately 10–2 hours

Drug Interactions
- May affect blood pressure and should be used cautiously with agents used to control blood pressure
- Gastrointestinal acidifying agents (guanethidine, reserpine, glutamic acid, ascorbic acid, fruit juices, etc.) and urinary acidifying agents (ammonium chloride, sodium phosphate, etc.) lower amphetamine plasma levels, so such agents can be useful to administer after an overdose but may also lower therapeutic efficacy of amphetamines
- Gastrointestinal alkalinizing agents (sodium bicarbonate, etc.) and urinary alkalinizing agents (acetazolamide, some thiazides) increase amphetamine plasma levels and potentiate amphetamine's actions
- Desipramine and protryptiline can cause striking and sustained increases in brain concentrations of d-amphetamine and may also add to d-amphetamine's cardiovascular effects
- Theoretically, other agents with norepinephrine reuptake blocking properties, such as venlafaxine, duloxetine, atomoxetine, milnacipran, and reboxetine, could also add to amphetamine's CNS and cardiovascular effects
- Amphetamines may counteract the sedative effects of antihistamines
- Haloperidol, chlorpromazine, and lithium may inhibit stimulatory effects of amphetamines
- Theoretically, atypical antipsychotics should also inhibit stimulatory effects of amphetamines

- Theoretically, amphetamines could inhibit the antipsychotic actions of antipsychotics
- Theoretically, amphetamines could inhibit the mood-stabilizing actions of atypical antipsychotics in some patients
- Combinations of amphetamines with mood stabilizers (lithium, anticonvulsants, atypical antipsychotics) is generally something for experts only, when monitoring patients closely and when other options fail
- Absorption of amphetamines is delayed by phenobarbital, phenytoin, ethosuximide
- Amphetamines inhibit adrenergic blockers and enhance adrenergic effects of norepinephrine
- Amphetamines may antagonize hypotensive effects of veratrum alkaloids and other antihypertensives
- Amphetamines increase the analgesic effects of meperidine
- Amphetamines contribute to excessive CNS stimulation if used with large doses of propoxyphene
- Amphetamines can raise plasma corticosteroid levels
- MAOIs slow absorption of amphetamines and thus potentiate their actions, which can cause headache, hypertension, and rarely hypertensive crisis and malignant hyperthermia, sometimes with fatal results
- Use with MAOIs, including within 14 days of MAOI use, is not advised, but this can sometimes be considered by experts who monitor depressed patients closely when other treatment options for depression fail

Other Warnings/ Precautions

- Use with caution in patients with any degree of hypertension, hyperthyroidism, or history of drug abuse
- Children who are not growing or gaining weight should stop treatment, at least temporarily
- May worsen motor and phonic tics
- May worsen symptoms of thought disorder and behavioral disturbance in psychotic patients
- Stimulants have a high potential for abuse and must be used with caution in anyone with a current or past history of substance abuse or alcoholism or in emotionally unstable patients
- Administration of stimulants for prolonged periods of time should be avoided whenever possible or done only with close monitoring, as it may lead to marked tolerance and drug dependence, including psychological dependence with varying degrees of abnormal behavior
- Particular attention should be paid to the possibility of subjects obtaining stimulants for nontherapeutic use or distribution to others and the drugs should in general be prescribed sparingly with documentation of appropriate use
- Unusual dosing has been associated with sudden death in children with structural cardiac abnormalities
- Not an appropriate first-line treatment for depression or for normal fatigue
- May lower the seizure threshold
- Emergence or worsening of activation and agitation may represent the induction of a bipolar state, especially a mixed dysphoric bipolar II condition sometimes associated with suicidal ideation, and require the addition of a mood stabilizer and/or discontinuation of d-amphetamine

Do Not Use

- If patient has extreme anxiety or agitation
- If patient has motor tics or Tourette's syndrome or if there is a family history of Tourette's, unless administered by an expert in cases when the potential benefits for ADHD outweigh the risks of worsening tics
- Should generally not be administered with an MAOI, including within 14 days of MAOI use, except in heroic circumstances and by an expert
- If patient has arteriosclerosis, cardiovascular disease, or severe hypertension
- If patient has glaucoma
- If patient has structural cardiac abnormalities
- If there is a proven allergy to any sympathomimetic agent

SPECIAL POPULATIONS

Renal Impairment

- No dose adjustment necessary

Hepatic Impairment
- Use with caution

Cardiac Impairment
- Use with caution, particularly in patients with recent myocardial infarction or other conditions that could be negatively affected by increased blood pressure
- Do not use in patients with structural cardiac abnormalities

Elderly
- Some patients may tolerate lower doses better

Children and Adolescents
- Safety and efficacy not established in children under age 3
- Use in young children should be reserved for the expert
- d-amphetamine may worsen symptoms of behavioral disturbance and thought disorder in psychotic children
- d-amphetamine has acute effects on growth hormone; long-term effects are unknown but weight and height should be monitored during long-term treatment
- Narcolepsy: ages 6–12: initial 5 mg/day; increase by 5 mg each week
- ADHD: ages 3–5: initial 2.5 mg/day; increase by 2.5 mg each week
- American Heart Association recommends EKG prior to initiating stimulant treatment in children, although not all experts agree

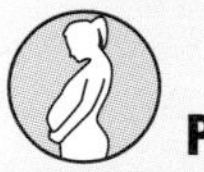

Pregnancy
- Risk Category C [some animal studies show adverse effects; no controlled studies in humans]
- There is a greater risk of premature birth and low birth weight in infants whose mothers take d-amphetamine during pregnancy
- Infants whose mothers take d-amphetamine during pregnancy may experience withdrawal symptoms
- Use in women of childbearing potential requires weighing potential benefits to the mother against potential risks to the fetus

✽ For ADHD patients, d-amphetamine should generally be discontinued before anticipated pregnancies

Breast Feeding
- Some drug is found in mother's breast milk

✽ Recommended either to discontinue drug or bottle feed

- If infant shows signs of irritability, drug may need to be discontinued

THE ART OF PSYCHOPHARMACOLOGY

Potential Advantages
- May work in ADHD patients unresponsive to other stimulants
- Established long-term efficacy of immediate-release and spansule formulations

Potential Disadvantages
- Patients with current or past substance abuse
- Patients with current or past bipolar disorder or psychosis

Primary Target Symptoms
- Concentration, attention span
- Motor hyperactivity
- Impulsiveness
- Physical and mental fatigue
- Daytime sleepiness
- Depression

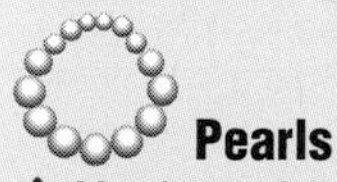

Pearls
✽ May be useful for treatment of depressive symptoms in medically ill elderly patients

✽ May be useful for treatment of post-stroke depression

✽ A classical augmentation strategy for treatment-refractory depression

✽ Specifically, may be useful for treatment of cognitive dysfunction and fatigue as residual symptoms of major depressive disorder unresponsive to multiple prior treatments

✽ May also be useful for the treatment of cognitive impairment, depressive symptoms, and severe fatigue in patients with HIV infection and in cancer patients

- Can be used to potentiate opioid analgesia and reduce sedation, particularly in end-of-life management
- Some patients respond to or tolerate d-amphetamine better than methylphenidate and vice versa

- Some patients may benefit from an occasional addition of 5–10 mg of immediate-release d-amphetamine to their daily base of sustained-release Dexedrine spansules
- ✱ Despite warnings, can be a useful adjunct to MAOIs for heroic treatment of highly refractory mood disorders when monitored with vigilance
- ✱ Can reverse sexual dysfunction caused by psychiatric illness and by some drugs such as SSRIs, including decreased libido, erectile dysfunction, delayed ejaculation, and anorgasmia
- Atypical antipsychotics may be useful in treating stimulant or psychotic consequences of overdose
- Taking with food may delay peak actions for 2–3 hours
- Half-life and duration of clinical action tend to be shorter in younger children
- Drug abuse may actually be lower in ADHD adolescents treated with stimulants than in ADHD adolescents who are not treated

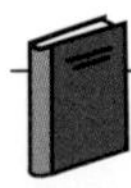

Suggested Reading

Fry JM. Treatment modalities for narcolepsy. Neurology 1998;50(2 Suppl 1):S43–8.

Greenhill LL, Pliszka S, Dulcan MK, Bernet W, Arnold V, Beitchman J, Benson RS, Bukstein O, Kinlan J, McClellan J, Rue D, Shaw JA, Stock S. Practice parameter for the use of stimulant medications in the treatment of children, adolescents, and adults. J Am Acad Child Adolesc Psychiatry 2002;41(2 Suppl):26S–49S.

Jadad AR, Boyle M, Cunningham C, Kim M, Schachar R. Treatment of attention-deficit/hyperactivity disorder. Evid Rep Technol Assess (Summ) 1999;(11):i–viii, 1–341.

Vinson DC. Therapy for attention-deficit hyperactivity disorder. Arch Fam Med 1994;3:445–51.

Wender PH, Wolf LE, Wasserstein J. Adults with ADHD. An overview. Ann N Y Acad Sci 2001;931:1–16.

THERAPEUTICS

Brands • Adderall
• Adderall XR

see index for additional brand names

Generic? No

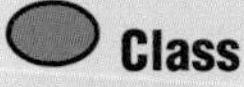

Class

• Stimulant

Commonly Prescribed for

(bold for FDA approved)

• **Attention deficit hyperactivity disorder (ADHD) in children ages 3–12 (Adderall)**
• **Attention-deficit hyperactivity disorder (ADHD) in children ages 6–17 and in adults (Adderall XR)**
• **Narcolepsy (Adderall)**
• Treatment-resistant depression

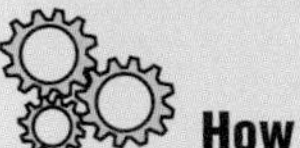

How the Drug Works

* Increases norepinephrine and especially dopamine actions by blocking their reuptake and facilitating their release
• Enhancement of dopamine and norepinephrine actions in certain brain regions (e.g., dorsolateral prefrontal cortex) may improve attention, concentration, executive function, and wakefulness
• Enhancement of dopamine actions in other brain regions (e.g., basal ganglia) may improve hyperactivity
• Enhancement of dopamine and norepinephrine in yet other brain regions (e.g., medial prefrontal cortex, hypothalamus) may improve depression, fatigue, and sleepiness

How Long Until It Works

• Some immediate effects can be seen with first dosing
• Can take several weeks to attain maximum therapeutic benefit

If It Works (for ADHD)

• The goal of treatment of ADHD is reduction of symptoms of inattentiveness, motor hyperactivity, and/or impulsiveness that disrupt social, school, and/or occupational functioning
• Continue treatment until all symptoms are under control or improvement is stable and then continue treatment indefinitely as long as improvement persists
• Reevaluate the need for treatment periodically
• Treatment for ADHD begun in childhood may need to be continued into adolescence and adulthood if continued benefit is documented

If It Doesn't Work (for ADHD)

• Consider adjusting dose or switching to another formulation of d,l-amphetamine or to another agent
• Consider behavioral therapy
• Consider the presence of noncompliance and counsel patient and parents
• Consider evaluation for another diagnosis or for a comorbid condition (e.g., bipolar disorder, substance abuse, medical illness, etc.)
* Some ADHD patients and some depressed patients may experience lack of consistent efficacy due to activation of latent or underlying bipolar disorder, and require either augmenting with a mood stabilizer or switching to a mood stabilizer

Best Augmenting Combos for Partial Response or Treatment Resistance

• Best to attempt other monotherapies prior to augmenting
• For the expert, can combine immediate-release formulation with a sustained-release formulation of d,l-amphetamine for ADHD
• For the expert, can combine with modafinil or atomoxetine for ADHD
• For the expert, can occasionally combine with atypical antipsychotics in highly treatment-resistant cases of bipolar disorder or ADHD
• For the expert, can combine with antidepressants to boost antidepressant efficacy in highly treatment-resistant cases of depression while carefully monitoring patient

Tests

• Blood pressure should be monitored regularly
• In children, monitor weight and height

SIDE EFFECTS

How Drug Causes Side Effects

- Increases in norepinephrine peripherally can cause autonomic side effects, including tremor, tachycardia, hypertension, and cardiac arrhythmias
- Increases in norepinephrine and dopamine centrally can cause CNS side effects such as insomnia, agitation, psychosis, and substance abuse

Notable Side Effects

✻ Insomnia, headache, exacerbation of tics, nervousness, irritability, overstimulation, tremor, dizziness
- Anorexia, nausea, dry mouth, constipation, diarrhea, weight loss
- Can temporarily slow normal growth in children (controversial)
- Sexual dysfunction long-term (impotence, libido changes) but can also improve sexual dysfunction short-term

Life-Threatening or Dangerous Side Effects

- Psychotic episodes, especially with parenteral abuse
- Seizures
- Palpitations, tachycardia, hypertension
- Rare activation of hypomania, mania, or suicidal ideation (controversial)
- Cardiovascular adverse effects, sudden death in patients with preexisting cardiac structural abnormalities

Weight Gain

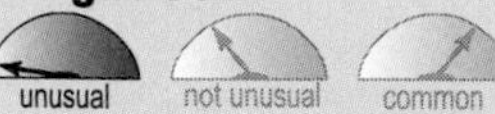

- Reported but not expected
- Some patients may experience weight loss

Sedation

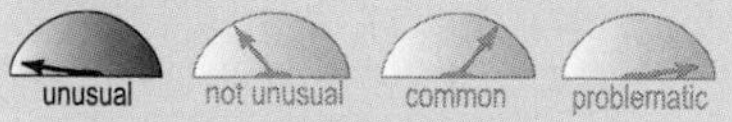

- Reported but not expected
- Activation much more common than sedation

What to Do About Side Effects

- Wait
- Adjust dose
- Switch to a long-acting stimulant
- Switch to another agent
- For insomnia, avoid dosing in afternoon/evening

Best Augmenting Agents for Side Effects

- Beta blockers for peripheral autonomic side effects
- Dose reduction or switching to another agent may be more effective since most side effects cannot be improved with an augmenting agent

DOSING AND USE

Usual Dosage Range

- Narcolepsy: 5–60 mg/day in divided doses
- ADHD: 5–40 mg/day (divided doses for immediate-release tablet, once-daily morning dose for extended-release tablet)

Dosage Forms

- Immediate-release tablet 5 mg double-scored, 7.5 mg double-scored, 10 mg double-scored, 12.5 mg double-scored, 15 mg double-scored, 20 mg double-scored, 30 mg double-scored
- Extended-release tablet 5 mg, 10 mg, 15 mg, 20 mg, 25 mg, 30 mg

How To Dose

- Immediate-release formulation in ADHD (ages 6 and older): initial 5 mg once or twice per day; can increase by 5 mg each week; maximum dose generally 40 mg/day; split daily dose with first dose on waking and every 4–6 hours thereafter
- Immediate-release formulation in narcolepsy (ages 12 and older): initial 10 mg/day; increase by 10 mg each week; give first dose on waking and every 4–6 hours thereafter
- Extended-release formulation in ADHD: initial 10 mg/day in the morning; can increase by 5–10 mg/day at weekly intervals; maximum dose generally 30 mg/day

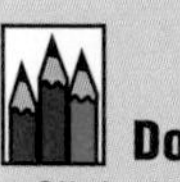

Dosing Tips

- Clinical duration of action often differs from pharmacokinetic half-life

✻ Immediate-release d,l-amphetamine has 3–6 hour duration of clinical action

* ✻ Extended-release d,l-amphetamine has up to 8-hour duration of clinical action
* Adderall XR is controlled-release and should therefore not be chewed but rather should only be swallowed whole
* ✻ Controlled-release delivery of d,l-amphetamine is sufficiently long in duration to allow elimination of lunchtime dosing
* ✻ This innovation can be an important practical element in stimulant utilization, eliminating the hassle and pragmatic difficulties of lunchtime dosing at school, including storage problems, potential diversion, and the need for a medical professional to supervise dosing away from home
* Avoid dosing late in the day because of the risk of insomnia
* May be possible to dose only during the school week for some ADHD patients
* Off-label uses are dosed the same as for ADHD
* ✻ May be able to give drug holidays over the summer in order to reassess therapeutic utility and effects on growth and to allow catch-up from any growth suppression as well as to assess any other side effects and the need to reinstitute stimulant treatment for the next school term
* Side effects are generally dose-related
* Taking with food may delay peak actions for 2–3 hours

Overdose

* Rarely fatal; panic, hyperreflexia, rhabdomyolysis, rapid respiration, confusion, coma, hallucinations, convulsions, arrhythmia, change in blood pressure, circulatory collapse

Long-Term Use

* Often used long-term for ADHD when ongoing monitoring documents continued efficacy
* Dependence and/or abuse may develop
* Tolerance to therapeutic effects may develop in some patients
* Long-term stimulant use may be associated with growth suppression in children (controversial)
* Periodic monitoring of weight, blood pressure, CBC, platelet counts, and liver function may be prudent

Habit Forming

* High abuse potential, Schedule II drug
* Patients may develop tolerance, psychological dependence

How to Stop

* Taper to avoid withdrawal effects
* Withdrawal following chronic therapeutic use may unmask symptoms of the underlying disorder and may require follow-up and reinstitution of treatment
* Careful supervision is required during withdrawal from abusive use since severe depression may occur

Pharmacokinetics

* Adderall and Adderall XR are a mixture of d-amphetamine and l-amphetamine salts in the ratio of 3:1
* A single dose of Adderall XR 20 mg gives drug levels of both d-amphetamine and l-amphetamine comparable to Adderall immediate-release 20 mg administered in 2 divided doses 4 hours apart
* In adults, half-life for d-amphetamine is 10 hours and for l-amphetamine is 13 hours
* For children ages 6–12, half-life for d-amphetamine is 9 hours and for l-amphetamine is 11 hours

Drug Interactions

* May affect blood pressure and should be used cautiously with agents used to control blood pressure
* Gastrointestinal acidifying agents (guanethidine, reserpine, glutamic acid, ascorbic acid, fruit juices, etc.) and urinary acidifying agents (ammonium chloride, sodium phosphate, etc.) lower amphetamine plasma levels, so such agents can be useful to administer after an overdose but may also lower therapeutic efficacy of amphetamines
* Gastrointestinal alkalinizing agents (sodium bicarbonate, etc.) and urinary alkalinizing agents (acetazolamide, some thiazides) increase amphetamine plasma levels and potentiate amphetamine's actions
* Desipramine and protryptiline can cause striking and sustained increases in brain concentrations of amphetamine and may also add to amphetamine's cardiovascular effects

- Theoretically, other agents with norepinephrine reuptake blocking properties, such as venlafaxine, duloxetine, atomoxetine, milnacipran, and reboxetine, could also add to amphetamine's CNS and cardiovascular effects
- Amphetamines may counteract the sedative effects of antihistamines
- Haloperidol, chlorpromazine, and lithium may inhibit stimulatory effects of amphetamines
- Theoretically, atypical antipsychotics should also inhibit stimulatory effects of amphetamines
- Theoretically, amphetamines could inhibit the antipsychotic actions of antipsychotics
- Theoretically, amphetamines could inhibit the mood-stabilizing actions of atypical antipsychotics in some patients
- Combinations of amphetamines with mood stabilizers (lithium, anticonvulsants, atypical antipsychotics) is generally something for experts only, when monitoring patients closely and when other options fail
- Absorption of amphetamine is delayed by phenobarbital, phenytoin, ethosuximide
- Amphetamines inhibit adrenergic blockers and enhance adrenergic effects of norepinephrine
- Amphetamines may antagonize hypotensive effects of veratrum alkaloids and other antihypertensives
- Amphetamines increase the analgesic effects of meperidine
- Amphetamines contribute to excessive CNS stimulation if used with large doses of propoxyphene
- Amphetamines can raise plasma corticosteroid levels
- MAOIs slow absorption of amphetamines and thus potentiate their actions, which can cause headache, hypertension, and rarely hypertensive crisis and malignant hyperthermia, sometimes with fatal results
- Use with MAOIs, including within 14 days of MAOI use, is not advised, but this can sometimes be considered by experts who monitor depressed patients closely when other treatment options for depression fail

Other Warnings/ Precautions

- Use with caution in patients with any degree of hypertension, hyperthyroidism, or history of drug abuse
- Children who are not growing or gaining weight should stop treatment, at least temporarily
- May worsen motor and phonic tics
- May worsen symptoms of thought disorder and behavioral disturbance in psychotic patients
- Stimulants have a high potential for abuse and must be used with caution in anyone with a current or past history of substance abuse or alcoholism or in emotionally unstable patients
- Administration of stimulants for prolonged periods of time should be avoided whenever possible or done only with close monitoring, as it may lead to marked tolerance and drug dependence, including psychological dependence with varying degrees of abnormal behavior
- Particular attention should be paid to the possibility of subjects obtaining stimulants for nontherapeutic use or distribution to others and the drugs should in general be prescribed sparingly with documentation of appropriate use
- Unusual dosing has been associated with sudden death in children with structural cardiac abnormalities
- Not an appropriate first-line treatment for depression or for normal fatigue
- May lower the seizure threshold
- Emergence or worsening of activation and agitation may represent the induction of a bipolar state, especially a mixed dysphoric bipolar II condition sometimes associated with suicidal ideation, and require the addition of a mood stabilizer and/or discontinuation of d,l-amphetamine

Do Not Use

- If patient has extreme anxiety or agitation
- If patient has motor tics or Tourette's syndrome or if there is a family history of Tourette's, unless administered by an expert in cases when the potential benefits for ADHD outweigh the risks of worsening tics
- Should generally not be administered with an MAOI, including within 14 days of MAOI

use, except in heroic circumstances and by an expert
- If patient has arteriosclerosis, cardiovascular disease, or severe hypertension
- If patient has glaucoma
- If patient has structural cardiac abnormalities
- If there is a proven allergy to any sympathomimetic agent

SPECIAL POPULATIONS

Renal Impairment
- No dose adjustment necessary

Hepatic Impairment
- No dose adjustment necessary

Cardiac Impairment
- Use with caution, particularly in patients with recent myocardial infarction or other conditions that could be negatively affected by increased blood pressure
- Do not use in patients with structural cardiac abnormalities

Elderly
- Some patients may tolerate lower doses better

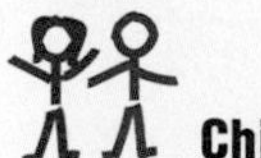

Children and Adolescents
- Safety and efficacy not established in children under age 3
- Use in young children should be reserved for the expert
- d,l-amphetamine may worsen symptoms of behavioral disturbance and thought disorder in psychotic children
- d,l-amphetamine has acute effects on growth hormone; long-term effects are unknown but weight and height should be monitored during long-term treatment
- ADHD: ages 3–5: initial 2.5 mg/day; can increase by 2.5 mg each week
- Narcolepsy: ages 6–12: initial 5 mg/day; increase by 5 mg each week
- American Heart Association recommends EKG prior to initiating stimulant treatment in children, although not all experts agree

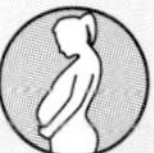

Pregnancy
- Risk Category C [some animal studies show adverse effects; no controlled studies in humans]
- Infants whose mothers take d,l-amphetamine during pregnancy may experience withdrawal symptoms
- Use in women of childbearing potential requires weighing potential benefits to the mother against potential risks to the fetus

✻ For ADHD patients, d,l-amphetamine should generally be discontinued before anticipated pregnancies

Breast Feeding
- Some drug is found in mother's breast milk

✻ Recommended either to discontinue drug or bottle feed

- If infant shows signs of irritability, drug may need to be discontinued

THE ART OF PSYCHOPHARMACOLOGY

Potential Advantages
- May work in ADHD patients unresponsive to other stimulants, including pure d-amphetamine sulfate
- New sustained-release option

Potential Disadvantages
- Patients with current or past substance abuse
- Patients with current or past bipolar disorder or psychosis

Primary Target Symptoms
- Concentration, attention span
- Motor hyperactivity
- Impulsiveness
- Physical and mental fatigue
- Daytime sleepiness
- Depression

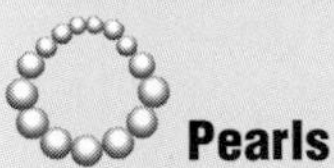

Pearls

✻ May be useful for treatment of depressive symptoms in medically ill elderly patients

✻ May be useful for treatment of post-stroke depression

✻ A classical augmentation strategy for treatment-refractory depression

* Specifically, may be useful for treatment of cognitive dysfunction and fatigue as residual symptoms of major depressive disorder unresponsive to multiple prior treatments
* May also be useful for the treatment of cognitive impairment, depressive symptoms, and severe fatigue in patients with HIV infection and in cancer patients
- Can be used to potentiate opioid analgesia and reduce sedation, particularly in end-of-life management
* Despite warnings, can be a useful adjunct to MAOIs for heroic treatment of highly refractory mood disorders when monitored with vigilance
* Can reverse sexual dysfunction caused by psychiatric illness and by some drugs such as SSRIs, including decreased libido, erectile dysfunction, delayed ejaculation, and anorgasmia
- Atypical antipsychotics may be useful in treating stimulant or psychotic consequences of overdose
- Taking with food may delay peak actions for 2–3 hours
- Half-life and duration of clinical action tend to be shorter in younger children
- Drug abuse may actually be lower in ADHD adolescents treated with stimulants than in ADHD adolescents who are not treated
- Some patients respond to or tolerate d,l-amphetamine better than methylphenidate and vice versa
* Adderall and Adderall XR are a mixture of d-amphetamine and l-amphetamine salts in the ratio of 3:1
* Specifically, Adderall and Adderall XR combine 1 part dextro-amphetamine saccharate, 1 part dextro-amphetamine sulfate, 1 part d,l-amphetamine aspartate, and 1 part d,l-amphetamine sulfate
* This mixture of salts may have a different pharmacologic profile, including mechanism of therapeutic action and duration of action, compared to pure dextro-amphetamine, which is given as the sulfate salt
* Specifically, d-amphetamine may have more profound action on dopamine than norepinephrine whereas l-amphetamine may have a more balanced action on both dopamine and norepinephrine
* Theoretically, this could lead to relatively more noradrenergic actions of the Adderall mixture of amphetamine salts than that of pure dextro-amphetamine sulfate, but this is unproven and of no clear clinical significance
- Nevertheless, some patients may respond to or tolerate Adderall/Adderall XR differently than they do pure dextro-amphetamine sulfate
- Adderall XR capsules also contain 2 types of drug-containing beads designed to give a double-pulsed delivery of amphetamines to prolong their release

Suggested Reading

Fry JM. Treatment modalities for narcolepsy. Neurology 1998;50(2 Suppl 1):S43–8.

Greenhill LL, Pliszka S, Dulcan MK, Bernet W, Arnold V, Beitchman J, Benson RS, Bukstein O, Kinlan J, McClellan J, Rue D, Shaw JA, Stock S. Practice parameter for the use of stimulant medications in the treatment of children, adolescents, and adults. J Am Acad Child Adolesc Psychiatry 2002;41(2 Suppl):26S–49S.

Jadad AR, Boyle M, Cunningham C, Kim M, Schachar R. Treatment of attention-deficit/hyperactivity disorder. Evid Rep Technol Assess (Summ) 1999;(11):i–viii,1–341.

Vinson DC. Therapy for attention-deficit hyperactivity disorder. Arch Fam Med 1994;3:445–51.

Wender PH, Wolf LE, Wasserstein J. Adults with ADHD. An overview. Ann N Y Acad Sci 2001;931:1–16.

THERAPEUTICS

Brands • Abilify
see index for additional brand names

Generic? Not in U.S., Europe, or Japan

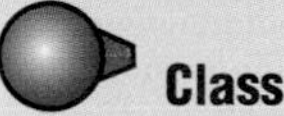

Class

- Dopamine partial agonist (dopamine stabilizer, atypical antipsychotic, third generation antipsychotic; sometimes included as a second-generation antipsychotic; also a mood stabilizer)

Commonly Prescribed for

(bold for FDA approved)

- **Schizophrenia (ages 13 and older)**
- **Maintaining stability in schizophrenia**
- **Acute mania/mixed mania (ages 10 and older)**
- **Bipolar maintenance**
- **Depression (adjunct)**
- Bipolar depression
- Other psychotic disorders
- Behavioral disturbances in dementias
- Behavioral disturbances in children and adolescents
- Disorders associated with problems with impulse control

How the Drug Works

✱ Partial agonism at dopamine 2 receptors
- Theoretically reduces dopamine output when dopamine concentrations are high, thus improving positive symptoms and mediating antipsychotic actions
- Theoretically increases dopamine output when dopamine concentrations are low, thus improving cognitive, negative, and mood symptoms
- Actions at dopamine 3 receptors could theoretically contribute to aripiprazole's efficacy
- Partial agonism at 5HT1A receptors may be relevant at clinical doses
- Blockade of serotonin type 2A receptors may contribute at clinical doses to cause enhancement of dopamine release in certain brain regions, thus reducing motor side effects and possibly improving cognitive and affective symptoms

How Long Until It Works

- Psychotic and manic symptoms can improve within 1 week, but it may take several weeks for full effect on behavior as well as on cognition and affective stabilization
- Classically recommended to wait at least 4–6 weeks to determine efficacy of drug, but in practice some patients require up to 16–20 weeks to show a good response, especially on cognitive symptoms

If It Works

- Most often reduces positive symptoms in schizophrenia but does not eliminate them
- Can improve negative symptoms, as well as aggressive, cognitive, and affective symptoms in schizophrenia
- Most schizophrenic patients do not have a total remission of symptoms but rather a reduction of symptoms by about a third
- Perhaps 5–15% of schizophrenic patients can experience an overall improvement of greater than 50–60%, especially when receiving stable treatment for more than a year
- Such patients are considered super-responders or "awakeners" since they may be well enough to be employed, live independently, and sustain long-term relationships
- Many bipolar patients may experience a reduction of symptoms by half or more
- Continue treatment until reaching a plateau of improvement
- After reaching a satisfactory plateau, continue treatment for at least a year after first episode of psychosis
- For second and subsequent episodes of psychosis, treatment may need to be indefinite
- Even for first episodes of psychosis, it may be preferable to continue treatment indefinitely to avoid subsequent episodes
- Treatment may not only reduce mania but also prevent recurrences of mania in bipolar disorder

If It Doesn't Work

- Try one of the other atypical antipsychotics (risperidone, olanzapine, quetiapine, ziprasidone, paliperidone, amisulpride)
- If two or more antipsychotic monotherapies do not work, consider clozapine

- If no first-line atypical antipsychotic is effective, consider higher doses or augmentation with valproate or lamotrigine
- Some patients may require treatment with a conventional antipsychotic
- Consider noncompliance and switch to another antipsychotic with fewer side effects or to an antipsychotic that can be given by depot injection
- Consider initiating rehabilitation and psychotherapy
- Consider presence of concomitant drug abuse

Best Augmenting Combos for Partial Response or Treatment Resistance

- Valproic acid (valproate, divalproex, divalproex ER)
- Other mood-stabilizing anticonvulsants (carbamazepine, oxcarbazepine, lamotrigine)
- Lithium
- Benzodiazepines

Tests

Before starting an atypical antipsychotic

* Weigh all patients and track BMI during treatment
- Get baseline personal and family history of diabetes, obesity, dyslipidemia, hypertension, and cardiovascular disease

* Get waist circumference (at umbilicus), blood pressure, fasting plasma glucose, and fasting lipid profile
- Determine if the patient is
  - overweight (BMI 25.0–29.9)
  - obese (BMI ≥30)
  - has pre-diabetes (fasting plasma glucose 100–25 mg/dL)
  - has diabetes (fasting plasma glucose >126 mg/dL)
  - has hypertension (BP >140/90 mm Hg)
  - has dyslipidemia (increased total cholesterol, LDL cholesterol, and triglycerides; decreased HDL cholesterol)
- Treat or refer such patients for treatment, including nutrition and weight management, physical activity counseling, smoking cessation, and medical management

Monitoring after starting an atypical antipsychotic

* BMI monthly for 3 months, then quarterly

* Consider monitoring fasting triglycerides monthly for several months in patients at high risk for metabolic complications and when initiating or switching antipsychotics

* Blood pressure, fasting plasma glucose, fasting lipids within 3 months and then annually, but earlier and more frequently for patients with diabetes or who have gained >5% of initial weight
- Treat or refer for treatment and consider switching to another atypical antipsychotic for patients who become overweight, obese, pre-diabetic, diabetic, hypertensive, or dyslipidemic while receiving an atypical antipsychotic

* Even in patients without known diabetes, be vigilant for the rare but life-threatening onset of diabetic ketoacidosis, which always requires immediate treatment, by monitoring for the rapid onset of polyuria, polydipsia, weight loss, nausea, vomiting, dehydration, rapid respiration, weakness and clouding of sensorium, even coma

SIDE EFFECTS

How Drug Causes Side Effects

- By blocking alpha 1 adrenergic receptors, it can cause dizziness, sedation, and hypotension
- Partial agonist actions at dopamine 2 receptors in the striatum can cause motor side effects, such as akathisia (occasionally)
- Partial agonist actions at dopamine 2 receptors can also cause nausea, occasional vomiting, and activating side effects

* Mechanism of any possible weight gain is unknown; weight gain is not common with aripiprazole and may thus have a different mechanism from atypical antipsychotics for which weight gain is common or problematic

* Mechanism of any possible increased incidence of diabetes or dyslipidemia is unknown; early experience suggests these complications are not clearly associated with aripiprazole and if present may therefore have a different mechanism from that of atypical antipsychotics associated with an increased incidence of diabetes and dyslipidemia

Notable Side Effects

✻ Dizziness, insomnia, akathisia, activation
✻ Nausea, vomiting
- Orthostatic hypotension, occasionally during initial dosing
- Constipation
- Headache, asthenia, sedation
- Theoretical risk of tardive dyskinesia

Life-Threatening or Dangerous Side Effects

- Rare neuroleptic malignant syndrome (much reduced risk compared to conventional antipsychotics)
- Rare seizures
- Increased risk of death and cerebrovascular events in elderly patients with dementia-related psychosis

Weight Gain

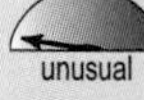

not unusual common problematic

- Reported in a few patients, especially those with low BMIs, but not expected
- Less frequent and less severe than for most other antipsychotics

Sedation

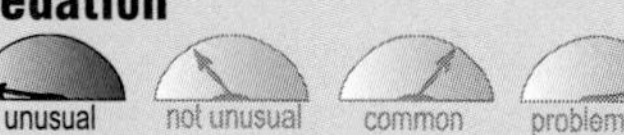

- Reported in a few patients but not expected
- May be less than for some other antipsychotics, but never say never
- Can be activating

What to Do About Side Effects

- Wait
- Wait
- Wait
- Reduce the dose
- Anticholinergics may reduce akathisia when present
- Weight loss, exercise programs, and medical management for high BMIs, diabetes, dyslipidemia
- Switch to another atypical antipsychotic

Best Augmenting Agents for Side Effects

- Benztropine or trihexyphenidyl for motor side effects and akathisia
- Many side effects cannot be improved with an augmenting agent

DOSING AND USE

Usual Dosage Range

- 15–30 mg/day

Dosage Forms

- Tablet 2 mg, 5 mg, 10 mg, 15 mg, 20 mg, 30 mg
- Orally disintegrating tablet 10 mg, 15 mg
- Oral solution 1 mg/mL
- Injection 9.75 mg/1.3 mL

How To Dose

- Initial approved recommendation is 10–15 mg/day; maximum approved dose 30 mg/day
- Oral solution: solution doses can be substituted for tablet doses on a mg-per-mg basis up to 25 mg; patients receiving 30-mg tablet should receive 25-mg solution

Dosing Tips

✻ **For some, less may be more:** frequently, patients not acutely psychotic may need to be dosed lower (e.g., 2.5–10 mg/day) in order to avoid akathisia and activation and for maximum tolerability
- **For others, more may be more:** rarely, patients may need to be dosed higher than 30 mg/day for optimum efficacy
- Consider cutting 5 mg tablet in half (tablets not scored) or administering 1–5 mg as the oral solution for children and adolescents, as well as for adults very sensitive to side effects

✻ Although studies suggest patients switching to aripiprazole from another antipsychotic can do well with rapid switch or with cross-titration, clinical experience suggests many patients may do best by adding a full dose of aripiprazole to the maintenance dose of the first antipsychotic for at least several days and possibly as long as 3 or 4 weeks prior to slow down-titration of the first antipsychotic
- Rather than raise the dose above these levels in acutely agitated patients requiring acute antipsychotic actions, consider augmentation with a benzodiazepine or conventional antipsychotic, either orally or intramuscularly
- Rather than raise the dose above these levels in partial responders, consider

augmentation with a mood-stabilizing anticonvulsant, such as valproate or lamotrigine
- Children and elderly should generally be dosed at the lower end of the dosage spectrum
- Less expensive than some antipsychotics, more expensive than others depending on dose administered
- Due to its very long half-life, aripiprazole will take longer to reach steady state when initiating dosing, and longer to wash out when stopping dosing, than other atypical antipsychotics

Overdose
- No fatalities have been reported; sedation, vomiting

Long-Term Use
- Approved to delay relapse in long-term treatment of schizophrenia
- Approved for long-term maintenance in bipolar disorder
- Often used for long-term maintenance in various behavioral disorders

Habit Forming
- No

How to Stop
- Slow down-titration (over 6–8 weeks), especially when simultaneously beginning a new antipsychotic while switching (i.e., cross-titration)
- Rapid discontinuation could theoretically lead to rebound psychosis and worsening of symptoms

Pharmacokinetics
- Metabolized primarily by CYP450 2D6 and CYP450 3A4
- Mean elimination half-life 75 hours (aripiprazole) and 94 hours (major metabolite dehydro-aripiprazole)

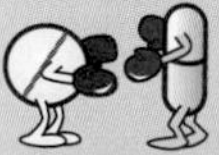

Drug Interactions
- Ketaconazole and possibly other CYP450 3A4 inhibitors such as nefazodone, fluvoxamine, and fluoxetine may increase plasma levels of aripiprazole
- Carbamazepine and possibly other inducers of CYP450 3A4 may decrease plasma levels of aripiprazole
- Quinidine and possibly other inhibitors of CYP40 2D6 such as paroxetine, fluoxetine, and duloxetine may increase plasma levels of aripiprazole
- Aripiprazole may enhance the effects of antihypertensive drugs
- Aripiprazole may antagonize levodopa, dopamine agonists

Other Warnings/ Precautions
- Use with caution in patients with conditions that predispose to hypotension (dehydration, overheating)
- Dysphagia has been associated with antipsychotic use, and aripiprazole should be used cautiously in patients at risk for aspiration pneumonia

Do Not Use
- If there is a proven allergy to aripiprazole

SPECIAL POPULATIONS

Renal Impairment
- Dose adjustment not necessary

Hepatic Impairment
- Dose adjustment not necessary

Cardiac Impairment
- Use in patients with cardiac impairment has not been studied, so use with caution because of risk of orthostatic hypotension

Elderly
- Dose adjustment generally not necessary, but some elderly patients may tolerate lower doses better
- Although atypical antipsychotics are commonly used for behavioral disturbances in dementia, no agent has been approved for treatment of elderly patients with dementia-related psychosis
- Elderly patients with dementia-related psychosis treated with atypical antipsychotics are at an increased risk of death compared to placebo, and also have an increased risk of cerebrovascular events

Children and Adolescents

- Approved for use in schizophrenia (ages 13 and older) and manic/mixed episodes (ages 10 and older)
- Clinical experience and early data suggest aripiprazole may be safe and effective for behavioral disturbances in children and adolescents, especially at lower doses
- Children and adolescents using aripiprazole may need to be monitored more often than adults and may tolerate lower doses better

Pregnancy

- Risk Category C [some animal studies show adverse effects; no controlled studies in humans]
- Psychotic symptoms may worsen during pregnancy and some form of treatment may be necessary
- Aripiprazole may be preferable to anticonvulsant mood stabilizers if treatment is required during pregnancy

Breast Feeding

- Unknown if aripiprazole is secreted in human breast milk, but all psychotropics assumed to be secreted in breast milk

✻ Recommended either to discontinue drug or bottle feed

- Infants of women who choose to breast feed while on aripiprazole should be monitored for possible adverse effects

THE ART OF PSYCHOPHARMACOLOGY

Potential Advantages

- Some cases of psychosis and bipolar disorder refractory to treatment with other antipsychotics

✻ Patients concerned about gaining weight and patients who are already obese or overweight

✻ Patients with diabetes

✻ Patients with dyslipidemia (especially elevated triglycerides)

- Patients requiring rapid onset of antipsychotic action without dosage titration

✻ Patients who wish to avoid sedation

Potential Disadvantages

- Patients in whom sedation is desired
- May be more difficult to dose for children, elderly, or "off label" uses

Primary Target Symptoms

- Positive symptoms of psychosis
- Negative symptoms of psychosis
- Cognitive symptoms
- Unstable mood
- Aggressive symptoms

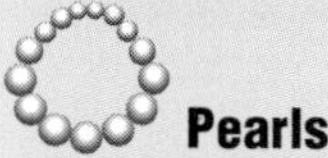

Pearls

✻ Only antipsychotic currently approved as an adjunct treatment for depression (e.g., to SSRIs, SNRIs)

✻ One of only two atypical antipsychotics with an indication in children

✻ Well accepted in clinical practice when wanting to avoid weight gain because less weight gain than most other antipsychotics

✻ Well accepted in clinical practice when wanting to avoid sedation because less sedation than most other antipsychotics at all doses

✻ Can even be activating, which can be reduced by lowering the dose or starting at a lower dose

- If sedation is desired, a benzodiazepine can be added short-term at the initiation of treatment until symptoms of agitation and insomnia are stabilized or intermittently as needed
- A moderately priced atypical antipsychotic within the therapeutic dosing range

✻ May not have diabetes or dyslipidemia risk, but monitoring is still indicated

- Anecdotal reports of utility in treatment-resistant cases
- Has a very favorable tolerability profile in clinical practice
- Favorable tolerability profile leading to "off-label" uses for many indications other than schizophrenia (e.g., bipolar II disorder, including hypomanic, mixed, rapid cycling, and depressed phases; treatment-resistant depression; anxiety disorders)

✻ An intramuscular formulation is currently in development

Suggested Reading

Andrezina R, Josiassen RC, Marcus RN, et al. Intramuscular aripiprazole for the treatment of acute agitation in patients with schizophrenia or schizoaffective disorder: a double-blind, placebo-controlled comparison with intramuscular haloperidol. Psychopharmacology 2006;188(3):281–92.

El-Sayeh HG, Morganti C. Aripiprazole for schizophrenia. Cochrane Databse Syst Rev 2006;(2):CD004578.

Marcus RN, McQuade RD, Carson WH, et al. The efficacy and safety of aripiprazole as adjunctive therapy in major depressive disorder: a second multicenter, randomized, double-blind, placebo-controlled study. J Clin Psychopharmacol 2008;28(2):156–65.

Nasrallah HA. Atypical antipsychotic-induced metabolic side effects: insights from receptor-binding profiles. Mol Psychiatry 2008;13(1):27–35.

Smith LA, Cornelius V, Warnock A, Tacchi MJ, Taylor D. Pharmacological interventions for acute bipolar mania: a systematic review of randomized placebo-controlled trials. Bipolar Disord 2007;9(6):551–60.

THERAPEUTICS

Brands • Strattera

see index for additional brand names

Generic? No

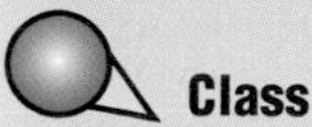

Class

- Selective norepinephrine reuptake inhibitor (NRI)

Commonly Prescribed for

(bold for FDA approved)

- **Attention deficit hyperactivity disorder (ADHD) in adults and children over 6**
- Treatment-resistant depression

How the Drug Works

- Boosts neurotransmitter norepinephrine/noradrenaline and may also increase dopamine in profrontal cortex
- Blocks norepinephrine reuptake pumps, also known as norepinephrine transporters
- Presumably this increases noradrenergic neurotransmission
- Since dopamine is inactivated by norepinephrine reuptake in frontal cortex, which largely lacks dopamine transporters, atomoxetine can also increase dopamine neurotransmission in this part of the brain

How Long Until It Works

* Onset of therapeutic actions in ADHD can be seen as early as the first day of dosing
- Therapeutic actions may continue to improve for 8–12 weeks
- If it is not working within 6–8 weeks, it may not work at all

If It Works

- The goal of treatment of ADHD is reduction of symptoms of inattentiveness, motor hyperactivity, and/or impulsiveness that disrupt social, school, and/or occupational functioning
- Continue treatment until all symptoms are under control or improvement is stable and then continue treatment indefinitely as long as improvement persists
- Reevaluate the need for treatment periodically
- Treatment for ADHD begun in childhood may need to be continued into adolescence and adulthood if continued benefit is documented

If It Doesn't Work

- Consider adjusting dose or switching to another agent
- Consider behavioral therapy
- Consider the presence of noncompliance and counsel patient and parents
- Consider evaluation for another diagnosis or for a comorbid condition (e.g., bipolar disorder, substance abuse, medical illness, etc.)
- Some patients may experience apparent lack of consistent efficacy due to activation of latent or underlying bipolar disorder, and require atomoxetine discontinuation and a switch to a mood stabilizer

Best Augmenting Combos for Partial Response or Treatment Resistance

* Best to attempt other monotherapies prior to augmenting
- SSRIs, SNRIs, or mirtazapine for treatment-resistant depression (use combinations of antidepressants with atomoxetine with caution as this may theoretically activate bipolar disorder and suicidal ideation)
- Mood stabilizers or atypical antipsychotics for comorbid bipolar disorder
- For the expert, can combine with modafinil, methylphenidate, or amphetamine for ADHD

Tests

- None recommended for healthy patients
- May be prudent to monitor blood pressure and pulse when initiating treatment and until dosage increments have stabilized

SIDE EFFECTS

How Drug Causes Side Effects

- Norepinephrine increases in parts of the brain and body and at receptors other than those that cause therapeutic actions (e.g., unwanted actions of norepinephrine on acetylcholine release causing decreased appetite, increased heart rate and blood pressure, dry mouth, urinary retention, etc.)

- Most side effects are immediate but often go away with time
- Lack of enhancing dopamine activity in limbic areas theoretically explains atomoxetine's lack of abuse potential

Notable Side Effects

❋ Sedation, fatigue (particularly in children)
❋ Decreased appetite
- Increased heart rate (6–9 beats/min)
- Increased blood pressure (2–4 mm Hg)
- Insomnia, dizziness, anxiety, agitation, aggression, irritability
- Dry mouth, constipation, nausea, vomiting, abdominal pain, dyspepsia
- Urinary hesitancy, urinary retention (older men)
- Dysmenorrhea, sweating
- Sexual dysfunction (men: decreased libido, erectile disturbance, impotence, ejaculatory dysfunction, abnormal orgasm; women: decreased libido, abnormal orgasm)

Life-Threatening or Dangerous Side Effects

- Increased heart rate and hypertension
- Orthostatic hypotension
- Severe liver damage (rare)
- Hypomania and, theoretically, rare induction of mania
- Rare activation of suicidal ideation and behavior (suicidality) (short-term studies did not show an increase in the risk of suicidality with antidepressants compared to placebo beyond age 24)

Weight Gain

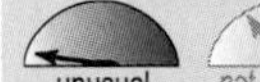

unusual not unusual common problematic

- Reported but not expected
- Patients may experience weight loss

Sedation

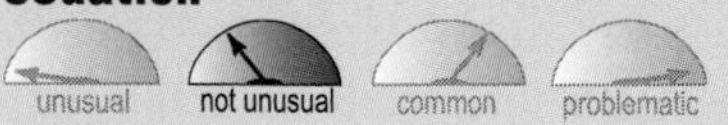

- Occurs in significant minority, particularly in children

What to Do About Side Effects

- Wait
- Wait
- Wait
- Lower the dose
- If giving once daily, can change to split dose twice daily
- If atomoxetine is sedating, take at night to reduce daytime drowsiness
- In a few weeks, switch or add other drugs

Best Augmenting Agents for Side Effects

- For urinary hesitancy, give an alpha 1 blocker such as tamsulosin
- Often best to try another monotherapy prior to resorting to augmentation strategies to treat side effects
- Many side effects are dose-dependent (i.e., they increase as dose increases, or they reemerge until tolerance redevelops)
- Many side effects are time-dependent (i.e., they start immediately upon dosing and upon each dose increase, but go away with time)
- Activation and agitation may represent the induction of a bipolar state, especially a mixed dysphoric bipolar II condition sometimes associated with suicidal ideation, and require the addition of lithium, a mood stabilizer or an atypical antipsychotic, and/or discontinuation of atomoxetine

DOSING AND USE

Usual Dosage Range

- 0.5–1.2 mg/kg per day in children up to 70 kg; 40–100 mg/day in adults

Dosage Forms

- Capsule 10 mg, 18 mg, 25 mg, 40 mg, 60 mg, 80 mg, 100 mg

How To Dose

- For children 70 kg or less: initial dose 0.5 mg/kg per day; after 7 days can increase to 1.2 mg/kg per day either once in the morning or divided; maximum dose 1.4 mg/kg per day or 100 mg per day, whichever is less
- For adults and children over 70 kg: initial dose 40 mg/day; after 7 days can increase to 80 mg/day once in the morning or divided; after 2–4 weeks can increase to

100 mg/day if necessary; maximum daily dose 100 mg

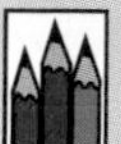

Dosing Tips

- Can be given once a day in the morning
- * Efficacy with once-daily dosing despite a half-life of 5 hours suggests therapeutic effects persist beyond direct pharmacologic effects, unlike stimulants whose effects are generally closely correlated with plasma drug levels
- Once-daily dosing may increase gastrointestinal side effects
- Lower starting dose allows detection of those patients who may be especially sensitive to side effects such as tachycardia and increased blood pressure
- Patients especially sensitive to the side effects of atomoxetine may include those individuals deficient in the enzyme that metabolizes atomoxetine, CYP450 2D6 (i.e., 7% of Caucasians and 2% of African Americans)
- In such individuals, drug should be titrated slowly to tolerability and effectiveness
- Other individuals may require up to 1.8 mg/kg total daily dose

Overdose

- No fatalities have been reported as monotherapy; sedation, agitation, hyperactivity, abnormal behavior, gastrointestinal symptoms

Long-Term Use

- Safe

Habit Forming

- No

How to Stop

- Taper not necessary

Pharmacokinetics

- Metabolized by CYP450 2D6
- Half-life approximately 5 hours

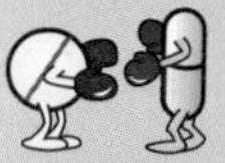

Drug Interactions

- Tramadol increases the risk of seizures in patients taking an antidepressant
- Plasma concentrations of atomoxetine may be increased by drugs that inhibit CYP450 2D6 (e.g., paroxetine, fluoxetine), so atomoxetine dose may need to be reduced if coadministered
- Coadministration of atomoxetine and oral or I.V. albuterol may lead to increases in heart rate and blood pressure
- Coadministration with methylphenidate does not increase cardiovascular side effects beyond those seen with methylphenidate alone
- Do not use with MAO inhibitors, including 14 days after MAOIs are stopped

Other Warnings/ Precautions

- Growth (height and weight) should be monitored during treatment with atomoxetine; for patients who are not growing or gaining weight satisfactorily, interruption of treatment should be considered
- Use with caution in patients with hypertension, tachycardia, cardiovascular disease, or cerebrovascular disease
- Use with caution in patients with bipolar disorder
- Use with caution in patients with urinary retention, benign prostatic hypertrophy
- Use with caution with antihypertensive drugs
- Increased risk of sudden death has been reported in children with structural cardiac abnormalities or other serious heart conditions
- When treating children, carefully weigh the risks and benefits of pharmacological treatment against the risks and benefits of nontreatment and make sure to document this in the patient's chart
- Distribute the brochures provided by the FDA and the drug companies
- Warn patients and their caregivers about the possibility of activating side effects and advise them to report such symptoms immediately
- Monitor patients for activation of suicidal ideation, especially children and adolescents

Do Not Use

- If patient is taking an MAO inhibitor
- If patient has narrow angle-closure glaucoma
- If there is a proven allergy to atomoxetine

SPECIAL POPULATIONS

Renal Impairment
- Dose adjustment not generally necessary

Hepatic Impairment
- For patients with moderate liver impairment, dose should be reduced to 50% of normal dose
- For patients with severe liver impairment, dose should be reduced to 25% of normal dose

Cardiac Impairment
- Use with caution because atomoxetine can increase heart rate and blood pressure
- Do not use in patients with structural cardiac abnormalities

Elderly
- Some patients may tolerate lower doses better
- Reduction in risk of suicidality with antidepressants compared to placebo in adults age 65 and older

Children and Adolescents
- Approved to treat ADHD in children over age 6
- Recommended target dose is 1.2 mg/kg per day
- Carefully weigh the risks and benefits of pharmacological treatment against the risks and benefits of nontreatment and make sure to document this in the patient's chart
- Monitor patients face-to-face regularly, particularly during the first several weeks of treatment
- Use with caution, observing for activation of known or unknown bipolar disorder and/or suicidal ideation, and inform parents or guardian of this risk so they can help observe child or adolescent patients

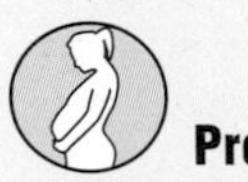

Pregnancy
- Risk Category C [some animal studies show adverse effects; no controlled studies in humans]
- Use in women of childbearing potential requires weighing potential benefits to the mother against potential risks to the fetus

✻ For women of childbearing potential, atomoxetine should generally be discontinued before anticipated pregnancies

Breast Feeding
- Unknown if atomoxetine is secreted in human breast milk, but all psychotropics assumed to be secreted in breast milk

✻ Recommend either to discontinue drug or bottle feed

THE ART OF PSYCHOPHARMACOLOGY

Potential Advantages
- No known abuse potential

Potential Disadvantages
- May not act as rapidly as stimulants when initiating treatment in some patients

Primary Target Symptoms
- Concentration, attention span
- Motor hyperactivity
- Depressed mood

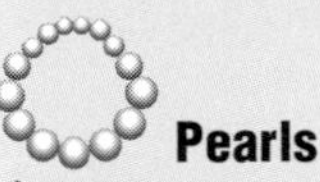

Pearls

✻ Unlike other agents approved for ADHD, atomoxetine does not have abuse potential and is not a scheduled substance

✻ Despite its name as a selective norepinephrine reuptake inhibitor, atomoxetine enhances both dopamine and norepinephrine in frontal cortex, presumably accounting for its therapeutic actions on attention and concentration

- Since dopamine is inactivated by norepinephrine reuptake in frontal cortex, which largely lacks dopamine transporters, atomoxetine can increase dopamine as well as norepinephrine in this part of the brain, presumably causing therapeutic actions in ADHD
- Since dopamine is inactivated by dopamine reuptake in nucleus accumbens, which largely lacks norepinephrine transporters, atomoxetine does not increase dopamine in this part of the brain, presumably explaining why atomoxetine lacks abuse potential
- Atomoxetine's known mechanism of action as a selective norepinephrine reuptake

inhibitor suggests its efficacy as an antidepressant
- Pro-noradrenergic actions may be theoretically useful for the treatment of chronic pain
- Atomoxetine's mechanism of action and its potential antidepressant actions suggest it has the potential to destabilize latent or undiagnosed bipolar disorder, similar to the known actions of proven antidepressants
- Thus, administer with caution to ADHD patients who may also have bipolar disorder
- Unlike stimulants, atomoxetine may not exacerbate tics in Tourette's syndrome patients with comorbid ADHD
- Urinary retention in men over 50 with borderline urine flow has been observed with other agents with potent norepinephrine reuptake blocking properties (e.g., reboxetine, milnacipran), so administer atomoxetine with caution to these patients
- Atomoxetine was originally called tomoxetine but the name was changed to avoid potential confusion with tamoxifen, which might lead to errors in drug dispensing

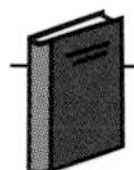

Suggested Reading

Kelsey D, Sumner C, Casat C, Coury D, Quintana H, Saylor K, et al. Once daily atomoxetine treatment for children with attention deficit hyperactivity behavior including an assessment of evening and morning behavior: a double-blind, placebo-controlled trial. Pediatrics 2004; 114: el-8.

Kratochvil CJ, Vaughan BS, Harrington MJ, Burke WJ. Atomoxetine: a selective noradrenaline reuptake inhibitor for the treatment of attention-deficit/hyperactivity disorder. Expert Opin Pharmacother 2003;4(7):1165–74.

Michelson D, Adler L, Spencer T, Reimherr FW, West SA, Allen AJ, Kelsey D, Wernicke J, Dietrich A, Milton D. Atomoxetine in adults with ADHD: two randomized, placebo-controlled studies. Biol Psychiatry 2003;53(2):112–20.

Michelson D, Buitelaar JK, Danckaerts M, Gillberg C, Spencer TJ, Zuddas A, et al. Relapse prevention in pediatric patients with ADHD treated with atomoxetine: a randomized, double-blind, placebo-controlled study. J Am Acad Child Adolesc Psychiatry 2004;43(7): 896–904.

Simpson D, Perry CM. Atomoxetine. Paediatr Drugs 2003;5(6):407–15.

Wernicke JF, Kratochvil CJ. Safety profile of atomoxetine in the treatment of children and adolescents with ADHD. J Clin Psychiatry 2002;63 Suppl 12:50–5.

THERAPEUTICS

Brands
- Wellbutrin, Wellbutrin SR, Wellbutrin XL
- Zyban
- Aplenzin

Generic? Yes

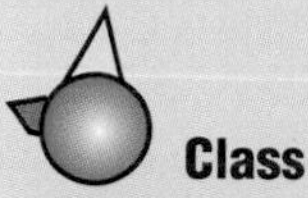

Class
- NDRI (norepinephrine dopamine reuptake inhibitor); antidepressant; smoking cessation treatment

Commonly Prescribed for
(bold for FDA approved)
- **Major depressive disorder (bupropion, bupropion SR, bupropion XL, bupropion hydrobromide)**
- **Seasonal affective disorder (bupropion XL)**
- **Nicotine addiction (bupropion SR)**
- Bipolar depression
- Attention deficit hyperactivity disorder (ADHD)
- Sexual dysfunction

How the Drug Works
- Boosts neurotransmitters norepinephrine/noradrenaline and dopamine
- Blocks norepinephrine reuptake pump (norepinephrine transporter), presumably increasing norepinephrine neurotransmission
- Since dopamine is inactivated by norepinephrine reuptake in frontal cortex, which largely lacks dopamine transporters, bupropion can increase dopamine neurotransmission in this part of the brain
- Blocks dopamine reuptake pump (dopamine transporter), presumably increasing dopaminergic neurotransmission

How Long Until It Works
- Onset of therapeutic actions usually not immediate, but often delayed 2–4 weeks
- If it is not working within 6–8 weeks for depression, it may require a dosage increase or it may not work at all
- May continue to work for many years to prevent relapse of symptoms

If It Works
- The goal of treatment of depression is complete remission of current symptoms as well as prevention of future relapses
- Treatment of depression most often reduces or even eliminates symptoms, but is not a cure since symptoms can recur after medicine stopped
- Continue treatment of depression until all symptoms are gone (remission)
- Once symptoms of depression are gone, continue treating for 1 year for the first episode of depression
- For second and subsequent episodes of depression, treatment may need to be indefinite
- Treatment for nicotine addiction should consist of a single treatment for 6 weeks

If It Doesn't Work
- Many patients have only a partial response where some symptoms are improved but others persist (especially insomnia, fatigue, and problems concentrating)
- Other patients may be nonresponders, sometimes called treatment-resistant or treatment-refractory
- Some patients who have an initial response may relapse even though they continue treatment, sometimes called "poop-out"
- Consider increasing dose, switching to another agent or adding an appropriate augmenting agent
- Consider psychotherapy
- Consider evaluation for another diagnosis or for a comorbid condition (e.g., medical illness, substance abuse, etc.)
- Some patients may experience apparent lack of consistent efficacy due to activation of latent or underlying bipolar disorder, and require antidepressant discontinuation and a switch to a mood stabilizer, although this may be a less frequent problem with bupropion than with other antidepressants

Best Augmenting Combos for Partial Response or Treatment Resistance
- Trazodone for residual insomnia
- Benzodiazepines for residual anxiety

✻ Can be added to SSRIs to reverse SSRI-induced sexual dysfunction, SSRI-induced apathy (use combinations of antidepressants with caution as this may activate bipolar disorder and suicidal ideation)

* Can be added to SSRIs to treat partial responders
* Often used as an augmenting agent to mood stabilizers and/or atypical antipsychotics in bipolar depression
- Mood stabilizers or atypical antipsychotics can also be added to bupropion for psychotic depression or treatment-resistant depression
- Hypnotics for insomnia
- Mirtazapine, modafinil, atomoxetine (add with caution and at lower doses since bupropion could theoretically raise atomoxetine levels) both for residual symptoms of depression and attention deficit disorder

Tests

- None for healthy individuals

SIDE EFFECTS

How Drug Causes Side Effects

- Side effects are probably caused in part by actions of norepinephrine and dopamine in brain areas with undesired effects (e.g., insomnia, tremor, agitation, headache, dizziness)
- Side effects are probably also caused in part by actions of norepinephrine in the periphery with undesired effects (e.g., sympathetic and parasympathetic effects such as dry mouth, constipation, nausea, anorexia, sweating)
- Most side effects are immediate but often go away with time

Notable Side Effects

- Dry mouth, constipation, nausea, weight loss, anorexia, myalgia
- Insomnia, dizziness, headache, agitation, anxiety, tremor, abdominal pain, tinnitus
- Sweating, rash
- Hypertension

Life-Threatening or Dangerous Side Effects

- Rare seizures (higher incidence for immediate-release than for sustained-release; risk increases with doses above the recommended maximums; risk increases for patients with predisposing factors)
- Hypomania (more likely in bipolar patients but perhaps less common than with some other antidepressants)
- Rare induction of mania
- Rare activation of suicidal ideation and behavior (suicidality) (short-term studies did not show an increase in the risk of suicidality with antidepressants compared to placebo beyond age 24)

Weight Gain

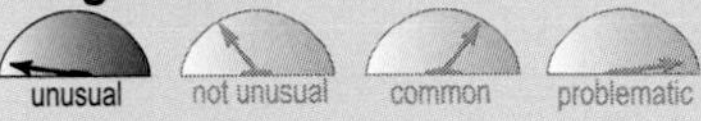

- Reported but not expected
* Patients may experience weight loss

Sedation

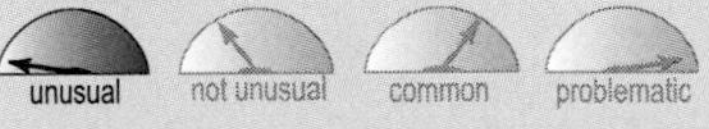

- Reported but not expected

What to Do About Side Effects

- Wait
- Wait
- Wait
- Keep dose as low as possible
- Take no later than mid-afternoon to avoid insomnia
- Switch to another drug

Best Augmenting Agents for Side Effects

- Often best to try another antidepressant monotherapy prior to resorting to augmentation strategies to treat side effects
- Trazodone or a hypnotic for drug-induced insomnia
- Mirtazapine for insomnia, agitation, and gastrointestinal side effects
- Benzodiazepines or buspirone for drug-induced anxiety, agitation
- Many side effects are dose-dependent (i.e., they increase as dose increases, or they reemerge until tolerance redevelops)
- Many side effects are time-dependent (i.e., they start immediately upon dosing and upon each dose increase, but go away with time)
- Activation and agitation may represent the induction of a bipolar state, especially a mixed dysphoric bipolar II condition

sometimes associated with suicidal ideation, and require the addition of lithium, a mood stabilizer or an atypical antipsychotic, and/or discontinuation of bupropion

DOSING AND USE

Usual Dosage Range

- Bupropion: 225–450 mg in 3 divided doses (maximum single dose 150 mg)
- Bupropion SR: 200–450 mg in 2 divided doses (maximum single dose 200 mg)
- Bupropion XL: 150–450 mg once daily (maximum single dose 450 mg)
- Bupropion hydrobromide: 174–522 mg once daily (maximum single dose 522 mg)

Dosage Forms

- Bupropion: tablet 75 mg, 100 mg
- Bupropion SR (sustained-release): tablet 100 mg, 150 mg, 200 mg
- Bupropion XL (extended-release): tablet 150 mg, 300 mg
- Bupropion hydrobromide (extended-release): tablet 174 mg, 378 mg, 522 mg

How To Dose

- Depression: for bupropion immediate-release, dosing should be in divided doses, starting at 75 mg twice daily, increasing to 100 mg twice daily, then to 100 mg 3 times daily; maximum dose 450 mg per day
- Depression: for bupropion SR, initial dose 100 mg twice a day, increase to 150 mg twice a day after at least 3 days; wait 4 weeks or longer to ensure drug effects before increasing dose; maximum dose 400 mg total per day
- Depression: for bupropion XL, initial dose 150 mg once daily in the morning; can increase to 300 mg once daily after 4 days; maximum single dose 450 mg once daily
- Depression: for bupropion hydrobromide, initial dose 174 mg once daily in the morning; can increase to 522 mg administered as a single dose
- Nicotine addiction [for bupropion SR]: Initial dose 150 mg/day once a day, increase to 150 mg twice a day after at least 3 days; maximum dose 300 mg/day; bupropion treatment should begin 1–2 weeks before smoking is discontinued

Dosing Tips

- XL formulation has replaced immediate-release and SR formulations as the preferred option
- XL is best dosed once a day, whereas SR is best dosed twice daily, and immediate-release is best dosed 3 times daily
- Dosing higher than 450 mg/day (400 mg/day SR) increases seizure risk
- Patients who do not respond to 450 mg/day should discontinue use or get blood levels of bupropion and its major active metabolite 6-hydroxy-bupropion
- If levels of parent drug and active metabolite are low despite dosing at 450 mg/day, experts can prudently increase dosing beyond the therapeutic range while monitoring closely, informing the patient of the potential risk of seizures and weighing risk-benefit ratios in difficult-to-treat patients
- When used for bipolar depression, it is usually as an augmenting agent to mood stabilizers, lithium, and/or atypical antipsychotics
- For smoking cessation, may be used in conjunction with nicotine replacement therapy
- Do not break or chew SR or XL tablets as this will alter controlled-release properties
- The more anxious and agitated the patient, the lower the starting dose, the slower the titration, and the more likely the need for a concomitant agent such as trazodone or a benzodiazepine
- If intolerable anxiety, insomnia, agitation, akathisia, or activation occur either upon dosing initiation or discontinuation, consider the possibility of activated bipolar disorder and switch to a mood stabilizer or an atypical antipsychotic

Overdose

- Rarely lethal; seizures, cardiac disturbances, hallucinations, loss of consciousness

Long-Term Use

- For smoking cessation, treatment for up to 6 months has been found effective
- For depression, treatment up to 1 year has been found to decrease rate of relapse

Habit Forming
- No

How to Stop
- Tapering is prudent to avoid withdrawal effects, but no well-documented tolerance, dependence, or withdrawal reactions

Pharmacokinetics
- Inhibits CYP450 2D6
- Parent half-life 10–4 hours
- Metabolite half-life 20–27 hours

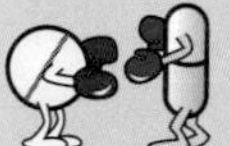

Drug Interactions
- Tramadol increases the risk of seizures in patients taking an antidepressant
- Can increase tricyclic antidepressant levels; use with caution with tricyclic antidepressants or when switching from a TCA to bupropion
- Can be fatal when combined with MAO inhibitors, so do not use with MAO inhibitors or for at least 14 days after MAOIs are stopped
- Do not start an MAO inhibitor for at least 2 weeks after discontinuing bupropion
- Via CYP450 2D6 inhibition, bupropion could theoretically interfere with the analgesic actions of codeine, and increase the plasma levels of some beta blockers and of atomoxetine
- Via CYP450 2D6 inhibition, bupropion could theoretically increase concentrations of thioridazine and cause dangerous cardiac arrhythmias

Other Warnings/ Precautions
- Use cautiously with other drugs that increase seizure risk (TCAs, lithium, phenothiazines, thioxanthenes, some antipsychotics)
- Bupropion should be used with caution in patients taking levodopa or amantadine, as these agents can potentially enhance dopamine neurotransmission and be activating
- Do not use if patient has severe insomnia
- Use with caution in patients with bipolar disorder unless treated with concomitant mood-stabilizing agent
- When treating children, carefully weigh the risks and benefits of pharmacological treatment against the risks and benefits of nontreatment and make sure to document this in the patient's chart
- Distribute the brochures provided by the FDA and the drug companies
- Warn patients and their caregivers about the possibility of activating side effects and advise them to report such symptoms immediately
- Monitor patients for activation of suicidal ideation, especially children and adolescents

Do Not Use
- Zyban or Aplenzin in combination with each other or with any formulation of Wellbutrin
- If patient has history of seizures
- If patient is anorexic or bulimic, either currently or in the past, but see Pearls
- If patient is abruptly discontinuing alcohol or sedative use
- If patient has had recent head injury
- If patient has a nervous system tumor
- If patient is taking an MAO inhibitor
- If patient is taking thioridazine
- If there is a proven allergy to bupropion

SPECIAL POPULATIONS

Renal Impairment
- Lower initial dose, perhaps give less frequently
- Drug concentration may be increased
- Patient should be monitored closely

Hepatic Impairment
- Lower initial dose, perhaps give less frequently
- Patient should be monitored closely
- In severe hepatic cirrhosis, bupropion XL should be administered at no more than 150 mg every other day

Cardiac Impairment
- Limited available data
- Evidence of rise in supine blood pressure
- Use with caution

Elderly
- Some patients may tolerate lower doses better
- Reduction in risk of suicidality with antidepressants compared to placebo in adults age 65 and older

Children and Adolescents

- Carefully weigh the risks and benefits of pharmacological treatment against the risks and benefits of nontreatment with antidepressants and make sure to document this in the patient's chart
- Monitor patients face-to-face regularly, particularly during the first several weeks of treatment
- Use with caution, observing for activation of known or unknown bipolar disorder and/or suicidal ideation, and inform parents or guardian of this risk so they can help observe child or adolescent patients
- Safety and efficacy have not been established
- May be used for ADHD in children or adolescents
- May be used for smoking cessation in adolescents
- Preliminary research suggests efficacy in comorbid depression and ADHD
- Dosage may follow adult pattern for adolescents
- Children may require lower doses initially, with a maximum dose of 300 mg/day

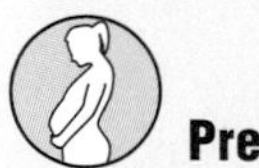

Pregnancy

- Risk Category C [some animal studies show adverse effects; no controlled studies in humans]
- Pregnant women wishing to stop smoking may consider behavioral therapy before pharmacotherapy
- Not generally recommended for use during pregnancy, especially during first trimester
- Must weigh the risk of treatment (first trimester fetal development, third trimester newborn delivery) to the child against the risk of no treatment (recurrence of depression, maternal health, infant bonding) to the mother and child
- For many patients this may mean continuing treatment during pregnancy

Breast Feeding

- Some drug is found in mother's breast milk
- If child becomes irritable or sedated, breast feeding or drug may need to be discontinued
- Immediate postpartum period is a high-risk time for depression, especially in women who have had prior depressive episodes, so drug may need to be reinstituted late in the third trimester or shortly after childbirth to prevent a recurrence during the postpartum period
- Must weigh benefits of breast feeding with risks and benefits of antidepressant treatment versus nontreatment to both the infant and the mother
- For many patients, this may mean continuing treatment during breast feeding

THE ART OF PSYCHOPHARMACOLOGY

Potential Advantages

- Retarded depression
- Atypical depression
- Bipolar depression
- Patients concerned about sexual dysfunction
- Patients concerned about weight gain

Potential Disadvantages

- Patients experiencing weight loss associated with their depression
- Patients who are excessively activated

Primary Target Symptoms

- Depressed mood
- Sleep disturbance, especially hypersomnia
- Cravings associated with nicotine withdrawal
- Cognitive functioning

Pearls

* May be effective if SSRIs have failed or for SSRI "poop-out"
- Less likely to produce hypomania than some other antidepressants
* May improve cognitive slowing/pseudodementia
* Reduces hypersomnia and fatigue
- Approved to help reduce craving during smoking cessation
- Anecdotal use in attention deficit disorder
- May cause sexual dysfunction only infrequently
- May exacerbate tics
- Bupropion may not be as effective in anxiety disorders as many other antidepressants

- Prohibition for use in eating disorders due to increased risk of seizures is related to past observations when bupropion immediate-release was dosed at especially high levels to low body weight patients with active anorexia nervosa
- Current practice suggests that patients of normal BMI without additional risk factors for seizures can benefit from bupropion, especially if given prudent doses of the XL formulation; such treatment should be administered by experts, and patients should be monitored closely and informed of the potential risks
- Recently approved hydrobromide salt formulation of bupropion may facilitate high dosing for difficult-to-treat patients, as it allows administration of single-pill doses up to 450 mg equivalency to bupropion hydrochloride salt (522 mg tablet), unlike bupropion hydrochloride controlled release formulations for which the biggest dose in a single pill is 300 mg
- As bromide salts have anticonvulsant properties, hydrobromide salts of bupropion could theoretically reduce risk of seizures, but this has not been proven
- The active enantiomer of the principal active metabolite [(+)-6-hydroxy-bupropion] is in clinical development as a novel antidepressant

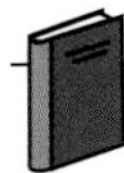

Suggested Reading

Clayton AH. Extended-release bupropion: an antidepressant with a broad spectrum of therapeutic activity? Expert Opin Pharmacother 2007;8(4):457–66.

Ferry L, Johnston JA. Efficacy and safety of bupropion SR for smoking cessation: data from clinical trials and five years of postmarketing experience. Int J Clin Pract 2003;57(3):224–30.

Foley KF, DeSanty KP, Kast RE. Bupropion: pharmacology and therapeutic applications. Expert Rev Neurother 2006;6(9)1249–65.

Jefferson JW, Pradko JF, Muir KT. Bupropion for major depressive disorder: pharmacokinetic and formulation considerations. Clin Ther 2005;27(11):1685–95.

Papakostas GI, Nutt DJ, Hallett LA et al. Resolution of sleepiness and fatigue in major depressive disorder: a comparison of bupropion and the selective serotonin reuptake inhibitors. Biol Psychiatry 2006;60(12):1350–5.

THERAPEUTICS

Brands • BuSpar

see index for additional brand names

Generic? Yes

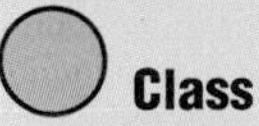

Class

- Anxiolytic (azapirone; serotonin 1A partial agonist; serotonin stabilizer)

Commonly Prescribed for

(bold for FDA approved)

- **Management of anxiety disorders**
- **Short-term treatment of symptoms of anxiety**
- Mixed anxiety and depression
- Treatment-resistant depression (adjunctive)

How the Drug Works

- Binds to serotonin type 1A receptors
- Partial agonist actions postsynaptically may theoretically diminish serotonergic activity and contribute to anxiolytic actions
- Partial agonist actions at presynaptic somatodendritic serotonin autoreceptors may theoretically enhance serotonergic activity and contribute to antidepressant actions

How Long Until It Works

- Generally takes within 2–4 weeks to achieve efficacy
- If it is not working within 6–8 weeks, it may require a dosage increase or it may not work at all

If It Works

- The goal of treatment is complete remission of symptoms as well as prevention of future relapses
- Treatment most often reduces or even eliminates symptoms, but not a cure since symptoms can recur after medicine stopped
- Chronic anxiety disorders may require long-term maintenance with buspirone to control symptoms

If It Doesn't Work

- Consider switching to another agent (a benzodiazepine or antidepressant)

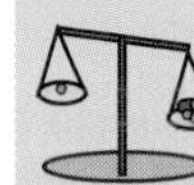

Best Augmenting Combos for Partial Response or Treatment Resistance

- Sedative hypnotic for insomnia
- Buspirone is often given as an augmenting agent to SSRIs or SNRIs

Tests

- None for healthy individuals

SIDE EFFECTS

How Drug Causes Side Effects

- Serotonin partial agonist actions in parts of the brain and body and at receptors other than those that cause therapeutic actions

Notable Side Effects

- ✱ Dizziness, headache, nervousness, sedation, excitement
- Nausea
- Restlessness

Life-Threatening or Dangerous Side Effects

- Rare cardiac symptoms

Weight Gain

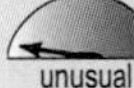

not unusual

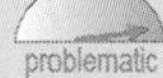

- Reported but not expected

Sedation

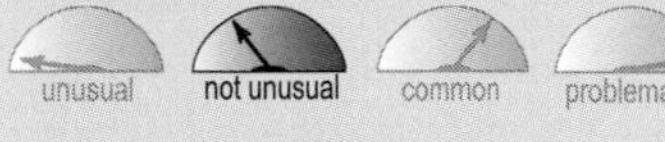

- Occurs in significant minority

What to Do About Side Effects

- Wait
- Wait
- Wait
- Lower the dose
- Give total daily dose divided into 3, 4, or more doses
- Switch to another agent

Best Augmenting Agents for Side Effects

- Many side effects cannot be improved with an augmenting agent

DOSING AND USE

Usual Dosage Range
- 20–30 mg/day

Dosage Forms
- Tablet 5 mg scored, 10 mg scored, 15 mg multiscored, 30 mg multiscored

How To Dose
- Initial 15 mg twice a day; increase in 5 mg/day increments every 2–3 days until desired efficacy is reached; maximum dose generally 60 mg/day

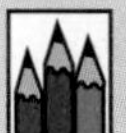

Dosing Tips
- Requires dosing 2–3 times a day for full effect

Overdose
- No deaths reported in monotherapy; sedation, dizziness, small pupils, nausea, vomiting

Long-Term Use
- Limited data suggest that it is safe

Habit Forming
- No

How to Stop
- Taper generally not necessary

Pharmacokinetics
- Metabolized primarily by CYP450 3A4
- Elimination half-life approximately 2–3 hours

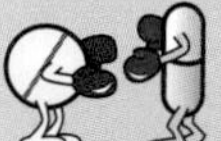

Drug Interactions
- Do not use with MAO inhibitors, including 14 days after MAOIs are stopped
- CYP450 3A4 inhibitors (e.g., fluxotine, fluvoxamine, nefazodone) may reduce clearance of buspirone and raise its plasma levels, so the dose of buspirone may need to be lowered when given concomitantly with these agents
- CYP450 3A4 inducers (e.g., carbamazepine) may increase clearance of buspirone, so the dose of buspirone may need to be raised
- Buspirone may increase plasma concentrations of haloperidol
- Buspirone may raise levels of nordiazepam, the active metabolite of diazepam, which may result in increased symptoms of dizziness, headache, or nausea

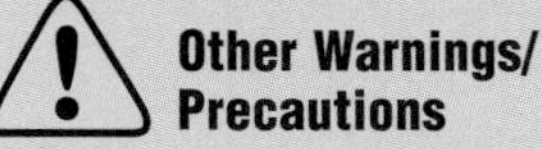

Other Warnings/ Precautions
- None

Do Not Use
- If patient is taking an MAO inhibitor
- If there is a proven allergy to buspirone

SPECIAL POPULATIONS

Renal Impairment
- Use with caution
- Not recommended for patients with severe renal impairment

Hepatic Impairment
- Use with caution
- Not recommended for patients with severe hepatic impairment

Cardiac Impairment
- Buspirone has been used to treat hostility in patients with cardiac impairment

Elderly
- Some patients may tolerate lower doses better

Children and Adolescents
- Studies in children age 6–17 do not show significant reduction in anxiety symptoms in GAD
- Safety profile in children encourages use

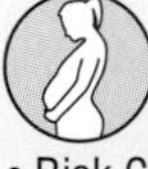

Pregnancy
- Risk Category B [animal studies do not show adverse effects; no controlled studies in humans]
- Not generally recommended in pregnancy, but may be safer than some other options

Breast Feeding
- Some drug is found in mother's breast milk
- Trace amounts may be present in nursing children whose mothers are on buspirone

- If child becomes irritable or sedated, breast feeding or drug may need to be discontinued

THE ART OF PSYCHOPHARMACOLOGY

Potential Advantages

- Safety profile
- Lack of dependence, withdrawal
- Lack of sexual dysfunction or weight gain

Potential Disadvantages

- Takes 4 weeks for results, whereas benzodiazepines have immediate effects

Primary Target Symptoms

- Anxiety

Pearls

✻ Buspirone does not appear to cause dependence and shows virtually no withdrawal symptoms

- May have less severe side effects than benzodiazepines

✻ Buspirone generally lacks sexual dysfunction

- Buspirone may reduce sexual dysfunction associated with generalized anxiety disorder and with serotonergic antidepressants
- Sedative effects may be more likely at doses above 20 mg/day
- May have less anxiolytic efficacy than benzodiazepines for some patients
- Buspirone is generally reserved as an augmenting agent to treat anxiety
- A new controlled-release azapirone related to buspirone is in late clinical testing as an antidepressant (gepirone ER)

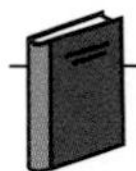

Suggested Reading

Apter JT, Allen LA. Buspirone: future directions. J Clin Psychopharmacol 1999; 19:86–93.

Mahmood I, Sahaiwalla C. Clinical pharmacokinetics and pharmacodynamics of buspirone, an anxiolytic drug. Clin Pharmacokinet 1999;36:277–87.

Pecknold JC. A risk-benefit assessment of buspirone in the treatment of anxiety disorders. Drug Saf 1997;16:118–32.

Sramek JJ, Hong WW, Hamid S, Nape B, Cutler NR. Meta-analysis of the safety and tolerability of two dose regimens of buspirone in patients with persistent anxiety. Depress Anxiety 1999;9:131–4.

THERAPEUTICS

Brands
- Tegretol
- Carbatrol
- Equetro

see index for additional brand names

Generic? Yes (not for extended-release formulation)

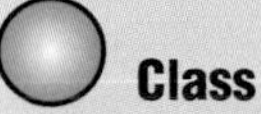

Class

- Anticonvulsant, antineuralgic for chronic pain, voltage-sensitive sodium channel antagonist

Commonly Prescribed for

(bold for FDA approved)
- **Partial seizures with complex symptomatology**
- **Generalized tonic-clonic seizures (grand mal)**
- **Mixed seizure patterns**
- **Pain associated with true trigeminal neuralgia**
- **Acute mania/mixed mania (Equetro)**
- Glossopharyngeal neuralgia
- Bipolar depression
- Bipolar maintenance
- Psychosis, schizophrenia (adjunctive)

How the Drug Works

✽ Acts as a use-dependent blocker of voltage-sensitive sodium channels
✽ Interacts with the open channel conformation of voltage-sensitive sodium channels
✽ Interacts at a specific site of the alpha pore-forming subunit of voltage-sensitive sodium channels
- Inhibits release of glutamate

How Long Until It Works

- For acute mania, effects should occur within a few weeks
- May take several weeks to months to optimize an effect on mood stabilization
- Should reduce seizures by 2 weeks

If It Works

- The goal of treatment is complete remission of symptoms (e.g., seizures, mania, pain)
- Continue treatment until all symptoms are gone or until improvement is stable and then continue treating indefinitely as long as improvement persists
- Continue treatment indefinitely to avoid recurrence of mania and seizures
- Treatment of chronic neuropathic pain most often reduces but does not eliminate pain and is not a cure since symptoms usually recur after medicine stopped

If It Doesn't Work (for bipolar disorder)

✽ Many patients only have a partial response where some symptoms are improved but others persist or continue to wax and wane without stabilization of mood
- Other patients may be nonresponders, sometimes called treatment-resistant or treatment-refractory
- Consider increasing dose, switching to another agent or adding an appropriate augmenting agent
- Consider adding psychotherapy
- Consider biofeedback or hypnosis for pain
- For bipolar disorder, consider the presence of noncompliance and counsel patient
- Switch to another mood stabilizer with fewer side effects or to extended-release carbamazepine
- Consider evaluation for another diagnosis or for a comorbid condition (e.g., medical illness, substance abuse, etc.)

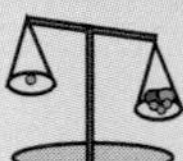

Best Augmenting Combos for Partial Response or Treatment Resistance

- Lithium
- Atypical antipsychotics (especially risperidone, olanzapine, quetiapine, ziprasidone, and aripiprazole)
- Valproate (carbamazepine can decrease valproate levels)
- Lamotrigine (carbamazepine can decrease lamotrigine levels)

✽ Antidepressants (with caution because antidepressants can destabilize mood in some patients, including induction of rapid cycling or suicidal ideation; in particular consider bupropion; also SSRIs, SNRIs, others; generally avoid TCAs, MAOIs)

Tests

✻ Before starting: blood count, liver, kidney, and thyroid function tests
- During treatment: blood count every 2–4 weeks for 2 months, then every 3–6 months throughout treatment
- During treatment: liver, kidney, and thyroid function tests every 6–12 months
- Consider monitoring sodium levels because of possibility of hyponatremia

✻ Before starting: individuals with ancestry across broad areas of Asia should consider screening for the presence of the HLA-B*1502 allele; those with HLA-B*1502 should not be treated with carbamazepine

SIDE EFFECTS

How Drug Causes Side Effects

- CNS side effects theoretically due to excessive actions at voltage-sensitive sodium channels
- Major metabolite (carbamazepine-10, 11 epoxide) may be the cause of many side effects
- Mild anticholinergic effects may contribute to sedation, blurred vision

Notable Side Effects

✻ Sedation, dizziness, confusion, unsteadiness, headache

✻ Nausea, vomiting, diarrhea
- Blurred vision

✻ Benign leukopenia (transient; in up to 10%)

✻ Rash

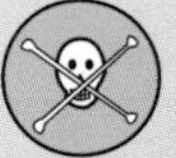

Life-Threatening or Dangerous Side Effects

✻ Rare aplastic anemia, agranulocytosis (unusual bleeding or bruising, mouth sores, infections, fever, sore throat)

✻ Rare severe dermatologic reactions (Stevens Johnson syndrome)
- Rare cardiac problems
- Rare induction of psychosis or mania

✻ SIADH (syndrome of inappropriate antidiuretic hormone secretion) with hyponatremia
- Increased frequency of generalized convulsions (in patients with atypical absence seizures)
- Rare activation of suicidal ideation and behavior (suicidality)

Weight Gain

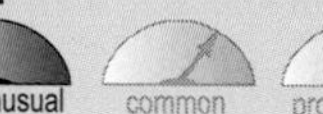

- Occurs in significant minority

Sedation

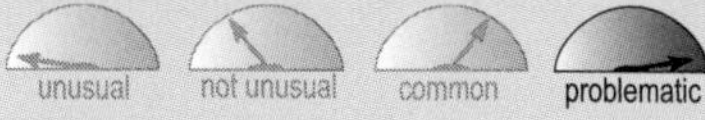

- Frequent and can be significant in amount
- Some patients may not tolerate it
- Dose-related
- Can wear off with time, but commonly does not wear off at high doses
- CNS side effects significantly lower with controlled-release formulation (e.g., Equetro, Carbatrol)

What to Do About Side Effects

- Wait
- Wait
- Wait
- Take with food or split dose to avoid gastrointestinal effects
- Extended-release carbamazepine can be sprinkled on soft food
- Take at night to reduce daytime sedation
- Switch to another agent or to extended-release carbamazepine

Best Augmenting Agents for Side Effects

- Many side effects cannot be improved with an augmenting agent

DOSING AND USE

Usual Dosage Range

- 400–1,200 mg/day
- Under age 6: 10–20 mg/kg per day

Dosage Forms

- Tablet 100 mg chewable, 200 mg chewable, 200 mg
- Extended-release tablet 100 mg, 200 mg, 400 mg
- Extended-release capsule 100 mg, 200 mg, 300 mg
- Oral suspension 100 mg/5 mL (450 mL)

How To Dose

- For bipolar disorder and seizures (ages 13 and older): initial 200 mg twice daily (tablet) or 1 teaspoon (100 mg) 4 times a day (suspension); each week increase by

up to 200 mg/day in divided doses (2 doses for extended-release formulation, 3–4 doses for other tablets); maximum dose generally 1,200 mg/day for adults and 1,000 mg/day for children under age 15; maintenance dose generally 800–1,200 mg/day for adults; some patients may require up to 1,600 mg/day
- Seizures (under age 13): see Children and Adolescents
- Trigeminal neuralgia: initial 100 mg twice daily (tablet) or 0.5 teaspoon (50 mg) 4 times a day; each week increase by up to 200 mg/day in divided doses (100 mg every 12 hours for tablet formulations, 50 mg 4 times a day for suspension formulation); maximum dose generally 1,200 mg/day
- Lower initial dose and slower titration should be used for carbamazepine suspension

Dosing Tips

- Higher peak levels occur with the suspension formulation than with the same dose of the tablet formulation, so suspension should generally be started at a lower dose and titrated slowly
- Take carbamazepine with food to avoid gastrointestinal effects

✻ Slow dose titration may delay onset of therapeutic action but enhance tolerability to sedating side effects
- Controlled-release formulations (e.g., Equetro, Carbatrol) can significantly reduce sedation and other CNS side effects
- Should titrate slowly in the presence of other sedating agents, such as other anticonvulsants, in order to best tolerate additive sedative side effects

✻ Can sometimes minimize the impact of carbamazepine upon the bone marrow by dosing slowly and monitoring closely when initiating treatment; initial trend to leukopenia/neutropenia may reverse with continued conservative dosing over time and allow subsequent dosage increases with careful monitoring

✻ Carbamazepine often requires a dosage adjustment upward with time, as the drug induces its own metabolism, thus lowering its own plasma levels over the first several weeks to months of treatment

- Do not break or chew carbamazepine extended-release tablets as this will alter controlled-release properties

Overdose

- Can be fatal (lowest known fatal dose in adults is 3.2 g, in adolescents is 4 g, and in children is 1.6 g); nausea, vomiting, involuntary movements, irregular heartbeat, urinary retention, trouble breathing, sedation, coma

Long-Term Use

- May lower sex drive
- Monitoring of liver, kidney, thyroid functions, blood counts and sodium may be required

Habit Forming

- No

How to Stop

- Taper; may need to adjust dosage of concurrent medications as carbamazepine is being discontinued

✻ Rapid discontinuation may increase the risk of relapse in bipolar disorder
- Epilepsy patients may seize upon withdrawal, especially if withdrawal is abrupt
- Discontinuation symptoms uncommon

Pharmacokinetics

- Metabolized in the liver, primarily by CYP450 3A4
- Renally excreted
- Active metabolite (carbamazepine-10,11 epoxide)
- Initial half-life 26–65 hours (35–40 hours for extended-release formulation); half-life 12–17 hours with repeated doses
- Half-life of active metabolite is approximately 34 hours

✻ Is not only a substrate for CYP450 3A4, but also an inducer of CYP450 3A4

✻ Thus, carbamazepine induces its own metabolism, often requiring an upward dosage adjustment

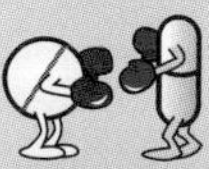

Drug Interactions

- Enzyme-inducing antiepileptic drugs (carbamazepine itself as well as phenobarbital, phenytoin, and primidone)

may increase the clearance of carbamazepine and lower its plasma levels
- CYP450 3A4 inducers, such as carbamazepine itself, can lower the plasma levels of carbamazepine
- CYP450 3A4 inhibitors, such as nefazodone, fluvoxamine, and fluoxetine, can increase plasma levels of carbamazepine
- Carbamazepine can increase plasma levels of clomipramine, phenytoin, primidone
- Carbamazepine can decrease plasma levels of acetaminophen, clozapine, benzodiazepines, dicumarol, doxycycline, theophylline, warfarin, and haloperidol as well as other anticonvulsants such as phensuximide, methsuximide, ethosuximide, phenytoin, tiagabine, topiramate, lamotrigine, and valproate
- Carbamazepine can decrease plasma levels of hormonal contraceptives and adversely affect their efficacy
- Combined use of carbamazepine with other anticonvulsants may lead to altered thyroid function
- Combined use of carbamazepine and lithium may increase risk of neurotoxic effects
- Depressive effects are increased by other CNS depressants (alcohol, MAOIs, other anticonvulsants, etc.)
- Combined use of carbamazepine suspension with liquid formulations of chlorpromazine has been shown to result in excretion of an orange rubbery precipitate; because of this, combined use of carbamazepine suspension with any liquid medicine is not recommended

Other Warnings/ Precautions

- ✱ Patients should be monitored carefully for signs of unusual bleeding or bruising, mouth sores, infections, fever, or sore throat, as the risk of aplastic anemia and agranulocytosis with carbamazepine use is 5–8 times greater than in the general population (risk in the untreated general population is 6 patients per 1 million per year for agranulocytosis and 2 patients per 1 million per year for aplastic anemia)
- Because carbamazepine has a tricyclic chemical structure, it is not recommended to be taken with MAOIs, including 14 days after MAOIs are stopped; do not start an MAOI until 2 weeks after discontinuing carbamazepine
- May exacerbate narrow angle-closure glaucoma
- Because carbamazepine can lower plasma levels of hormonal contraceptives, it may also reduce their effectiveness
- May need to restrict fluid intake because of risk of developing syndrome of inappropriate antidiuretic hormone secretion, hyponatremia and its complications
- Use with caution in patients with mixed seizure disorders that include atypical absence seizures because carbamazepine has been associated with increased frequency of generalized convulsions in such patients
- Individuals with the HLA-B*1502 allele are at increased risk of developing Stevens Johnson syndrome and toxic epidermal necrolysis
- Warn patients and their caregivers about the possibility of activation of suicidal ideation and advise them to report such side effects immediately

Do Not Use

- If patient is taking an MAOI
- If patient has history of bone marrow suppression
- If patient tests positive for the HLA-B*1502 allele
- If there is a proven allergy to any tricyclic compound
- If there is a proven allergy to carbamazepine

SPECIAL POPULATIONS

Renal Impairment

- Carbamazepine is renally secreted, so the dose may need to be lowered

Hepatic Impairment

- Drug should be used with caution
- Rare cases of hepatic failure have occurred

Cardiac Impairment

- Drug should be used with caution

Elderly

- Some patients may tolerate lower doses better
- Elderly patients may be more susceptible to adverse effects

Children and Adolescents

- Approved use for epilepsy; therapeutic range of total carbamazepine in plasma is considered the same for children and adults
- Ages 6–12: initial dose 100 mg twice daily (tablets) or 0.5 teaspoon (50 mg) 4 times a day (suspension); each week increase by up to 100 mg/day in divided doses (2 doses for extended-release formulation, 3–4 doses for all other formulations); maximum dose generally 1,000 mg/day; maintenance dose generally 400–800 mg/day
- Ages 5 and younger: initial 10–20 mg/kg per day in divided doses (2–3 doses for tablet formulations, 4 doses for suspension); increase weekly as needed; maximum dose generally 35 mg/kg/day

Pregnancy

- Risk Category D [positive evidence of risk to human fetus; potential benefits may still justify its use during pregnancy]
- ✻ Use during first trimester may raise risk of neural tube defects (e.g., spina bifida) or other congenital anomalies
- Use in women of childbearing potential requires weighing potential benefits to the mother against the risks to the fetus
- ✻ If drug is continued, perform tests to detect birth defects
- ✻ If drug is continued, start on folate 1 mg/day early in pregnancy to reduce risk of neural tube defects
- Antiepileptic Drug Pregnancy Registry: (888) 233-2334
- Use of anticonvulsants in combination may cause a higher prevalence of teratogenic effects than anticonvulsant monotherapy
- Taper drug if discontinuing
- Seizures, even mild seizures, may cause harm to the embryo/fetus
- ✻ For bipolar patients, carbamazepine should generally be discontinued before anticipated pregnancies
- Recurrent bipolar illness during pregnancy can be quite disruptive
- For bipolar patients, given the risk of relapse in the postpartum period, some form of mood stabilizer treatment may need to be restarted immediately after delivery if patient is unmedicated during pregnancy
- ✻ Atypical antipsychotics may be preferable to lithium or anticonvulsants such as carbamazepine if treatment of bipolar disorder is required during pregnancy
- Bipolar symptoms may recur or worsen during pregnancy and some form of treatment may be necessary

Breast Feeding

- Some drug is found in mother's breast milk
- ✻ Recommended either to discontinue drug or bottle feed
- If drug is continued while breast feeding, infant should be monitored for possible adverse effects, including hematological effects
- If infant shows signs of irritability or sedation, drug may need to be discontinued
- Some cases of neonatal seizures, respiratory depression, vomiting, and diarrhea have been reported in infants whose mothers received carbamazepine during pregnancy
- ✻ Bipolar disorder may recur during the postpartum period, particularly if there is a history of prior postpartum episodes of either depression or psychosis
- Relapse rates may be lower in women who receive prophylactic treatment for postpartum episodes of bipolar disorder
- Atypical antipsychotics and anticonvulsants such as valproate may be safer than carbamazepine during the postpartum period when breast feeding

THE ART OF PSYCHOPHARMACOLOGY

Potential Advantages

- Treatment-resistant bipolar and psychotic disorders

Potential Disadvantages

- Patients who do not wish to or cannot comply with blood testing and close monitoring

- Patients who cannot tolerate sedation
- Pregnant patients

Primary Target Symptoms

- Incidence of seizures
- Unstable mood, especially mania
- Pain

Pearls

- Carbamazepine was the first anticonvulsant widely used for the treatment of bipolar disorder and is now formally approved for acute mania and mixed mania

* An extended-release formulation has better evidence of efficacy and improved tolerability in bipolar disorder than does immediate-release carbamazepine

- Dosage frequency as well as sedation, diplopia, confusion, and ataxia may be reduced with extended-release carbamazepine
- Risk of serious side effects is greatest in the first few months of treatment
- Common side effects such as sedation often abate after a few months

* May be effective in patients who fail to respond to lithium or other mood stabilizers

- May be effective for the depressed phase of bipolar disorder and for maintenance in bipolar disorder
- Can be complicated to use with concomitant medications

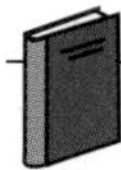

Suggested Reading

Leucht S, McGrath J, White P, Kissling W. Carbamazepine for schizophrenia and schizoaffective psychoses. Cochrane Database Syst Rev 2002;(3):CD001258.

Marson AG, Williamson PR, Hutton JL, Clough HE, Chadwick DW. Carbamazepine versus valproate monotherapy for epilepsy. Cochrane Database Syst Rev 2000; (3): CD001030.

Smith LA, Cornelius V, Warnock A, Tacchi MJ, Taylor D. Pharmacological interventions for acute bipolar mania: a systematic review of randomized placebo-controlled trials. Bipolar Disord 2007;9(6):551–60.

Weisler RH, Kalali AH, Ketter TA. A multicenter, randomized, double-blind, placebo-controlled trial of extended-release carbamazepine capsules as monotherapy for bipolar disorder patients with manic or mixed episodes. J Clin Psychiatry 2004; 65:478–84.

THERAPEUTICS

Brands
- Limbitrol
- Librium
- Librax

see index for additional brand names

Generic? Yes

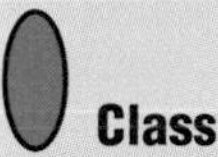

Class
- Benzodiazepine (anxiolytic)

Commonly Prescribed for
(bold for FDA approved)
- **Anxiety disorders**
- **Symptoms of anxiety**
- **Preoperative apprehension and anxiety**
- **Withdrawal symptoms of acute alcoholism**

How the Drug Works
- Binds to benzodiazepine receptors at the GABA-A ligand-gated chloride channel complex
- Enhances the inhibitory effects of GABA
- Boosts chloride conductance through GABA-regulated channels
- Inhibits neuronal activity presumably in amygdala-centered fear circuits to provide therapeutic benefits in anxiety disorders

How Long Until It Works
- Some immediate relief with first dosing is common; can take several weeks with daily dosing for maximal therapeutic benefit

If It Works
- For short-term symptoms of anxiety – after a few weeks, discontinue use or use on an "as-needed" basis
- For chronic anxiety disorders, the goal of treatment is complete remission of symptoms as well as prevention of future relapses
- For chronic anxiety disorders, treatment most often reduces or even eliminates symptoms, but not a cure since symptoms can recur after medicine stopped
- For long-term symptoms of anxiety, consider switching to an SSRI or SNRI for long-term maintenance
- If long-term maintenance with a benzodiazepine is necessary, continue treatment for 6 months after symptoms resolve, and then taper dose slowly
- If symptoms reemerge, consider treatment with an SSRI or SNRI, or consider restarting the benzodiazepine; sometimes benzodiazepines have to be used in combination with SSRIs or SNRIs for best results

If It Doesn't Work
- Consider switching to another agent or adding an appropriate augmenting agent
- Consider psychotherapy, especially cognitive behavioral psychotherapy
- Consider presence of concomitant substance abuse
- Consider presence of chlordiazepoxide abuse
- Consider another diagnosis, such as a comorbid medical condition

Best Augmenting Combos for Partial Response or Treatment Resistance
- Benzodiazepines are frequently used as augmenting agents for antipsychotics and mood stabilizers in the treatment of psychotic and bipolar disorders
- Benzodiazepines are frequently used as augmenting agents for SSRIs and SNRIs in the treatment of anxiety disorders
- Not generally rational to combine with other benzodiazepines
- Caution if using as an anxiolytic concomitantly with other sedative hypnotics for sleep

Tests
- In patients with seizure disorders, concomitant medical illness, and/or those with multiple concomitant long-term medications, periodic liver tests and blood counts may be prudent

SIDE EFFECTS

How Drug Causes Side Effects
- Same mechanism for side effects as for therapeutic effects – namely due to excessive actions at benzodiazepine receptors
- Long-term adaptations in benzodiazepine receptors may explain the development of dependence, tolerance, and withdrawal

- Side effects are generally immediate, but immediate side effects often disappear in time

Notable Side Effects

✽ Sedation, fatigue, depression
✽ Dizziness, ataxia, slurred speech, weakness
✽ Forgetfulness, confusion
✽ Hyperexcitability, nervousness
✽ Pain at injection site
- Rare hallucinations, mania
- Rare hypotension
- Hypersalivation, dry mouth

Life-Threatening or Dangerous Side Effects

- Respiratory depression, especially when taken with CNS depressants in overdose
- Rare hepatic dysfunction, renal dysfunction, blood dyscrasias

Weight Gain

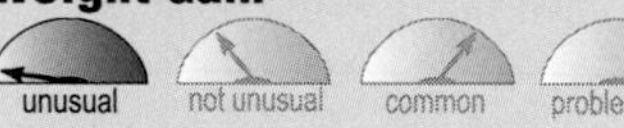

- Reported but not expected

Sedation

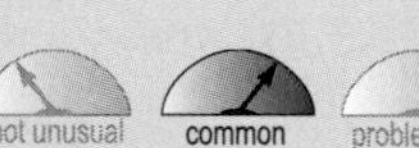

- Many experience and/or can be significant in amount
- Especially at initiation of treatment or when dose increases
- Tolerance often develops over time

What to Do About Side Effects

- Wait
- Wait
- Wait
- Lower the dose
- Take largest dose at bedtime to avoid sedative effects during the day
- Switch to another agent
- Administer flumazenil if side effects are severe or life-threatening

Best Augmenting Agents for Side Effects

- Many side effects cannot be improved with an augmenting agent

DOSING AND USE

Usual Dosage Range

- Oral: mild to moderate anxiety: 15–40 mg/day in 3–4 doses
- Oral: severe anxiety: 60–100 mg/day in 3–4 doses

Dosage Forms

- Capsule 5 mg, 10 mg, 25 mg
- Injectable 100 mg/5 mL

How To Dose

- Injectable: acute/severe anxiety: initial 50–100 mg; 25–50 mg 3–4 times/day if necessary
- Injectable: alcohol withdrawal: initial 50–100 mg; repeat after 2 hours if necessary
- Injectable: preoperative: 50–100 mg 1 hour before surgery
- Patients who receive injectable chlordiazepoxide should be observed for up to 3 hours

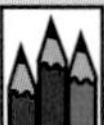

Dosing Tips

✽ One of the few benzodiazepines available in an injectable formulation
- Chlordiazepoxide injection is intended for acute use; patients who require longer treatment should be switched to the oral formulation
- Use lowest possible effective dose for the shortest possible period of time (a benzodiazepine-sparing strategy)
- Assess need for continued treatment regularly
- Risk of dependence may increase with dose and duration of treatment
- For interdose symptoms of anxiety, can either increase dose or maintain same total daily dose but divide into more frequent doses
- Can also use an as-needed occasional "top up" dose for interdose anxiety
- Because anxiety disorders can require higher doses, the risk of dependence may be greater in these patients
- Some severely ill patients may require doses higher than the generally recommended maximum dose
- Frequency of dosing in practice is often greater than predicted from half-life, as duration of biological activity is often shorter than pharmacokinetic terminal half-life

Overdose
- Fatalities can occur; hypotension, tiredness, ataxia, confusion, coma

Long-Term Use
- Evidence of efficacy for up to 16 weeks
- Risk of dependence, particularly for treatment periods longer than 12 weeks, and especially in patients with past or current polysubstance abuse

Habit Forming
- Chlordiazepoxide is a Schedule IV drug
- Patients may develop dependence and/or tolerance with long-term use

How to Stop
- Patients with history of seizure may seize upon withdrawal, especially if withdrawal is abrupt
- Taper by 10 mg every 3 days to reduce chances of withdrawal effects
- For difficult to taper patients, consider reducing dose much more slowly after reaching 20 mg/day, perhaps by as little as 5 mg per week or less
- For other patients with severe problems discontinuing a benzodiazepine, dosing may need to be tapered over many months (i.e., reduce dose by 1% every 3 days by crushing tablet and suspending or dissolving in 100 mL of fruit juice and then disposing of 1 mL while drinking the rest; 3–7 days later, dispose of 2 mL, and so on). This is both a form of very slow biological tapering and a form of behavioral desensitization
- Be sure to differentiate reemergence of symptoms requiring reinstitution of treatment from withdrawal symptoms
- Benzodiazepine-dependent anxiety patients and insulin-dependent diabetics are not addicted to their medications. When benzodiazepine-dependent patients stop their medication, disease symptoms can reemerge, disease symptoms can worsen (rebound), and/or withdrawal symptoms can emerge

Pharmacokinetics
- Elimination half-life 24–48 hours

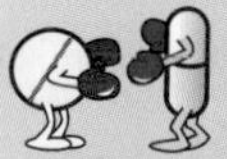

Drug Interactions
- Increased depressive effects when taken with other CNS depressants

Other Warnings/ Precautions
- Dosage changes should be made in collaboration with prescriber
- Use with caution in patients with pulmonary disease; rare reports of death after initiation of benzodiazepines in patients with severe pulmonary impairment
- History of drug or alcohol abuse often creates greater risk for dependency
- Some depressed patients may experience a worsening of suicidal ideation
- Some patients may exhibit abnormal thinking or behavioral changes similar to those caused by other CNS depressants (i.e., either depressant actions or disinhibiting actions)

Do Not Use
- If patient has narrow angle-closure glaucoma
- If there is a proven allergy to chlordiazepoxide or any benzodiazepine

SPECIAL POPULATIONS

Renal Impairment
- Oral: Initial 10–20 mg/day in 2–4 doses; increase as needed
- Injectable: 25–50 mg

Hepatic Impairment
- Oral: Initial 10–20 mg/day in 2–4 doses; increase as needed
- Injectable: 25–50 mg

Cardiac Impairment
- Benzodiazepines have been used to treat anxiety associated with acute myocardial infarction

Elderly
- Oral: Initial 10–20 mg/day in 2–4 doses; increase as needed
- Injectable: 25–50 mg
- Elderly patients may be more sensitive to sedative effects

Children and Adolescents
- Oral: Not recommended in children under age 6
- Oral: Initial 10–20 mg/day in 2–4 doses; may increase to 20–30 mg/day in 2–3 doses if ineffective

- Injectable: Not recommended in children under age 12
- Injectable: 25–50 mg
- Hyperactive children should be monitored for paradoxical effects
- Long-term effects of chlordiazepoxide in children/adolescents are unknown
- Should generally receive lower doses and be more closely monitored

Pregnancy

- Risk Category D [positive evidence of risk to human fetus; potential benefits may still justify its use during pregnancy]
- Possible increased risk of birth defects when benzodiazepines taken during pregnancy
- Because of the potential risks, chlordiazepoxide is not generally recommended as treatment for anxiety during pregnancy, especially during the first trimester
- Drug should be tapered if discontinued
- Infants whose mothers received a benzodiazepine late in pregnancy may experience withdrawal effects
- Neonatal flaccidity has been reported in infants whose mothers took a benzodiazepine during pregnancy
- Seizures, even mild seizures, may cause harm to the embryo/fetus

Breast Feeding

- Unknown if chlordiazepoxide is secreted in human breast milk, but all psychotropics assumed to be secreted in breast milk

✻ Recommended either to discontinue drug or bottle feed

- Effects of benzodiazepines on nursing infants have been reported and include feeding difficulties, sedation, and weight loss

THE ART OF PSYCHOPHARMACOLOGY

Potential Advantages

- Rapid onset of action

Potential Disadvantages

- Euphoria may lead to abuse
- Abuse especially risky in past or present substance abusers

Primary Target Symptoms

- Panic attacks
- Anxiety

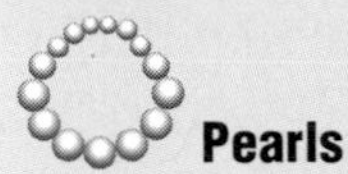

Pearls

- Can be a useful adjunct to SSRIs and SNRIs in the treatment of numerous anxiety disorders, but not used as frequently as some other benzodiazepines
- Not effective for treating psychosis as a monotherapy, but can be used as an adjunct to antipsychotics
- Not effective for treating bipolar disorder as a monotherapy, but can be used as an adjunct to mood stabilizers and antipsychotics
- Can both cause depression and treat depression in different patients
- When using to treat insomnia, remember that insomnia may be a symptom of some other primary disorder itself, and thus warrant evaluation for comorbid psychiatric and/or medical conditions

✻ Remains a viable treatment option for alcohol withdrawal

Suggested Reading

Baskin SI, Esdale A. Is chlordiazepoxide the rational choice among benzodiazepines? Pharmacotherapy 1982;2:110–9.

Erstad BL, Cotugno CL. Management of alcohol withdrawal. Am J Health Syst Pharm 1995;52:697–709.

Fraser AD. Use and abuse of the benzodiazepines. Ther Drug Monit 1998; 20:481–9.

Murray JB. Effects of valium and librium on human psychomotor and cognitive functions. Genet Psychol Monogr 1984;109(2D Half):167–97.

THERAPEUTICS

Brands • Thorazine

see index for additional brand names

Generic? Yes

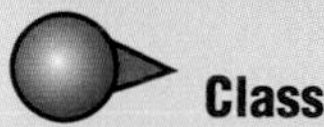

Class

- Conventional antipsychotic (neuroleptic, phenothiazine, dopamine 2 antagonist, antiemetic)

Commonly Prescribed for

(bold for FDA approved)

- **Schizophrenia**
- **Nausea, vomiting**
- **Restlessness and apprehension before surgery**
- **Acute intermittent porphyria**
- **Manifestations of manic type of manic-depressive illness**
- **Tetanus (adjunct)**
- **Intractable hiccups**
- **Combativeness and/or explosive hyperexcitable behavior (in children)**
- **Hyperactive children who show excessive motor activity with accompanying conduct disorders consisting of some or all of the following symptoms: impulsivity, difficulty sustaining attention, aggressivity, mood lability, and poor frustration tolerance**
- **Psychosis**
- Bipolar disorder

How the Drug Works

- Blocks dopamine 2 receptors, reducing positive symptoms of psychosis and improving other behaviors
- Combination of dopamine D2, histamine H1, and cholinergic M1 blockade in the vomiting center may reduce nausea and vomiting

How Long Until It Works

- Psychotic symptoms can improve within 1 week, but it may take several weeks for full effect on behavior
- Actions on nausea and vomiting are immediate

If It Works

- Most often reduces positive symptoms in schizophrenia but does not eliminate them
- Most schizophrenic patients do not have a total remission of symptoms but rather a reduction of symptoms by about a third
- Continue treatment in schizophrenia until reaching a plateau of improvement
- After reaching a satisfactory plateau, continue treatment for at least a year after first episode of psychosis in schizophrenia
- For second and subsequent episodes of psychosis in schizophrenia, treatment may need to be indefinite
- Reduces symptoms of acute psychotic mania but not proven as a mood stabilizer or as an effective maintenance treatment in bipolar disorder
- After reducing acute psychotic symptoms in mania, switch to a mood stabilizer and/or an atypical antipsychotic for mood stabilization and maintenance

If It Doesn't Work

- Consider trying one of the first-line atypical antipsychotics (risperidone, olanzapine, quetiapine, ziprasidone, aripiprazole, paliperidone, amisulpride)
- Consider trying another conventional antipsychotic
- If 2 or more antipsychotic monotherapies do not work, consider clozapine

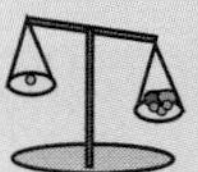

Best Augmenting Combos for Partial Response or Treatment-Resistance

- Augmentation of conventional antipsychotics has not been systematically studied
- Addition of a mood-stabilizing anticonvulsant such as valproate, carbamazepine, or lamotrigine may be helpful in both schizophrenia and bipolar mania
- Augmentation with lithium in bipolar mania may be helpful
- Addition of a benzodiazepine, especially short-term for agitation

Tests

✻ Since conventional antipsychotics are frequently associated with weight gain, before starting treatment, weigh all patients and determine if the patient is already

overweight (BMI 25.0–29.9) or obese (BMI ≥30)
- Before giving a drug that can cause weight gain to an overweight or obese patient, consider determining whether the patient already has pre-diabetes (fasting plasma glucose 100–25 mg/dL), diabetes (fasting plasma glucose >126 mg/dL), or dyslipidemia (increased total cholesterol, LDL cholesterol and triglycerides; decreased HDL cholesterol), and treat or refer such patients for treatment, including nutrition and weight management, physical activity counseling, smoking cessation, and medical management
- ✽ Monitor weight and BMI during treatment
- ✽ Consider monitoring fasting triglycerides monthly for several months in patients at high risk for metabolic complications and when initiating or switching antipsychotics
- ✽ While giving a drug to a patient who has gained >5% of initial weight, consider evaluating for the presence of pre-diabetes, diabetes, or dyslipidemia, or consider switching to a different antipsychotic
- Should check blood pressure in the elderly before starting and for the first few weeks of treatment
- Monitoring elevated prolactin levels of dubious clinical benefit
- Phenothiazines may cause false-positive phenylketonuria results

SIDE EFFECTS

How Drug Causes Side Effects

- By blocking dopamine 2 receptors in the striatum, it can cause motor side effects
- By blocking dopamine 2 receptors in the pituitary, it can cause elevations in prolactin
- By blocking dopamine 2 receptors excessively in the mesocortical and mesolimbic dopamine pathways, especially at high doses, it can cause worsening of negative and cognitive symptoms (neuroleptic-induced deficit syndrome)
- Anticholinergic actions may cause sedation, blurred vision, constipation, dry mouth
- Antihistaminic actions may cause sedation, weight gain
- By blocking alpha 1 adrenergic receptors, it can cause dizziness, sedation, and hypotension
- Mechanism of weight gain and any possible increased incidence of diabetes or dyslipidemia with conventional antipsychotics is unknown

Notable Side Effects

- ✽ Neuroleptic-induced deficit syndrome
- ✽ Akathisia
- ✽ Priapism
- ✽ Extrapyramidal symptoms, Parkinsonism, tardive dyskinesia
- ✽ Galactorrhea, amenorrhea
- Dizziness, sedation, impaired memory
- Dry mouth, constipation, urinary retention, blurred vision
- Decreased sweating
- Sexual dysfunction
- Hypotension, tachycardia, syncope
- Weight gain

Life-Threatening or Dangerous Side Effects

- Rare neuroleptic malignant syndrome
- Rare jaundice, agranulocytosis
- Rare seizures
- Increased risk of death and cerebrovascular events in elderly patients with dementia-related psychosis

Weight Gain

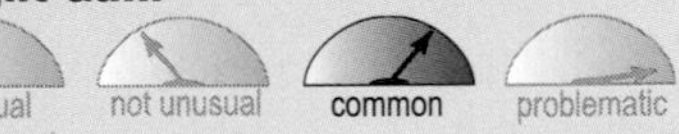

- Many experience and/or can be significant in amount

Sedation

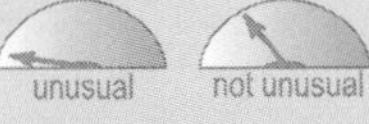

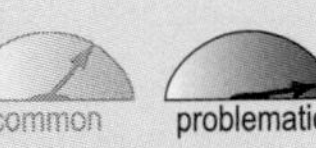

- Tolerance to sedation can develop over time

What to Do About Side Effects

- Wait
- Wait
- Wait
- For motor symptoms, add an anticholinergic agent
- Reduce the dose
- For sedation, give at night
- Switch to an atypical antipsychotic

- Weight loss, exercise programs, and medical management for high BMIs, diabetes dyslipidemia

Best Augmenting Agents for Side Effects

- Benztropine or trihexyphenidyl for motor side effects
- Sometimes amantadine can be helpful for motor side effects
- Benzodiazepines may be helpful for akathisia
- Many side effects cannot be improved with an augmenting agent

DOSING AND USE

Usual Dosage Range

- 200–800 mg/day

Dosage Forms

- Tablet 10 mg, 25 mg, 50 mg, 100 mg, 200 mg
- Capsule 30 mg, 75 mg, 150 mg
- Ampul 25 mg/mL; 1 mL, 2 mL
- Vial 25 mg/mL; 10 mL
- Liquid 10 mg/5 mL
- Suppository 25 mg, 100 mg

How to Dose

- Psychosis: increase dose until symptoms are controlled; after 2 weeks reduce to lowest effective dose
- Psychosis (intramuscular): varies by severity of symptoms and inpatient/outpatient status

Dosing Tips

- Low doses may have more sedative actions than antipsychotic actions
- Low doses have been used to provide short-term relief of daytime agitation and anxiety and to enhance sedative hypnotic actions in nonpsychotic patients, but other treatment options such as atypical antipsychotics are now preferred
- Higher doses may induce or worsen negative symptoms of schizophrenia
- Ampuls and vials contain sulfites that may cause allergic reactions, particularly in patients with asthma
- One of the few antipsychotics available as a suppository

Overdose

- Extrapyramidal symptoms, sedation, hypotension, coma, respiratory depression

Long-Term Use

- Some side effects may be irreversible (e.g., tardive dyskinesia)

Habit Forming

- No

How to Stop

- Slow down-titration of oral formulation (over 6–8 weeks), especially when simultaneously beginning a new antipsychotic while switching (i.e., cross-titration)
- Rapid oral discontinuation may lead to rebound psychosis and worsening of symptoms
- If antiparkinson agents are being used, they should be continued for a few weeks after chlorpromazine is discontinued

Pharmacokinetics

- Half-life approximately 8–33 hours

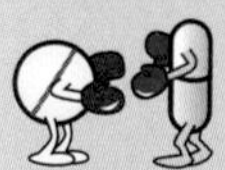

Drug Interactions

- May decrease the effects of levodopa, dopamine agonists
- May increase the effects of antihypertensive drugs except for guanethidine, whose antihypertensive actions chlorpromazine may antagonize
- Additive effects may occur if used with CNS depressants
- Some pressor agents (e.g., epinephrine) may interact with chlorpromazine to lower blood pressure
- Alcohol and diuretics may increase the risk of hypotension
- Reduces effects of anticoagulants
- May reduce phenytoin metabolism and increase phenytoin levels
- Plasma levels of chlorpromazine and propranolol may increase if used concomitantly
- Some patients taking a neuroleptic and lithium have developed an encephalopathic syndrome similar to neuroleptic malignant syndrome

Other Warnings/ Precautions

- If signs of neuroleptic malignant syndrome develop, treatment should be immediately discontinued
- Use cautiously in patients with alcohol withdrawal or convulsive disorders because of possible lowering of seizure threshold
- Use with caution in patients with respiratory disorders, glaucoma, or urinary retention
- Avoid extreme heat exposure
- Avoid undue exposure to sunlight
- Antiemetic effect of chlorpromazine may mask signs of other disorders or overdose; suppression of cough reflex may cause asphyxia
- Use only with caution if at all in Parkinson's disease or Lewy body dementia

Do Not Use

- If patient is in a comatose state
- If patient is taking metrizamide or large doses of CNS depressants
- If there is a proven allergy to chlorpromazine
- If there is a known sensitivity to any phenothiazine

SPECIAL POPULATIONS

Renal Impairment

- Use with caution

Hepatic Impairment

- Use with caution

Cardiac Impairment

- Cardiovascular toxicity can occur, especially orthostatic hypotension

Elderly

- Lower doses should be used and patient should be monitored closely
- Often do not tolerate sedating actions of chlorpromazine
- Although conventional antipsychotics are commonly used for behavioral disturbances in dementia, no agent has been approved for treatment of elderly patients with dementia-related psychosis
- Elderly patients with dementia-related psychosis treated with antipsychotics are at an increased risk of death compared to placebo, and also have an increased risk of cerebrovascular events

Children and Adolescents

- Can be used cautiously in children or adolescents over age 1 with severe behavioral problems
- Oral – 0.25 mg/lb every 4–6 hours as needed; rectal – 0.5 mg/lb every 6–8 hours as needed; IM – 0.25 mg/lb every 6–8 hours as needed; maximum 40 mg/day (under 5), 75 mg/day (5–12)
- Do not use if patient shows signs of Reye's syndrome
- Generally consider second-line after atypical antipsychotics

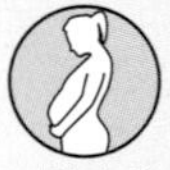

Pregnancy

- Risk Category C [some animal studies show adverse effects; no controlled studies in humans]
- Reports of extrapyramidal symptoms, jaundice, hyperreflexia, hyporeflexia in infants whose mothers took a phenothiazine during pregnancy
- Chlorpromazine should generally not be used during the first trimester
- Chlorpromazine should be used during pregnancy only if clearly needed
- Psychotic symptoms may worsen during pregnancy and some form of treatment may be necessary
- Atypical antipsychotics may be preferable to conventional antipsychotics or anticonvulsant mood stabilizers if treatment is required during pregnancy

Breast Feeding

- Some drug is found in mother's breast milk
- Effects on infant have been observed (dystonia, tardive dyskinesia, sedation)

✻ Recommended either to discontinue drug or bottle feed

THE ART OF PSYCHOPHARMACOLOGY

Potential Advantages
- Intramuscular formulation for emergency use
- Patients who require sedation for behavioral control

Potential Disadvantages
- Patients with tardive dyskinesia
- Children
- Elderly
- Patients who wish to avoid sedation

Primary Target Symptoms
- Positive symptoms of psychosis
- Motor and autonomic hyperactivity
- Violent or aggressive behavior

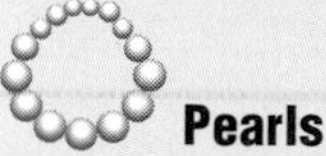

Pearls
- Chlorpromazine is one of the earliest classical conventional antipsychotics
- Chlorpromazine has a broad spectrum of efficacy, but risk of tardive dyskinesia and the availability of alternative treatments make its utilization outside of psychosis a short-term and second-line treatment option
- Chlorpromazine is a low-potency phenothiazine
- Sedative actions of low-potency phenothiazines are an important aspect of their therapeutic actions in some patients and side effect profile in others
- Conventional antipsychotics are much less expensive than atypical antipsychotics
- Low-potency phenothiazines like chlorpromazine have a greater risk of cardiovascular side effects
- Patients have very similar antipsychotic responses to any conventional antipsychotic, which is different from atypical antipsychotics, where antipsychotic responses of individual patients can occasionally vary greatly from one atypical antipsychotic to another
- Patients with inadequate responses to atypical antipsychotics may benefit from a trial of augmentation with a conventional antipsychotic such as chlorpromazine or from switching to a conventional antipsychotic such as chlorpromazine
- However, long-term polypharmacy with a combination of a conventional antipsychotic such as chlorpromazine with an atypical antipsychotic may combine their side effects without clearly augmenting the efficacy of either

Suggested Reading

Davis JM, Chen N, Glick ID. A meta-analysis of the efficacy of second-generation antipsychotics. Arch Gen Psychiatry 2003;60:553–64.

Frankenburg FR. Choices in antipsychotic therapy in schizophrenia. Harv Rev Psychiatry 1999;6:241–49.

Gocke E. Review of the genotoxic properties of chlorpromazine and related phenothiazines. Mutat Res 1996;366:9–21.

Leucht S, Wahlbeck K, Hamann J, Kissling W. New generation antipsychotics versus low-potency conventional antipsychotics: a systematic review and meta-analysis. The Lancet 2003;361:1581–89.

ThomLey B, Adams CE, Awad G. Chlorpromazine versus placebo for schizophrenia. Cochrane Database Syst Rev 2000;(2):CD000284.

Tohen M, Jacobs TG, Feldman PD. Onset of action of antipsychotics in the treatment of mania. Bipolar Disord 2000;2(3 Pt 2):261–68.

THERAPEUTICS

Brands • Celexa

see index for additional brand names

Generic? Yes

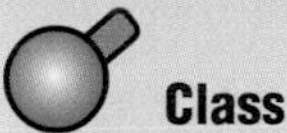

Class

- SSRI (selective serotonin reuptake inhibitor); often classified as an antidepressant, but it is not just an antidepressant

Commonly Prescribed for

(bold for FDA approved)

- **Depression**
- Premenstrual dysphoric disorder (PMDD)
- Obsessive-compulsive disorder (OCD)
- Panic disorder
- Generalized anxiety disorder
- Posttraumatic stress disorder (PTSD)
- Social anxiety disorder (social phobia)

How the Drug Works

- Boosts neurotransmitter serotonin
- Blocks serotonin reuptake pump (serotonin transporter)
- Desensitizes serotonin receptors, especially serotonin 1A autoreceptors
- Presumably increases serotonergic neurotransmission

✻ Citalopram also has mild antagonist actions at H1 histamine receptors

✻ Citalopram's inactive R enantiomer may interfere with the therapeutic actions of the active S enantiomer at serotonin reuptake pumps

How Long Until It Works

- Onset of therapeutic actions usually not immediate, but often delayed 2–4 weeks
- If it is not working within 6–8 weeks, it may require a dosage increase or it may not work at all
- May continue to work for many years to prevent relapse of symptoms

If It Works

- The goal of treatment is complete remission of current symptoms as well as prevention of future relapses
- Treatment most often reduces or even eliminates symptoms, but not a cure since symptoms can recur after medicine stopped
- Continue treatment until all symptoms are gone (remission) or significantly reduced (e.g., OCD, PTSD)
- Once symptoms are gone, continue treating for 1 year for the first episode of depression
- For second and subsequent episodes of depression, treatment may need to be indefinite
- Use in anxiety disorders may also need to be indefinite

If It Doesn't Work

- Many patients have only a partial response where some symptoms are improved but others persist (especially insomnia, fatigue, and problems concentrating in depression)
- Other patients may be nonresponders, sometimes called treatment-resistant or treatment-refractory
- Some patients who have an initial response may relapse even though they continue treatment, sometimes called "poop-out"
- Consider increasing dose, switching to another agent or adding an appropriate augmenting agent
- Consider psychotherapy
- Consider evaluation for another diagnosis or for a comorbid condition (e.g., medical illness, substance abuse, etc.)
- Some patients may experience apparent lack of consistent efficacy due to activation of latent or underlying bipolar disorder, and require antidepressant discontinuation and a switch to a mood stabilizer

Best Augmenting Combos for Partial Response or Treatment-Resistance

- Trazodone, especially for insomnia
- Bupropion, mirtazapine, reboxetine, or atomoxetine (add with caution and at lower doses since citalopram could theoretically raise atomoxetine levels); use combinations of antidepressants with caution as this may activate bipolar disorder and suicidal ideation
- Modafinil, especially for fatigue, sleepiness, and lack of concentration
- Mood stabilizers or atypical antipsychotics for bipolar depression, psychotic depression, treatment-resistant depression, or treatment-resistant anxiety disorders

- Benzodiazepines
- If all else fails for anxiety disorders, consider gabapentin or tiagabine
- Hypnotics for insomnia
- Classically, lithium, buspirone, or thyroid hormone

Tests

- None for healthy individuals

SIDE EFFECTS

How Drug Causes Side Effects

- Theoretically due to increases in serotonin concentrations at serotonin receptors in parts of the brain and body other than those that cause therapeutic actions (e.g., unwanted actions of serotonin in sleep centers causing insomnia, unwanted actions of serotonin in the gut causing diarrhea, etc.)
- Increasing serotonin can cause diminished dopamine release and might contribute to emotional flattening, cognitive slowing, and apathy in some patients
- Most side effects are immediate but often go away with time, in contrast to most therapeutic effects which are delayed and are enhanced over time

✻ Citalopram's unique mild antihistamine properties may contribute to sedation and fatigue in some patients

Notable Side Effects

- Sexual dysfunction (men: delayed ejaculation, erectile dysfunction; men and women: decreased sexual desire, anorgasmia)
- Gastrointestinal (decreased appetite, nausea, diarrhea, constipation, dry mouth)
- Mostly central nervous system (insomnia but also sedation, agitation, tremors, headache, dizziness)
- Note: patients with diagnosed or undiagnosed bipolar or psychotic disorders may be more vulnerable to CNS-activating actions of SSRIs
- Autonomic (sweating)
- Bruising and rare bleeding
- Rare hyponatremia (mostly in elderly patients and generally reversible on discontinuation of citalopram)
- SIADH (syndrome of inappropriate antidiuretic hormone secretion)

Life-Threatening or Dangerous Side Effects

- Rare seizures
- Rare induction of mania
- Rare activation of suicidal ideation and behavior (suicidality) (short-term studies did not show an increase in the risk of suicidality with antidepressants compared to placebo beyond age 24)

Weight Gain

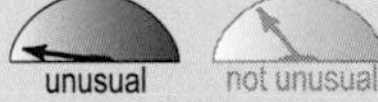

- Reported but not expected
- Citalopram has been associated with both weight gain and weight loss in various studies, but is relatively weight neutral overall

Sedation

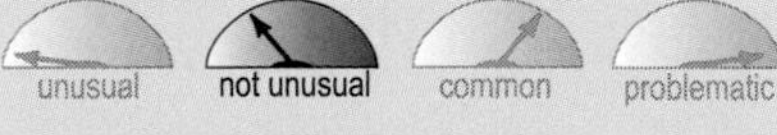

- Occurs in significant minority

What to Do About Side Effects

- Wait
- Wait
- Wait
- Take in the morning if nighttime insomnia
- Take at night if daytime sedation
- In a few weeks, switch to another agent or add other drugs

Best Augmenting Agents for Side Effects

- Often best to try another SSRI or another antidepressant monotherapy prior to resorting to augmentation strategies to treat side effects
- Trazodone or a hypnotic for insomnia
- Bupropion, sildenafil, vardenafil, or tadalafil for sexual dysfunction
- Bupropion for emotional flattening, cognitive slowing, or apathy
- Mirtazapine for insomnia, agitation, and gastrointestinal side effects
- Benzodiazepines for jitteriness and anxiety, especially at initiation of treatment and especially for anxious patients
- Many side effects are dose-dependent (i.e., they increase as dose increases, or they reemerge until tolerance redevelops)

- Many side effects are time-dependent (i.e., they start immediately upon dosing and upon each dose increase, but go away with time)
- Activation and agitation may represent the induction of a bipolar state, especially a mixed dysphoric bipolar II condition sometimes associated with suicidal ideation, and require the addition of lithium, a mood stabilizer or an atypical antipsychotic, and/or discontinuation of citalopram

DOSING AND USE

Usual Dosage Range
- 20–60 mg/day

Dosage Forms
- Tablets 10 mg, 20 mg scored, 40 mg scored
- Orally disintegrating tablet 10 mg, 20 mg, 40 mg
- Capsule 10 mg, 20 mg, 40 mg

How to Dose
- Initial 20 mg/day; increase by 20 mg/day after 1 or more weeks until desired efficacy is reached; maximum usually 60 mg/day; single dose administration, morning or evening

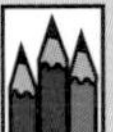

Dosing Tips
- Tablets are scored, so to save costs, give 10 mg as half of 20-mg tablet or 20 mg as half of 40-mg tablet, since the tablets cost about the same in many markets
- Many patients respond better to 40 mg than to 20 mg
- Given once daily, any time of day when best tolerated by the individual
- If intolerable anxiety, insomnia, agitation, akathisia, or activation occur either upon dosing initiation or discontinuation, consider the possibility of activated bipolar disorder and switch to a mood stabilizer or an atypical antipsychotic

Overdose
- Rare fatalities have been reported with citalopram overdose, both alone and in combination with other drugs
- Vomiting, sedation, heart rhythm disturbances, dizziness, sweating, nausea, tremor
- Rarely amnesia, confusion, coma, convulsions

Long-Term Use
- Safe

Habit Forming
- No

How to Stop
- Taper not usually necessary
- However, tapering to avoid potential withdrawal reactions generally prudent
- Many patients tolerate 50% dose reduction for 3 days, then another 50% reduction for 3 days, then discontinuation
- If withdrawal symptoms emerge during discontinuation, raise dose to stop symptoms and then restart withdrawal much more slowly

Pharmacokinetics
- Parent drug has 23–45 hour half-life
- Weak inhibitor of CYP450 2D6

Drug Interactions
- Tramadol increases the risk of seizures in patients taking an antidepressant
- Can increase tricyclic antidepressant levels; use with caution with tricyclic antidepressants
- Can cause a fatal "serotonin syndrome" when combined with MAO inhibitors, so do not use with MAO inhibitors or at least for 14 days after MAOIs are stopped
- Do not start an MAO inhibitor for at least 2 weeks after discontinuing citalopram
- May displace highly protein bound drugs (e.g., warfarin)
- Can rarely cause weakness, hyperreflexia, and incoordination when combined with sumatriptan or possibly other triptans, requiring careful monitoring of patient
- Possible increased risk of bleeding, especially when combined with anticoagulants (e.g., warfarin, NSAIDs)
- Via CYP450 2D6 inhibition, citalopram could theoretically interfere with the analgesic actions of codeine, and increase the plasma levels of some beta blockers and of atomoxetine

- Via CYP450 2D6 inhibition, citalopram could theoretically increase concentrations of thioridazine and cause dangerous cardiac arrhythmias

Other Warnings/ Precautions

- Use with caution in patients with history of seizures
- Use with caution in patients with bipolar disorder unless treated with concomitant mood-stabilizing agent
- When treating children, carefully weigh the risks and benefits of pharmacological treatment against the risks and benefits of nontreatment with antidepressants and make sure to document this in the patient's chart
- Distribute the brochures provided by the FDA and the drug companies
- Warn patients and their caregivers about the possibility of activating side effects and advise them to report such symptoms immediately
- Monitor patients for activation of suicidal ideation, especially children and adolescents

Do Not Use

- If patient is taking an MAO inhibitor
- If patient is taking thioridazine
- If there is a proven allergy to citalopram or escitalopram

SPECIAL POPULATIONS

Renal Impairment

- No dose adjustment for mild to moderate impairment
- Use cautiously in patients with severe impairment

Hepatic Impairment

- Recommended dose 20 mg/day; can be raised to 40 mg/day for nonresponders
- May need to dose cautiously at the lower end of the dose range in some patients for maximal tolerability

Cardiac Impairment

- Clinical experience suggests that citalopram is safe in these patients
- Treating depression with SSRIs in patients with acute angina or following myocardial infarction may reduce cardiac events and improve survival as well as mood

Elderly

- 20 mg/day; 40 mg/day for nonresponders
- May need to dose at the lower end of the dose range in some patients for maximal tolerability
- Citalopram may be an especially well-tolerated SSRI in the elderly
- Reduction in risk of suicidality with antidepressants compared to placebo in adults age 65 and older

Children and Adolescents

- Carefully weigh the risks and benefits of pharmacological treatment against the risks and benefits of nontreatment with antidepressants and make sure to document this in the patient's chart
- Monitor patients face-to-face regularly, particularly during the first several weeks of treatment
- Use with caution, observing for activation of known or unknown bipolar disorder and/or suicidal ideation, and inform parents or guardian of this risk so they can help observe child or adolescent patients
- Not specifically approved, but preliminary data suggest citalopram is safe and effective in children and adolescents with OCD and with depression

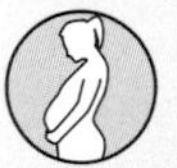

Pregnancy

- Risk Category C [some animal studies show adverse effects; no controlled studies in humans]
- Not generally recommended for use during pregnancy, especially during first trimester
- Nonetheless, continuous treatment during pregnancy may be necessary and has not been proven to be harmful to the fetus
- At delivery there may be more bleeding in the mother and transient irritability or sedation in the newborn
- Must weigh the risk of treatment (first trimester fetal development, third trimester newborn delivery) to the child against the risk of no treatment (recurrence of

depression, maternal health, infant bonding) to the mother and child
- For many patients, this may mean continuing treatment during pregnancy
- SSRI use beyond the 20th week of pregnancy may be associated with increased risk of pulmonary hypertension in newborns
- Neonates exposed to SSRIs or SNRIs late in the third trimester have developed complications requiring prolonged hospitalization, respiratory support, and tube feeding; reported symptoms are consistent with either a direct toxic effect of SSRIs and SNRIs or, possibly, a drug discontinuation syndrome, and include respiratory distress, cyanosis, apnea, seizures, temperature instability, feeding difficulty, vomiting, hypoglycemia, hypotonia, hypertonia, hyperreflexia, tremor, jitteriness, irritability, and constant crying

Breast Feeding

- Some drug is found in mother's breast milk
- Trace amounts may be present in nursing children whose mothers are on citalopram
- If child becomes irritable or sedated, breast feeding or drug may need to be discontinued
- Immediate postpartum period is a high-risk time for depression, especially in women who have had prior depressive episodes, so drug may need to be reinstituted late in the third trimester or shortly after childbirth to prevent a recurrence during the postpartum period
- Must weigh benefits of breast feeding with risks and benefits of antidepressant treatment versus nontreatment to both the infant and the mother
- For many patients, this may mean continuing treatment during breast feeding

THE ART OF PSYCHOPHARMACOLOGY

Potential Advantages

- Elderly patients
- Patients excessively activated or sedated by other SSRIs

Potential Disadvantages

- May require dosage titration to attain optimal efficacy
- Can be sedating in some patients

Primary Target Symptoms

- Depressed mood
- Anxiety
- Panic attacks, avoidant behavior, re-experiencing, hyperarousal
- Sleep disturbance, both insomnia and hypersomnia

Pearls

✻ May be more tolerable than some other antidepressants
- May have less sexual dysfunction than some other SSRIs
- May be especially well tolerated in the elderly

✻ May be less well tolerated than escitalopram
- Documentation of efficacy in anxiety disorders is less comprehensive than for escitalopram and other SSRIs
- Can cause cognitive and affective "flattening"
- Some evidence suggests that citalopram treatment during only the luteal phase may be more effective than continuous treatment for patients with PMDD
- SSRIs may be less effective in women over 50, especially if they are not taking estrogen
- SSRIs may be useful for hot flushes in perimenopausal women
- Nonresponse to citalopram in elderly may require consideration of mild cognitive impairment or Alzheimer disease

Suggested Reading

Bezchlibnyk-Butler K, Aleksic I, Kennedy SH. Citalopram – a review of pharmacological and clinical effects. J Psychiatry and Neurosci 2000;25:241–54.

Edwards JG, Anderson I. Systematic review and guide to selection of selective serotonin reuptake inhibitors. Drugs 1999;57:507–33.

Keller MB. Citalopram therapy for depression: a review of 10 years of European experience and data from U.S. clinical trials. J Clin Psychiatry 2000;61:896–908.

Pollock BG. Citalopram: a comprehensive review. Expert Opin Pharmacother 2001;2:681–98.

Rush AJ, Trivedi MH, Wisniewski SR. Acute and longer-term outcomes in depressed outpatients requiring one or several treatment steps:a STAR*D report. Am J Psychiatry 2006;163(11):1905–17.

THERAPEUTICS

Brands • Anafranil

see index for additional brand names

Generic? Yes

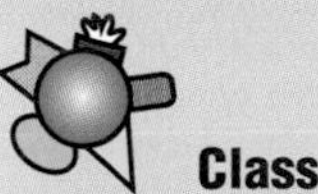

Class

- Tricyclic antidepressant (TCA)
- Parent drug is a potent serotonin reuptake inhibitor
- Active metabolite is a potent norepinephrine/noradrenaline reuptake inhibitor

Commonly Prescribed for

(bold for FDA approved)

* **Obsessive-compulsive disorder**
- Depression
* Severe and treatment-resistant depression
* Cataplexy syndrome
- Anxiety
- Insomnia
- Neuropathic pain/chronic pain

How the Drug Works

- Boosts neurotransmitters serotonin and norepinephrine/noradrenaline
- Blocks serotonin reuptake pump (serotonin transporter), presumably increasing serotonergic neurotransmission
- Blocks norepinephrine reuptake pump (norepinephrine transporter), presumably increasing noradrenergic neurotransmission
- Presumably desensitizes both serotonin 1A receptors and beta adrenergic receptors
- Since dopamine is inactivated by norepinephrine reuptake in frontal cortex, which largely lacks dopamine transporters, clomipramine can increase dopamine neurotransmission in this part of the brain

How Long Until It Works

- May have immediate effects in treating insomnia or anxiety
- Onset of therapeutic actions in depression usually not immediate, but often delayed 2 to 4 weeks
- Onset of therapeutic action in OCD can be delayed 6–12 weeks
- If it is not working for depression within 6–8 weeks, it may require a dosage increase or it may not work at all
- If it is not working for OCD within 12 weeks, it may not work at all
- May continue to work for many years to prevent relapse of symptoms

If It Works

- The goal of treatment of depression is complete remission of current symptoms as well as prevention of future relapses
- Treatment most often reduces or even eliminates symptoms, but not a cure since symptoms can recur after medicine stopped
- Although the goal of treatment of OCD is also complete remission of symptoms, this may be less likely than in depression
- The goal of treatment of chronic neuropathic pain is to reduce symptoms as much as possible, especially in combination with other treatments
- Continue treatment of depression until all symptoms are gone (remission)
- Once symptoms of depression are gone, continue treating for 1 year for the first episode of depression
- For second and subsequent episodes of depression, treatment may need to be indefinite
- Use in OCD may also need to be indefinite, starting from the time of initial treatment
- Use in other anxiety disorders and chronic pain may also need to be indefinite, but long-term treatment is not well studied in these conditions

If It Doesn't Work

- Many patients have only a partial response where some symptoms are improved but others persist (especially insomnia, fatigue, and problems concentrating)
- Other patients may be nonresponders, sometimes called treatment-resistant or treatment-refractory
- Consider increasing dose, switching to another agent, or adding an appropriate augmenting agent
- Consider psychotherapy, especially behavioral therapy in OCD
- Consider evaluation for another diagnosis or for a comorbid condition (e.g., medical illness, substance abuse, etc.)
- Some patients may experience apparent lack of consistent efficacy due to activation

of latent or underlying bipolar disorder, and require antidepressant discontinuation and a switch to a mood stabilizer

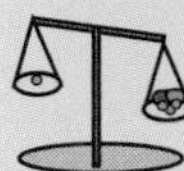

Best Augmenting Combos for Partial Response or Treatment-Resistance

- Lithium, buspirone, hormone (for depression and OCD)
- For the expert: consider cautious addition of fluvoxamine for treatment-resistant OCD
- Thyroid hormone (for depression)
- Atypical antipsychotics (for OCD)

Tests

✻ None for healthy individuals, although monitoring of plasma drug levels is potentially available at specialty laboratories for the expert

✻ Since tricyclic and tetracyclic antidepressants are frequently associated with weight gain, before starting treatment, weigh all patients and determine if the patient is already overweight (BMI 25.0–29.9) or obese (BMI ≥30)

- Before giving a drug that can cause weight gain to an overweight or obese patient, consider determining whether the patient already has pre-diabetes (fasting plasma glucose 100–25 mg/dL), diabetes (fasting plasma glucose >126 mg/dL), or dyslipidemia (increased total cholesterol, LDL cholesterol and triglycerides; decreased HDL cholesterol), and treat or refer such patients for treatment, including nutrition and weight management, physical activity counseling, smoking cessation, and medical management

✻ Monitor weight and BMI during treatment

✻ While giving a drug to a patient who has gained >5% of initial weight, consider evaluating for the presence of pre-diabetes, diabetes, or dyslipidemia, or consider switching to a different antidepressant

- EKGs may be useful for selected patients (e.g., those with personal or family history of QTc prolongation; cardiac arrhythmia; recent myocardial infarction; uncompensated heart failure; or taking agents that prolong QTc interval such as pimozide, thioridazine, selected antiarrhythmics, moxifloxacin, sparfloxacin, etc.)
- Patients at risk for electrolyte disturbances (e.g., patients on diuretic therapy) should have baseline and periodic serum potassium and magnesium measurements

SIDE EFFECTS

How Drug Causes Side Effects

- Anticholinergic activity may explain sedative effects, dry mouth, constipation, and blurred vision
- Sedative effects and weight gain may be due to antihistamine properties
- Blockade of alpha adrenergic 1 receptors may explain dizziness, sedation, and hypotension
- Cardiac arrhythmias and seizures, especially in overdose, may be caused by blockade of ion channels

Notable Side Effects

- Blurred vision, constipation, urinary retention, increased appetite, dry mouth, nausea, diarrhea, heartburn, unusual taste in mouth, weight gain
- Fatigue, weakness, dizziness, sedation, headache, anxiety, nervousness, restlessness
- Sexual dysfunction, sweating

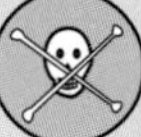

Life-Threatening or Dangerous Side Effects

- Paralytic ileus, hyperthermia (TCAs + anticholinergic agents)
- Lowered seizure threshold and rare seizures
- Orthostatic hypotension, sudden death, arrhythmias, tachycardia
- QTc prolongation
- Hepatic failure, extrapyramidal symptoms
- Increased intraocular pressure
- Rare induction of mania
- Rare activation of suicidal ideation and behavior (suicidality) (short-term studies did not show an increase in the risk of suicidality with antidepressants compared to placebo beyond age 24)

Weight Gain

unusual | not unusual | **common** | problematic

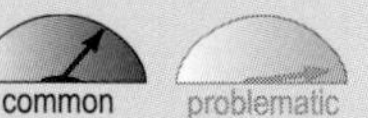

- Many experience and/or can be significant in amount
- Can increase appetite and carbohydrate craving

Sedation

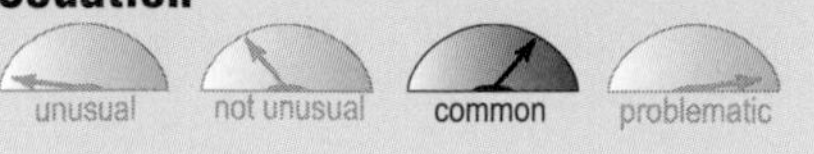

- Many experience and/or can be significant in amount
- Tolerance to sedative effect may develop with long-term use

What to Do About Side Effects
- Wait
- Wait
- Wait
- Lower the dose
- Switch to an SSRI or newer antidepressant

Best Augmenting Agents for Side Effects
- Many side effects cannot be improved with an augmenting agent

DOSING AND USE

Usual Dosage Range
- 100 mg/day–200 mg/day

Dosage Forms
- Capsule 25 mg, 50 mg, 75 mg

How to Dose
- Initial 25 mg/day; increase over 2 weeks to 100 mg/day; maximum dose generally 250 mg/day

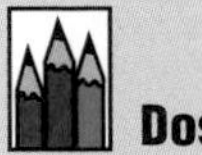

Dosing Tips
- If given in a single dose, should generally be administered at bedtime because of its sedative properties
- If given in split doses, largest dose should generally be given at bedtime because of its sedative properties
- If patients experience nightmares, split dose and do not give large dose at bedtime
- Patients treated for chronic pain may only require lower doses

✻ Patients treated for OCD may often require doses at the high end of the range (e.g., 200–250 mg/day)

- Risk of seizure increases with dose, especially with clomipramine at doses above 250 mg/day

✻ Dose of 300 mg may be associated with up to 7/1,000 incidence of seizures, a generally unacceptable risk

- If intolerable anxiety, insomnia, agitation, akathisia, or activation occur either upon dosing initiation or discontinuation, consider the possibility of activated bipolar disorder, and switch to a mood stabilizer or an atypical antipsychotic

Overdose
- Death may occur; convulsions, cardiac dysrhythmias, severe hypotension, CNS depression, coma, changes in EKG

Long-Term Use
- Limited data but appears to be efficacious and safe long-term

Habit Forming
- No

How to Stop
- Taper to avoid withdrawal effects
- Even with gradual dose reduction some withdrawal symptoms may appear within the first 2 weeks
- Many patients tolerate 50% dose reduction for 3 days, then another 50% reduction for 3 days, then discontinuation
- If withdrawal symptoms emerge during discontinuation, raise dose to stop symptoms and then restart withdrawal much more slowly

Pharmacokinetics
- Substrate for CYP450 2D6 and 1A2
- Metabolized to an active metabolite, desmethyl-clomipramine, a predominantly norepinephrine reuptake inhibitor, by demethylation via CYP450 1A2
- Half-life approximately 17–28 hours

Drug Interactions
- Tramadol increases the risk of seizures in patients taking TCAs
- Use of TCAs with anticholinergic drugs may result in paralytic ileus or hyperthermia
- Fluoxetine, paroxetine, bupropion, duloxetine, and other CYP450 2D6 inhibitors may increase TCA concentrations
- Fluvoxamine, a CYP450 1A2 inhibitor, can decrease the conversion of clomipramine to desmethyl-clomipramine, and increase clomipramine plasma concentrations
- Cimetidine may increase plasma concentrations of TCAs and cause anticholinergic symptoms

- Phenothiazines or haloperidol may raise TCA blood concentrations
- May alter effects of antihypertensive drugs
- Use of TCAs with sympathomimetic agents may increase sympathetic activity
- TCAs may inhibit hypotensive effects of clonidine
- Methylphenidate may inhibit metabolism of TCAs
- Activation and agitation, especially following switching or adding antidepressants, may represent the induction of a bipolar state, especially a mixed dysphoric bipolar II condition sometimes associated with suicidal ideation, and require the addition of lithium, a mood stabilizer or an atypical antipsychotic, and/or discontinuation of clomipramine

Other Warnings/ Precautions

- Add or initiate other antidepressants with caution for up to 2 weeks after discontinuing clomipramine
- Generally, do not use with MAO inhibitors, including 14 days after MAOIs are stopped; do not start an MAOI until 2 weeks after discontinuing clomipramine, but see Pearls
- Use with caution in patients with history of seizures, urinary retention, narrow angle-closure glaucoma, hyperthyroidism
- TCAs can increase QTc interval, especially at toxic doses, which can be attained not only by overdose but also by combining with drugs that inhibit TCA metabolism via CYP450 2D6, potentially causing torsade de pointes-type arrhythmia or sudden death
- Because TCAs can prolong QTc interval, use with caution in patients who have bradycardia or who are taking drugs that can induce bradycardia (e.g., beta blockers, calcium channel blockers, clonidine, digitalis)
- Because TCAs can prolong QTc interval, use with caution in patients who have hypokalemia and/or hypomagnesemia or who are taking drugs that can induce hypokalemia and/or magnesemia (e.g., diuretics, stimulant laxatives, intravenous amphotericin B, glucocorticoids, tetracosactide)
- When treating children, carefully weigh the risks and benefits of pharmacological treatment against the risks and benefits of nontreatment with antidepressants and make sure to document this in the patient's chart
- Distribute the brochures provided by the FDA and the drug companies
- Warn patients and their caregivers about the possibility of activating side effects and advise them to report such symptoms immediately
- Monitor patients for activation of suicidal ideation, especially children and adolescents

Do Not Use

- If patient is recovering from myocardial infarction
- If patient is taking agents capable of significantly prolonging QTc interval (e.g., pimozide, thioridazine, selected antiarrhythmics, moxifloxacin, sparfloxacin)
- If there is a history of QTc prolongation or cardiac arrhythmia, recent acute myocardial infarction, uncompensated heart failure
- If patient is taking drugs that inhibit TCA metabolism, including CYP450 2D6 inhibitors, except by an expert
- If there is reduced CYP450 2D6 function, such as patients who are poor 2D6 metabolizers, except by an expert and at low doses
- If there is a proven allergy to clomipramine

SPECIAL POPULATIONS

Renal Impairment

- Use with caution

Hepatic Impairment

- Use with caution

Cardiac Impairment

- TCAs have been reported to cause arrhythmias, prolongation of conduction time, orthostatic hypotension, sinus tachycardia, and heart failure, especially in the diseased heart
- Myocardial infarction and stroke have been reported with TCAs

- TCAs produce QTc prolongation, which may be enhanced by the existence of bradycardia, hypokalemia, congenital or acquired long QTc interval, which should be evaluated prior to administering clomipramine
- Use with caution if treating concomitantly with a medication likely to produce prolonged bradycardia, hypokalemia, slowing of intracardiac conduction, or prolongation of the QTc interval
- Avoid TCAs in patients with a known history of QTc prolongation, recent acute myocardial infarction, and uncompensated heart failure
- TCAs may cause a sustained increase in heart rate in patients with ischemic heart disease and may worsen (decrease) heart rate variability, an independent risk of mortality in cardiac populations
- Since SSRIs may improve (increase) heart rate variability in patients following a myocardial infarct and may improve survival as well as mood in patients with acute angina or following a myocardial infarction, these are more appropriate agents for cardiac population than tricyclic/tetracyclic antidepressants

✽ Risk/benefit ratio may not justify use of TCAs in cardiac impairment

Elderly

- May be more sensitive to anticholinergic, cardiovascular, hypotensive, and sedative effects
- Dose may need to be lower than usual adult dose, at least initially
- Reduction in risk of suicidality with antidepressants compared to placebo in adults age 65 and older

Children and Adolescents

- Carefully weigh the risks and benefits of pharmacological treatment against the risks and benefits of nontreatment with antidepressants and make sure to document this in the patient's chart
- Monitor patients face-to-face regularly, particularly during the first several weeks of treatment
- Use with caution, observing for activation of known or unknown bipolar disorder and/or suicidal ideation, and inform parents or guardian of this risk so they can help observe child or adolescent patients
- Not recommended for use in children under age 10
- Several studies show lack of efficacy of TCAs for depression
- May be used to treat enuresis or hyperactive/impulsive behaviors
- Effective for OCD in children
- Some cases of sudden death have occurred in children taking TCAs
- Dose in children/adolescents should be titrated to a maximum of 100 mg/day or 3 mg/kg per day after 2 weeks, after which dose can then be titrated up to a maximum of 200 mg/day or 3 mg/kg per day

Pregnancy

- Risk Category C [some animal studies show adverse effects; no controlled studies in humans]
- Clomipramine crosses the placenta
- Adverse effects have been reported in infants whose mothers took a TCA (lethargy, withdrawal symptoms, fetal malformations)
- Must weigh the risk of treatment (first trimester fetal development, third trimester newborn delivery) to the child against the risk of no treatment (recurrence of depression, worsening of OCD, maternal health, infant bonding) to the mother and child
- For many patients this may mean continuing treatment during pregnancy

Breast Feeding

- Some drug is found in mother's breast milk

✽ Recommended either to discontinue drug or bottle feed

- Immediate postpartum period is a high-risk time for depression and worsening of OCD, especially in women who have had prior depressive episodes or OCD symptoms, so drug may need to be reinstituted late in the third trimester or shortly after childbirth to prevent a recurrence or exacerbation during the postpartum period
- Must weigh benefits of breast feeding with risks and benefits of antidepressant treatment versus nontreatment to both the infant and the mother
- For many patients this may mean continuing treatment during breast feeding

THE ART OF PSYCHOPHARMACOLOGY

Potential Advantages

- Patients with insomnia
- Severe or treatment-resistant depression
- Patients with comorbid OCD and depression
- Patients with cataplexy

Potential Disadvantages

- Pediatric and geriatric patients
- Patients concerned with weight gain
- Cardiac patients
- Patients with seizure disorders

Primary Target Symptoms

- Depressed mood
- Obsessive thoughts
- Compulsive behaviors

Pearls

✻ The only TCA with proven efficacy in OCD
- Normally, clomipramine (CMI), a potent serotonin reuptake blocker, at steady state is metabolized extensively to its active metabolite desmethyl-clomipramine (de-CMI), a potent nonadrenaline reuptake blocker, by the enzyme CYP450 1A2
- Thus, at steady state, plasma drug activity is generally more noradrenergic (with higher de-CMI levels) than serotonergic (with lower parent CMI levels)
- Addition of the SSRI and CYP450 1A2 inhibitor fluvoxamine blocks this conversion and results in higher CMI levels than de-CMI levels
- For the expert only: addition of the SSRI fluvoxamine to CMI in treatment-resistant OCD can powerfully enhance serotonergic activity, not only due to the inherent additive pharmacodynamic serotonergic activity of fluvoxamine added to CMI, but also due to a favorable pharmacokinetic interaction inhibiting CYP450 1A2 and thus converting CMI's metabolism to a more powerful serotonergic portfolio of parent drug

✻ One of the most favored TCAs for treating severe depression
- Tricyclic antidepressants are no longer generally considered a first-line treatment option for depression because of their side effect profile
- Tricyclic antidepressants continue to be useful for severe or treatment-resistant depression
- Tricyclic antidepressants are often a first-line treatment option for chronic pain

✻ Unique among TCAs, clomipramine has a potentially fatal interaction with MAOIs in addition to the danger of hypertension characteristic of all MAOI-TCA combinations

✻ A potentially fatal serotonin syndrome with high fever, seizures, and coma, analogous to that caused by SSRIs and MAOIs, can occur with clomipramine and SSRIs, presumably due to clomipramine's potent serotonin reuptake blocking properties
- TCAs may aggravate psychotic symptoms
- Alcohol should be avoided because of additive CNS effects
- Underweight patients may be more susceptible to adverse cardiovascular effects
- Children, patients with inadequate hydration, and patients with cardiac disease may be more susceptible to TCA-induced cardiotoxicity than healthy adults
- Patients on TCAs should be aware that they may experience symptoms such as photosensitivity or blue-green urine
- SSRIs may be more effective than TCAs in women, and TCAs may be more effective than SSRIs in men
- Since tricyclic/tetracyclic antidepressants are substrates for CYP450 2D6, and 7% of the population (especially Caucasians) may have a genetic variant leading to reduced activity of 2D6, such patients may not safely tolerate normal doses of tricyclic/tetracyclic antidepressants and may require dose reduction
- Phenotypic testing may be necessary to detect this genetic variant prior to dosing with a tricyclic/tetracyclic antidepressant, especially in vulnerable populations such as children, elderly, cardiac populations, and those on concomitant medications
- Patients who seem to have extraordinarily severe side effects at normal or low doses may have this phenotypic CYP450 2D6 variant and require low doses or switching to another antidepressant not metabolized by 2D6

Suggested Reading

Anderson IM. Meta-analytical studies on new antidepressants. Br Med Bull 2001; 57:161–78.

Anderson IM. Selective serotonin reuptake inhibitors versus tricyclic antidepressants: a meta-analysis of efficacy and tolerability. J Aff Disorders 2000;58:19–36.

Cox BJ, Swinson RP, Morrison B, Lee PS. Clomipramine, fluoxetine, and behavior therapy in the treatment of obsessive-compulsive disorder: a meta-analysis. J Behav Ther Exp Psychiatry 1993;24:149–53.

Feinberg M. Clomipramine for obsessive-compulsive disorder. Am Fam Physician 1991; 43:1735–38.

THERAPEUTICS

Brands • Klonopin

see index for additional brand names

Generic? Yes

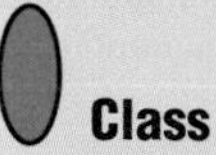

Class

• Benzodiazepine (anxiolytic, anticonvulsant)

Commonly Prescribed for

(bold for FDA approved)

- **Panic disorder, with or without agoraphobia**
- **Lennox-Gastaut syndrome (petit mal variant)**
- **Akinetic seizure**
- **Myoclonic seizure**
- **Absence seizure (petit mal)**
- Atonic seizures
- Other seizure disorders
- Other anxiety disorders
- Acute mania (adjunctive)
- Acute psychosis (adjunctive)
- Insomnia

How the Drug Works

- Binds to benzodiazepine receptors at the GABA-A ligand-gated chloride channel complex
- Enhances the inhibitory effects of GABA
- Boosts chloride conductance through GABA-regulated channels
- Inhibits neuronal activity presumably in amygdala-centered fear circuits to provide therapeutic benefits in anxiety disorders
- Inhibitory actions in cerebral cortex may provide therapeutic benefits in seizure disorders

How Long Until It Works

- Some immediate relief with first dosing is common; can take several weeks with daily dosing for maximal therapeutic benefit

If It Works

- For short-term symptoms of anxiety – after a few weeks, discontinue use or use on an "as-needed" basis
- For chronic anxiety disorders, the goal of treatment is complete remission of symptoms as well as prevention of future relapses
- For chronic anxiety disorders, treatment most often reduces or even eliminates symptoms, but not a cure since symptoms can recur after medicine stopped
- For long-term symptoms of anxiety, consider switching to an SSRI or SNRI for long-term maintenance
- If long-term maintenance with a benzodiazepine is necessary, continue treatment for 6 months after symptoms resolve, and then taper dose slowly
- If symptoms reemerge, consider treatment with an SSRI or SNRI, or consider restarting the benzodiazepine; sometimes benzodiazepines have to be used in combination with SSRIs or SNRIs for best results
- For long-term treatment of seizure disorders, development of tolerance dose escalation and loss of efficacy necessitating adding or switching to other anticonvulsants is not uncommon

If It Doesn't Work

- Consider switching to another agent or adding an appropriate augmenting agent
- Consider psychotherapy, especially cognitive behavioral psychotherapy
- Consider presence of concomitant substance abuse
- Consider presence of clonazepam abuse
- Consider another diagnosis such as a comorbid medical condition

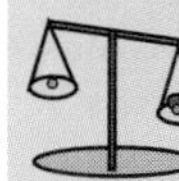

Best Augmenting Combos for Partial Response or Treatment-Resistance

- Benzodiazepines are frequently used as augmenting agents for antipsychotics and mood stabilizers in the treatment of psychotic and bipolar disorders
- Benzodiazepines are frequently used as augmenting agents for SSRIs and SNRIs in the treatment of anxiety disorders
- Not generally rational to combine with other benzodiazepines
- Caution if using as an anxiolytic concomitantly with other sedative hypnotics for sleep
- Clonazepam is commonly combined with other anticonvulsants for the treatment of seizure disorders

Tests

- In patients with seizure disorders, concomitant medical illness, and/or those with multiple concomitant long-term medications, periodic liver tests and blood counts may be prudent

SIDE EFFECTS

How Drug Causes Side Effects

- Same mechanism for side effects as for therapeutic effects – namely due to excessive actions at benzodiazepine receptors
- Long-term adaptations in benzodiazepine receptors may explain the development of dependence, tolerance, and withdrawal
- Side effects are generally immediate, but immediate side effects often disappear in time

Notable Side Effects

✻ Sedation, fatigue, depression
✻ Dizziness, ataxia, slurred speech, weakness
✻ Forgetfulness, confusion
✻ Hyperexcitability, nervousness
- Rare hallucinations, mania
- Rare hypotension
- Hypersalivation, dry mouth

Life-Threatening or Dangerous Side Effects

- Respiratory depression, especially when taken with CNS depressants in overdose
- Rare hepatic dysfunction, renal dysfunction, blood dyscrasias
- Grand mal seizures

Weight Gain

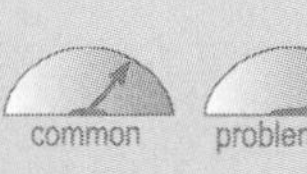

- Reported but not expected

Sedation

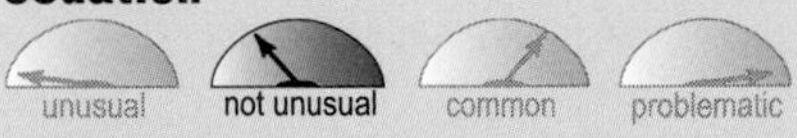

- Occurs in significant minority
- Especially at initiation of treatment or when dose increases
- Tolerance often develops over time

What to Do About Side Effects

- Wait
- Wait
- Wait
- Lower the dose
- Take largest dose at bedtime to avoid sedative effects during the day
- Switch to another agent
- Administer flumazenil if side effects are severe or life-threatening

Best Augmenting Agents for Side Effects

- Many side effects cannot be improved with an augmenting agent

DOSING AND USE

Usual Dosage Range

- Seizures: dependent on individual response of patient, up to 20 mg/day
- Panic: 0.5–2 mg/day either as divided doses or once at bedtime

Dosage Forms

- Tablet 0.5 mg scored, 1 mg, 2 mg
- Disintegrating (wafer): 0.125 mg, 0.25 mg, 0.5 mg, 1 mg, 2 mg

How to Dose

- Seizures – 1.5 mg divided into 3 doses, raise by 0.5 mg every 3 days until desired effect is reached; divide into 3 even doses or else give largest dose at bedtime; maximum dose generally 20 mg/day
- Panic – 1 mg/day; start at 0.25 mg divided into 2 doses, raise to 1 mg after 3 days; dose either twice daily or once at bedtime; maximum dose generally 4 mg/day

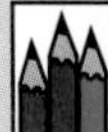

Dosing Tips

- For anxiety disorders, use lowest possible effective dose for the shortest possible period of time (a benzodiazepine sparing strategy)
- Assess need for continuous treatment regularly
- Risk of dependence may increase with dose and duration of treatment
- For interdose symptoms of anxiety, can either increase dose or maintain same daily dose but divide into more frequent doses

- Can also use an as-needed occasional "top-up" dose for interdose anxiety
- Because seizure disorder can require doses much higher than 2 mg/day, the risk of dependence may be greater in these patients
- Because panic disorder can require doses somewhat higher than 2 mg/day, the risk of dependence may be greater in these patients than in anxiety patients maintained at lower doses
- Some severely ill seizure patients may require more than 20 mg/day
- Some severely ill panic patients may require 4 mg/day or more
- Frequency of dosing in practice is often greater than predicted from half-life, as duration of biological activity is often shorter than pharmacokinetic terminal half-life

✱ Clonazepam is generally dosed half the dosage of alprazolam

- Escalation of dose may be necessary if tolerance develops in seizure disorders
- Escalation of dose usually not necessary in anxiety disorders, as tolerance to clonazepam does not generally develop in the treatment of anxiety disorders

✱ Available as an oral disintegrating wafer

Overdose

- Rarely fatal in monotherapy; sedation, confusion, coma, diminished reflexes

Long-Term Use

- May lose efficacy for seizures; dose increase may restore efficacy
- Risk of dependence, particularly for treatment periods longer than 12 weeks and especially in patients with past or current polysubstance abuse

Habit Forming

- Clonazepam is a Schedule IV drug
- Patients may develop dependence and/or tolerance with long-term use

How to Stop

- Patients with history of seizures may seize upon withdrawal, especially if withdrawal is abrupt
- Taper by 0.25 mg every 3 days to reduce chances of withdrawal effects
- For difficult to taper cases, consider reducing dose much more slowly after reaching 1.5 mg/day, perhaps by as little as 0.125 mg per week or less
- For other patients with severe problems discontinuing a benzodiazepine, dosing may need to be tapered over many months (i.e., reduce dose by 1% every 3 days by crushing tablet and suspending or dissolving in 100 mL of fruit juice and then disposing of 1 mL while drinking the rest; 3–7 days later, dispose of 2 mL, and so on). This is both a form of very slow biological tapering and a form of behavioral desensitization
- Be sure to differentiate reemergence of symptoms requiring reinstitution of treatment from withdrawal symptoms
- Benzodiazepine-dependent anxiety patients and insulin-dependent diabetics are not addicted to their medications. When benzodiazepine-dependent patients stop their medication, disease symptoms can reemerge, disease symptoms can worsen (rebound), and/or withdrawal symptoms can emerge

Pharmacokinetics

- Long half-life compared to other benzodiazepine anxiolytics (elimination half-life approximately 30–40 hours)

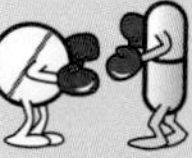

Drug Interactions

- Increased depressive effects when taken with other CNS depressants
- Inhibitors of CYP450 3A4 may affect the clearance of clonazepam, but dosage adjustment usually not necessary
- Flumazenil (used to reverse the effects of benzodiazepines) may precipitate seizures and should not be used in patients treated for seizure disorders with clonazepam
- Use of clonazepam with valproate may cause absence status

Other Warnings/ Precautions

- Dosage changes should be made in collaboration with prescriber
- Use with caution in patients with pulmonary disease; rare reports of death after initiation of benzodiazepines in patients with severe pulmonary impairment
- History of drug or alcohol abuse often creates greater risk for dependency

- Clonazepam may induce grand mal seizures in patients with multiple seizure disorders
- Use only with extreme caution if patient has obstructive sleep apnea
- Some depressed patients may experience a worsening of suicidal ideation
- Some patients may exhibit abnormal thinking or behavioral changes similar to those caused by other CNS depressants (i.e., either depressant actions or disinhibiting actions)

Do Not Use
- If patient has narrow angle-closure glaucoma
- If patient has severe liver disease
- If there is a proven allergy to clonazepam or any benzodiazepine

SPECIAL POPULATIONS

Renal Impairment
- Dose should be reduced

Hepatic Impairment
- Dose should be reduced

Cardiac Impairment
- Benzodiazepines have been used to treat anxiety associated with acute myocardial infarction

Elderly
- Should receive lower doses and be monitored

Children and Adolescents
- Seizures – up to 10 years or 30 kg – 0.01–0.03 mg/kg per day divided into 2–3 doses; maximum dose 0.05 mg/kg per day
- Safety and efficacy not established in panic disorder
- For anxiety, children and adolescents should generally receive lower doses and be more closely monitored
- Long-term effects of clonazepam in children/adolescents are unknown

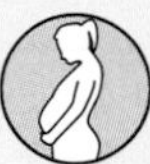

Pregnancy
- Risk Category D [positive evidence of risk to human fetus; potential benefits may still justify its use during pregnancy, especially for seizure disorders]
- Possible increased risk of birth defects when benzodiazepines taken during pregnancy
- Because of the potential risks, clonazepam is not generally recommended as treatment for anxiety during pregnancy, especially during the first trimester
- Drug should be tapered if discontinued
- Infants whose mothers received a benzodiazepine late in pregnancy may experience withdrawal effects
- Neonatal flaccidity has been reported in infants whose mothers took a benzodiazepine during pregnancy
- Seizures, even mild seizures, may cause harm to the embryo/fetus

Breast Feeding
- Some drug is found in mother's breast milk
- ✻ Recommended either to discontinue drug or bottle feed
- Effects on infant have been observed and include feeding difficulties, sedation, and weight loss

THE ART OF PSYCHOPHARMACOLOGY

Potential Advantages
- Rapid onset of action
- Less sedation than some other benzodiazepines
- Longer duration of action than some other benzodiazepines
- Availability of oral disintegrating wafer

Potential Disadvantages
- Development of tolerance may require dose increases, especially in seizure disorders
- Abuse especially risky in past or present substance abusers

Primary Target Symptoms
- Frequency and duration of seizures
- Spike and wave discharges in absence seizures (petit mal)
- Panic attacks
- Anxiety

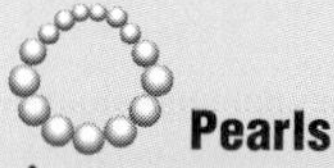

Pearls

- ✻ One of the most popular benzodiazepines for anxiety, especially among psychiatrists
- Is a very useful adjunct to SSRIs and SNRIs in the treatment of numerous anxiety disorders
- Not effective for treating psychosis as a monotherapy, but can be used as an adjunct to antipsychotics
- Not effective for treating bipolar disorder as a monotherapy, but can be used as an adjunct to mood stabilizers and antipsychotics
- Generally used as second-line treatment for petit mal seizures if succinimides are ineffective
- Can be used as an adjunct or as monotherapy for seizure disorders
- Clonazepam is the only benzodiazepine that is used as a solo maintenance treatment for seizure disorders
- ✻ Easier to taper than some other benzodiazepines because of long half-life
- ✻ May have less abuse potential than some other benzodiazepines
- ✻ May cause less depression, euphoria, or dependence than some other benzodiazepines
- ✻ Clonazepan is often considered a "longer-acting alprazolam-like anxiolytic" with improved tolerability features in terms of less euphoria, abuse, dependence, and withdrawal problems, but this has not been proven
- When using to treat insomnia, remember that insomnia may be a symptom of some other primary disorder itself, and thus warrant evaluation for comorbid psychiatric and/or medical conditions

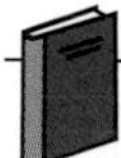

Suggested Reading

Davidson JR, Moroz G. Pivotal studies of clonazepam in panic disorder. Psychopharmacol Bull 1998;34:169–74.

DeVane CL, Ware MR, Lydiard RB. Pharmacokinetics, pharmacodynamics, and treatment issues of benzodiazepines: alprazolam, adinazolam, and clonazepam. Psychopharmacol Bull 1991;27:463–73.

Iqbal MM, Sobhan T, Ryals T. Effects of commonly used benzodiazepines on the fetus, the neonate, and the nursing infant. Psychiatr Serv 2002;53:39–49.

Panayiotopoulos CP. Treatment of typical absence seizures and related epileptic syndromes. Paediatr Drugs 2001;3:379–403.

THERAPEUTICS

Brands
- Duraclon (injection)
- Catapres
- Catapres-TTS (Clonidine Transdermal Therapeutic System)
- Clorpres

see index for additional brand names

Generic? Yes (not for transdermal)

Class
- Antihypertensive; centrally acting alpha 2 agonist hypotensive agent

Commonly Prescribed for
(bold for FDA approved)
- **Hypertension**
- Attention deficit hyperactivity disorder (ADHD)
- Tourette's syndrome
- Substance withdrawal, including opiates and alcohol
- Anxiety disorders, including Posttraumatic stress disorder (PTSD) and social anxiety disorder
- Clozapine-induced hypersalivation
- Menopausal flushing
- Severe pain in cancer patients that is not adequately relieved by opioid analgesics alone (combination with opiates)

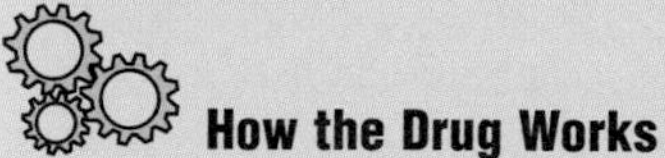

How the Drug Works
- For hypertension, stimulates alpha 2 adrenergic receptors in the brain stem, reducing sympathetic outflow from the CNS and decreasing peripheral resistance, renal vascular resistance, heart rate, and blood pressure
- An imidazoline, so also interacts at imidazoline receptors
- ✻ For CNS uses, presumably has central actions on either pre- or postsynaptic alpha 2 receptors, and/or actions at imidazoline receptors may cause behavioral changes in numerous conditions (unknown and speculative)

How Long Until It Works
- Blood pressure may be lowered 30–60 minutes after first dose; greatest reduction seen after 2–4 hours
- May take several weeks to control blood pressure adequately
- For CNS uses, can take a few weeks to see therapeutic benefits

If It Works
- For hypertension, continue treatment indefinitely and check blood pressure regularly
- For CNS uses, continue to monitor continuing benefits as well as blood pressure

If It Doesn't Work (for CNS indications)
- ✻ Since clonidine is a second-line and experimental treatment for CNS disorders, many patients may not respond
- Consider adjusting dose or switching to another agent with better evidence for CNS efficacy

Best Augmenting Combos for Partial Response or Treatment-Resistance
- Best to attempt another monotherapy prior to augmenting for CNS uses
- Chlorthalidone, thiazide-type diuretics, and furosemide for hypertension
- Possibly combination with stimulants (with caution as benefits of combination poorly documented and there are some reports of serious adverse events)
- Combinations for CNS uses should be for the expert, while monitoring the patient closely, and when other treatment options have failed

Tests
- Blood pressure should be checked regularly during treatment

SIDE EFFECTS

How Drug Causes Side Effects
- Excessive actions on alpha 2 receptors and/or on imidazoline receptors

Notable Side Effects
- ✻ Dry mouth
- ✻ Dizziness, constipation, sedation
- Weakness, fatigue, impotence, loss of libido, insomnia, headache
- Major depression
- Dermatologic reactions (especially with transdermal clonidine)

- Hypotension, occasional syncope
- Tachycardia
- Nervousness, agitation
- Nausea, vomiting

Life-Threatening or Dangerous Side Effects

- Sinus bradycardia, atrioventricular block
- During withdrawal, hypertensive encephalopathy, cerebrovascular accidents, and death (rare)

Weight Gain

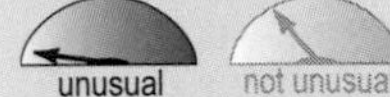

- Reported but not expected

Sedation

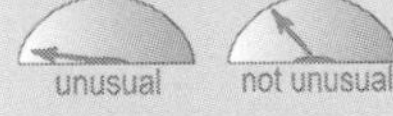

- Many experience and/or can be significant in amount
- Some patients may not tolerate it
- Can abate with time

What to Do About Side Effects

- Wait
- Take larger dose at bedtime to avoid daytime sedation
- Switch to another medication with better evidence of efficacy

✻ For withdrawal and discontinuation reactions, may need to reinstate clonidine and taper very slowly when stabilized

Best Augmenting Agents for Side Effects

- Dose reduction or switching to another agent may be more effective since most side effects cannot be improved with an augmenting agent

DOSING AND USE

Usual Dosage Range

- 0.2–0.6 mg/day in divided doses

Dosage Forms

- Tablet 0.1 mg scored, 0.2 mg scored, 0.3 mg scored
- Topical (7 day administration) 0.1 mg/24 hours, 0.2 mg/24 hours, 0.3 mg/24 hours
- Injection 100 mg/mL, 500 mg/mL

How to Dose

- Oral: initial 0.1 mg in 2 divided doses, morning and night; can increase by 0.1 mg/day each week; maximum dose generally 2.4 mg/day
- Topical: apply once every 7 days in hairless area; change location with each application
- Injection: initial 30 mcg/hr; maximum 40 mcg/hr; 500 mg/mL must be diluted

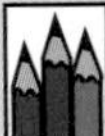

Dosing Tips

- Adverse effects are dose-related and usually transient
- The last dose of the day should occur at bedtime so that blood pressure is controlled overnight
- If clonidine is terminated abruptly, rebound hypertension may occur within 2–4 days
- Using clonidine in combination with another antihypertensive agent may attenuate the development of tolerance to clonidine's antihypertensive effects
- The likelihood of severe discontinuation reactions with CNS and cardiovascular symptoms may be greater after administration of high doses of clonidine

✻ In patients who have developed localized contact sensitization to transdermal clonidine, continuing transdermal dosing on other skin areas or substituting with oral clonidine may be associated with the development of a generalized skin rash, urticaria, or angioedema

✻ If administered with a beta blocker, stop the beta blocker first for several days before the gradual discontinuation of clonidine in cases of planned discontinuation

Overdose

- Hypotension, hypertension, miosis, respiratory depression, seizures, bradycardia, hypothermia, coma, sedation, decreased reflexes, weakness, irritability, dysrhythmia

Long-Term Use

- Patients may develop tolerance to the antihypertensive effects

✻ Studies have not established the utility of clonidine for long-term CNS uses

✽ Be aware that forgetting to take clonidine or running out of medication can lead to abrupt discontinuation and associated withdrawal reactions and complications

Habit Forming

- Reports of some abuse by opiate addicts
- Reports of some abuse by non-opioid-dependent patients

How to Stop

✽ Discontinuation reactions are common and sometimes severe

- Sudden discontinuation can result in nervousness, agitation, headache, and tremor, with rapid rise in blood pressure
- Rare instances of hypertensive encephalopathy, cerebrovascular accident, and death have been reported after clonidine withdrawal
- Taper over 2–4 days or longer to avoid rebound effects (nervousness, increased blood pressure)
- If administered with a beta blocker, stop the beta blocker first for several days before the gradual discontinuation of clonidine

Pharmacokinetics

- Half-life 12–16 hours
- Metabolized by the liver
- Excreted renally

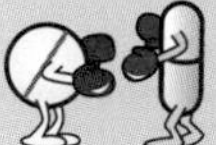

Drug Interactions

- The likelihood of severe discontinuation reactions with CNS and cardiovascular symptoms may be greater when clonidine is combined with beta blocker treatment
- Increased depressive and sedative effects when taken with other CNS depressants
- Tricyclic antidepressants may reduce the hypotensive effects of clonidine
- Corneal lesions in rats increased by use of clonidine with amitriptyline
- Use of clonidine with agents that affect sinus node function or AV nodal function (e.g., digitalis, calcium channel blockers, beta blockers) may result in bradycardia or AV block

Other Warnings/ Precautions

- There have been cases of hypertensive encephalopathy, cerebrovascular accidents, and death after abrupt discontinuation
- If used with a beta blocker, the beta blocker should be stopped several days before tapering clonidine
- In patients who have developed localized contact sensitization to transdermal clonidine, continuing transdermal dosing on other skin areas or substituting with oral clonidine may be associated with the development of a generalized skin rash, urticaria, or angioedema
- Injection is not recommended for use in managing obstetrical, postpartum or peri-operative pain

Do Not Use

- If there is a proven allergy to clonidine

SPECIAL POPULATIONS

Renal Impairment

- Use with caution and possibly reduce dose

Hepatic Impairment

- Use with caution

Cardiac Impairment

- Use with caution in patients with recent myocardial infarction, severe coronary insufficiency, cerebrovascular disease

Elderly

- Elderly patients may tolerate a lower initial dose better
- Elderly patients may be more sensitive to sedative effects

Children and Adolescents

- Safety and efficacy not established for children under age 12
- Children may be more sensitive to hypertensive effects of withdrawing treatment

✽ Because children commonly have gastrointestinal illnesses that lead to vomiting, they may be more likely to abruptly discontinue clonidine and therefore be more susceptible to

hypertensive episodes resulting from abrupt inability to take medication
- Children may be more likely to experience CNS depression with overdose and may even exhibit signs of toxicity with 0.1 mg of clonidine
- ADHD: initial 0.05 mg at bedtime; titrate over 2–4 weeks; usual dose 0.05–4 mg/day
- Injection may be used in pediatric cancer patients with severe pain unresponsive to other medications

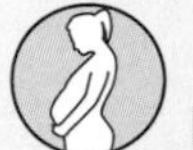

Pregnancy
- Risk Category C [some animal studies show adverse effects; no controlled studies in humans]
- Use in women of childbearing potential requires weighing potential benefits to the mother against potential risks to the fetus
- ✻ For ADHD patients, clonidine should generally be discontinued before anticipated pregnancies

Breast Feeding
- Some drug is found in mother's breast milk
- No adverse effects have been reported in nursing infants
- If irritability or sedation develop in nursing infant, may need to discontinue drug or bottle feed

THE ART OF PSYCHOPHARMACOLOGY

Potential Advantages
- For numerous CNS indications when conventional treatments have failed (investigational)

Potential Disadvantages
- Poor documentation of efficacy for most off-label uses
- Withdrawal reactions
- Noncompliant patients
- Patients on concomitant CNS medications

Primary Target Symptoms
- High blood pressure
- Miscellaneous CNS, behavioral, and psychiatric symptoms

Pearls
- ✻ Although not approved for ADHD, clonidine has been shown to be effective treatment for this disorder in several published studies
- ✻ As monotherapy for ADHD, may be inferior to other options, including stimulants and desipramine
- As monotherapy or in combination with methylphenidate for ADHD with conduct disorder or oppositional defiant disorder, may improve aggression, oppositional, and conduct disorder symptoms
- Clonidine is sometimes used in combination with stimulants to reduce side effects and enhance therapeutic effects on motor hyperactivity
- Doses of 0.1 mg in 3 divided doses have been reported to reduce stimulant-induced insomnia as well as impulsivity
- Considered a third-line treatment option now for ADHD
- ✻ Clonidine may also be effective for treatment of tic disorders, including Tourette's syndrome
- May suppress tics, especially in severe Tourette's syndrome, and may be even better at reducing explosive violent behaviors in Tourette's syndrome
- Sedation is often unacceptable in various patients despite improvement in CNS symptoms and leads to discontinuation of treatment, especially for ADHD and Tourette's syndrome
- Considered an investigational treatment for most other CNS applications
- May block the autonomic symptoms in anxiety and panic disorders (e.g., palpitations, sweating) and improve subjective anxiety as well
- May be useful in decreasing the autonomic arousal of PTSD
- May be useful as an as needed medication for stage fright or other predictable socially phobic situations
- May also be useful when added to SSRIs for reducing arousal and dissociative symptoms in PTSD
- May block autonomic symptoms of opioid withdrawal (e.g., palpitations, sweating) especially in inpatients, but muscle aches, irritability, and insomnia may not be well suppressed by clonidine

- May be useful in decreasing the hypertension, tachycardia, and tremulousness associated with alcohol withdrawal, but not the seizures or delirium tremens in complicated alcohol withdrawal
- Clonidine may improve social relationships, affectual responses, and sensory responses in autistic disorder
- Clonidine may reduce the incidence of menopausal flushing
- Growth hormone response to clonidine may be reduced during menses
- Clonidine stimulates growth hormone secretion (no chronic effects have been observed)
- Alcohol may reduce the effects of clonidine on growth hormone

✻ Guanfacine is a related centrally active alpha 2 agonist hypotensive agent that has been used for similar CNS applications but has not been as widely investigated or used as clonidine

✻ Guanfacine may be tolerated better than clonidine in some patients (e.g., sedation) or it may work better in some patients for CNS applications than clonidine, but no head-to-head trials

Suggested Reading

Burris JF. The USA experience with the clonidine transdermal therapeutic system. Clin Auton Res 1993;3:391–96.

Gavras I, Manolis AJ, Gayras H. The alpha2-adrenergic receptors in hypertension and heart failure: experimental and clinical studies. J Hypertens 2001;19:2115–24.

Guay DR. Adjunctive agents in the management of chronic pain. Pharmacotherapy 2001;21:1070–81.

Silver LB. Alternative (nonstimulant) medications in the treatment of attention-deficit/hyperactivity disorder in children. Pediatr Clin North Am 1999;46: 965–75.

THERAPEUTICS

Brands
- Azene
- Tranxene

see index for additional brand names

Generic? Yes

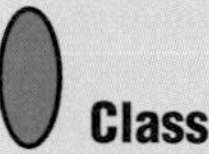

Class
- Benzodiazepine (anxiolytic)

Commonly Prescribed for
(bold for FDA approved)
- **Anxiety disorder**
- **Symptoms of anxiety**
- **Acute alcohol withdrawal**
- Partial seizures (adjunct)

How the Drug Works
- Binds to benzodiazepine receptors at the GABA-A ligand-gated chloride channel complex
- Enhances the inhibitory effects of GABA
- Boosts chloride conductance through GABA-regulated channels
- Inhibits neuronal activity presumably in amygdala-centered fear circuits to provide therapeutic benefits in anxiety disorders

How Long Until It Works
- Some immediate relief with first dosing is common; can take several weeks with daily dosing for maximal therapeutic benefit

If It Works
- For short-term symptoms of anxiety – after a few weeks, discontinue use or use on an "as-needed" basis
- For chronic anxiety disorders, the goal of treatment is complete remission of symptoms as well as prevention of future relapses
- For chronic anxiety disorders, treatment most often reduces or even eliminates symptoms, but not a cure since symptoms can recur after medicine stopped
- For long-term symptoms of anxiety, consider switching to an SSRI or SNRI for long-term maintenance
- If long-term maintenance with a benzodiazepine is necessary, continue treatment for 6 months after symptoms resolve, and then taper dose slowly
- If symptoms reemerge, consider treatment with an SSRI or SNRI, or consider restarting the benzodiazepine; sometimes benzodiazepines have to be used in combination with SSRIs or SNRIs for best results

If It Doesn't Work
- Consider switching to another agent or adding an appropriate augmenting agent
- Consider psychotherapy, especially cognitive behavioral psychotherapy
- Consider presence of concomitant substance abuse
- Consider presence of clorazepate abuse
- Consider another diagnosis, such as a comorbid medical condition

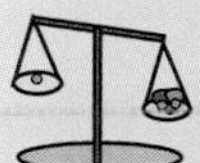

Best Augmenting Combos for Partial Response or Treatment-Resistance
- Benzodiazepines are frequently used as augmenting agents for antipsychotics and mood stabilizers in the treatment of psychotic and bipolar disorders
- Benzodiazepines are frequently used as augmenting agents for SSRIs and SNRIs in the treatment of anxiety disorders
- Not generally rational to combine with other benzodiazepines
- Caution if using as an anxiolytic concomitantly with other sedative hypnotics for sleep

Tests
- In patients with seizure disorders, concomitant medical illness, and/or those with multiple concomitant long-term medications, periodic liver tests and blood counts may be prudent

SIDE EFFECTS

How Drug Causes Side Effects
- Same mechanism for side effects as for therapeutic effects – namely due to excessive actions at benzodiazepine receptors
- Long-term adaptations in benzodiazepine receptors may explain the development of dependence, tolerance, and withdrawal
- Side effects are generally immediate, but immediate side effects often disappear in time

Notable Side Effects

- ✻ Sedation, fatigue, depression
- ✻ Dizziness, ataxia, slurred speech, weakness
- ✻ Forgetfulness, confusion
- ✻ Hyperexcitability, nervousness
- Rare hallucinations, mania
- Rare hypotension
- Hypersalivation, dry mouth

Life-Threatening or Dangerous Side Effects

- Respiratory depression, especially when taken with CNS depressants in overdose
- Rare hepatic dysfunction, renal dysfunction, blood dyscrasias

Weight Gain

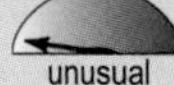

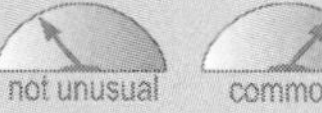

common problematic

- Reported but not expected

Sedation

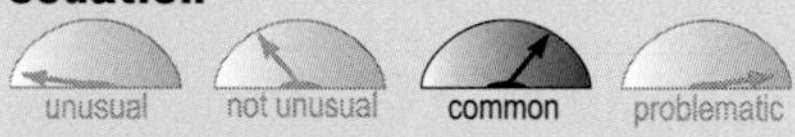

- Many experience and/or can be significant in amount
- Especially at initiation of treatment or when dose increases
- Tolerance often develops over time

What to Do About Side Effects

- Wait
- Wait
- Wait
- Lower the dose
- Take largest dose at bedtime to avoid sedative effects during the day
- Switch to another agent
- Administer flumazenil if side effects are severe or life-threatening

Best Augmenting Agents for Side Effects

- Many side effects cannot be improved with an augmenting agent

DOSING AND USE

Usual Dosage Range

- Anxiety: 15–60 mg/day in divided doses
- Alcohol withdrawal: 30–60 mg/day in divided doses

Dosage Forms

- Tablet 3.75 mg scored, 7.5 mg scored, 15 mg scored, 22.5 mg single dose, 11.25 mg single dose half strength

How to Dose

- Anxiety: Initial 15 mg/day in divided doses; adjust dose as needed on subsequent days; single-dose tablet may be given once daily at bedtime after patient is stable; maximum generally 90 mg/day
- Alcohol withdrawal: Initial 30 mg, then 30–60 mg in divided doses; second day 45–90 mg in divided doses; third day 22.5–45 mg in divided doses; fourth day 15–30 mg in divided doses; after fourth day decrease dose gradually and discontinue when patient is stable; maximum generally 90 mg/day
- Epilepsy: Initial 7.5 mg 3 times/day; increase by 7.5 mg weekly; maximum generally 90 mg/day

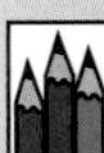

Dosing Tips

- Use lowest possible effective dose for the shortest possible period of time (a benzodiazepine-sparing strategy)
- Assess need for continued treatment regularly
- Risk of dependence may increase with dose and duration of treatment
- For interdose symptoms of anxiety, can either increase dose or maintain same total daily dose but divide into more frequent doses
- Can also use an as-needed occasional “top up” dose for interdose anxiety
- Because anxiety disorders can require higher doses, the risk of dependence may be greater in these patients
- Frequency of dosing in practice is often greater than predicted from half-life, as duration of biological activity is often shorter than pharmacokinetic terminal half-life

Overdose

- Fatalities can occur; hypotension, tiredness, ataxia, confusion, coma

Long-Term Use

- Evidence of efficacy for up to 16 weeks
- Risk of dependence, particularly for periods longer than 12 weeks and especially in patients with past or current polysubstance abuse

Habit Forming

- Clorazepate is a Schedule IV drug
- Patients may develop dependence and/or tolerance with long-term use

How to Stop

- Patients with history of seizure may seize upon withdrawal, especially if withdrawal is abrupt
- Taper by 7.5 mg every 3 days to reduce chances of withdrawal effects
- For difficult to taper cases, consider reducing dose much more slowly after reaching 30 mg/day, perhaps by as little as 3.75 mg per week or less
- For other patients with severe problems discontinuing a benzodiazepine, dosing may need to be tapered over many months (i.e., reduce dose by 1% every 3 days by crushing tablet and suspending or dissolving in 100 mL of fruit juice and then disposing of 1 mL while drinking the rest; 3–7 days later, dispose of 2 mL, and so on). This is both a form of very slow biological tapering and a form of behavioral desensitization
- Be sure to differentiate reemergence of symptoms requiring reinstitution of treatment from withdrawal symptoms
- Benzodiazepine-dependent anxiety patients and insulin-dependent diabetics are not addicted to their medications. When benzodiazepine-dependent patients stop their medication, disease symptoms can reemerge, disease symptoms can worsen (rebound), and/or withdrawal symptoms can emerge

Pharmacokinetics

- Elimination half-life 40–50 hours

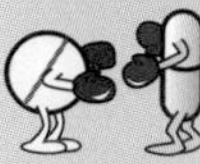

Drug Interactions

- Increased depressive effects when taken with other CNS depressants

Other Warnings/ Precautions

- Dosage changes should be made in collaboration with prescriber
- Use with caution in patients with pulmonary disease; rare reports of death after initiation of benzodiazepines in patients with severe pulmonary impairment
- History of drug or alcohol abuse often creates greater risk for dependency
- Some depressed patients may experience a worsening of suicidal ideation
- Some patients may exhibit abnormal thinking or behavioral changes similar to those caused by other CNS depressants (i.e., either depressant actions or disinhibiting actions)

Do Not Use

- If patient has narrow angle-closure glaucoma
- If there is a proven allergy to clorazepate or any benzodiazepine

SPECIAL POPULATIONS

Renal Impairment

- Initial 7.5–15 mg/day in divided doses or in 1 dose at bedtime

Hepatic Impairment

- Initial 7.5–15 mg/day in divided doses or in 1 dose at bedtime

Cardiac Impairment

- Benzodiazepines have been used to treat anxiety associated with acute myocardial infarction

Elderly

- Initial 7.5–15 mg/day in divided doses or in 1 dose at bedtime

Children and Adolescents

- Not recommended for use in children under age 9
- Recommended initial dose: 7.5 mg twice a day

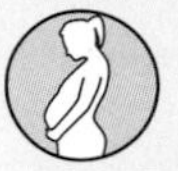

Pregnancy

- Risk Category D [positive evidence of risk to human fetus; potential benefits may still justify its use during pregnancy]
- Possible increased risk of birth defects when benzodiazepines taken during pregnancy
- Because of the potential risks, clorazepate is not generally recommended as treatment for anxiety during pregnancy, especially during the first trimester
- Drug should be tapered if discontinued
- Infants whose mothers received a benzodiazepine late in pregnancy may experience withdrawal effects
- Neonatal flaccidity has been reported in infants whose mothers took a benzodiazepine during pregnancy
- Seizures, even mild seizures, may cause harm to the embryo/fetus

Breast Feeding

- Some drug is found in mother's breast milk

✱ Recommended either to discontinue drug or bottle feed

- Effects of benzodiazepines on nursing infants have been reported and include feeding difficulties, sedation, and weight loss

THE ART OF PSYCHOPHARMACOLOGY

Potential Advantages

- Rapid onset of action

Potential Disadvantages

- Euphoria may lead to abuse
- Abuse especially risky in past or present substance abusers

Primary Target Symptoms

- Panic attacks
- Anxiety
- Incidence of seizures (adjunct)

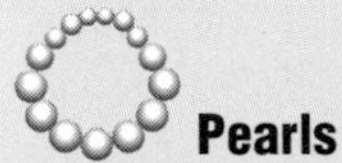

Pearls

- Can be very useful as an adjunct to SSRIs and SNRIs in the treatment of numerous anxiety disorders
- Not effective for treating psychosis as a monotherapy, but can be used as an adjunct to antipsychotics
- Not effective for treating bipolar disorder as a monotherapy, but can be used as an adjunct to mood stabilizers and antipsychotics

✱ More commonly used than some other benzodiazepines for treating alcohol withdrawal

- May both cause depression and treat depression in different patients
- When using to treat insomnia, remember that insomnia may be a symptom of some other primary disorder itself, and thus warrant evaluation for comorbid psychiatric and/or medical conditions

Suggested Reading

Griffith JL, Murray GB. Clorazepate in the treatment of complex partial seizures with psychic symptomatology. J Nerv Ment Dis 1985;173:185–86.

Kiejna A, Kantorska-Janiec M, Malyszczak K. [The use of chlorazepate dipotassium (Tranxene) in the states of restlessness and agitation]. Psychiatr Pol 1997;31:753–60.

Mielke L, Breinbauer B, Schubert M, Kling M, Entolzner E, Hargasser S, Hipp R. [Comparison of the effectiveness of orally administered clorazepate dipotassium and nordiazepam on preoperative anxiety]. Anaesthesiol Reanim 1995;20:144–8.

Rickels K, Schweizer E, Csanalosi I, Case WG, Chung H. Long-term treatment of anxiety and risk of withdrawal. Prospective comparison of clorazepate and buspirone. Arch Gen Psychiatry 1988;45:444–50.

THERAPEUTICS

Brands
- Clozaril
- Leponex

see index for additional brand names

Generic? Yes

Class

- Atypical antipsychotic (serotonin-dopamine antagonist; second generation antipsychotic; also a mood stabilizer)

Commonly Prescribed for

(bold for FDA approved)

- **Treatment-resistant schizophrenia**
- **Reduction in risk of recurrent suicidal behavior in patients with schizophrenia or schizoaffective disorder**
- Treatment-resistant bipolar disorder
- Violent aggressive patients with psychosis and other brain disorders not responsive to other treatments

How the Drug Works

- Blocks dopamine 2 receptors, reducing positive symptoms of psychosis and stabilizing affective symptoms
- Blocks serotonin 2A receptors, causing enhancement of dopamine release in certain brain regions and thus reducing motor side effects and possibly improving cognitive and affective symptoms
- Interactions at a myriad of other neurotransmitter receptors may contribute to clozapine's efficacy

✻ Specifically, interactions at 5HT2C and 5HT1A receptors may contribute to efficacy for cognitive and affective symptoms in some patients

- Mechanism of efficacy for psychotic patients who do not respond to conventional antipsychotics is unknown

How Long Until It Works

- Psychotic and manic symptoms can improve within 1 week, especially with first-line use, but often takes several weeks for full effect on behavior as well as on cognition and affective stabilization, especially in treatment-resistant cases
- Classically recommended to wait at least 4–6 weeks to determine efficacy of drug, but in practice patients often require up to 16–20 weeks to show a good response, especially in treatment-resistant cases

If It Works

- As for other antipsychotics, most often reduces positive symptoms in schizophrenia but does not eliminate them

✻ However, clozapine may reduce positive symptoms in patients who do not respond to other antipsychotics, especially other conventional antipsychotics

- Can improve negative symptoms, as well as aggressive, cognitive, and affective symptoms in schizophrenia
- Most schizophrenic patients do not have a total remission of symptoms but rather a reduction of symptoms by about a third
- Many patients with bipolar disorder and other disorders with psychotic, aggressive, violent, impulsive, and other types of behavioral disturbances may respond to clozapine when other agents have failed
- Perhaps 5–15% of schizophrenic patients can experience an overall improvement of greater than 50–60%, especially when receiving stable treatment for more than a year

✻ Such patients are considered super-responders or "awakeners" since they may be well enough to be employed, live independently, and sustain long-term relationships; super-responders are anecdotally reported more often with clozapine than with some other antipsychotics

- Continue treatment until reaching a plateau of improvement
- After reaching a satisfactory plateau, continue treatment for at least a year after first episode of psychosis
- For second and subsequent episodes of psychosis, treatment may need to be indefinite
- Even for first episodes of psychosis, it may be preferable to continue treatment indefinitely to avoid subsequent episodes
- Treatment may not only reduce mania but also prevent recurrences of mania in bipolar disorder

If It Doesn't Work

- Some patients may respond better if switched to a conventional antipsychotic

* Some patients may require augmentation with a conventional antipsychotic or with an atypical antipsychotic (especially risperidone or amisulpride), but these are the most refractory of all psychotic patients and such treatment is very expensive
* Consider augmentation with valproate or lamotrigine
- Consider noncompliance and switch to another antipsychotic with fewer side effects or to an antipsychotic that can be given by depot injection
- Consider initiating rehabilitation and psychotherapy
- Consider presence of concomitant drug abuse

Best Augmenting Combos for Partial Response or Treatment-Resistance

- Valproic acid (valproate, divalproex, divalproex ER)
- Lamotrigine
- Other mood stabilizing anticonvulsants (carbamazepine, oxcarbazepine)
- Conventional antipsychotics
- Benzodiazepines
- Lithium

Tests

* Complete blood count before treatment, weekly for 6 months of treatment, biweekly for months 6–12, and every 4 weeks thereafter
- Weekly monitoring of white blood cell count and absolute neurotrophil count for a period of 12 months is required in patients who are rechallenged with clozapine after recovery from an initial episode of moderate leukopenia (white blood cell count between 2,000/mm^3 and 3,000/mm^3, absolute neutrophil count between 1,000/mm^3 and 1,500/mm^3)

Before starting an atypical antipsychotic

* Weigh all patients and track BMI during treatment
- Get baseline personal and family history of diabetes, obesity, dyslipidemia, hypertension, and cardiovascular disease
* Get waist circumference (at umbilicus), blood pressure, fasting plasma glucose, and fasting lipid profile
- Determine if the patient is
  - overweight (BMI 25.0–29.9)
  - obese (BMI ≥30)
  - has pre-diabetes (fasting plasma glucose 100–25 mg/dL)
  - has diabetes (fasting plasma glucose >126 mg/dL)
  - has hypertension (BP >140/90 mm Hg)
  - has dyslipidemia (increased total cholesterol, LDL cholesterol, and triglycerides; decreased HDL cholesterol)
- Treat or refer such patients for treatment, including nutrition and weight management, physical activity counseling, smoking cessation, and medical management

Monitoring after starting an atypical antipsychotic

* BMI monthly for 3 months, then quarterly
* Consider monitoring fasting triglycerides monthly for several months in patients at high risk for metabolic complications and when initiating or switching antipsychotics
* Blood pressure, fasting plasma glucose, fasting lipids within 3 months and then annually, but earlier and more frequently for patients with diabetes or who have gained >5% of initial weight
- Treat or refer for treatment and consider switching to another atypical antipsychotic for patients who become overweight, obese, pre-diabetic, diabetic, hypertensive, or dyslipidemic while receiving an atypical antipsychotic
* Even in patients without known diabetes, be vigilant for the rare but life-threatening onset of diabetic ketoacidosis, which always requires immediate treatment, by monitoring for the rapid onset of polyuria, polydipsia, weight loss, nausea, vomiting, dehydration, rapid respiration, weakness and clouding of sensorium, even coma
- Liver function testing, electrocardiogram, general physical exam, and assessment of baseline cardiac status before starting treatment
- Liver tests may be necessary during treatment in patients who develop nausea, vomiting, or anorexia
* Electrocardiograms and cardiac evaluation to rule out myocarditis may be necessary during treatment in patients who develop shortness of breath or chest pain

SIDE EFFECTS

How Drug Causes Side Effects

- By blocking histamine 1 receptors in the brain, it can cause sedation and possibly weight gain
- By blocking alpha 1 adrenergic receptors, it can cause dizziness, sedation, and hypotension
- By blocking muscarinic 1 receptors, it can cause dry mouth, constipation, and sedation
- By blocking dopamine 2 receptors in the striatum, it can cause motor side effects (very rare)
- Mechanism of weight gain and increased incidence of diabetes and dyslipidemia with atypical antipsychotics is unknown but insulin regulation may be impaired by blocking pancreatic M3 muscarinic receptors

Notable Side Effects

✻ Probably increases risk for diabetes and dyslipidemia
✻ Increased salivation (can be severe)
✻ Sweating

- Dizziness, sedation, headache, tachycardia, hypotension
- Nausea, constipation, dry mouth, weight gain
- Rare tardive dyskinesia (no reports have directly implicated clozapine in the development of tardive dyskinesia)

Life-Threatening or Dangerous Side Effects

- Hyperglycemia, in some cases extreme and associated with ketoacidosis or hyperosmolar coma or death, has been reported in patients taking atypical antipsychotics
- Agranulocytosis (includes flu-like symptoms or signs of infection)
- Seizures (risk increases with dose)
- Neuroleptic malignant syndrome (more likely when clozapine is used with another agent)
- Pulmonary embolism (may include deep vein thrombosis or respiratory symptoms)
- Myocarditis
- Increased risk of death and cerebrovascular events in elderly patients with dementia-related psychosis

Weight Gain

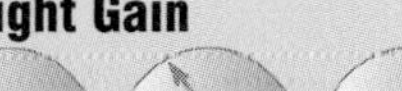

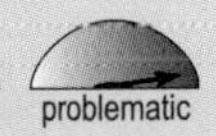

- Frequent and can be significant in amount
- Can become a health problem in some
- More than for some other antipsychotics, but never say always as not a problem in everyone

Sedation

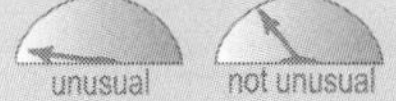

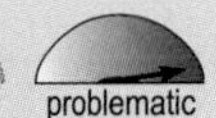

- Frequent and can be significant in amount
- Some patients may not tolerate it
- More than for some other antipsychotics, but never say always as not a problem in everyone
- Can wear off over time
- Can reemerge as dose increases and then wear off again over time

What to Do About Side Effects

- Patients must inform prescriber immediately of any flu-like symptoms, muscle rigidity, altered mental status, irregular pulse or blood pressure
- Take at bedtime to help reduce daytime sedation
- Sedation may wear off with time
- Start dosing low and increase slowly as side effects wear off at each dosing increment
- Weight loss, exercise programs, and medical management for high BMIs, diabetes, dyslipidemia
- Switch to another agent

Best Augmenting Agents for Side Effects

- Many side effects cannot be improved with an augmenting agent

DOSING AND USE

Usual Dosage Range

- 300–450 mg/day

Dosage Forms

- Tablet 12.5 mg, 25 mg scored, 50 mg, 100 mg scored
- Orally disintegrating tablet 12.5 mg, 25 mg, 50 mg, 100 mg

How to Dose

- Initial 25 mg in 2 divided doses; increase by 25–50 mg/day each day until desired efficacy is reached; maintenance dose 300–450 mg/day; doses above 300 mg/day should be divided; increases in doses above 450 mg/day should be made weekly; maximum dose generally 900 mg/day

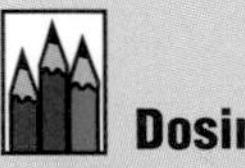

Dosing Tips

- Prescriptions are generally given 1 week at a time for the first 6 months of treatment because of the risk of agranulocytosis; for months 6–12 prescriptions can generally be given 2 weeks at a time; after 12 months prescriptions can generally be given monthly

✻ Treatment should be suspended if absolute neutrophil count falls below 1,000/mm^3

- Treatment should be suspended if white blood cell count falls below 2,000/mm^3
- Treatment should be suspended if eosinophil count rises above 4,000/mm^3, and continued once it falls below 3,000/mm^3
- If treatment is discontinued for more than 2 days, it may need to be reinitiated at a lower dose and slowly increased in order to maximize tolerability
- Plasma half-life suggests twice daily administration, but in practice it may be given once a day at night
- Doses over 550 mg/day may require concomitant anticonvulsant administration to reduce the chances of a seizure

✻ Rebound psychosis may occur unless dose is very slowly tapered, by 100 mg/week or less

Overdose

- Sometimes lethal; changes in heart rhythm, excess salivation, respiratory depression, altered state of consciousness

Long-Term Use

- Treatment to reduce risk of suicidal behavior should be continued for at least 2 years
- Often used for long-term maintenance in treatment-resistant schizophrenia

Habit Forming

- No

How to Stop

- Slow down-titration (over 6–8 weeks), especially when simultaneously beginning a new antipsychotic while switching (i.e., cross-titration)
- Blood testing is necessary every week for 4 weeks following discontinuation, or until WBC ≥3,500/mm^3 and ANC ≥2,000/mm^3

✻ Rapid discontinuation may lead to rebound psychosis and worsening of symptoms

Pharmacokinetics

- Half-life 5–16 hours
- Metabolized by multiple CYP450 enzymes, including 1A2, 2D6, and 3A4

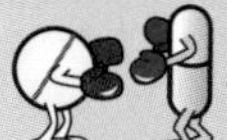

Drug Interactions

- Dose may need to be reduced if given in conjunction with CYP450 1A2 inhibitors (e.g., fluvoxamine)
- Dose may need to be raised if given in conjunction with CYP450 1A2 inducers (e.g., cigarette smoke)
- CYP450 2D6 inhibitors (e.g., paroxetine, fluoxetine, duloxetine) can raise clozapine levels, but dosage adjustment usually not necessary
- CYP450 3A4 inhibitors (e.g., nefazodone, fluvoxamine, fluoxetine) can raise clozapine levels, but dosage adjustment usually not necessary
- Clozapine may enhance effects of antihypertensive drugs

Other Warnings/ Precautions

- Possible association between myocarditis and cardiomyopathy and clozapine use, even in physically healthy individuals
- Should not be used in conjunction with agents that are known to cause agranulocytosis
- Use with caution in patients with glaucoma
- Use with caution in patients with enlarged prostate

Do Not Use

- In patients with myeloproliferative disorder
- In patients with uncontrolled epilepsy
- In patients with granulocytopenia
- In patients with paralytic ileus
- In patients with CNS depression
- If there is a proven allergy to clozapine

SPECIAL POPULATIONS

Renal Impairment
- Should be used with caution

Hepatic Impairment
- Should be used with caution

Cardiac Impairment
- Should be used with caution, particularly if patient is taking concomitant medication

Elderly
- Some patients may tolerate lower doses better
- Although atypical antipsychotics are commonly used for behavioral disturbances in dementia, no agent has been approved for treatment of elderly patients with dementia-related psychosis
- Elderly patients with dementia-related psychosis treated with atypical antipsychotics are at an increased risk of death compared to placebo, and also have an increased risk of cerebrovascular events

Children and Adolescents
- Safety and efficacy have not been established
- Preliminary research has suggested efficacy in early-onset treatment-resistant schizophrenia
- Children and adolescents taking clozapine should be monitored more often than adults

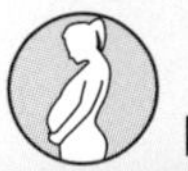

Pregnancy
- Risk Category B [animal studies do not show adverse effects; no controlled studies in humans]
- Psychotic symptoms may worsen during pregnancy and some form of treatment may be necessary
- Clozapine should be used only when the potential benefits outweigh potential risks to the fetus

Breast Feeding
- Unknown if clozapine is secreted in human breast milk, but all psychotropics assumed to be secreted in breast milk
- ✻ Recommended either to discontinue drug or bottle feed
- Infants of women who choose to breast feed while on clozapine should be monitored for possible adverse effects

THE ART OF PSYCHOPHARMACOLOGY

Potential Advantages
- ✻ Treatment-resistant schizophrenia
- ✻ Violent, aggressive patients
- ✻ Patients with tardive dyskinesia
- ✻ Patients with suicidal behavior

Potential Disadvantages
- ✻ Patients with diabetes, obesity, and/or dyslipidemia
- Patients with cardiac impairment

Primary Target Symptoms
- Positive symptoms of psychosis
- Negative symptoms of psychosis
- Cognitive symptoms
- Affective symptoms
- Suicidal behavior
- Violence and aggression

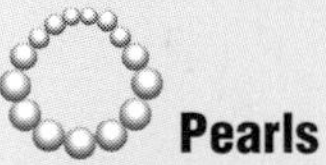

Pearls
- ✻ Not a first-line treatment choice in most countries
- ✻ Most efficacious but most dangerous
- ✻ Documented efficacy in treatment-refractory schizophrenia
- May reduce violence and aggression in difficult cases, including forensic cases
- ✻ Reduces suicide in schizophrenia
- May reduce substance abuse
- May improve tardive dyskinesia
- Little or no prolactin elevation, motor side effects, or tardive dyskinesia
- Clinical improvements often continue slowly over several years
- Cigarette smoke can decrease clozapine levels and patients may be at risk for relapse if they begin or increase smoking
- More weight gain than many other antipsychotics – does not mean every patient gains weight

Suggested Reading

Iqbal MM, Rahman A, Husain Z, Mahmud SZ, Ryan WG, Feldman JM. Clozapine: a clinical review of adverse effects and management. Ann Clin Psychiatry 2003;15:33–48.

Lieberman JA. Maximizing clozapine therapy: managing side effects. J Clin Psychiatry 1998;59 (suppl 3):38–43.

Schulte P. What is an adequate trial with clozapine?: therapeutic drug monitoring and time to response in treatment-refractory schizophrenia. Clin Pharmacokinet 2003;42:607–18.

Wagstaff A, Perry C. Clozapine: in prevention of suicide in patients with schizophrenia or schizoaffective disorder. CNS Drugs 2003;17:273–80.

Wahlbeck K, Cheine M, Essali A, Adams C. Evidence of clozapine's effectiveness in schizophrenia: a systematic review and meta-analysis of randomized trials. Am J Psychiatry 1999;156:990–99.

THERAPEUTICS

Brands • Tercian

see index for additional brand names

Generic? Not in the U.S.

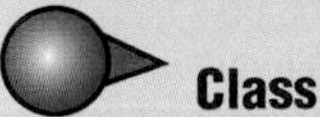

Class

- Conventional antipsychotic (neuroleptic, phenothiazine, dopamine 2 antagonist, serotonin dopamine antagonist)

Commonly Prescribed for

(bold for FDA approved)

- Schizophrenia
- ✻ Anxiety associated with psychosis (short-term)
- Anxiety associated with nonpsychotic disorders, including mood disorders and personality disorders (short-term)
- Severe depression
- Bipolar disorder
- Other psychotic disorders
- Acute agitation/aggression (injection)
- Benzodiazepine withdrawal

How the Drug Works

- Blocks dopamine 2 receptors, reducing positive symptoms of psychosis
- ✻ Although classified as a conventional antipsychotic, cyamemazine is a potent serotonin 2A antagonist
- Affinity at a myriad of other neurotransmitter receptors may contribute to cyamemazine's efficacy
- ✻ Specifically, antagonist actions at 5HT2C receptors may contribute to notable anxiolytic effects in many patients
- 5HT2C antagonist actions may also contribute to antidepressant actions in severe depression and to improvement of cognitive and negative symptoms of schizophrenia in some patients

How Long Until It Works

- Psychotic symptoms can improve with high doses within 1 week, but it may take several weeks for full effect on behavior
- Anxiolytic actions can improve with low doses within 1 week, but it may take several days to weeks for full effect on behavior

If It Works

- High doses most often reduce positive symptoms in schizophrenia but do not eliminate them
- Low doses most often reduce anxiety symptoms in psychotic and nonpsychotic disorders
- Most schizophrenia patients do not have a total remission of symptoms but rather a reduction of symptoms by about a third
- Continue treatment in schizophrenia until reaching a plateau of improvement
- After reaching a satisfactory plateau, continue treatment for at least a year, after first episode of psychosis in schizophrenia
- For second and subsequent episodes of psychosis in schizophrenia, treatment may need to be indefinite
- For symptomatic treatment of anxiety in psychotic and nonpsychotic disorders, treatment may also need to be indefinite while monitoring the risks versus the benefits of long-term treatment
- Reduces symptoms of acute psychotic mania but not proven as a mood stabilizer or as an effective maintenance treatment in bipolar disorder
- After reducing acute psychotic symptoms in mania, consider switching to a mood stabilizer and/or an atypical antipsychotic for long-term mood stabilization and maintenance

If It Doesn't Work

- For treatment of psychotic symptoms, consider trying one of the first-line atypical antipsychotics (risperidone, olanzapine, quetiapine, ziprasidone, aripiprazole, paliperidone, amisulpiride)
- Consider trying another conventional antipsychotic
- If 2 or more antipsychotic monotherapies do not work, consider clozapine
- For treatment of anxiety symptoms, consider adding a benzodiazepine or switching to a benzodiazepine

Best Augmenting Combos for Partial Response or Treatment-Resistance

- Generally, best to switch to another agent
- Augmentation of conventional antipsychotics has not been systematically studied

- Addition of a mood-stabilizing anticonvulsant such as valproate, carbamazepine, or lamotrigine may be helpful in both schizophrenia and bipolar mania
- Augmentation with lithium in bipolar mania may be helpful
- Addition of a benzodiazepine, especially for short-term agitation
- Addition of antidepressants for severe depression

Tests

✻ Since conventional antipsychotics are frequently associated with weight gain, before starting treatment, weigh all patients and determine if the patient is already overweight (BMI 25.0–29.9) or obese BMI ≥30)
- Before giving a drug that can cause weight gain to an overweight or obese patient, consider determining whether the patient already has pre-diabetes (fasting glucose 100–25 mg/dL), diabetes (fasting plasma glucose >125 mg/dL) or dyslipidemia (increased total cholesterol, LDL cholesterol and triglycerides; decreased HDL cholesterol), and treat or refer such patients for treatment, including nutrition and weight management, physical activity counseling, smoking cessation and medical management

✻ Monitor weight, and BMI during treatment

✻ Consider monitoring fasting triglycerides monthly for several months in patients at high risk for metabolic complications and when initiating or switching antipsychotics

✻ While giving a drug to a patient who has gained >5% of initial weight, consider evaluating for the presence of pre-diabetes, diabetes or dyslipidemia, or consider switching to a different antipsychotic
- Should check blood pressure in the elderly before starting and for the first few weeks of treatment
- Monitoring elevated prolactin levels of dubious clinical benefit

SIDE EFFECTS

How Drug Causes Side Effects

- By blocking dopamine 2 receptors in the striatum, it can cause motor side effects at antipsychotic (high) doses
- Much lower propensity to cause motor side effects at low doses used to treat anxiety
- By blocking dopamine 2 receptors in the pituitary, it can cause elevations in prolactin, but unlike other conventional antipsychotics, prolactin elevations at low doses of cyamemazine are uncommon or transient
- By blocking dopamine 2 receptors excessively in the mesocortical and mesolimbic dopamine pathways, especially at high doses, it can cause worsening of negative and cognitive symptoms (neuroleptic-induced deficit syndrome)
- Anticholinergic actions, especially at high doses, may cause sedation, blurred vision, constipation, dry mouth
- Antihistamine actions may contribute to anxiolytic actions at low doses and to sedation and weight gain at high doses
- By blocking alpha 1 adrenergic receptors, cyamemazine can cause dizziness, sedation and hypotension especially at high doses
- Mechanism of weight gain and any possible increased incidence of diabetes and dyslipidemia with conventional antipsychotics is unknown

Notable Side Effects

✻ Neuroleptic-induced deficit syndrome (unusual at low doses)
- Akathisia
- Extrapyramidal symptoms, Parkinsonism, tardive dyskinesia (unusual at low doses)
- Galactorrhea, amenorrhea (unusual at low doses)
- Hypotension, tachycardia (unusual at low doses)
- Dry mouth, constipation, vision disturbance, urinary retention
- Sedation
- Decreased sweating
- Weight gain (may be unusual at low doses)
- Sexual dysfunction
- Metabolic effects, glucose tolerance

Life-Threatening or Dangerous Side Effects

- Rare neuroleptic malignant syndrome
- Rare seizures
- Rare jaundice, agranulocytosis
- Increased risk of death and cerebrovascular events in elderly patients with dementia-related psychosis
- Increased risk of death and cerebrovascular events in elderly patients with dementia-related psychosis

Weight Gain

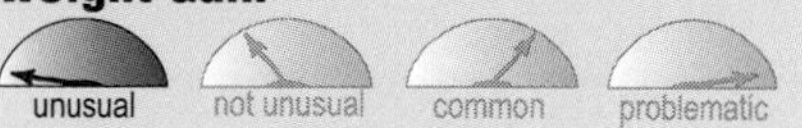

- Reported but not expected especially at low doses

Sedation

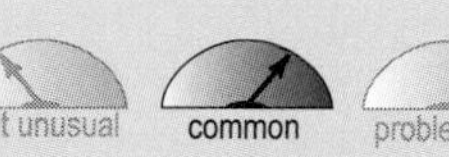

- Many experience and/or can be significant in amount, especially at high doses
- Sedation is usually dose-dependent and may not be experienced as sedation but as anxiolytic actions on anxiety and aggression at low doses where cyamemazine may function as an atypical antipsychotic (e.g., <300 mg/day; especially 25–100 mg/day)

What to Do About Side Effects

- Wait
- Wait
- Wait
- For motor symptoms, add an anticholinergic agent
- Reduce the dose
- For sedation, give at night
- Switch to an atypical antipsychotic
- Weight loss, exercise programs, and medical management for high BMIs, diabetes, dyslipidemia

Best Augmenting Agents for Side Effects

- Benztropine or trihexyphenidyl for motor side effects
- Benzodiazepines may be helpful for akathisia
- Many side effects cannot be improved with an augmenting agent

DOSING AND USE

Usual Dosage Range

- 50–300 mg at bedtime for treatment of psychosis
- 25–100 mg for anxiety; duration of treatment 4 weeks
- Children (ages 6 and older): 1–4 mg/kg per day
- Injection: 25–100 mg/day

Dosage Forms

- Tablet 25 mg, 100 mg
- Oral solution 40 mg/mL
- Injection 50 mg/5 mL

How to Dose

- Psychosis: usual maintenance dose 50–300 mg at bedtime; maximum dose 600 mg/day divided into 2 or 3 doses; after 2 weeks consider reducing to lowest effective dose
- Anxiety (adults): usual dose 25–100 mg/day; reduce dose if unacceptable sedation; maximum duration of treatment 4 weeks
- Anxiety (children): usual dose 1–4 mg/kg per day

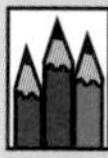

Dosing Tips

- Has conventional antipsychotic properties at originally recommended high doses (300–600 mg/day)

✽ Binding studies, PET studies and clinical observations suggest that cyamemazine may be "atypical" with low motor side effects or prolactin elevations at low doses (below 300 mg/day)

✽ Clinical evidence suggests substantial anxiolytic benefits at 25–100 mg/day in many patients

✽ Clinical evidence suggests low extrapyramidal side effects, little prolactin elevation yet demonstrable anxiolytic, anti-aggression and antidepressant actions at doses below 300 mg/day

- Robust antipsychotic actions on positive symptoms may require dosing above 300 mg/day
- Low doses up to 100 mg/day may be used to augment partial responders to other conventional or atypical antipsychotics, especially for anxiolytic actions

Overdose

- Extrapyramidal symptoms, sedation, hypotension, coma, respiratory depression

Long-Term Use

- Some side effects may be irreversible (e.g., tardive dyskinesia)

Habit Forming

- No

How to Stop

- Slow down titration (over 6–8 weeks), especially when simultaneously beginning a new antipsychotic while switching (i.e., cross titration)
- Rapid oral discontinuation of high doses of phenothiazines in psychotic patients may lead to rebound psychosis and worsening of symptoms
- If antiparkinsonian agents are being used, they should generally be continued for a few weeks after high dose cyamemazine is discontinued

Pharmacokinetics

- Half-life 10 hours

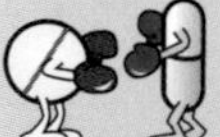

Drug Interactions

- May decrease the effects of levodopa; contraindicated for use with dopamine agonists other than levodopa
- May increase the effects of antihypertensive drugs except for guanethidine, whose antihypertensive actions phenothiazines may antagonize
- May enhance QTc prolongation of other drugs capable of prolonging QTc interval
- Additive effects may occur if used with CNS depressants
- Anticholinergic effects may occur if used with atropine or related compounds
- Some patients taking a neuroleptic and lithium have developed an encephalopathic syndrome similar to neuroleptic malignant syndrome
- Epinephrine may lower blood pressure; diuretics and alcohol may increase risk of hypotension when administered with a phenothiazine

Other Warnings/ Precautions

- If signs of neuroleptic malignant syndrome develop, treatment should be immediately discontinued
- Use cautiously in patients with respiratory disorders
- Use cautiously in patients with alcohol withdrawal or convulsive disorders because phenothiazines can lower seizure threshold
- Do not use epinephrine in event of overdose as interaction with some pressor agents may lower blood pressure
- Avoid undue exposure to sunlight
- Avoid extreme heat exposure
- Use with caution in patients with respiratory disorders, glaucoma, or urinary retention
- Antiemetic effects of phenothiazines may mask signs of other disorders or overdose; suppression of cough reflex may cause asphyxia
- Observe for signs of ocular toxicity (corneal and lenticular deposits) as for other phenothiazines
- Use only with caution or at low doses, if at all, in Parkinson's disease or Lewy body dementia
- Because cyamemazine may dose-dependently prolong QTc interval, use with caution in patients who have bradycardia or who are taking drugs that can induce bradycardia (e.g., beta blockers, calcium channel blockers, clonidine, digitalis)
- Because cyamemazine may dose-dependently prolong QTc interval, use with caution in patients who have hyperkalemia and/or hypomagnesemia or who are taking drugs that can induce hypokalemia and/or magnesemia (e.g., diuretics, stimulant laxatives, intravenous amphotericin B, glucocorticoids, tetracosaclides)
- Cyamemazine can increase the QTc interval, potentially causing torsades de pointes-type arrhythmia or sudden death

Do Not Use

- If there is a history of QTc prolongation or cardiac arrhythmia, recent acute myocardial infarction, uncompensated heart failure
- ✱ If QTc interval greater than 450 msec or if taking an agent capable of prolonging the QTc interval

- If patient is taking sultopride
- If patient is in a comatose state or has CNS depression
- If there is the presence of blood dyscrasias, bone marrow depression, or liver disease
- If there is subcortical brain damage
- If patient has sensitivity to or intolerance of gluten (tablets contain gluten)
- If patient has congenital galactosemy, does not adequately absorb glucose/galactose, or has lactase deficit (tablets contain lactose)
- If patient is intolerant of fructose, does not adequately absorb glucose/galactose, or has sugar-isomaltase deficit (oral solution only; oral solution contains saccharose)
- If there is a proven allergy to cyamemazine
- If there is a known sensitivity to any phenothiazine

SPECIAL POPULATIONS

Renal Impairment

- Use with caution

Hepatic Impairment

- Use with caution

Cardiac Impairment

- Cardiovacular toxicity can occur, especially orthostatic hypotension

Elderly

- Elderly patients may be more susceptible to adverse effects
- Lower doses should be used and patient should be monitored closely
- Generally, doses above 100 mg/day are not recommended
- Elderly patients with dementia-related psychosis treated with antipsychotics are at an increased risk of death compared to placebo, and also have an increased risk of cerebrovascular events
- Elderly patients with dementia-related psychosis treated with antipsychotics are at an increased risk of death compared to placebo, and also have an increased risk of cerebrovascular events

Children and Adolescents

- Sometimes used for severe behavioral disturbances in children ages 6 and older
- Oral solution is preferable to the other formulations

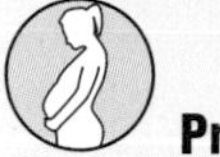

Pregnancy

- Phenothiazines are considered Risk Category C [some animal studies show adverse effects; no controlled studies in humans]
- Reports of extrapyramidal symptoms, jaundice, hyperreflexia, hyporeflexia in infants whose mothers took a phenothiazine during pregnancy
- Phenothiazines should only be used during pregnancy if clearly needed
- Psychotic symptoms may worsen during pregnancy and some form of treatment may be necessary
- Atypical antipsychotics may be preferable to phenothiazines or anticonvulsant mood stabilizers if treatment is required during pregnancy

Breast Feeding

- Unknown if cyamemazine is secreted in human breast milk, but all psychotropics assumed to be secreted in breast milk
- ✻ Recommended either to discontinue drug or bottle feed

THE ART OF PSYCHOPHARMACOLOGY

Potential Advantages

- For anxiety in patients with psychotic illnesses
- For anxiety in patients with nonpsychotic illnesses
- For severe depression

Potential Disadvantages

- Patients with tardive dyskinesia
- Children
- Elderly

Primary Target Symptoms

- Anxiety associated with psychosis
- Anxiety
- Aggression
- Agitation
- Positive symptoms of psychosis
- Severe depression

Pearls

- One of the most frequently prescribed antipsychotics in France, especially as a low dose anxiolytic for psychotic patients
- ✻ Appears to have unique anxiolytic actions at low doses without rebound anxiety following discontinuation
- ✻ Low doses rarely associated with motor side effects or with prolactin elevation
- ✻ Recently discovered to be a serotonin dopamine antagonist with more potent binding of 5HT2A and 5HT2C receptors than D2 receptors (binding studies and PET scans)
- Low doses appear to saturate 5HT2A receptors in frontal cortex while not saturating D2 receptors in the striatum, accounting for apparent atypical antipsychotic and anxiolytic properties at low doses
- May be useful second-line therapy in facilitating benzodiazepine withdrawal for those patients in whom substitution with another benzodiazepine is not effective or is not appropriate

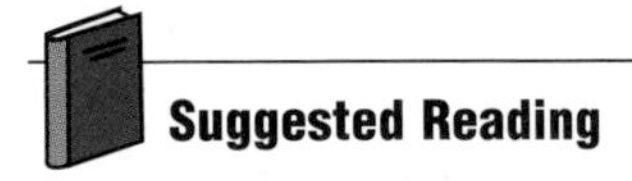

Suggested Reading

Lemoine P, Kermadi I, Garcia-Acosta S, Garay RP, Dib M. Double-blind, comparative study of cyamemazine vs. bromazepam in the benzodiazepine withdrawal syndrome. Prog Neuropsychopharmacol Biol Psychiatry 2006;30(1):131–7.

Hameg A, Bayle F, Nuss P, Dupuis P, Garay RP, Dib M. Affinity of cyamemazine, an anxiolytic antipsychotic drug, for human recombinant dopamine vs. serotonin receptor subtypes. Biochem Pharmacol 2003;65(3):435–40.

Hode Y, Reimold M, Demazieres A, Reischl G, Bayle F, Nuss P. et al. A positron emission tomography (PET) study of cerebral dopamine D2 and serotonine 5-HT2A receptor occupancy in patients treated with cyamemazine (Tercian). Psychopharmacology (Berl) 2005;180(2):377–84.

THERAPEUTICS

Brands • Norpramin
see index for additional brand names

Generic? Yes

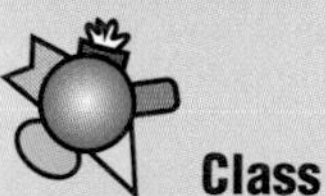

Class
- Tricyclic antidepressant (TCA)
- Predominantly a norepinephrine/noradrenaline reuptake inhibitor

Commonly Prescribed for
(bold for FDA approved)
- **Depression**
- Anxiety
- Insomnia
- Neuropathic pain/chronic pain
- Treatment-resistant depression

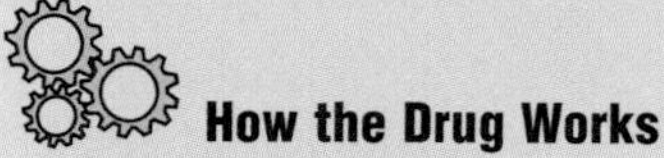

How the Drug Works
- Boosts neurotransmitter norepinephrine/noradrenaline
- Blocks norepinephrine reuptake pump (norepinephrine transporter), presumably increasing noradrenergic neurotransmission
- Since dopamine is inactivated by norepinephrine reuptake in frontal cortex, which largely lacks dopamine transporters, desipramine can thus increase dopamine neurotransmission in this part of the brain
- A more potent inhibitor of norepinephrine reuptake pump than serotonin reuptake pump (serotonin transporter)
- At high doses may also boost neurotransmitter serotonin and presumably increase serotonergic neurotransmission

How Long Until It Works
- May have immediate effects in treating insomnia or anxiety
- Onset of therapeutic actions usually not immediate, but often delayed 2–4 weeks
- If it is not working within 6–8 weeks for depression, it may require a dosage increase or it may not work at all
- May continue to work for many years to prevent relapse of symptoms

If It Works
- The goal of treatment of depression is complete remission of current symptoms as well as prevention of future relapses
- The goal of treatment of chronic neuropathic pain is to reduce symptoms as much as possible, especially in combination with other treatments
- Treatment of depression most often reduces or even eliminates symptoms, but not a cure since symptoms can recur after medicine stopped
- Treatment of chronic neuropathic pain may reduce symptoms, but rarely eliminates them completely, and is not a cure since symptoms can recur after medicine is stopped
- Continue treatment of depression until all symptoms are gone (remission)
- Once symptoms of depression are gone, continue treating for 1 year for the first episode of depression
- For second and subsequent episodes of depression, treatment may need to be indefinite
- Use in anxiety disorders and chronic pain may also need to be indefinite, but long-term treatment is not well studied in these conditions

If It Doesn't Work
- Many depressed patients only have a partial response where some symptoms are improved but others persist (especially insomnia, fatigue, and problems concentrating)
- Other depressed patients may be nonresponders, sometimes called treatment-resistant or treatment-refractory
- Consider increasing dose, switching to another agent or adding an appropriate augmenting agent
- Consider psychotherapy
- Consider evaluation for another diagnosis or for a comorbid condition (e.g., medical illness, substance abuse, etc.)
- Some patients may experience apparent lack of consistent efficacy due to activation of latent or underlying bipolar disorder, and require antidepressant discontinuation and a switch to a mood stabilizer

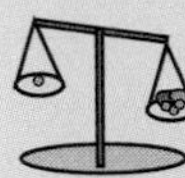

Best Augmenting Combos for Partial Response or Treatment-Resistance

- Lithium, buspirone, thyroid hormone (for depression)
- Gabapentin, tiagabine, other anticonvulsants, even opiates if done by experts while monitoring carefully in difficult cases (for chronic pain)

Tests

✻ None for healthy individuals, although monitoring of plasma drug levels is available

✻ Since tricyclic and tetracyclic antidepressants are frequently associated with weight gain, before starting treatment, weigh all patients and determine if the patient is already overweight (BMI 25.0–29.9) or obese (BMI ≥30)

- Before giving a drug that can cause weight gain to an overweight or obese patient, consider determining whether the patient already has pre-diabetes (fasting plasma glucose 100–25 mg/dL), diabetes (fasting plasma glucose >126 mg/dL), or dyslipidemia (increased total cholesterol, LDL cholesterol and triglycerides; decreased HDL cholesterol), and treat or refer such patients for treatment, including nutrition and weight management, physical activity counseling, smoking cessation, and medical management

✻ Monitor weight and BMI during treatment

✻ While giving a drug to a patient who has gained >5% of initial weight, consider evaluating for the presence of pre-diabetes, diabetes, or dyslipidemia, or consider switching to a different antidepressant

- EKGs may be useful for selected patients (e.g., those with personal or family history of QTc prolongation; cardiac arrhythmia; recent myocardial infarction; uncompensated heart failure; or taking agents that prolong QTc interval such as pimozide, thioridazine, selected antiarrhythmics, moxifloxacin, sparfloxacin, etc.)
- Patients at risk for electrolyte disturbances (e.g., patients on diuretic therapy) should have baseline and periodic serum potassium and magnesium measurements

SIDE EFFECTS

How Drug Causes Side Effects

✻ Anticholinergic activity for desipramine may be somewhat less than for some other TCAs, yet can still explain the presence, if lower incidence, of sedative effects, dry mouth, constipation, and blurred vision

- Sedative effects and weight gain may be due to antihistamine properties
- Blockade of alpha adrenergic 1 receptors may explain dizziness, sedation, and hypotension
- Cardiac arrhythmias and seizures, especially in overdose, may be caused by blockade of ion channels

Notable Side Effects

- Blurred vision, constipation, urinary retention, increased appetite, dry mouth, nausea, diarrhea, heartburn, unusual taste in mouth, weight gain
- Fatigue, weakness, dizziness, sedation, headache, anxiety, nervousness, restlessness
- Sexual dysfunction, sweating

Life-Threatening or Dangerous Side Effects

- Paralytic ileus, hyperthermia (TCAs + anticholinergic agents)
- Lowered seizure threshold and rare seizures
- Orthostatic hypotension, sudden death, arrhythmias, tachycardia
- QTc prolongation
- Hepatic failure, extrapyramidal symptoms
- Increased intraocular pressure
- Blood dyscrasias
- Rare induction of mania
- Rare activation of suicidal ideation and behavior (suicidality) (short-term studies did not show an increase in the risk of suicidality with antidepressants compared to placebo beyond age 24)

Weight Gain

unusual | not unusual | **common** | problematic

- Many experience and/or can be significant in amount
- Can increase appetite and carbohydrate craving

Sedation

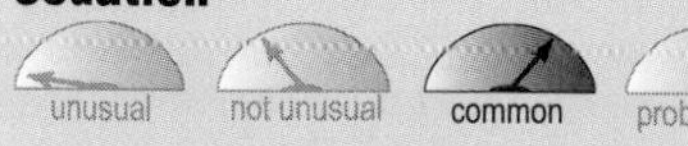

- Many experience and/or can be significant in amount
- Tolerance to sedative effects may develop with long-term use

What to Do About Side Effects

- Wait
- Wait
- Wait
- Lower the dose
- Switch to an SSRI or newer antidepressant

Best Augmenting Agents for Side Effects

- Many side effects cannot be improved with an augmenting agent

DOSING AND USE

Usual Dosage Range

- 100–200 mg/day (for depression)
- 50–150 mg/day (for chronic pain)

Dosage Forms

- Tablets 10 mg, 25 mg, 50 mg, 75 mg, 100 mg, 150 mg

How to Dose

- Initial 25 mg/day at bedtime; increase by 25 mg every 3–7 days
- 75 mg/day once daily or in divided doses; gradually increase dose to achieve desired therapeutic effect; maximum dose 300 mg/day

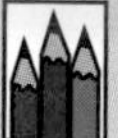

Dosing Tips

- If given in a single dose, should generally be administered at bedtime because of its sedative properties
- If given in split doses, largest dose should generally be given at bedtime because of its sedative properties
- If patients experience nightmares, split dose and do not give large dose at bedtime
- Patients treated for chronic pain may only require lower doses (e.g., 50–75 mg/day)
- Risk of seizure increases with dose

❋ Monitoring plasma levels of desipramine is recommended in patients who do not respond to the usual dose or whose treatment is regarded as urgent

- If intolerable anxiety, insomnia, agitation, akathisia, or activation occur either upon dosing initiation or discontinuation, consider the possibility of activated bipolar disorder, and switch to a mood stabilizer or an atypical antipsychotic

Overdose

- Death may occur; convulsions, cardiac dysrhythmias, severe hypotension, CNS depression, coma, changes in EKG

Long-Term Use

- Safe

Habit Forming

- No

How to Stop

- Taper to avoid withdrawal effects
- Even with gradual dose reduction some withdrawal symptoms may appear within the first 2 weeks
- Many patients tolerate 50% dose reduction for 3 days, then another 50% reduction for 3 days, then discontinuation
- If withdrawal symptoms emerge during discontinuation, raise dose to stop symptoms and then restart withdrawal much more slowly

Pharmacokinetics

- Substrate for CYP450 2D6 and 1A2
- Is the active metabolite of imipramine, formed by demethylation via CYP450 1A2
- Half-life approximately 24 hours

Drug Interactions

- Tramadol increases the risk of seizures in patients taking TCAs
- Use of TCAs with anticholinergic drugs may result in paralytic ileus or hyperthermia
- Fluoxetine, paroxetine, bupropion, duloxetine, and other CYP450 2D6 inhibitors may increase TCA concentrations
- Cimetidine may increase plasma concentrations of TCAs and cause anticholinergic symptoms
- Phenothiazines or haloperidol may raise TCA blood concentrations

- May alter effects of antihypertensive drugs; may inhibit hypotensive effects of clonidine
- Use of TCAs with sympathomimetic agents may increase sympathetic activity
- Methylphenidate may inhibit metabolism of TCAs
- Activation and agitation, especially following switching or adding antidepressants, may represent the induction of a bipolar state, especially a mixed dysphoric bipolar II condition sometimes associated with suicidal ideation, and require the addition of lithium, a mood stabilizer or an atypical antipsychotic, and/or discontinuation of desipramine

Other Warnings/ Precautions

- Add or initiate other antidepressants with caution for up to 2 weeks after discontinuing desipramine
- Generally, do not use with MAO inhibitors, including 14 days after MAOIs are stopped; do not start an MAOI until 2 weeks after discontinuing desipramine, but see Pearls
- Use with caution in patients with history of seizures, urinary retention, narrow angle-closure glaucoma, hyperthyroidism
- TCAs can increase QTc interval, especially at toxic doses, which can be attained not only by overdose but also by combining with drugs that inhibit TCA metabolism via CYP450 2D6, potentially causing torsade de pointes-type arrhythmia or sudden death
- Because TCAs can prolong QTc interval, use with caution in patients who have bradycardia or who are taking drugs that can induce bradycardia (e.g., beta blockers, calcium channel blockers, clonidine, digitalis)
- Because TCAs can prolong QTc interval, use with caution in patients who have hypokalemia and/or hypomagnesemia or who are taking drugs that can induce hypokalemia and/or magnesemia (e.g., diuretics, stimulant laxatives, intravenous amphotericin B, glucocorticoids, tetracosactide)
- When treating children, carefully weigh the risks and benefits of pharmacological treatment against the risks and benefits of nontreatment with antidepressants and make sure to document this in the patient's chart
- Distribute the brochures provided by the FDA and the drug companies
- Warn patients and their caregivers about the possibility of activating side effects and advise them to report such symptoms immediately
- Monitor patients for activation of suicidal ideation, especially children and adolescents

Do Not Use

- If patient is recovering from myocardial infarction
- If patient is taking agents capable of significantly prolonging QTc interval (e.g., pimozide, thioridazine, selected antiarrhythmics, moxifloxacin, sparfloxacin)
- If there is a history of QTc prolongation or cardiac arrhythmia, recent acute myocardial infarction, uncompensated heart failure
- If patient is taking drugs that inhibit TCA metabolism, including CYP450 2D6 inhibitors, except by an expert
- If there is reduced CYP450 2D6 function, such as patients who are poor 2D6 metabolizers, except by an expert and at low doses
- If there is a proven allergy to desipramine, imipramine, or lofepramine

SPECIAL POPULATIONS

Renal Impairment

- Use with caution; may need to lower dose
- May need to monitor plasma levels

Hepatic Impairment

- Use with caution; may need to lower dose
- May need to monitor plasma levels

Cardiac Impairment

- TCAs have been reported to cause arrhythmias, prolongation of conduction time, orthostatic hypotension, sinus tachycardia, and heart failure, especially in the diseased heart
- Myocardial infarction and stroke have been reported with TCAs
- TCAs produce QTc prolongation, which may be enhanced by the existence of

bradycardia, hypokalemia, congenital or acquired long QTc interval, which should be evaluated prior to administering desipramine

- Use with caution if treating concomitantly with a medication likely to produce prolonged bradycardia, hypokalemia, slowing of intracardiac conduction, or prolongation of the QTc interval
- Avoid TCAs in patients with a known history of QTc prolongation, recent acute myocardial infarction, and uncompensated heart failure
- TCAs may cause a sustained increase in heart rate in patients with ischemic heart disease and may worsen (decrease) heart rate variability, an independent risk of mortality in cardiac populations
- Since SSRIs may improve (increase) heart rate variability in patients following a myocardial infarct and may improve survival as well as mood in patients with acute angina or following a myocardial infarction, these are more appropriate agents for cardiac population than tricyclic/tetracyclic antidepressants

* Risk/benefit ratio may not justify use of TCAs in cardiac impairment

Elderly

- May be more sensitive to anticholinergic, cardiovascular, hypotensive, and sedative effects
- Initial dose 25–50 mg/day, raise to 100 mg/day; maximum 150 mg/day
- May be useful to monitor plasma levels in elderly patients
- Reduction in risk of suicidality with antidepressants compared to placebo in adults age 65 and older

Children and Adolescents

- Carefully weigh the risks and benefits of pharmacological treatment against the risks and benefits of nontreatment with antidepressants and make sure to document this in the patient's chart
- Monitor patients face-to-face regularly, particularly during the first several weeks of treatment
- Use with caution, observing for activation of known or unknown bipolar disorder and/or suicidal ideation, and inform parents or guardian of this risk so they can help observe child or adolescent patients
- Not recommended for use in children under age 12
- Several studies show lack of efficacy of TCAs for depression
- May be used to treat enuresis or hyperactive/impulsive behaviors
- May reduce tic symptoms
- Some cases of sudden death have occurred in children taking TCAs
- Adolescents: initial dose 25–50 mg/day, increase to 100 mg/day; maximum dose 150 mg/day
- May be useful to monitor plasma levels in children and adolescents

Pregnancy

- Risk Category C [some animal studies show adverse effects; no controlled studies in humans]
- Crosses the placenta
- Adverse effects have been reported in infants whose mothers took a TCA (lethargy, withdrawal symptoms, fetal malformations)
- Must weigh the risk of treatment (first trimester fetal development, third trimester newborn delivery) to the child against the risk of no treatment (recurrence of depression, maternal health, infant bonding) to the mother and child
- For many patients this may mean continuing treatment during pregnancy

Breast Feeding

- Some drug is found in mother's breast milk

* Recommended either to discontinue drug or bottle feed

- Immediate postpartum period is a high-risk time for depression, especially in women who have had prior depressive episodes, so drug may need to be reinstituted late in the third trimester or shortly after childbirth to prevent a recurrence during the postpartum period
- Must weigh benefits of breast feeding with risks and benefits of antidepressant treatment versus nontreatment to both the infant and the mother
- For many patients this may mean continuing treatment during breast feeding

THE ART OF PSYCHOPHARMACOLOGY

Potential Advantages

- Patients with insomnia
- Severe or treatment-resistant depression
- Patients for whom therapeutic drug monitoring is desirable

Potential Disadvantages

- Pediatric and geriatric patients
- Patients concerned with weight gain
- Cardiac patients

Primary Target Symptoms

- Depressed mood
- Chronic pain

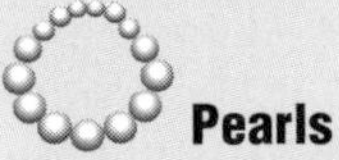

Pearls

- Tricyclic antidepressants are often a first-line treatment option for chronic pain
- Tricyclic antidepressants are no longer generally considered a first-line option for depression because of their side effect profile
- Tricyclic antidepressants continue to be useful for severe or treatment-resistant depression
- Noradrenergic reuptake inhibitors such as desipramine can be used as a second-line treatment for smoking cessation, cocaine dependence, and attention deficit disorder
- TCAs may aggravate psychotic symptoms
- Alcohol should be avoided because of additive CNS effects
- Underweight patients may be more susceptible to adverse cardiovascular effects
- Children, patients with inadequate hydration, and patients with cardiac disease may be more susceptible to TCA-induced cardiotoxicity than healthy adults
- For the expert only: although generally prohibited, a heroic but potentially dangerous treatment for severely treatment-resistant patients is to give a tricyclic/tetracyclic antidepressant other than clomipramine simultaneously with an MAO inhibitor for patients who fail to respond to numerous other antidepressants
- If this option is elected, start the MAOI with the tricyclic/tetracyclic antidepressant simultaneously at low doses after appropriate drug washout, then alternately increase doses of these agents every few days to a week as tolerated
- Although very strict dietary and concomitant drug restrictions must be observed to prevent hypertensive crises and serotonin syndrome, the most common side effects of MAOI/ tricyclic or tetracyclic combinations may be weight gain and orthostatic hypotension
- Patients on TCAs should be aware that they may experience symptoms such as photosensitivity or blue-green urine
- SSRIs may be more effective than TCAs in women, and TCAs may be more effective than SSRIs in men
- Not recommended for first-line use in children with ADHD because of the availability of safer treatments with better documented efficacy and because of desipramine's potential for sudden death in children

✱ Desipramine is one of the few TCAs where monitoring of plasma drug levels has been well studied

✱ Fewer anticholinergic side effects than some other TCAs

- Since tricyclic/tetracyclic antidepressants are substrates for CYP450 2D6, and 7% of the population (especially Caucasians) may have a genetic variant leading to reduced activity of 2D6, such patients may not safely tolerate normal doses of tricyclic/tetracyclic antidepressants and may require dose reduction
- Phenotypic testing may be necessary to detect this genetic variant prior to dosing with a tricyclic/tetracyclic antidepressant, especially in vulnerable populations such as children, elderly, cardiac populations, and those on concomitant medications
- Patients who seem to have extraordinarily severe side effects at normal or low doses may have this phenotypic CYP450 2D6 variant and require low doses or switching to another antidepressant not metabolized by 2D6

Suggested Reading

Anderson IM. Meta-analytical studies on new antidepressants. Br Med Bull 2001; 57:161–78.

Anderson IM. Selective serotonin reuptake inhibitors versus tricyclic antidepressants: a meta-analysis of efficacy and tolerability. J Aff Disorders 2000;58:19–36.

Janowsky DS, Byerley B. Desipramine: an overview. J Clin Psychiatry 1984;45:3–9.

Levin FR, Lehman AF. Meta-analysis of desipramine as an adjunct in the treatment of cocaine addiction. J Clin Psychopharmacol 1991;11:374–8.

THERAPEUTICS

Brands • Pristiq

see index for additional brand names

Generic? No

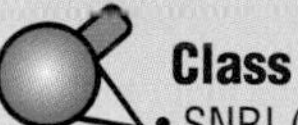

Class

- SNRI (dual serotonin and norepinephrine reuptake inhibitor); often classified as an antidepressant, but it is not just an antidepressant

Commonly Prescribed for

(bold for FDA approved)

- **Major depressive disorder**
- Vasomotor symptoms
- Fibromyalgia
- Generalized anxiety disorder (GAD)
- Social anxiety disorder (social phobia)
- Panic disorder
- Posttraumatic stress disorder (PTSD)
- Premenstrual dysphoric disorder (PMDD)

How the Drug Works

- Boosts neurotransmitters serotonin, norepinephrine/noradrenaline, and dopamine
- Blocks serotonin reuptake pump (serotonin transporter), presumably increasing serotonergic neurotransmission
- Blocks norepinephrine reuptake pump (norepinephrine transporter), presumably increasing noradrenergic neurotransmission
- Presumably desensitizes both serotonin 1A receptors and beta adrenergic receptors
- Since dopamine is inactivated by norepinephrine reuptake in frontal cortex, which largely lacks dopamine transporters, desvenlafaxine can increase dopamine neurotransmission in this part of the brain

How Long Until It Works

- Onset of therapeutic actions usually not immediate, but often delayed 2–4 weeks
- If it is not working within 6 or 8 weeks for depression, it may require a dosage increase or it may not work at all
- May continue to work for many years to prevent relapse of depressive symptoms
- Vasomotor symptoms in perimenopausal women with or without depression may improve within 1 week

If It Works

- The goal of treatment is complete remission of current symptoms as well as prevention of future relapses
- Treatment most often reduces or even eliminates symptoms, but not a cure since symptoms can recur after medicine stopped
- Continue treatment until all symptoms are gone (remission) or significantly reduced
- Once symptoms are gone, continue treating for 1 year for the first episode of depression
- For second and subsequent episodes of depression, treatment may need to be indefinite

If It Doesn't Work

- Many patients only have a partial response where some symptoms are improved but others persist (especially insomnia, fatigue, and problems concentrating)
- Other patients may be nonresponders, sometimes called treatment-resistant or treatment-refractory
- Some patients who have an initial response may relapse even though they continue treatment, sometimes called "poop-out"
- Consider increasing dose, switching to another agent, or adding an appropriate augmenting agent
- Consider psychotherapy
- Consider evaluation for another diagnosis or for a comorbid condition (e.g., medical illness, substance abuse, etc.)
- Some patients may experience apparent lack of consistent efficacy due to activation of latent or underlying bipolar disorder, and require antidepressant discontinuation and switch to a mood stabilizer

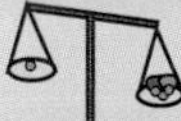

Best Augmenting Combos for Partial Response or Treatment-Resistance

- Mirtazapine ("California rocket fuel"; a potentially powerful dual serotonin and norepinephrine combination, but observe for activation of bipolar disorder and suicidal ideation)
- Bupropion, reboxetine, nortriptyline, desipramine, maprotiline, atomoxetine (all potentially powerful enhancers of noradrenergic action, but observe for

activation of bipolar disorder and suicidal ideation)
- Modafinil, especially for fatigue, sleepiness, and lack of concentration
- Mood stabilizers or atypical antipsychotics for bipolar depression, psychotic depression, or treatment-resistant depression
- Benzodiazepines
- If all else fails for anxiety disorders, consider gabapentin or tiagabine
- Hypnotics or trazodone for insomnia
- Classically, lithium, buspirone, or thyroid hormone

Tests

- Check blood pressure before initiating treatment and regularly during treatment

SIDE EFFECTS

How Drug Causes Side Effects

- Theoretically due to increases in serotonin and norepinephrine concentrations at receptors in parts of the brain and body other than those that cause therapeutic actions (e.g., unwanted actions of serotonin in sleep centers causing insomnia, unwanted actions of norepinephrine on acetylcholine release causing constipation and dry mouth, etc.)
- Most side effects are immediate but often go away with time

Notable Side Effects

- Most side effects increase with higher doses, at least transiently
- Insomnia, sedation, anxiety, dizziness
- Nausea, vomiting, constipation, decreased appetite
- Sexual dysfunction (abnormal ejaculation/orgasm, impotence)
- Sweating
- SIADH (syndrome of inappropriate antidiuretic hormone secretion)
- Hyponatremia
- Increase in blood pressure

Life-Threatening or Dangerous Side Effects

- Rare seizures
- Rare induction of hypomania
- Rare activation of suicidal ideation and behavior (suicidality) (short-term studies did not show an increase in the risk of suicidality with antidepressants compared to placebo beyond age 24)

Weight Gain

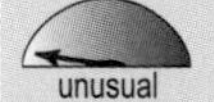
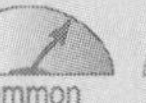

- Reported but not expected

Sedation

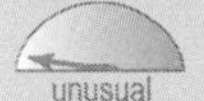
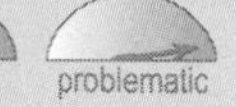

- Occurs in significant minority
- May also be activating in some patients

What to Do About Side Effects

- Wait
- Wait
- Wait
- Lower the dose
- In a few weeks, switch or add other drugs

Best Augmenting Agents for Side Effects

- Often best to try another antidepressant monotherapy prior to resorting to augmentation strategies to treat side effects
- Trazodone or a hypnotic for insomnia
- Bupropion, sildenafil, vardenafil, or tadalafil for sexual dysfunction
- Benzodiazepines for jitteriness and anxiety, especially at initiation of treatment and especially for anxious patients
- Mirtazapine for insomnia, agitation, and gastrointestinal side effects
- Many side effects are dose-dependent (i.e., they increase as dose increases, or they reemerge until tolerance redevelops)
- Many side effects are time-dependent (i.e., they start immediately upon dosing and upon each dose increase, but go away with time)
- Activation and agitation may represent the induction of a bipolar state, especially a mixed dysphoric bipolar II condition sometimes associated with suicidal ideation, and require the addition of lithium, a mood stabilizer or an atypical antipsychotic, and/or discontinuation of desvenlafaxine

DOSING AND USE

Usual Dosage Range
- Depression: 50 mg once daily

Dosage Forms
- Tablet (extended-release) 50 mg, 100 mg

How to Dose
- Initial dose 50 mg once daily; maximum recommended dose generally 100 mg once daily; doses up to 400 mg once daily have been shown to be effective but higher doses are associated with increased side effects

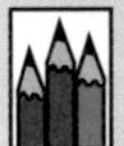

Dosing Tips
- Desvenlafaxine is the active metabolite O-desmethylvenlafaxine (ODV) of venlafaxine, and is formed as the result of CYP450 2D6
- More potent at the serotonin transporter (SERT) than at the norepinephrine transporter (NET), but has greater inhibition of NET relative to SERT compared to venlafaxine
- Nonresponders at lower doses may try higher doses to be assured of the benefits of dual SNRI action
- For vasomotor symptoms, current data suggest that a dose of 100 mg/day is effective
- Do not break or chew tablets, as this will alter controlled-release properties
- For patients with severe problems discontinuing desvenlafaxine, dosing may need to be tapered over many months (i.e., reduce dose by 1% every 3 days by crushing tablet and suspending or dissolving in 100 mL of fruit juice, and then disposing of 1 mL while drinking the rest; 3–7 days later, dispose of 2 mL, and so on). This is both a form of very slow biological tapering and a form of behavioral desensitization
- For some patients with severe problems discontinuing desvenlafaxine, it may be useful to add an SSRI with a long half-life, especially fluoxetine, prior to taper of desvenlafaxine. While maintaining fluoxetine dosing, first slowly taper desvenlafaxine and then taper fluoxetine
- Be sure to differentiate between re-emergence of symptoms requiring re-institution of treatment and withdrawal symptoms
- May dose up to 400 mg/day in patients who do not respond t lower doses, if tolerated

Overdose
- No fatalities have been reported as monotherapy; headache, vomiting, agitation, dizziness, nausea, constipation, diarrhea, dry mouth, paresthesia, tachycardia
- Desvenlafaxine is the active metabolite of venlafaxine; fatal toxicity index data from the U.K. suggest a higher rate of deaths from overdose with venlafaxine than with SSRIs; it is unknown whether this is related to differences in patients who receive venlafaxine or to potential cardiovascular toxicity of venlafaxine

Long Term Use
- See doctor regularly to monitor blood pressure

Habit Forming
- No

How to Stop
- Taper to avoid withdrawal effects (dizziness, nausea, diarrhea, sweating, anxiety, irritability)
- Recommended taper schedule is to give a fully daily dose (50 mg) less frequently
- If withdrawal symptoms emerge during discontinuation, raise dose to stop symptoms and then restart withdrawal much more slowly

Pharmacokinetics
- Active metabolite of venlafaxine
- Half-life 9–13 hours
- Minimally metabolized by CYP450 3A4

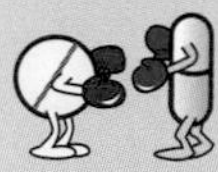

Drug Interactions
- Tramadol increases the risk of seizures in patients taking an antidepressant
- Can cause a fatal "serotonin syndrome" when combined with MAO inhibitors, so do not use with MAO inhibitors or for at least 14 days after MAOIs are stopped
- Do not start an MAO inhibitor for at least 2 weeks after discontinuing desvenlafaxine

- Possible increased risk of bleeding, especially when combined with anticoagulants (e.g., warfarin, NSAIDs)
- Potent inhibitors of CYP450 3A4 may increase plasma levels of desvenlafaxine, but the clinical significance of this is unknown
- Few known adverse drug interactions

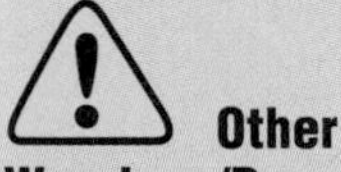

Other Warnings/Precautions

- Use with caution in patients with history of seizure
- Use with caution in patients with heart disease
- Use with caution in patients with bipolar disorder unless treated with concomitant mood-stabilizing agent
- When treating children, carefully weight the risks and benefits of pharmacological treatment against the risks and benefits of nontreatment with antidepressants and make sure to document this in the patient's chart
- Distribute the brochures provided by the FDA and the drug companies
- Warn patients and their caregivers about the possibility of activating side effects and advise them to report such symptoms immediately
- Monitor patients for activation of suicidal ideation, especially children and adolescents

Do Not Use

- If patient has uncontrolled narrow angle-closure glaucoma
- If patient is taking an MAO inhibitor
- If there is a proven allergy to desvenlafaxine or venlafaxine

SPECIAL POPULATIONS

Renal Impairment

- For moderate impairment, recommended dose is 50 mg/day
- For severe impairment, recommended dose is 50 mg every other day
- Patients on dialysis should not receive subsequent dose until dialysis is completed

Hepatic Impairment

- Doses greater than 100 mg/day not recommended

Cardiac Impairment

- Drug should be used with caution
- Hypertension should be controlled prior to initiation of desvenlafaxine and should be monitored regularly during treatment
- Desvenlafaxine has a dose-dependent effect on increasing blood pressure
- Desvenlafaxine is the active metabolite of venlafaxine, which is contraindicated in patients with heart disease in the U.K.
- Venlafaxine can block cardiac ion channels in vitro and worsens (i.e., reduces) heart rate variability in depression, perhaps due to norepinephrine reuptake inhibition

Elderly

- Some patients may tolerate lower doses better
- Reduction in risk of suicidality with antidepressants compared to placebo in adults age 65 and older

Children and Adolescents

- Carefully weigh the risks and benefits of pharmacological treatment against the risks and benefits of nontreatment with antidepressants and make sure to document this in the patient's chart
- Monitor patients face-to-face regularly, particularly during the first several weeks of treatment
- Use with caution, observing for activation of known or unknown bipolar disorder and/or suicidal ideation, and inform parents or guardian of this risk so they can help observe child or adolescent patients

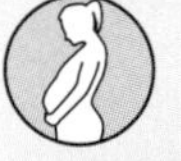

Pregnancy

- Risk Category C [some animal studies show adverse effects; no controlled studies in humans]
- Not generally recommended for use during pregnancy, especially during first trimester
- Nonetheless, continuous treatment during pregnancy may be necessary and has not been proven to be harmful to the fetus
- Must weigh the risk of treatment (first trimester fetal development, third trimester newborn delivery) to the child against the risk of no treatment (recurrence of

depression, maternal health, infant bonding) to the mother and child
- For many patients this may mean continuing treatment during pregnancy
- SSRI use beyond the 20th week of pregnancy may be associated with increased risk of pulmonary hypertension in newborns
- Neonates exposed to SSRIs or SNRIs late in the third trimester have developed complications requiring prolonged hospitalization, respiratory support, and tube feeding; reported symptoms are consistent with either a direct toxic effect of SSRIs and SNRIs or, possibly, a drug discontinuation syndrome, and include respiratory distress, cyanosis, apnea, seizures, temperature instability, feeding difficulty, vomiting, hypoglycemia, hypotonia, hypertonia, hyperreflexia, tremor, jitteriness, irritability, and constant crying

Breast Feeding
- Some drug is found in mother's breast milk
- Trace amounts may be present in nursing children whose mothers are on desvenlafaxine
- If child becomes irritable or sedated, breast feeding or drug may need to be discontinued
- Immediate postpartum period is a high-risk time for depression, especially in women who have had prior depressive episodes, so drug may need to be reinstituted late in the third trimester or shortly after childbirth to prevent a recurrence during the postpartum period
- Must weigh benefits of breast feeding with risks and benefits of antidepressant treatment versus nontreatment to both the infant and the mother
- For many patients, this may mean continuing treatment during breast feeding

THE ART OF PSYCHOPHARMACOLOGY

Potential Advantages
- Patients with retarded depression
- Patients with atypical depression
- Patients with depression may have higher remission rates on SNRIs than on SSRIs
- Depressed patients with somatic symptoms, fatigue, and pain
- Depressed patients with vasomotor symptoms
- Patients who do not respond or remit on treatment with SSRIs

Potential Disadvantages
- Patients sensitive to nausea
- Patients with borderline or uncontrolled hypertension
- Patients with cardiac disease

Primary Target Symptoms
- Depressed mood
- Energy, motivation, and interest
- Sleep disturbance
- Physical symptoms
- Pain

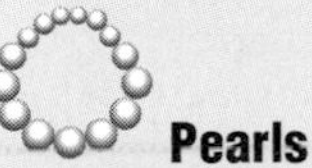

Pearls
- Because desvenlafaxine is only minimally metabolized by CYP450 3A4 and is not metabolized at all by CYP450 2D6, as venlafaxine is, it should have more consistent plasma levels than venlafaxine
- In addition, although desvenlafaxine, like venlafaxine, is more potent at the serotonin transporter (SERT) than the norepinephrine transporter (NET), it has relatively greater actions on NET versus SERT than venlafaxine does at comparable doses
- The greater potency for NET may make it a preferable agent for conditions theoretically associated with targeting norepinephrine actions, such as vasomotor symptoms and fibromyalgia
- May be particularly helpful for hot flushes in perimenopausal women
- May be effective in patients who fail to respond to SSRIs
- May be used in combination with other antidepressants for treatment-refractory cases
- May be effective in a broad array of anxiety disorders and possibly adult ADHD, although it has not been studied in these conditions
- May be associated with higher depression remission rates than SSRIs
- Because of recent studies from the U.K. that suggest a higher rate of deaths from overdose with venlafaxine than with SSRIs, and because of its potential to affect heart function, venlafaxine can only be

prescribed in the U.K. by specialist doctors and is contraindicated there in patients with heart disease
- Overdose data are from fatal toxicity index studies, which do not take into account patient characteristics or whether drug use was first- or second-line
- Venlafaxine's toxicity in overdose is less that that for tricyclic antidepressants

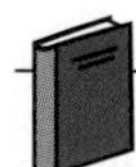

Suggested Reading

Deecher DC, Beyer CE, Johnston G, et al. Desvenlafaxine succinate: A new serotonin and norepinephrine reuptake inhibitor. J Pharmacol Exp Ther 2006;318(2):657–65.

Lieberman DZ, Montgomery SA, Tourian KA et al. A pooled analysis of two placebo-controlled trials of desvenlafaxine in major depressive disorder. Int Clin Psychopharmacol 2008;23(4):188–97.

Speroff L, Gass M, Constantine G. Efficacy and tolerability of desvenlafaxine succinate treatment for menopausal vasomotor symptoms: a randomized controlled trial. Obstet Gynecol 2008;111(1):77–87.

THERAPEUTICS

Brands
- Valium
- Diastat

see index for additional brand names

Generic? Yes (not Diastat)

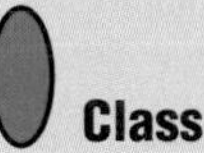

Class
- Benzodiazepine (anxiolytic, muscle relaxant, anticonvulsant)

Commonly Prescribed for
(bold for FDA approved)
- **Anxiety disorder**
- **Symptoms of anxiety (short-term)**
- **Acute agitation, tremor, impending or acute delirium tremens and hallucinosis in acute alcohol withdrawal**
- **Skeletal muscle spasm due to reflex spasm to local pathology**
- **Spasticity caused by upper motor neuron disorder**
- **Athetosis**
- **Stiffman syndrome**
- **Convulsive disorder (adjunctive)**
- **Anxiety during endoscopic procedures (adjunctive) (injection only)**
- **Preoperative anxiety (injection only)**
- **Anxiety relief prior to cardioversion (intravenous)**
- **Initial treatment of status epilepticus (injection only)**
- Insomnia

How the Drug Works
- Binds to benzodiazepine receptors at the GABA-A ligand-gated chloride channel complex
- Enhances the inhibitory effects of GABA
- Boosts chloride conductance through GABA-regulated channels
- Inhibits neuronal activity presumably in amygdala-centered fear circuits to provide therapeutic benefits in anxiety disorders
- Inhibiting actions in cerebral cortex may provide therapeutic benefits in seizure disorders
- Inhibitory actions in spinal cord may provide therapeutic benefits for muscle spasms

How Long Until It Works
- Some immediate relief with first dosing is common; can take several weeks with daily dosing for maximal therapeutic benefit

If It Works
- For short-term symptoms of anxiety or muscle spasms – after a few weeks, discontinue use or use on an "as-needed" basis
- Chronic muscle spasms may require chronic diazepam treatment
- For chronic anxiety disorders, the goal of treatment is complete remission of symptoms as well as prevention of future relapses
- For chronic anxiety disorders, treatment most often reduces or even eliminates symptoms, but not a cure since symptoms can recur after medicine stopped
- For long-term symptoms of anxiety, consider switching to an SSRI or SNRI for long-term maintenance
- If long-term maintenance with a benzodiazepine is necessary, continue treatment for 6 months after symptoms resolve, and then taper dose slowly
- If symptoms reemerge, consider treatment with an SSRI or SNRI, or consider restarting the benzodiazepine; sometimes benzodiazepines have to be used in combination with SSRIs or SNRIs for best results

If It Doesn't Work
- Consider switching to another agent or adding an appropriate augmenting agent
- Consider psychotherapy, especially cognitive behavioral psychotherapy
- Consider presence of concomitant substance abuse
- Consider presence of diazepam abuse
- Consider another diagnosis, such as a comorbid medical condition

Best Augmenting Combos for Partial Response or Treatment-Resistance
- Benzodiazepines are frequently used as augmenting agents for antipsychotics and mood stabilizers in the treatment of psychotic and bipolar disorders
- Benzodiazepines are frequently used as augmenting agents for SSRIs and SNRIs in the treatment of anxiety disorders

- Not generally rational to combine with other benzodiazepines
- Caution if using as an anxiolytic concomitantly with other sedative hypnotics for sleep

Tests

- In patients with seizure disorders, concomitant medical illness, and/or those with multiple concomitant long-term medications, periodic liver tests and blood counts may be prudent

SIDE EFFECTS

How Drug Causes Side Effects

- Same mechanism for side effects as for therapeutic effects – namely due to excessive actions at benzodiazepine receptors
- Long-term adaptations in benzodiazepine receptors may explain the development of dependence, tolerance, and withdrawal
- Side effects are generally immediate, but immediate side effects often disappear in time

Notable Side Effects

✻ Sedation, fatigue, depression
✻ Dizziness, ataxia, slurred speech, weakness
✻ Forgetfulness, confusion
✻ Hyperexcitability, nervousness
✻ Pain at injection site
- Rare hallucinations, mania
- Rare hypotension
- Hypersalivation, dry mouth

Life-Threatening or Dangerous Side Effects

- Respiratory depression, especially when taken with CNS depressants in overdose
- Rare hepatic dysfunction, renal dysfunction, blood dyscrasias

Weight Gain

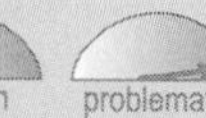

unusual not unusual common problematic

- Reported but not expected

Sedation

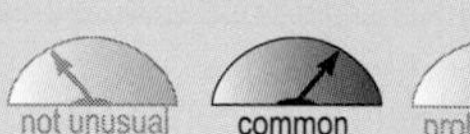

unusual not unusual common problematic

- Many experience and/or can be significant in amount
- Especially at initiation of treatment or when dose increases
- Tolerance often develops over time

What to Do About Side Effects

- Wait
- Wait
- Wait
- Lower the dose
- Take largest dose at bedtime to avoid sedative effects during the day
- Switch to another agent
- Administer flumazenil if side effects are severe or life-threatening

Best Augmenting Agents for Side Effects

- Many side effects cannot be improved with an augmenting agent

DOSING AND USE

Usual Dosage Range

- Oral: 4–40 mg/day in divided doses
- Intravenous (adults): 5 mg/minute
- Intravenous (children): 0.25 mg/kg every 3 minutes

Dosage Forms

- Tablet 2 mg scored, 5 mg scored, 10 mg scored
- Liquid 5 mg/5 mL, concentrate 5 mg/mL
- Injection vial 5 mg/mL; 10 mL, boxes of 1; 2 mL boxes of 10
- Rectal gel 5 mg/mL; 2.5 mg, 5 mg, 10 mg, 15 mg, 20 mg

How to Dose

- Oral (anxiety, muscle spasm, seizure): 2–10 mg, 2–4 times/day
- Oral (alcohol withdrawal): Initial 10 mg, 3–4 times/day for 1 day; reduce to 5 mg, 3–4 times/day; continue treatment as needed
- Liquid formulation should be mixed with water or fruit juice, applesauce, or pudding
- Because of risk of respiratory depression, rectal diazepam treatment should not be

given more than once in 5 days or more than twice during a treatment course, especially for alcohol withdrawal or status epilepticus

Dosing Tips

* ✻ Only benzodiazepine with a formulation specifically for rectal administration
* ✻ One of the few benzodiazepines available in an oral liquid formulation
* ✻ One of the few benzodiazepines available in an injectable formulation
* Diazepam injection is intended for acute use; patients who require long-term treatment should be switched to the oral formulation
* Use lowest possible effective dose for the shortest possible period of time (a benzodiazepine-sparing strategy)
* Assess need for continued treatment regularly
* Risk of dependence may increase with dose and duration of treatment
* For interdose symptoms of anxiety, can either increase dose or maintain same total daily dose but divide into more frequent doses
* Can also use an as-needed occasional "top up" dose for interdose anxiety
* Because some anxiety disorder patients and muscle spasm patients can require doses higher than 40 mg/day or more, the risk of dependence may be greater in these patients
* Frequency of dosing in practice is often greater than predicted from half-life, as duration of biological activity is often shorter than pharmacokinetic terminal half-life

Overdose

* Fatalities can occur; hypotension, tiredness, ataxia, confusion, coma

Long-Term Use

* Evidence of efficacy up to 16 weeks
* Risk of dependence, particularly for treatment periods longer than 12 weeks and especially in patients with past or current polysubstance abuse
* Not recommended for long-term treatment of seizure disorders

Habit Forming

* Diazepam is a Schedule IV drug
* Patients may develop dependence and/or tolerance with long-term use

How to Stop

* Patients with history of seizure may seize upon withdrawal, especially if withdrawal is abrupt
* Taper by 2 mg every 3 days to reduce chances of withdrawal effects
* For difficult to taper cases, consider reducing dose much more slowly after reaching 20 mg/day, perhaps by as little as 0.5–1 mg every week or less
* For other patients with severe problems discontinuing a benzodiazepine, dosing may need to be tapered over many months (i.e., reduce dose by 1% every 3 days by crushing tablet and suspending or dissolving in 100 mL of fruit juice and then disposing of 1 mL while drinking the rest; 3–7 days later, dispose of 2 mL, and so on). This is both a form of very slow biological tapering and a form of behavioral desensitization
* Be sure to differentiate reemergence of symptoms requiring reinstitution of treatment from withdrawal symptoms
* Benzodiazepine-dependent anxiety patients and insulin-dependent diabetics are not addicted to their medications. When benzodiazepine-dependent patients stop their medication, disease symptoms can reemerge, disease symptoms can worsen (rebound), and/or withdrawal symptoms can emerge

Pharmacokinetics

* Elimination half-life 20–50 hours

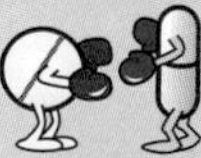

Drug Interactions

* Increased depressive effects when taken with other CNS depressants
* Cimetidine may reduce the clearance and raise the levels of diazepam
* Flumazenil (used to reverse the effects of benzodiazepines) may precipitate seizures and should not be used in patients treated for seizure disorders with diazepam

Other Warnings/ Precautions

- Dosage changes should be made in collaboration with prescriber
- Use with caution in patients with pulmonary disease; rare reports of death after initiation of benzodiazepines in patients with severe pulmonary impairment
- History of drug or alcohol abuse often creates greater risk for dependency
- Some depressed patients may experience a worsening of suicidal ideation
- Some patients may exhibit abnormal thinking or behavioral changes similar to those caused by other CNS depressants (i.e., either depressant actions or disinhibiting actions)

Do Not Use

- If narrow angle-closure glaucoma
- If there is a proven allergy to diazepam or any benzodiazepine

SPECIAL POPULATIONS

Renal Impairment

- Initial 2–2.5 mg, 1–2 times/day; increase gradually as needed

Hepatic Impairment

- Initial 2–2.5 mg, 1–2 times/day; increase gradually as needed

Cardiac Impairment

- Benzodiazepines have been used to treat anxiety associated with acute myocardial infarction
- Diazepam may be used as an adjunct during cardiovascular emergencies

Elderly

- Initial 2–2.5 mg, 1–2 times/day; increase gradually as needed

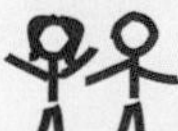

Children and Adolescents

- 6 months and up: Initial 1–2.5 mg, 3–4 times/day; increase gradually as needed
- Parenteral: 30 days or older
- Rectal: 2 years or older
- Long-term effects of diazepam in children/adolescents are unknown
- Should generally receive lower doses and be more closely monitored

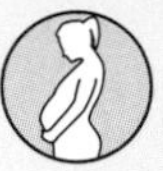

Pregnancy

- Risk Category D [positive evidence of risk to human fetus; potential benefits may still justify its use during pregnancy]
- Possible increased risk of birth defects when benzodiazepines taken during pregnancy
- Because of the potential risks, diazepam is not generally recommended as treatment for anxiety during pregnancy, especially during the first trimester
- Drug should be tapered if discontinued
- Infants whose mothers received a benzodiazepine late in pregnancy may experience withdrawal effects
- Neonatal flaccidity has been reported in infants whose mothers took a benzodiazepine during pregnancy
- Seizures, even mild seizures, may cause harm to the embryo/fetus

Breast Feeding

- Unknown if diazepam is secreted in human breast milk, but all psychotropics assumed to be secreted in breast milk

* Recommended either to discontinue drug or bottle feed

- Effects of benzodiazepines on nursing infants have been reported and include feeding difficulties, sedation, and weight loss

THE ART OF PSYCHOPHARMACOLOGY

Potential Advantages

- Rapid onset of action
- Availability of oral liquid, rectal, and injectable dosage formulations

Potential Disadvantages

- Euphoria may lead to abuse
- Abuse especially risky in past or present substance abusers
- Can be sedating at doses necessary to treat moderately severe anxiety disorders

Primary Target Symptoms

- Panic attacks
- Anxiety

- Incidence of seizures (adjunct)
- Muscle spasms

Pearls

- Can be a useful adjunct to SSRIs and SNRIs in the treatment of numerous anxiety disorders, but not used as frequently as other benzodiazepines for this purpose
- Not effective for treating psychosis as a monotherapy, but can be used as an adjunct to antipsychotics
- Not effective for treating bipolar disorder as a monotherapy, but can be used as an adjunct to mood stabilizers and antipsychotics
- ✻ Diazepam is often the first choice benzodiazepine to treat status epilepticus, and is administered either intravenously or rectally
- Because diazepam suppresses stage 4 sleep, it may prevent night terrors in adults
- May both cause depression and treat depression in different patients
- Was once one of the most commonly prescribed drugs in the world and the most commonly prescribed benzodiazepine
- ✻ Remains a popular benzodiazepine for treating muscle spasms
- A commonly used benzodiazepine to treat sleep disorders
- ✻ Remains a popular benzodiazepine to treat acute alcohol withdrawal
- Not especially useful as an oral anticonvulsant
- ✻ Multiple dosage formulations (oral tablet, oral liquid, rectal gel, injectable) allow more flexibility of administration compared to most other benzodiazepines
- When using to treat insomnia, remember that insomnia may be a symptom of some other primary disorder itself, and thus warrant evaluation for comorbid psychiatric and/or medical conditions

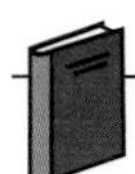

Suggested Reading

Ashton H. Guidelines for the rational use of benzodiazepines. When and what to use. Drugs 1994;48:25–40.

De Negri M, Baglietto MG. Treatment of status epilepticus in children. Paediatr Drugs 2001; 3:411–20.

Mandelli M, Tognoni G, Garattini S. Clinical pharmacokinetics of diazepam. Clin Pharmacokinet 1978;3:72–91.

Rey E. Treluver JM, Pons G. Pharmacokinetic optimization of benzodiazepine therapy for acute seizures. Focus on delivery routes. Clin Pharmacokinet 1999;36:409–24.

THERAPEUTICS

Brands • Aricept
• Memac

see index for additional brand names

Generic? No

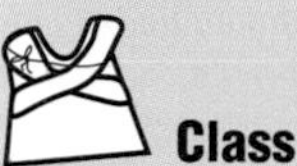

Class

- Cholinesterase inhibitor (selective acetylcholinesterase inhibitor); cognitive enhancer

Commonly Prescribed for

(bold for FDA approved)

- **Alzheimer disease (mild, moderate, and severe)**
- Memory disorders in other conditions
- Mild cognitive impairment

How the Drug Works

✻ Reversibly but noncompetitively inhibits centrally active acetylcholinesterase (AChE), making more acetylcholine available
- Increased availability of acetylcholine compensates in part for degenerating cholinergic neurons in neocortex that regulate memory
- Does not inhibit butyrylcholinesterase
- May release growth factors or interfere with amyloid deposition

How Long Until It Works

- May take up to 6 weeks before any improvement in baseline memory or behavior is evident
- May take months before any stabilization in degenerative course is evident

If It Works

- May improve symptoms and slow progression of disease, but does not reverse the degenerative process

If It Doesn't Work

- Consider adjusting dose, switching to a different cholinesterase inhibitor or adding an appropriate augmenting agent
- Reconsider diagnosis and rule out other conditions such as depression or a dementia other than Alzheimer disease

Best Augmenting Combos for Partial Response or Treatment Resistance

✻ Atypical antipsychotics to reduce behavioral disturbances
✻ Antidepressants if concomitant depression, apathy, or lack of interest
✻ Memantine for moderate to severe Alzheimer disease
- Divalproex, carbamazepine, or oxcarbazepine for behavioral disturbances
- Not rational to combine with another cholinesterase inhibitor

Tests

- None for healthy individuals

SIDE EFFECTS

How Drug Causes Side Effects

- Peripheral inhibition of acetylcholinesterase can cause gastrointestinal side effects
- Central inhibition of acetylcholinesterase may contribute to nausea, vomiting, weight loss, and sleep disturbances

Notable Side Effects

✻ Nausea, diarrhea, vomiting, appetite loss, increased gastric acid secretion, weight loss
- Insomnia, dizziness
- Muscle cramps, fatigue, depression, abnormal dreams

Life-Threatening or Dangerous Side Effects

- Rare seizures
- Rare syncope

Weight Gain

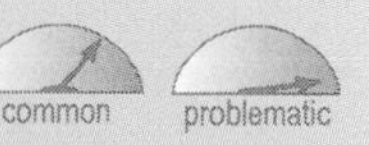

- Reported but not expected
- Some patients may experience weight loss

Sedation

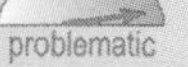

- Reported but not expected

What to Do About Side Effects

- Wait
- Wait

- Wait
- Take in daytime to reduce insomnia
- Use slower dose titration
- Consider lowering dose, switching to a different agent or adding an appropriate augmenting agent

Best Augmenting Agents for Side Effects

- Hypnotics or trazodone may improve insomnia
- Many side effects cannot be improved with an augmenting agent

DOSING AND USE

Usual Dosage Range

- 5–10 mg at night

Dosage Forms

- Tablet 5 mg, 10 mg
- Orally disintegrating tablet 5 mg, 10 mg

How To Dose

- Initial 5 mg/day; may increase to 10 mg/day after 4–6 weeks

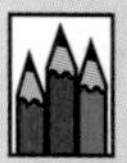

Dosing Tips/

- Side effects occur more frequently at 10 mg/day than at 5 mg/day
- Slower titration (e.g., 6 weeks to 10 mg/day) may reduce the risk of side effects
- Food does not affect the absorption of donepezil
- Probably best to utilize highest tolerated dose within the usual dosage range
- Some off-label uses for cognitive disturbances other than Alzheimer disease have anecdotally utilized doses higher than 10 mg/day

✻ When switching to another cholinesterase inhibitor, probably best to cross-titrate from one to the other to prevent precipitous decline in function if the patient washes out of one drug entirely

Overdose

- Can be lethal; nausea, vomiting, excess salivation, sweating, hypotension, bradycardia, collapse, convulsions, muscle weakness (weakness of respiratory muscles can lead to death)

Long-Term Use

- Drug may lose effectiveness in slowing degenerative course of Alzheimer disease after 6 months
- Can be effective in some patients for several years

Habit Forming

- No

How to Stop

- Taper to avoid withdrawal effects
- Discontinuation may lead to notable deterioration in memory and behavior, which may not be restored when drug is restarted or another cholinesterase inhibitor is initiated

Pharmacokinetics

- Metabolized by CYP450 2D6 and CYP450 3A4
- Elimination half-life approximately 70 hours

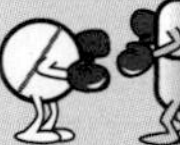

Drug Interactions

- Donepezil may increase the effects of anesthetics and should be discontinued prior to surgery
- Inhibitors of CYP450 2D6 and CYP450 3A4 may inhibit donepezil metabolism and increase its plasma levels
- Inducers of CYP450 2D6 and CYP450 3A4 may increase clearance of donepezil and decrease its plasma levels
- Donepezil may interact with anticholinergic agents and the combination may decrease the efficacy of both
- May have synergistic effect if administered with cholinomimetics (e.g., bethanechol)
- Bradycardia may occur if combined with beta blockers
- Theoretically, could reduce the efficacy of levodopa in Parkinson's disease
- Not rational to combine with another cholinesterase inhibitor

Other Warnings/ Precautions

- May exacerbate asthma or other pulmonary disease
- Increased gastric acid secretion may increase the risk of ulcers
- Bradycardia or heart block may occur in patients with or without cardiac impairment

Do Not Use
- If there is a proven allergy to donepezil

SPECIAL POPULATIONS

Renal Impairment
- Few data available but dose adjustment is most likely unnecessary

Hepatic Impairment
- Few data available; may need to lower dose

Cardiac Impairment
- Should be used with caution
- Syncopal episodes have been reported with the use of donepezil

Elderly
- Some patients may tolerate lower doses better

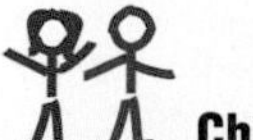

Children and Adolescents
- Safety and efficacy have not been established
- Preliminary reports of efficacy as an adjunct in attention deficit hyperactivity disorder (ADHD) (ages 8–17)

Pregnancy
- Risk Category C [some animal studies show adverse effects; no controlled studies in humans]

✻ Not recommended for use in pregnant women or women of childbearing potential

Breast Feeding
- Unknown if donepezil is secreted in human breast milk, but all psychotropics assumed to be secreted in breast milk

✻ Recommended either to discontinue drug or bottle feed

- Donepezil is not recommended for use in nursing women

THE ART OF PSYCHOPHARMACOLOGY

Potential Advantages
- Once a day dosing
- May be used in vascular dementia
- May work in some patients who do not respond to other cholinesterase inhibitors
- May work in some patients who do not tolerate other cholinesterase inhibitors

Potential Disadvantages
- Patients with insomnia

Primary Target Symptoms
- Memory loss in Alzheimer disease
- Behavioral symptoms in Alzheimer disease
- Memory loss in other dementias

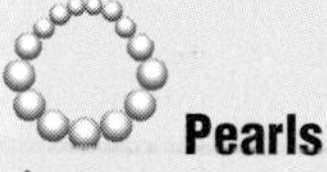

Pearls

✻ One of only two drugs indicated for moderate to severe Alzheimer disease

- Dramatic reversal of symptoms of Alzheimer disease is not generally seen with cholinesterase inhibitors
- Can lead to therapeutic nihilism among prescribers and lack of an appropriate trial of a cholinesterase inhibitor

✻ Perhaps only 50% of Alzheimer patients are diagnosed, and only 50% of those diagnosed are treated, and only 50% of those treated are given a cholinesterase inhibitor, and then only for 200 days in a disease that lasts 7–10 years

- Must evaluate lack of efficacy and loss of efficacy over months, not weeks

✻ Treats behavioral and psychological symptoms of Alzheimer dementia as well as cognitive symptoms (i.e., especially apathy, disinhibition, delusions, anxiety, cooperation, pacing)

- Patients who complain themselves of memory problems may have depression, whereas patients whose spouses or children complain of the patient's memory problems may have Alzheimer disease
- Treat the patient but ask the caregiver about efficacy
- What you see may depend upon how early you treat
- The first symptoms of Alzheimer disease are generally mood changes; thus, Alzheimer disease may initially be diagnosed as depression

- Women may experience cognitive symptoms in perimenopause as a result of hormonal changes that are not a sign of dementia or Alzheimer disease
- Aggressively treat concomitant symptoms with augmentation (e.g., atypical antipsychotics for agitation, antidepressants for depression)
- If treatment with antidepressants fails to improve apathy and depressed mood in the elderly, it is possible that this represents early Alzheimer disease and a cholinesterase inhibitor like donepezil may be helpful
- What to expect from a cholinesterase inhibitor:
  - Patients do not generally improve dramatically although this can be observed in a significant minority of patients
  - Onset of behavioral problems and nursing home placement can be delayed
  - Functional outcomes, including activities of daily living, can be preserved
  - Caregiver burden and stress can be reduced
- Delay in progression in Alzheimer disease is not evidence of disease-modifying actions of cholinesterase inhibition
- Cholinesterase inhibitors like donepezil depend upon the presence of intact targets for acetylcholine for maximum effectiveness and thus may be most effective in the early stages of Alzheimer disease
- The most prominent side effects of donepezil are gastrointestinal effects, which are usually mild and transient

✱ May cause more sleep disturbances than some other cholinesterase inhibitors

- For patients with intolerable side effects, generally allow a washout period with resolution of side effects prior to switching to another cholinesterase inhibitor
- Weight loss can be a problem in Alzheimer patients with debilitation and muscle wasting
- Women over 85, particularly with low body weights, may experience more adverse effects
- Use with caution in underweight or frail patients
- Cognitive improvement may be linked to substantial (>65%) inhibition of acetylcholinesterase
- Donepezil has greater action on CNS acetylcholinesterase than on peripheral acetylcholinesterase
- Some Alzheimer patients who fail to respond to donepezil may respond to another cholinesterase inhibitor
- Some Alzheimer patients who fail to respond to another cholinesterase inhibitor may respond when switched to donepezil
- To prevent potential clinical deterioration, generally switch from long-term treatment with one cholinesterase inhibitor to another without a washout period

✱ Donepezil may slow the progression of mild cognitive impairment to Alzheimer disease

✱ May be useful for dementia with Lewy bodies (DLB, constituted by early loss of attentiveness and visual perception with possible hallucinations, Parkinson-like movement problems, fluctuating cognition such as daytime drowsiness and lethargy, staring into space for long periods, episodes of disorganized speech)

- May decrease delusions, apathy, agitation, and hallucinations in dementia with Lewy bodies

✱ May be useful for vascular dementia (e.g., acute onset with slow stepwise progression that has plateaus, often with gait abnormalities, focal signs, imbalance, and urinary incontinence)

- May be helpful for dementia in Down's syndrome
- Suggestions of utility in some cases of treatment-resistant bipolar disorder
- Theoretically, may be useful for ADHD, but not yet proven
- Theoretically, could be useful in any memory condition characterized by cholinergic deficiency (e.g., some cases of brain injury, cancer chemotherapy-induced cognitive changes, etc.)

Suggested Reading

Bentue-Ferrer D, Tribut O, Polard E, Allain H. Clinically significant drug interactions with cholinesterase inhibitors: a guide for neurologists. CNS Drugs 2003;17:947–63.

Birks, JS, Harvey R. Donepezil for dementia due to Alzheimer's disease. Cochrane Database Syst Rev 2003;CD001190.

Bonner LT, Peskind ER. Pharmacologic treatments of dementia. Med Clin North Am 2002;86:657–74.

Jones RW. Have cholinergic therapies reached their clinical boundary in Alzheimer's disease? Int J Geriatr Psychiatry 2003;18(Suppl 1): S7–S13.

Seltzer B. Donepezil: an update. Expert Opin Pharmacother 2007;8(7):1011–23.

THERAPEUTICS

Brands • Prothiaden

see index for additional brand names

Generic? In United Kingdom

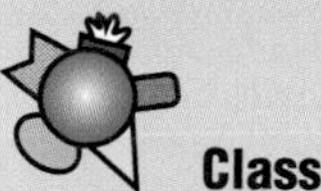

Class

- Tricyclic antidepressant (TCA)
- Serotonin and norepinephrine/noradrenaline reuptake inhibitor

Commonly Prescribed for

(bold for FDA approved)

- Major depressive disorder
- Anxiety
- Insomnia
- Neuropathic pain/chronic pain
- Treatment-resistant depression

How the Drug Works

- Boosts neurotransmitters serotonin and norepinephrine/noradrenaline
- Blocks serotonin reuptake pump (serotonin transporter), presumably increasing serotonergic neurotransmission
- Blocks norepinephrine reuptake pump (norepinephrine transporter), presumably increasing noradrenergic neurotransmission
- Presumably by desensitizes both serotonin 1A receptors and beta adrenergic receptors
- Since dopamine is inactivated by norepinephrine reuptake in frontal cortex, which largely lacks dopamine transporters, dothiepin can increase dopamine neurotransmission in this part of the brain

How Long Until It Works

- May have immediate effects in treating insomnia or anxiety
- Onset of therapeutic actions usually not immediate, but often delayed 2–4 weeks
- If it is not working within 6–8 weeks for depression, it may require a dosage increase or it may not work at all
- May continue to work for many years to prevent relapse of symptoms

If It Works

- The goal of treatment of depression is complete remission of current symptoms as well as prevention of future relapses
- The goal of treatment of chronic neuropathic pain is to reduce symptoms as much as possible, especially in combination with other treatments
- Treatment of depression most often reduces or even eliminates symptoms, but not a cure since symptoms can recur after medicine stopped
- Treatment of chronic neuropathic pain may reduce symptoms, but rarely eliminates them completely, and is not a cure since symptoms can recur after medicine is stopped
- Continue treatment of depression until all symptoms are gone (remission)
- Once symptoms of depression are gone, continue treating for 1 year for the first episode of depression
- For second and subsequent episodes of depression, treatment may need to be indefinite
- Use in anxiety disorders and chronic pain may also need to be indefinite, but long-term treatment is not well studied in these conditions

If It Doesn't Work

- Many depressed patients only have a partial response where some symptoms are improved but others persist (especially insomnia, fatigue, and problems concentrating)
- Other depressed patients may be nonresponders, sometimes called treatment-resistant or treatment-refractory
- Consider increasing dose, switching to another agent or adding an appropriate augmenting agent
- Consider psychotherapy
- Consider evaluation for another diagnosis or for a comorbid condition (e.g, medical illness, substance abuse, etc.)
- Some patients may experience apparent lack of consistent efficacy due to activation of latent or underlying bipolar disorder, and require antidepressant discontinuation and a switch to a mood stabilizer

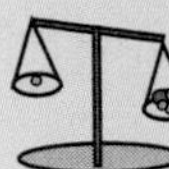

Best Augmenting Combos for Partial Response or Treatment Resistance

- Lithium, buspirone, thyroid hormone (for depression)
- Gabapentin, tiagabine, other anticonvulsants, even opiates if done by experts while monitoring carefully in difficult cases (for chronic pain)

Tests

- None for healthy individuals

✻ Since tricyclic and tetracyclic antidepressants are frequently associated with weight gain, before starting treatment, weigh all patients and determine if the patient is already overweight (BMI 25.0–29.9) or obese (BMI ≥30)

- Before giving a drug that can cause weight gain to an overweight or obese patient, consider determining whether the patient already has pre-diabetes (fasting plasma glucose 100–25 mg/dL), diabetes (fasting plasma glucose >126 mg/dL), or dyslipidemia (increased total cholesterol, LDL cholesterol and triglycerides; decreased HDL cholesterol), and treat or refer such patients for treatment including nutrition and weight management, physical activity counseling, smoking cessation, and medical management

✻ Monitor weight and BMI during treatment

✻ While giving a drug to a patient who has gained >5% of initial weight, consider evaluating for the presence of pre-diabetes, diabetes, or dyslipidemia, or consider switching to a different antidepressant

- EKGs may be useful for selected patients (e.g., those with personal or family history of QTc prolongation; cardiac arrhythmia; recent myocardial infarction; uncompensated heart failure; or taking agents that prolong QTc interval such as pimozide, thioridazine, selected antiarrhythmics, moxifloxacin, sparfloxacin, etc.)
- Patients at risk for electrolyte disturbances (e.g., patients on diuretic therapy) should have baseline and periodic serum potassium and magnesium measurements

SIDE EFFECTS

How Drug Causes Side Effects

- Anticholinergic activity may explain sedative effects, dry mouth, constipation, and blurred vision
- Sedative effects and weight gain may be due to antihistamine properties
- Blockade of alpha adrenergic 1 receptors may explain dizziness, sedation, and hypotension
- Cardiac arrhythmias and seizures, especially in overdose, may be caused by blockade of ion channels

Notable Side Effects

- Blurred vision, constipation, urinary retention, increased appetite, dry mouth, nausea, diarrhea, heartburn, unusual taste in mouth, weight gain
- Fatigue, weakness, dizziness, sedation, headache, anxiety, nervousness, restlessness
- Sexual dysfunction, sweating

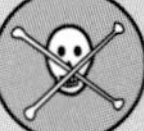

Life-Threatening or Dangerous Side Effects

- Paralytic ileus, hyperthermia (TCAs + anticholinergic agents)
- Lowered seizure threshold and rare seizures
- Orthostatic hypotension, sudden death, arrhythmias, tachycardia
- QTc prolongation
- Hepatic failure, extrapyramidal symptoms
- Increased intraocular pressure
- Rare induction of mania
- Rare activation of suicidal ideation and behavior (suicidality) (short-term studies did not show an increase in the risk of suicidality with antidepressants compared to placebo beyond age 24)

Weight Gain

unusual not unusual **common** problematic

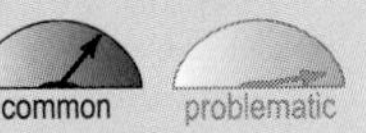

- Many experience and/or can be significant in amount
- Can increase appetite and carbohydrate craving

Sedation

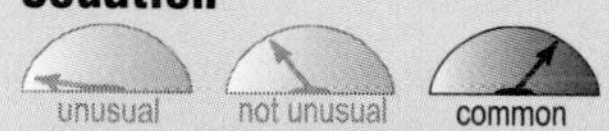

- Many experience and/or can be significant in amount
- Tolerance to sedative effect may develop with long-term use

What to Do About Side Effects

- Wait
- Wait
- Wait
- Lower the dose
- Switch to an SSRI or newer antidepressant

Best Augmenting Agents for Side Effects

- Many side effects cannot be improved with an augmenting agent

DOSING AND USE

Usual Dosage Range

- 75–150 mg/day

Dosage Forms

- Capsule 25 mg
- Tablet 75 mg

How To Dose

- 75 mg/day once daily or in divided doses; gradually increase dose to achieve desired therapeutic effect; maximum dose 300 mg/day

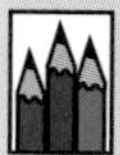

Dosing Tips

- If given in a single dose, should generally be administered at bedtime because of its sedative properties
- If given in split doses, largest dose should generally be given at bedtime because of its sedative properties
- If patients experience nightmares, split dose and do not give large dose at bedtime
- Patients treated for chronic pain may only require lower doses
- Risk of seizure increases with dose
- If intolerable anxiety, insomnia, agitation, akathisia, or activation occur either upon dosing initiation or discontinuation, consider the possibility of activated bipolar disorder, and switch to a mood stabilizer or an atypical antipsychotic

Overdose

- Death may occur; convulsions, cardiac dysrhythmias, severe hypotension, CNS depression, coma, changes in EKG

Long-Term Use

- Safe

Habit Forming

- No

How to Stop

- Taper to avoid withdrawal effects
- Even with gradual dose reduction some withdrawal symptoms may appear within the first 2 weeks
- Many patients tolerate 50% dose reduction for 3 days, then another 50% reduction for 3 days, then discontinuation
- If withdrawal symptoms emerge during discontinuation, raise dose to stop symptoms and then restart withdrawal much more slowly

Pharmacokinetics

- Substrate for CYP450 2D6
- Half-life approximately 14–40 hours

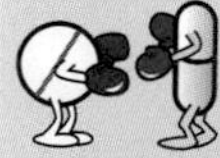

Drug Interactions

- Tramadol increases the risk of seizures in patients taking TCAs
- Use of TCAs with anticholinergic drugs may result in paralytic ileus or hyperthermia
- Fluoxetine, paroxetine, bupropion, duloxetine, and other CYP450 2D6 inhibitors may increase TCA concentrations
- Cimetidine may increase plasma concentrations of TCAs and cause anticholinergic symptoms
- Phenothiazines or haloperidol may raise TCA blood concentrations
- May alter effects of antihypertensive drugs; may inhibit hypotensive effects of clonidine
- Use of TCAs with sympathomimetic agents may increase sympathetic activity
- Methylphenidate may inhibit metabolism of TCAs
- Activation and agitation, especially following switching or adding antidepressants, may represent the

induction of a bipolar state, especially a mixed dysphoric bipolar II condition sometimes associated with suicidal ideation, and require the addition of lithium, a mood stabilizer or an atypical antipsychotic, and/or discontinuation of dothiepin

Other Warnings/ Precautions

- Add or initiate other antidepressants with caution for up to 2 weeks after discontinuing dothiepin
- Generally, do not use with MAO inhibitors, including 14 days after MAOIs are stopped; do not start an MAOI until 2 weeks after discontinuing dothiepin, but see Pearls
- Use with caution in patients with history of seizures, urinary retention, narrow angle-closure glaucoma, hyperthyroidism, and in patients recovering from myocardial infarction
- TCAs can increase QTc interval, especially at toxic doses, which can be attained not only by overdose but also by combining with drugs that inhibit TCA metabolism via CYP450 2D6, potentially causing torsade de pointes-type arrhythmia or sudden death
- Because TCAs can prolong QTc interval, use with caution in patients who have bradycardia or who are taking drugs that can induce bradycardia (e.g., beta blockers, calcium channel blockers, clonidine, digitalis)
- Because TCAs can prolong QTc interval, use with caution in patients who have hypokalemia and/or hypomagnesemia or who are taking drugs that can induce hypokalemia and/or magnesemia (e.g., diuretics, stimulant laxatives, intravenous amphotericin B, glucocorticoids, tetracosactide)
- When treating children, carefully weigh the risks and benefits of pharmacological treatment against the risks and benefits of nontreatment with antidepressants and make sure to document this in the patient's chart
- Distribute the brochures provided by the FDA and the drug companies
- Warn patients and their caregivers about the possibility of activating side effects and advise them to report such symptoms immediately
- Monitor patients for activation of suicidal ideation, especially children and adolescents

Do Not Use

- If patient is recovering from myocardial infarction
- If patient is taking agents capable of significantly prolonging QTc interval (e.g., pimozide, thioridazine, selected antiarrhythmics, moxifloxacin, sparfloxacin)
- If there is a history of QTc prolongation or cardiac arrhythmia, recent acute myocardial infarction, uncompensated heart failure
- If patient is taking drugs that inhibit TCA metabolism, including CYP450 2D6 inhibitors, except by an expert
- If there is reduced CYP450 2D6 function, such as patients who are poor 2D6 metabolizers, except by an expert and at low doses
- If there is a proven allergy to dothiepin

SPECIAL POPULATIONS

Renal Impairment

- Use with caution

Hepatic Impairment

- Use with caution

Cardiac Impairment

- TCAs have been reported to cause arrhythmias, prolongation of conduction time, orthostatic hypotension, sinus tachycardia, and heart failure, especially in the diseased heart
- Myocardial infarction and stroke have been reported with TCAs
- TCAs produce QTc prolongation, which may be enhanced by the existence of bradycardia, hypokalemia, congenital or acquired long QTc interval, which should be evaluated prior to administering dothiepin
- Use with caution if treating concomitantly with a medication likely to produce prolonged bradycardia, hypokalemia, slowing of intracardiac conduction, or prolongation of the QTc interval

- Avoid TCAs in patients with a known history of QTc prolongation, recent acute myocardial infarction, and uncompensated heart failure
- TCAs may cause a sustained increase in heart rate in patients with ischemic heart disease and may worsen (decrease) heart rate variability, an independent risk of mortality in cardiac populations
- Since SSRIs may improve (increase) heart rate variability in patients following a myocardial infarct and may improve survival as well as mood in patients with acute angina or following a myocardial infarction, these are more appropriate agents for cardiac population than tricyclic/tetracyclic antidepressants
- ✻ Risk/benefit ratio may not justify use of TCAs in cardiac impairment

Elderly

- May be more sensitive to anticholinergic, cardiovascular, hypotensive, and sedative effects
- Reduction in risk of suicidality with antidepressants compared to placebo in adults age 65 and older

Children and Adolescents

- Carefully weigh the risks and benefits of pharmacological treatment against the risks and benefits of nontreatment with antidepressants and make sure to document this in the patient's chart
- Monitor patients face-to-face regularly, particularly during the first several weeks of treatment
- Use with caution, observing for activation of known or unknown bipolar disorder and/or suicidal ideation, and inform parents or guardian of this risk so they can help observe child or adolescent patients
- Not recommended for use in children under age 18
- Several studies show lack of efficacy of TCAs for depression
- May be used to treat enuresis or hyperactive/impulsive behaviors
- Some cases of sudden death have occurred in children taking TCAs

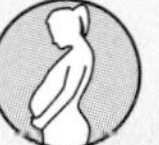

Pregnancy

- Risk Category C [some animal studies show adverse effects; no controlled studies in humans]
- Crosses the placenta
- Adverse effects have been reported in infants whose mothers took a TCA (lethargy, withdrawal symptoms, fetal malformations)
- Not generally recommended for use during pregnancy, especially during first trimester
- Must weigh the risk of treatment (first trimester fetal development, third trimester newborn delivery) to the child against the risk of no treatment (recurrence of depression, maternal health, infant bonding) to the mother and child
- For many patients this may mean continuing treatment during pregnancy

Breast Feeding

- Some drug is found in mother's breast milk
- ✻ Recommended either to discontinue drug or bottle feed
- Immediate postpartum period is a high-risk time for depression, especially in women who have had prior depressive episodes, so drug may need to be reinstituted late in the third trimester or shortly after childbirth to prevent a recurrence during the postpartum period
- Must weigh benefits of breast feeding with risks and benefits of antidepressant treatment versus nontreatment to both the infant and the mother
- For many patients this may mean continuing treatment during breast feeding

THE ART OF PSYCHOPHARMACOLOGY

Potential Advantages

- Patients with insomnia
- Severe or treatment-resistant depression
- Anxious depression

Potential Disadvantages

- Pediatric and geriatric patients
- Patients concerned with weight gain
- Cardiac patients

Primary Target Symptoms

- Depressed mood
- Chronic pain

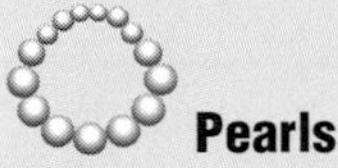

Pearls

* ✻ Close structural similarity to amitriptyline
* Tricyclic antidepressants are often a first-line treatment option for chronic pain
* Tricyclic antidepressants are no longer generally considered a first-line option for depression because of their side effect profile
* Tricyclic antidepressants continue to be useful for severe or treatment-resistant depression
* TCAs may aggravate psychotic symptoms
* Alcohol should be avoided because of additive CNS effects
* Underweight patients may be more susceptible to adverse cardiovascular effects
* Children, patients with inadequate hydration, and patients with cardiac disease may be more susceptible to TCA-induced cardiotoxicity than healthy adults
* For the expert only: a heroic treatment (but potentially dangerous) for severely treatment-resistant patients is to give simultaneously with monoamine oxidase inhibitors for patients who fail to respond to numerous other antidepressants, but generally recommend a different TCA than dothiepin for this use
* If this option is elected, start the MAOI with the tricyclic/tetracyclic antidepressant simultaneously at low doses after appropriate drug washout, then alternately increase doses of these agents every few days to a week as tolerated
* Although very strict dietary and concomitant drug restrictions must be observed to prevent hypertensive crises and serotonin syndrome, the most common side effects of MAOI and tricyclic/tetracyclic antidepressant combinations may be weight gain and orthostatic hypotension
* Patients on TCAs should be aware that they may experience symptoms such as photosensitivity or blue-green urine
* SSRIs may be more effective than TCAs in women, and TCAs may be more effective than SSRIs in men
* Since tricyclic/tetracyclic antidepressants are substrates for CYP450 2D6, and 7% of the population (especially Caucasians) may have a genetic variant leading to reduced activity of 2D6, such patients may not safely tolerate normal doses of tricyclic/tetracyclic antidepressants and may require dose reduction
* Phenotypic testing may be necessary to detect this genetic variant prior to dosing with a tricyclic/tetracyclic antidepressant, especially in vulnerable populations such as children, elderly, cardiac populations, and those on concomitant medications
* Patients who seem to have extraordinarily severe side effects at normal or low doses may have this phenotypic CYP450 2D6 variant and require low doses or switching to another antidepressant not metabolized by 2D6

Suggested Reading

Anderson IM. Meta-analytical studies on new antidepressants. Br Med Bull 2001;57:161–78.

Anderson IM. Selective serotonin reuptake inhibitors versus tricyclic antidepressants: a meta-analysis of efficacy and tolerability. J Aff Disorders 2000;58:19–36.

Donovan S, Dearden L, Richardson L. The tolerability of dothiepin: a review of clinical studies between 1963 and 1990 in over 13,000 depressed patients. Prog Neuropsychopharmacol Biol Psychiatry 1994; 18:1143–62.

Lancaster SG, Gonzalez JP. Dothiepin. A review of its pharmacodynamic and pharmacokinetic properties, and therapeutic efficacy in depressive illness. Drugs 1989; 38:123–47.

THERAPEUTICS

Brands • Sinequan

see index for additional brand names

Generic? Yes

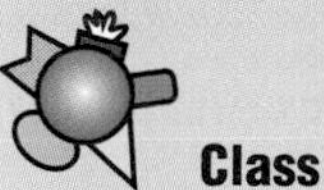

Class

- Tricyclic antidepressant (TCA)
- Serotonin and norepinephrine/noradrenaline reuptake inhibitor

Commonly Prescribed for

(bold for FDA approved)

- **Psychoneurotic patient with depression and/or anxiety**
- **Depression and/or anxiety associated with alcoholism**
- **Depression and/or anxiety associated with organic disease**
- **Psychotic depressive disorders with associated anxiety**
- **Involutional depression**
- **Manic-depressive disorder**
- Insomnia

✻ Pruritus/itching (topical)
- Dermatitis, atopic (topical)
- Lichen simplex chronicus (topical)
- Anxiety
- Neuropathic pain/chronic pain
- Treatment-resistant depression

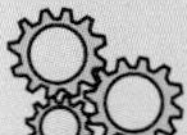

How the Drug Works

At antidepressant doses:
- Boosts neurotransmitters serotonin and norepinephrine/noradrenaline
- Blocks serotonin reuptake pump (serotonin transporter), presumably increasing serotonergic neurotransmission
- Blocks norepinephrine reuptake pump (norepinephrine transporter), presumably increasing noradrenergic neurotransmission
- Presumably by desensitizes both serotonin 1A receptors and beta adrenergic receptors
- Since dopamine is inactivated by norepinephrine reuptake in frontal cortex, which largely lacks dopamine transporters, doxepin can thus increase dopamine neurotransmission in this part of the brain
- May be effective in treating skin conditions because of its strong antihistamine properties

At low doses (1–6 mg/day):
- Selectively and potently blocks histamine 1 receptors, presumably decreasing wakefulness and thus promoting sleep

How Long Until It Works

- May have immediate effects in treating insomnia or anxiety
- Onset of therapeutic actions usually not immediate, but often delayed 2–4 weeks
- If it is not working within 6–8 weeks for depression, it may require a dosage increase or it may not work at all
- May continue to work for many years to prevent relapse of symptoms

If It Works

- The goal of treatment of depression is complete remission of current symptoms as well as prevention of future relapses
- The goal of treatment of insomnia is to improve quality of sleep, including effects on total wake time and number of nighttime awakenings
- The goal of treatment of chronic neuropathic pain is to reduce symptoms as much as possible, especially in combination with other treatments
- Treatment of depression most often reduces or even eliminates symptoms, but not a cure since symptoms can recur after medicine stopped
- Treatment of chronic neuropathic pain may reduce symptoms, but rarely eliminates them completely, and is not a cure since symptoms can recur after medicine is stopped
- Continue treatment of depression until all symptoms are gone (remission)
- Once symptoms of depression are gone, continue treating for 1 year for the first episode of depression
- For second and subsequent episodes of depression, treatment may need to be indefinite
- Use in insomia, anxiety disorders, chronic pain, and skin conditions may also need to

be indefinite, but long-term treatment is not well studied in these conditions

If It Doesn't Work

- Many depressed patients only have a partial response where some symptoms are improved but others persist (especially insomnia, fatigue, and problems concentrating)
- Other depressed patients may be nonresponders, sometimes called treatment-resistant or treatment-refractory
- Consider increasing dose, switching to another agent or adding an appropriate augmenting agent
- Consider psychotherapy
- Consider evaluation for another diagnosis or for a comorbid condition (e.g., medical illness, substance abuse, etc.)
- Some patients may experience apparent lack of consistent efficacy due to activation of latent or underlying bipolar disorder, and require antidepressant discontinuation and a switch to a mood stabilizer
- If insomnia does not improve after 7–10 days, it may be a manifestation of a primary psychiatric or physical illness such as obstructive sleep apnea or restless leg syndrome, which requires independent evaluation

Best Augmenting Combos for Partial Response or Treatment Resistance

- Lithium, buspirone, thyroid hormone (for depression)
- Trazodone, GABA-ergic sedative hypnotics (for insomnia)
- Gabapentin, tiagabine, other anticonvulsants, even opiates if done by experts while monitoring carefully in difficult cases (for chronic pain)

Tests

- None for healthy individuals
- ✱ Since tricyclic and tetracyclic antidepressants are frequently associated with weight gain, before starting treatment, weigh all patients and determine if the patient is already overweight (BMI 25.0–29.9) or obese (BMI ≥30)
- Before giving a drug that can cause weight gain to an overweight or obese patient, consider determining whether the patient already has pre-diabetes (fasting plasma glucose 100–25 mg/dL), diabetes (fasting plasma glucose >126 mg/dL), or dyslipidemia (increased total cholesterol, LDL cholesterol and triglycerides; decreased HDL cholesterol), and treat or refer such patients for treatment including nutrition and weight management, physical activity counseling, smoking cessation, and medical management
- ✱ Monitor weight and BMI during treatment
- ✱ While giving a drug to a patient who has gained >5% of initial weight, consider evaluating for the presence of pre-diabetes, diabetes, or dyslipidemia, or consider switching to a different antidepressant
- EKGs may be useful for selected patients (e.g., those with personal or family history of QTc prolongation; cardiac arrhythmia; recent myocardial infarction; uncompensated heart failure; or taking agents that prolong QTc interval such as pimozide, thioridazine, selected antiarrhythmics, moxifloxacin, sparfloxacin, etc.)
- Patients at risk for electrolyte disturbances (e.g., patients on diuretic therapy) should have baseline and periodic serum potassium and magnesium measurements

SIDE EFFECTS

How Drug Causes Side Effects

- At antidepressant doses, anticholinergic activity may explain sedative effects, dry mouth, constipation, and blurred vision
- Sedative effects and weight gain may be due to antihistamine properties
- At antidepressant doses, blockade of alpha adrenergic 1 receptors may explain dizziness, sedation, and hypotension
- Cardiac arrhythmias and seizures, especially in overdose, may be caused by blockade of ion channels

Notable Side Effects

- Blurred vision, constipation, urinary retention, increased appetite, dry mouth, nausea, diarrhea, heartburn, unusual taste in mouth, weight gain
- Fatigue, weakness, dizziness, sedation, headache, anxiety, nervousness, restlessness
- Sexual dysfunction, sweating
- Topical: burning, stinging, itching, or swelling at application site
- Few side effects at low doses (1–6 mg/day)

Life-Threatening or Dangerous Side Effects

- Paralytic ileus, hyperthermia (TCAs + anticholinergic agents)
- Lowered seizure threshold and rare seizures
- Orthostatic hypotension, sudden death, arrhythmias, tachycardia
- QTc prolongation
- Hepatic failure, extrapyramidal symptoms
- Increased intraocular pressure, increased psychotic symptoms
- Rare induction of mania
- Rare activation of suicidal ideation and behavior (suicidality) (short-term studies did not show an increase in the risk of suicidality with antidepressants compared to placebo beyond age 24)

Weight Gain

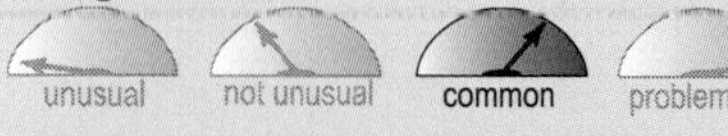

- Many experience and/or can be significant in amount (antidepressant doses)
- Can increase appetite and carbohydrate craving

Sedation

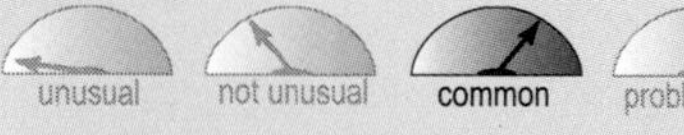

- Many experience and/or can be significant in amount
- Tolerance to sedative effect may develop with long-term use

What to Do About Side Effects

- Wait
- Wait
- Wait
- Lower the dose
- Switch to an SSRI or newer antidepressant

Best Augmenting Agents for Side Effects

- Many side effects cannot be improved with an augmenting agent

DOSING AND USE

Usual Dosage Range

- 75–150 mg/day for depression
- 1–6 mg at bedtime for insomnia (possible with liquid formulation)

Dosage Forms

- Capsule 10 mg, 25 mg, 50 mg, 75 mg, 100 mg, 150 mg
- Solution 10 mg/mL
- Topical 5%

How To Dose

- Initial 25 mg/day at bedtime; increase by 25 mg every 3–7 days
- 75 mg/day; increase gradually until desired efficacy is achieved; can be dosed once a day at bedtime or in divided doses; maximum dose 300 mg/day
- Topical: apply thin film 4 times a day (or every 3–4 hours while awake)

Dosing Tips

- If given in a single antidepressant dose, should generally be administered at bedtime because of its sedative properties
- If given in split antidepressant doses, largest dose should generally be given at bedtime because of its sedative properties
- If patients experience nightmares, split antidepressant dose and do not give large dose at bedtime
- Patients treated for chronic pain may only require lower doses
- Patients treated for insomnia may benefit from doses of 1–6 mg at bedtime
- 1 mg, 3 mg, and 6 mg doses are in late-stage clinical development for the treatment of insomnia
- Liquid formulation should be diluted with water or juice, excluding grape juice
- 150-mg capsule available only for maintenance use, not initial therapy

✱ Topical administration is absorbed systematically and can cause the same systematic side effects as oral administration

- If intolerable anxiety, insomnia, agitation, akathisia, or activation occur either upon dosing initiation or discontinuation, consider the possibility of activated bipolar disorder, and switch to a mood stabilizer or an atypical antipsychotic

Overdose

- Death may occur; convulsions, cardiac dysrhythmias, severe hypotension, CNS depression, coma, changes in EKG

Long-Term Use
- Safe

Habit Forming
- No

How to Stop
- At antidepressant doses, taper to avoid withdrawal effects
- Even with gradual dose reduction some withdrawal symptoms may appear within the first 2 weeks
- Many patients tolerate 50% dose reduction for 3 days, then another 50% reduction for 3 days, then discontinuation
- If withdrawal symptoms emerge during discontinuation, raise dose to stop symptoms and then restart withdrawal much more slowly
- Taper not necessary for low doses (1–6 mg/day)

Pharmacokinetics
- Substrate for CYP450 2D6
- Half-life approximately 8–24 hours

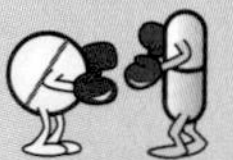

Drug Interactions
- Tramadol increases the risk of seizures in patients taking TCAs
- Use of TCAs with anticholinergic drugs may result in paralytic ileus or hyperthermia
- Fluoxetine, paroxetine, bupropion, duloxetine, and other CYP450 2D6 inhibitors may increase TCA concentrations
- Cimetidine may increase plasma concentrations of TCAs and cause anticholinergic symptoms
- Phenothiazines or haloperidol may raise TCA blood concentrations
- May alter effects of antihypertensive drugs; may inhibit hypotensive effects of clonidine
- Use with sympathomimetic agents may increase sympathetic activity
- Methylphenidate may inhibit metabolism of TCAs
- Most drug interactions may be less likely at low doses (1–6 mg/day) due to the lack of effects on receptors other than the histamine 1 receptors

- Activation and agitation, especially following switching or adding antidepressants, may represent the induction of a bipolar state, especially a mixed dysphoric bipolar II condition sometimes associated with suicidal ideation, and require the addition of lithium, a mood stabilizer or an atypical antipsychotic, and/or discontinuation of doxepin

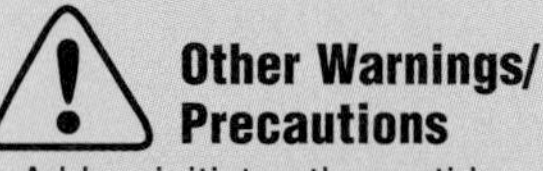

- Add or initiate other antidepressants with caution for up to 2 weeks after discontinuing doxepin
- Generally, do not use with MAO inhibitors, including 14 days after MAOIs are stopped; do not start an MAOI until 2 weeks after discontinuing doxepin, but see Pearls
- Use with caution in patients with history of seizures, urinary retention, narrow angle-closure glaucoma, hyperthyroidism
- TCAs can increase QTc interval, especially at toxic doses, which can be attained not only by overdose but also by combining with drugs that inhibit TCA metabolism via CYP450 2D6, potentially causing torsade de pointes-type arrhythmia or sudden death
- Because TCAs can prolong QTc interval, use with caution in patients who have bradycardia or who are taking drugs that can induce bradycardia (e.g., beta blockers, calcium channel blockers, clonidine, digitalis)
- Because TCAs can prolong QTc interval, use with caution in patients who have hypokalemia and/or hypomagnesemia or who are taking drugs that can induce hypokalemia and/or magnesemia (e.g., diuretics, stimulant laxatives, intravenous amphotericin B, glucocorticoids, tetracosactide)
- When treating children, carefully weigh the risks and benefits of pharmacological treatment against the risks and benefits of nontreatment with antidepressants and make sure to document this in the patient's chart
- Distribute the brochures provided by the FDA and the drug companies
- Warn patients and their caregivers about the possibility of activating side effects and

advise them to report such symptoms immediately
- Monitor patients for activation of suicidal ideation, especially children and adolescents

Do Not Use

- If patient is recovering from myocardial infarction
- If patient is taking agents capable of significantly prolonging QTc interval (e.g., pimozide, thioridazine, selected antiarrhythmics, moxifloxacin, sparfloxacin)
- If there is a history of QTc prolongation or cardiac arrhythmia, recent acute myocardial infarction, uncompensated heart failure
- If patient is taking drugs that inhibit TCA metabolism, including CYP450 2D6 inhibitors, except by an expert
- If there is reduced CYP450 2D6 function, such as patients who are poor 2D6 metabolizers, except by an expert and at low doses
- If patient has narrow angle-closure glaucoma
- If there is a proven allergy to doxepin

SPECIAL POPULATIONS

Renal Impairment

- Use with caution

Hepatic Impairment

- Use with caution – may need lower than usual adult dose

Cardiac Impairment

- TCAs have been reported to cause arrhythmias, prolongation of conduction time, orthostatic hypotension, sinus tachycardia, and heart failure, especially in the diseased heart
- Myocardial infarction and stroke have been reported with TCAs
- TCAs produce QTc prolongation, which may be enhanced by the existence of bradycardia, hypokalemia, congenital or acquired long QTc interval, which should be evaluated prior to administering doxepin
- Use with caution if treating concomitantly with a medication likely to produce prolonged bradycardia, hypokalemia, slowing of intracardiac conduction, or prolongation of the QTc interval
- Avoid TCAs in patients with a known history of QTc prolongation, recent acute myocardial infarction, and uncompensated heart failure
- TCAs may cause a sustained increase in heart rate in patients with ischemic heart disease and may worsen (decrease) heart rate variability, an independent risk of mortality in cardiac populations
- Since SSRIs may improve (increase) heart rate variability in patients following a myocardial infarct and may improve survival as well as mood in patients with acute angina or following a myocardial infarction, these are more appropriate agents for cardiac population than tricyclic/tetracyclic antidepressants

✻ Risk/benefit ratio may not justify use of TCAs in cardiac impairment

Elderly

- May be more sensitive to anticholinergic, cardiovascular, hypotensive, and sedative effects
- Low-dose doxepin (1–6 mg/day) has been studied and found effective for insomnia in elderly patients and is in late-stage clinical development
- Reduction in risk of suicidality with antidepressants compared to placebo in adults age 65 and older

Children and Adolescents

- Carefully weigh the risks and benefits of pharmacological treatment against the risks and benefits of nontreatment with antidepressants and make sure to document this in the patient's chart
- Monitor patients face-to-face regularly, particularly during the first several weeks of treatment
- Use with caution, observing for activation of known or unknown bipolar disorder and/or suicidal ideation, and inform parents or guardian of this risk so they can help observe child or adolescent patients
- Not recommended for use in children under age 12
- Several studies show lack of efficacy of TCAs for depression
- May be used to treat enuresis or hyperactive/impulsive behaviors

- Some cases of sudden death have occurred in children taking TCAs
- Initial dose 25–50 mg/day; maximum 100 mg/day

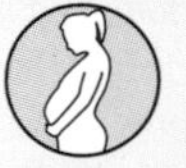

Pregnancy

- Risk Category C [some animal studies show adverse effects; no controlled studies in humans]
- Crosses the placenta
- Adverse effects have been reported in infants whose mothers took a TCA (lethargy, withdrawal symptoms, fetal malformations)
- Not generally recommended for use during pregnancy, especially during first trimester
- Must weigh the risk of treatment (first trimester fetal development, third trimester newborn delivery) to the child against the risk of no treatment (recurrence of depression, maternal health, infant bonding) to the mother and child
- For many patients this may mean continuing treatment during pregnancy

Breast Feeding

- Some drug is found in mother's breast milk
- Significant drug levels have been detected in some nursing infants

✻ Recommended either to discontinue drug or bottle feed

- Immediate postpartum period is a high-risk time for depression, especially in women who have had prior depressive episodes, so drug may need to be reinstituted late in the third trimester or shortly after childbirth to prevent a recurrence during the postpartum period
- Must weigh benefits of breast feeding with risks and benefits of antidepressant treatment versus nontreatment to both the infant and the mother
- For many patients this may mean continuing treatment during breast feeding

THE ART OF PSYCHOPHARMACOLOGY

Potential Advantages

- Patients with insomnia
- Severe or treatment-resistant depression
- Patients with neurodermatitis and itching

Potential Disadvantages

- Pediatric and geriatric patients
- Patients concerned with weight gain
- Cardiac patients

Primary Target Symptoms

- Depressed mood
- Anxiety
- Disturbed sleep, energy
- Somatic symptoms
- Itching skin

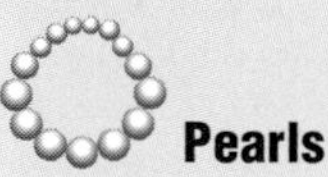

Pearls

✻ Only TCA available in topical formulation

✻ Topical administration may reduce symptoms in patients with various neurodermatitis syndromes, especially itching

- Tricyclic antidepressants are often a first-line treatment option for chronic pain
- Tricyclic antidepressants are no longer generally considered a first-line option for depression because of their side effect profile
- Tricyclic antidepressants continue to be useful for severe or treatment-resistant depression
- TCAs may aggravate psychotic symptoms
- Alcohol should be avoided because of additive CNS effects
- Underweight patients may be more susceptible to adverse cardiovascular effects
- Children, patients with inadequate hydration, and patients with cardiac disease may be more susceptible to TCA-induced cardiotoxicity than healthy adults
- Phase III trials of low dose doxepin (1–6 mg/day) for insomnia have been completed and show effectiveness in adult and elderly populations
- At these low doses doxepin is selective for the histamine 1 receptor and thus can improve sleep without causing side effects associated with other neurotransmitter systems

- In particular, low-dose doxepin does not appear to cause anticholinergic symptoms, memory impairment, or weight gain, nor is there evidence of tolerance, rebound insomnia, or withdrawal effects
- For the expert only: although generally prohibited, a heroic but potentially dangerous treatment for severely treatment-resistant patients is to give a tricyclic/tetracyclic antidepressant other than clomipramine simultaneously with an MAO inhibitor for patients who fail to respond to numerous other antidepressants
- If this option is elected, start the MAOI with the tricyclic/tetracyclic antidepressant simultaneously at low doses after appropriate drug washout, then alternately increase doses of these agents every few days to a week as tolerated
- Although very strict dietary and concomitant drug restrictions must be observed to prevent hypertensive crises and serotonin syndrome, the most common side effects of MAOI/tricyclic or tetracyclic combinations may be weight gain and orthostatic hypotension
- Patients on TCAs should be aware that they may experience symptoms such as photosensitivity or blue-green urine
- SSRIs may be more effective than TCAs in women, and TCAs may be more effective than SSRIs in men
- Since tricyclic/tetracyclic antidepressants are substrates for CYP450 2D6, and 7% of the population (especially Caucasians) may have a genetic variant leading to reduced activity of 2D6, such patients may not safely tolerate normal doses of tricyclic/tetracyclic antidepressants and may require dose reduction
- Phenotypic testing may be necessary to detect this genetic variant prior to dosing with a tricyclic/tetracyclic antidepressant, especially in vulnerable populations such as children, elderly, cardiac populations, and those on concomitant medications
- Patients who seem to have extraordinarily severe side effects at normal or low doses may have this phenotypic CYP450 2D6 variant and require low doses or switching to another antidepressant not metabolized by 2D6

Suggested Reading

Anderson IM. Meta-analytical studies on new antidepressants. Br Med Bull 2001; 57:161–78.

Anderson IM. Selective serotonin reuptake inhibitors versus tricyclic antidepressants: a meta-analysis of efficacy and tolerability. J Aff Disorders 2000;58:19–36.

Godfrey RG. A guide to the understanding and use of tricyclic antidepressants in the overall management of fibromyalgia and other chronic pain syndromes. Arch Intern Med 1996; 156:1047–52.

Singh H, Becker PM. Novel therapeutic usage of low-dose doxepin hydrochloride. Expert Opin Investig Drugs 2007;16(8):1295–305.

Stahl SM. Selective histamine 1 antagonism: novel hypnotic and pharmacologic actions challenge classical notions of antihistamines. CNS Spectrums 2008;13(12):855–65.

THERAPEUTICS

Brands • Cymbalta
see index for additional brand names

Generic? No

Class

- SNRI (dual serotonin and norepinephrine reuptake inhibitor); may be classified as an antidepressant, but it is not just an antidepressant

Commonly Prescribed for

(bold for FDA approved)

- **Major depressive disorder**
- **Diabetic peripheral neuropathic pain (DPNP)**
- **Fibromyalgia**
- **Generalized anxiety disorder**
- Stress urinary incontinence
- Neuropathic pain/chronic pain
- Other anxiety disorders

How the Drug Works

- Boosts neurotransmitters serotonin, norepinephrine/noradrenaline, and dopamine
- Blocks serotonin reuptake pump (serotonin transporter), presumably increasing serotonergic neurotransmission
- Blocks norepinephrine reuptake pump (norepinephrine transporter), presumably increasing noradrenergic neurotransmission
- Presumably desensitizes both serotonin 1A receptors and beta adrenergic receptors
- Since dopamine is inactivated by norepinephrine reuptake in frontal cortex, which largely lacks dopamine transporters, duloxetine can increase dopamine neurotransmission in this part of the brain
- Weakly blocks dopamine reuptake pump (dopamine transporter), and may increase dopamine neurotransmission

How Long Until It Works

- Onset of therapeutic actions usually not immediate, but often delayed 2–4 weeks for depression
- If it is not working within 6–8 weeks for depression, it may require a dosage increase or it may not work at all
- Can reduce neuropathic pain within a week, but onset can take longer
- May continue to work for many years to prevent relapse of depressive symptoms or prevent worsening of painful symptoms
- Vasomotor symptoms in perimenopausal women with or without depression may improve within 1 week

If It Works

- The goal of treatment of depression and anxiety disorders is complete remission of current symptoms as well as prevention of future relapses
- The goal of treatment of diabetic peripheral neuropathic pain and fibromyalgia and chronic neuropathic pain is to reduce symptoms as much as possible, especially in combination with other treatments
- Treatment of depression most often reduces or even eliminates symptoms, but is not a cure since symptoms can recur after medicine stopped
- Treatment of diabetic peripheral neuropathic pain, fibromyalgia, and chronic neuropathic pain may reduce symptoms, but rarely eliminates them completely, and is not a cure since symptoms can recur after medicine is stopped
- Continue treatment of depression and anxiety disorders until all symptoms are gone (remission)
- Once symptoms of depression are gone, continue treating for 1 year for the first episode of depression
- For second and subsequent episodes of depression, treatment may need to be indefinite
- Use in anxiety disorders may also need to be indefinite
- Use in diabetic peripheral neuropathic pain, fibromyalgia, and chronic neuropathic pain may also need to be indefinite, but long-term treatment is not well studied in these conditions

If It Doesn't Work

- Many patients only have a partial response where some symptoms are improved but others persist (especially insomnia, fatigue, and problems concentrating)
- Other patients may be nonresponders, sometimes called treatment-resistant or treatment-refractory

- Some depressed patients who have an initial response may relapse even though they continue treatment, sometimes called "poop-out"
- Consider increasing dose, switching to another agent or adding an appropriate augmenting agent
- Consider psychotherapy for depression or biofeedback or hypnosis for pain
- Consider evaluation for another diagnosis or for a comorbid condition (e.g., medical illness, substance abuse, etc.)
- Consider the presence of noncompliance and counsel the patient
- Some patients may experience apparent lack of consistent efficacy due to activation of latent or underlying bipolar disorder, and require antidepressant discontinuation and a switch to a mood stabilizer

Best Augmenting Combos for Partial Response or Treatment Resistance

✱ Augmentation experience is limited compared to other antidepressants and treatments for neuropathic pain

✱ Adding other agents to duloxetine for treating depression could follow the same practice for augmenting SSRIs or other SNRIs if done by experts while monitoring carefully in difficult cases

- Although no controlled studies and little clinical experience, adding other agents for treating diabetic peripheral neuropathic pain and fibromyalgia and neuropathic pain could theoretically include gabapentin, pregabalin, and tiagabine, if done by experts while monitoring carefully in difficult cases
- Mirtazapine ("California rocket fuel" for depression; a potentially powerful dual serotonin and norepinephrine combination, but observe for activation of bipolar disorder and suicidal ideation)
- Bupropion, reboxetine, nortriptyline, desipramine, maprotiline, atomoxetine (all potentially powerful enhancers of noradrenergic action for depression, but observe for activation of bipolar disorder and suicidal ideation)
- Modafinil, especially for fatigue, sleepiness, and lack of concentration
- Mood stabilizers or atypical antipsychotics for bipolar depression, psychotic depression or treatment-resistant depression
- Benzodiazepines
- If all else fails for anxiety disorders, consider gabapentin, pregabalin, or tiagabine
- Hypnotics or trazodone for insomnia
- Classically, lithium, buspirone, or thyroid hormone for depression

Tests

- Check blood pressure before initiating treatment and regularly during treatment

SIDE EFFECTS

How Drug Causes Side Effects

- Theoretically due to increases in serotonin and norepinephrine concentrations at receptors in parts of the brain and body other than those that cause therapeutic actions (e.g., unwanted actions of serotonin in sleep centers causing insomnia, unwanted actions of norepinephrine on acetylcholine release causing decreased appetite, increased blood pressure, urinary retention, etc.)
- Most side effects are immediate but often go away with time

Notable Side Effects

- Nausea, diarrhea, decreased appetite, dry mouth, constipation
- Insomnia, sedation, dizziness
- Sexual dysfunction (men: abnormal ejaculation/orgasm, impotence, decreased libido; women: abnormal orgasm)
- Sweating
- Increase in blood pressure (up to 2 mm Hg)
- Urinary retention

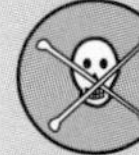

Life-Threatening or Dangerous Side Effects

- Rare seizures
- Rare induction of hypomania
- Rare activation of suicidal ideation, suicide attempts, and completed suicide
- Short-term studies did not show an increase in the risk of suicidality with antidepressants compared to placebo beyond age 24

Weight Gain

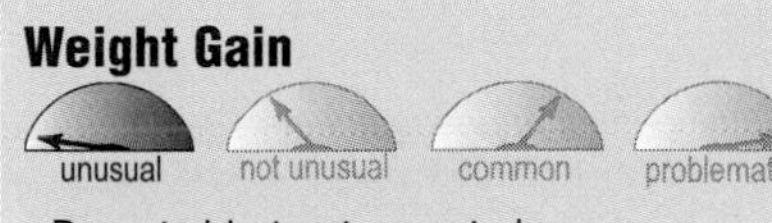

- Reported but not expected

Sedation

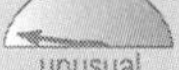

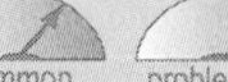

common problematic

- Occurs in significant minority
- May also be activating in some patients

What to Do About Side Effects

- Wait
- Wait
- Wait
- Lower the dose
- In a few weeks, switch or add other drugs

Best Augmenting Agents for Side Effects

- For urinary hesitancy, give an alpha 1 blocker such as tamsulosin
- Often best to try another antidepressant monotherapy prior to resorting to augmentation strategies to treat side effects
- Trazodone or a hypnotic for insomnia
- Bupropion, sildenafil, vardenafil, or tadalafil for sexual dysfunction
- Benzodiazepines for jitteriness and anxiety, especially at initiation of treatment and especially for anxious patients
- Mirtazapine for insomnia, agitation, and gastrointestinal side effects
- Many side effects are dose-dependent (i.e., they increase as dose increases, or they reemerge until tolerance re-develops)
- Many side effects are time-dependent (i.e., they start immediately upon dosing and upon each dose increase, but go away with time)
- Activation and agitation may represent the induction of a bipolar state, especially a mixed dysphoric bipolar II condition sometimes associated with suicidal ideation, and require the addition of lithium, a mood stabilizer or an atypical antipsychotic, and/or discontinuation of duloxetine

DOSING AND USE

Usual Dosage Range

- 40–60 mg/day in 1–2 doses for depression
- 60 mg once daily for diabetic peripheral neuropathic pain and fibromyalgia
- 60 mg once daily for generalized anxiety disorder
- 40 mg twice daily for stress urinary incontinence

Dosage Forms

- Capsule 20 mg, 30 mg, 60 mg

How To Dose

- For depression, initial 40 mg/day in 2 doses; can increase to 60 mg/day in 1–2 doses if necessary; maximum dose generally 120 mg/day
- For neuropathic pain and fibromyalgia, initial 30 mg once daily; increase to 60 mg once daily after one week; maximum dose generally 60 mg/day
- For generalized anxiety, initial 60 mg once daily; maximum dose generally 120 mg/day

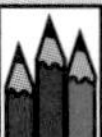

Dosing Tips

- Studies have not demonstrated increased efficacy beyond 60 mg/day

✻ Some patients may require up to or more than 120 mg/day, but clinical experience is quite limited with high dosing

- In relapse prevention studies in depression, a significant percentage of patients who relapsed on 60 mg/day responded and remitted when the dose was increased to 120 mg/day
- In neuropathic pain and fibromyalgia, doses above 60 mg/day have been associated with increased side effects without an increase in efficacy
- Some studies suggest that both serotonin and norepinephrine reuptake blockade are present at 40–60 mg/day
- Do not chew or crush and do not sprinkle on food or mix with food, but rather always swallow whole to avoid affecting enteric coating
- Some patients may require dosing above 120 mg/day in 2 divided doses, but this should be done with caution and by experts

Overdose
- Rare fatalities have been reported; serotonin syndrome, sedation, vomiting, seizures, coma, change in blood pressure

Long-Term Use
- Blood pressure should be monitored regularly

Habit Forming
- No

How to Stop
- Taper to avoid withdrawal effects (dizziness, nausea, vomiting, headache, paresthesias, irritability)
- Many patients tolerate 50% dose reduction for 3 days, then another 50% reduction for 3 days, then discontinuation

✻ If withdrawal symptoms emerge during discontinuation, raise dose to stop symptoms and then restart withdrawal much more slowly

Pharmacokinetics
- Elimination half-life approximately 12 hours
- Metabolized mainly by CYP450 2D6 and CYP450 1A2
- Inhibitor of CYP450 2D6 (probably clinically significant) and CYP450 1A2 (probably not clinically significant)
- Absorption may be delayed by up to 3 hours and clearance may be increased by one-third after an evening dose as compared to a morning dose

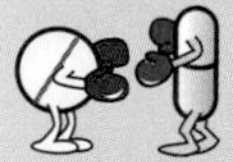

Drug Interactions
- Can increase tricyclic antidepressant levels; use with caution with tricyclic antidepressants or when switching from a TCA to duloxetine
- Can cause a fatal "serotonin syndrome" when combined with MAO inhibitors, so do not use with MAO inhibitors or for at least 14 days after MAOIs are stopped
- Possible increased risk of bleeding, especially when combined with anticoagulants (e.g., warfarin, NSAIDs)
- Do not start an MAO inhibitor for at least 5 days after discontinuing duloxetine
- Inhibitors of CYP450 1A2, such as fluvoxamine, increase plasma levels of duloxetine and may require a dosage reduction of duloxetine
- Cigarette smoking induces CYP450 1A2 and may reduce plasma levels of duloxetine, but dosage modifications are not recommended for smokers

✻ Inhibitors of CYP450 2D6, such as paroxetine, fluoxetine, and quinidine, may increase plasma levels of duloxetine and require a dosage reduction of duloxetine

- Via CYP450 1A2 inhibition, duloxetine could theoretically reduce clearance of theophylline and clozapine; however, studies of coadministration with theophylline did not demonstrate significant effects of duloxetine on theophylline pharmacokinetics
- Via CYP450 2D6 inhibition, duloxetine could theoretically interfere with the analgesic actions of codeine, and increase the plasma levels of some beta blockers and of atomoxetine
- Via CYP450 2D6 inhibition, duloxetine could theoretically increase concentrations of thioridazine and cause dangerous cardiac arrhythmias

⚠ Other Warnings/ Precautions
- Use with caution in patients with history of seizures
- Use with caution in patients with bipolar disorder unless treated with concomitant mood-stabilizing agent
- Rare reports of hepatotoxicity; although causality has not been established, duloxetine should be discontinued in patients who develop jaundice or other evidence of significant liver dysfunction
- When treating children, carefully weigh the risks and benefits of pharmacological treatment against the risks and benefits of nontreatment with antidepressants and make sure to document this in the patient's chart
- Distribute the brochures provided by the FDA and the drug companies
- Warn patients and their caregivers about the possibility of activating side effects and advise them to report such symptoms immediately
- Monitor patients for activation of suicidal ideation, especially children and adolescents

- Duloxetine may increase blood pressure, so blood pressure should be monitored during treatment

Do Not Use

- If patient has uncontrolled narrow angle-closure glaucoma
- If patient has substantial alcohol use
- If patient is taking an MAO inhibitor
- If patient is taking thioridazine
- If there is a proven allergy to duloxetine

SPECIAL POPULATIONS

Renal Impairment

- Dose adjustment generally not necessary for mild to moderate impairment
- Not recommended for use in patients with end-stage renal disease (requiring dialysis) or severe renal impairment

Hepatic Impairment

- Not to be administered to patients with any hepatic insufficiency
- Not recommended for use in patients with substantial alcohol use
- Increased risk of elevation of serum transaminase levels

Cardiac Impairment

- Drug should be used with caution
- Duloxetine may raise blood pressure

Elderly

- Some patients may tolerate lower doses better
- Reduction in risk of suicidality with antidepressants compared to placebo in adults age 65 and older

Children and Adolescents

- Carefully weigh the risks and benefits of pharmacological treatment against the risks and benefits of nontreatment with antidepressants and make sure to document this in the patient's chart
- Monitor patients face-to-face regularly, particularly during the first several weeks of treatment
- Use with caution, observing for activation of known or unknown bipolar disorder and/or suicidal ideation, and inform parents or guardian of this risk so they can help observe child or adolescent patients
- Not studied, but can be used by experts

Pregnancy

- Risk Category C [some animal studies show adverse effects; no controlled studies in humans]
- Not generally recommended for use during pregnancy, especially during first trimester
- Nonetheless, continuous treatment during pregnancy may be necessary and has not been proven to be harmful to the fetus
- Must weigh the risk of treatment (first trimester fetal development, third trimester newborn delivery) to the child against the risk of no treatment (recurrence of depression, maternal health, infant bonding) to the mother and child
- For many patients this may mean continuing treatment during pregnancy
- Neonates exposed to SSRIs or SNRIs late in the third trimester have developed complications requiring prolonged hospitalization, respiratory support, and tube feeding; reported symptoms are consistent with either a direct toxic effect of SSRIs and SNRIs or, possibly, a drug discontinuation syndrome, and include respiratory distress, cyanosis, apnea, seizures, temperature instability, feeding difficulty, vomiting, hypoglycemia, hypotonia, hypertonia, hyperreflexia, tremor, jitteriness, irritability, and constant crying

Breast Feeding

- Some drug is found in mother's breast milk
- If child becomes irritable or sedated, breast feeding or drug may need to be discontinued
- Immediate postpartum period is a high-risk time for depression, especially in women who have had prior depressive episodes, so drug may need to be reinstituted late in the third trimester or shortly after childbirth to prevent a recurrence during the postpartum period

- Must weigh benefits of breast feeding with risks and benefits of antidepressant treatment versus nontreatment to both the infant and the mother
- For many patients, this may mean continuing treatment during breast feeding

THE ART OF PSYCHOPHARMACOLOGY

Potential Advantages

- Patients with physical symptoms of depression
- Patients with retarded depression
- Patients with atypical depression
- Patients with comorbid anxiety
- Patients with depression may have higher remission rates on SNRIs than on SSRIs
- Depressed patients with somatic symptoms, fatigue, and pain
- Patients who do not respond or do not remit on treatment with SSRIs

Potential Disadvantages

- Patients with urologic disorders, prostate disorders (e.g., older men)
- Patients sensitive to nausea

Primary Target Symptoms

- Depressed mood
- Energy, motivation, and interest
- Sleep disturbance
- Anxiety
- Physical symptoms
- Pain

Pearls

✻ Duloxetine has well-documented efficacy for the painful physical symptoms of depression
- Duloxetine has only somewhat greater potency for serotonin reuptake blockade than for norepinephrine reuptake blockade, but this is of unclear clinical significance as a differentiator from other SNRIs
- No head-to-head studies, but may have less hypertension than venlafaxine XR
- Powerful pro-noradrenergic actions may occur at doses greater than 60 mg/day
- Not well-studied in ADHD, but may be effective

✻ Approved in many countries for stress urinary incontinence
- Patients may have higher remission rate for depression on SNRIs than on SSRIs
- Add or switch to or from pro-noradrenergic agents (e.g., atomoxetine, reboxetine, other SNRIs, mirtazapine, maprotiline, nortriptyline, desipramine, bupropion) with caution
- Add or switch to or from CYP450 2D6 substrates with caution (e.g., atomoxetine, maprotiline, nortriptyline, desipramine)
- Mechanism of action as SNRI suggests it may be effective in some patients who fail to respond to SSRIs

Suggested Reading

Arnold LM, Pritchett YL, D'Souza DN et al. Duloxetine for the treatment of fibromyalgia in women: pooled results from two randomized, placebo-controlled trials. J Womens Health (Larchmt) 2007;16(8):1145–56.

Bymaster FP, Dreshfield-Ahmad LJ, Threlkeld PG, Shaw JL, Thompson L, Nelson DL, Hemrick-Luecke SK, Wong DT. Comparative affinity of duloxetine and venlafaxine for serotonin and norepinephrine transporters in vitro and in vivo, human serotonin receptor subtypes, and other neuronal receptors. Neuropsychopharmacology 2001; 25(6):871–80.

Hartford J, Kornstein S, Liebowitz M, et al. Duloxetine as an SNRI treatment for generalized anxiety disorder: results from a placebo and active-controlled trial. Int Clin Psychopharmacol 2007;22(3):167–74.

Muller N, Schennach R, Riedel M, Moller HJ. Duloxetine in the treatment of major psychiatric and neuropathic disorders. Expert Rev Neurother 2008;8(4):527–36.

Zinner NR. Duloxetine: a serotonin-noradrenaline re-uptake inhibitor for the treatment of stress urinary incontinence. Expert Opin Investig Drugs 2003; 12(9):1559–66.

ESCITALOPRAM

THERAPEUTICS

Brands • Lexapro

see index for additional brand names

Generic? Yes

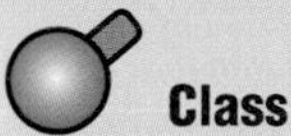

Class

- SSRI (selective serotonin reuptake inhibitor); often classified as an antidepressant, but it is not just an antidepressant

Commonly Prescribed for

(bold for FDA approved)

- **Major depressive disorder**
- **Generalized anxiety disorder**
- Panic disorder
- Obsessive-compulsive disorder (OCD)
- Posttraumatic stress disorder (PTSD)
- Social anxiety disorder (social phobia)
- Premenstrual dysphoric disorder (PMDD)

How the Drug Works

- Boosts neurotransmitter serotonin
- Blocks serotonin reuptake pump (serotonin transporter)
- Desensitizes serotonin receptors, especially serotonin 1A autoreceptors
- Presumably increases serotonergic neurotransmission

How Long Until It Works

- Onset of therapeutic actions usually not immediate, but often delayed 2–4 weeks
- If it is not working within 6–8 weeks, it may require a dosage increase or it may not work at all
- May continue to work for many years to prevent relapse of symptoms

If It Works

- The goal of treatment is complete remission of current symptoms as well as prevention of future relapses
- Treatment most often reduces or even eliminates symptoms, but not a cure since symptoms can recur after medicine stopped
- Continue treatment until all symptoms are gone (remission) or significantly reduced (e.g., OCD, PTSD)
- Once symptoms gone, continue treating for 1 year for the first episode of depression
- For second and subsequent episodes of depression, treatment may need to be indefinite
- Use in anxiety disorders may also need to be indefinite

If It Doesn't Work

- Many patients only have a partial response where some symptoms are improved but others persist (especially insomnia, fatigue, and problems concentrating in depression)
- Other patients may be nonresponders, sometimes called treatment-resistant or treatment-refractory
- Some patients who have an initial response may relapse even though they continue treatment, sometimes called "poop-out"
- Consider increasing dose, switching to another agent or adding an appropriate augmenting agent
- Consider psychotherapy
- Consider evaluation for another diagnosis or for a comorbid condition (e.g., medical illness, substance abuse, etc.)
- Some patients may experience apparent lack of consistent efficacy due to activation of latent or underlying bipolar disorder, and require antidepressant discontinuation and a switch to a mood stabilizer

Best Augmenting Combos for Partial Response or Treatment Resistance

- Trazodone, especially for insomnia
- Bupropion, mirtazapine, reboxetine, or atomoxetine (use combinations of antidepressants with caution as this may activate bipolar disorder and suicidal ideation)
- Modafinil, especially for fatigue, sleepiness, and lack of concentration
- Mood stabilizers or atypical antipsychotics for bipolar depression, psychotic depression, treatment-resistant depression, or treatment-resistant anxiety disorders
- Benzodiazepines
- If all else fails for anxiety disorders, consider gabapentin or tiagabine
- Hypnotics for insomnia
- Classically, lithium, buspirone, or thyroid hormone

Tests

- None for healthy individuals

SIDE EFFECTS

How Drug Causes Side Effects

- Theoretically due to increases in serotonin concentrations at serotonin receptors in parts of the brain and body other than those that cause therapeutic actions (e.g., unwanted actions of serotonin in sleep centers causing insomnia, unwanted actions of serotonin in the gut causing diarrhea, etc.)
- Increasing serotonin can cause diminished dopamine release and might contribute to emotional flattening, cognitive slowing, and apathy in some patients
- Most side effects are immediate but often go away with time, in contrast to most therapeutic effects which are delayed and are enhanced over time

✻ As escitalopram has no known important secondary pharmacologic properties, its side effects are presumably all mediated by its serotonin reuptake blockade

Notable Side Effects

- Sexual dysfunction (men: delayed ejaculation, erectile dysfunction; men and women: decreased sexual desire, anorgasmia)
- Gastrointestinal (decreased appetite, nausea, diarrhea, constipation, dry mouth)
- Mostly central nervous system (insomnia but also sedation, agitation, tremors, headache, dizziness)
- Note: patients with diagnosed or undiagnosed bipolar or psychotic disorders may be more vulnerable to CNS-activating actions of SSRIs
- Autonomic (sweating)
- Bruising and rare bleeding
- Rare hyponatremia (mostly in elderly patients and generally reversible on discontinuation of escitalopram

Life-Threatening or Dangerous Side Effects

- Rare seizures
- Rare induction of mania
- Rare activation of suicidal ideation and behavior (suicidality) (short-term studies did not show an increase in the risk of suicidality with antidepressants compared to placebo beyond age 24)

Weight Gain

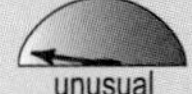
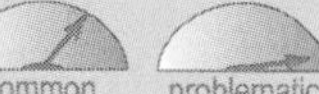

- Reported but not expected

Sedation

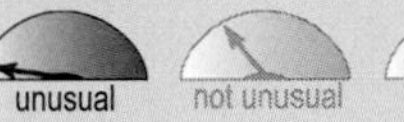

- Reported but not expected

What to Do About Side Effects

- Wait
- Wait
- Wait
- In a few weeks, switch to another agent or add other drugs

Best Augmenting Agents for Side Effects

- Often best to try another SSRI or another antidepressant monotherapy prior to resorting to augmentation strategies to treat side effects
- Trazodone or a hypnotic for insomnia
- Bupropion, sildenafil, vardenafil, or tadalafil for sexual dysfunction
- Bupropion for emotional flattening, cognitive slowing, or apathy
- Mirtazapine for insomnia, agitation, and gastrointestinal side effects
- Benzodiazepines for jitteriness and anxiety, especially at initiation of treatment and especially for anxious patients
- Many side effects are dose-dependent (i.e., they increase as dose increases, or they reemerge until tolerance redevelops)
- Many side effects are time-dependent (i.e., they start immediately upon dosing and upon each dose increase, but go away with time)
- Activation and agitation may represent the induction of a bipolar state, especially a mixed dysphoric bipolar II condition sometimes associated with suicidal ideation, and require the addition of lithium, a mood stabilizer or an atypical antipsychotic, and/or discontinuation of escitalopram

DOSING AND USE

Usual Dosage Range
- 10–20 mg/day
- Oral solution 5 mg/5 mL

Dosage Forms
- Tablets 5 mg, 10 mg, 20 mg
- Capsule 5 mg, 10 mg, 20 mg
- Oral solution 5 mg/5 mL

How To Dose
- Initial 10 mg/day; increase to 20 mg/day if necessary; single-dose administration, morning or evening

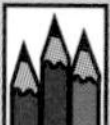

Dosing Tips
- Given once daily, any time of day tolerated
- ✻ 10 mg of escitalopram may be comparable in efficacy to 40 mg of citalopram with fewer side effects
- Thus, give an adequate trial of 10 mg prior to giving 20 mg
- Some patients require dosing with 30 or 40 mg
- If intolerable anxiety, insomnia, agitation, akathisia, or activation occur either upon dosing initiation or discontinuation, consider the possibility of activated bipolar disorder and switch to a mood stabilizer or an atypical antipsychotic

Overdose
- Few reports of escitalopram overdose, but probably similar to citalopram overdose
- Rare fatalities have been reported in citalopram overdose, both in combination with other drugs and alone
- Symptoms associated with citalopram overdose include vomiting, sedation, heart rhythm disturbances, dizziness, sweating, nausea, tremor, and rarely amnesia, confusion, coma, convulsions

Long-Term Use
- Safe

Habit Forming
- No

How to Stop
- Taper not usually necessary
- However, tapering to avoid potential withdrawal reactions generally prudent
- Many patients tolerate 50% dose reduction for 3 days, then another 50% reduction for 3 days, then discontinuation
- If withdrawal symptoms emerge during discontinuation, raise dose to stop symptoms and then restart withdrawal much more slowly

Pharmacokinetics
- Mean terminal half-life 27–32 hours
- Steady-state plasma concentrations achieved within 1 week
- No significant actions on CYP450 enzymes

Drug Interactions
- Tramadol increases the risk of seizures in patients taking an antidepressant
- Can cause a fatal "serotonin syndrome" when combined with MAO inhibitors, so do not use with MAO inhibitors or for at least 14 days after MAOIs are stopped
- Do not start an MAO inhibitor for at least 2 weeks after discontinuing escitalopram
- Could theoretically cause weakness, hyperreflexia, and incoordination when combined with sumatriptan or possibly other triptans, requiring careful monitoring of patient
- Possible increased risk of bleeding, especially when combined with anticoagulants (e.g., warfarin, NSAIDs)
- Few known adverse drug interactions

Other Warnings/ Precautions
- Use with caution in patients with history of seizures
- Use with caution in patients with bipolar disorder unless treated with concomitant mood-stabilizing agent
- When treating children, carefully weigh the risks and benefits of pharmacological treatment against the risks and benefits of nontreatment with antidepressants and make sure to document this in the patient's chart
- Distribute the brochures provided by the FDA and the drug companies
- Warn patients and their caregivers about the possibility of activating side effects and advise them to report such symptoms immediately

- Monitor patients for activation of suicidal ideation, especially children and adolescents

Do Not Use

- If patient is taking an MAO inhibitor
- If there is a proven allergy to escitalopram or citalopram

SPECIAL POPULATIONS

Renal Impairment

- Few data available for use in patients with renal impairment, but start with 10 mg/day

Hepatic Impairment

- Recommended dose 10 mg/day

Cardiac Impairment

- Not systematically evaluated in patients with cardiac impairment
- Preliminary data suggest that citalopram is safe in patients with cardiac impairment, suggesting that escitalopram is also safe
- Treating depression with SSRIs in patients with acute angina or following myocardial infarction may reduce cardiac events and improve survival as well as mood

Elderly

- Recommended dose 10 mg/day
- Reduction in risk of suicidality with antidepressants compared to placebo in adults age 65 and older

Children and Adolescents

- Safety and efficacy have not been established
- Carefully weigh the risks and benefits of pharmacological treatment against the risks and benefits of nontreatment with antidepressants and make sure to document this in the patient's chart
- Monitor patients face-to-face regularly, particularly during the first several weeks of treatment
- Use with caution, observing for activation of known or unknown bipolar disorder and/or suicidal ideation, and inform parents or guardian of this risk so they can help observe child or adolescent patients

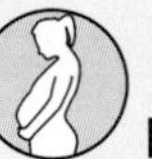

Pregnancy

- Risk Category C [some animal studies show adverse effects; no controlled studies in humans]
- Not generally recommended for use during pregnancy, especially during first trimester
- Nonetheless, continuous treatment during pregnancy may be necessary and has not been proven to be harmful to the fetus
- At delivery there may be more bleeding in the mother and transient irritability or sedation in the newborn
- Must weigh the risk of treatment (first trimester fetal development, third trimester newborn delivery) to the child against the risk of no treatment (recurrence of depression, maternal health, infant bonding) to the mother and child
- For many patients, this may mean continuing treatment during pregnancy
- SSRI use beyond the 20th week of pregnancy may be associated with increased risk of pulmonary hypertension in newborns
- Neonates exposed to SSRIs or SNRIs late in the third trimester have developed complications requiring prolonged hospitalization, respiratory support, and tube feeding; reported symptoms are consistent with either a direct toxic effect of SSRIs and SNRIs or, possibly, a drug discontinuation syndrome, and include respiratory distress, cyanosis, apnea, seizures, temperature instability, feeding difficulty, vomiting, hypoglycemia, hypotonia, hypertonia, hyperreflexia, tremor, jitteriness, irritability, and constant crying

Breast Feeding

- Some drug is found in mother's breast milk
- Trace amounts may be present in nursing children whose mothers are on escitalopram
- If child becomes irritable or sedated, breast feeding or drug may need to be discontinued
- Immediate postpartum period is a high-risk time for depression, especially in women who have had prior depressive episodes, so drug may need to be reinstituted late in the third trimester or shortly after

childbirth to prevent a recurrence during the postpartum period
- Must weigh benefits of breast feeding with risks and benefits of antidepressant treatment versus nontreatment to both the infant and the mother
- For many patients, this may mean continuing treatment during breast feeding

THE ART OF PSYCHOPHARMACOLOGY

Potential Advantages
- Patients taking concomitant medications (few drug interactions and fewer even than with citalopram)
- Patients requiring faster onset of action

Potential Disadvantages
- More expensive than citalopram in markets where citalopram is generic

Primary Target Symptoms
- Depressed mood
- Anxiety
- Panic attacks, avoidant behavior, re-experiencing, hyperarousal
- Sleep disturbance, both insomnia and hypersomnia

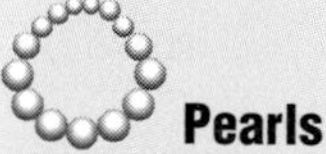

Pearls
✻ May be among the best-tolerated antidepressants
- May have less sexual dysfunction than some other SSRIs
- May be better tolerated than citalopram
- Can cause cognitive and affective "flattening"

✻ R-citalopram may interfere with the binding of S-citalopram at the serotonin transporter

✻ For this reason, S-citalopram may be more than twice as potent as R,S-citalopram (i.e., citalopram)
- Thus, 10 mg starting dose of S-citalopram may have the therapeutic efficacy of 40 mg of R,S-citalopram
- Thus, escitalopram may have faster onset and better efficacy with reduced side effects compared to R,S-citalopram
- Some data may actually suggest remission rates comparable to dual serotonin and norepinephrine reuptake inhibitors, but this is not proven

✻ Escitalopram is commonly used with augmenting agents, as it is the SSRI with the least interaction at either CYP450 2D6 or 3A4, therefore causing fewer pharmacokinetically mediated drug interactions with augmenting agents than other SSRIs
- SSRIs may be less effective in women over 50, especially if they are not taking estrogen
- SSRIs may be useful for hot flushes in perimenopausal women
- Some postmenopausal women's depression will respond better to escitalopram plus estrogen augmentation than to escitalopram alone
- Nonresponse to escitalopram in elderly may require consideration of mild cognitive impairment or Alzheimer disease

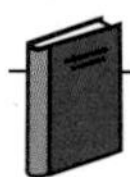

Suggested Reading

Baldwin DS, Reines EH, Guiton C, Weiller E. Escitalopram therapy for major depression and anxiety disorders. Ann Pharmacother 2007;41(10):1583–92.

Bareggi SR, Mundo E, Dell-Osso B, Altamura AC. The use of escitalopram beyond major depression: pharmacological aspects, efficacy and tolerability in anxiety disorders. Expert Opin Drug Metab Toxicol 2007;3(5):741–53.

Burke WJ. Escitalopram. Expert Opin Investig Drugs 2002;11(10):1477–86.

THERAPEUTICS

Brands • ProSom

see index for additional brand names

Generic? Yes

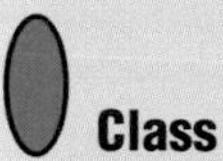

Class

- Benzodiazepine (hypnotic)

Commonly Prescribed for

(bold for FDA approved)

- **Insomnia characterized by difficulty in falling asleep, frequent nocturnal awakenings, and/or early morning awakenings**

How the Drug Works

- Binds to benzodiazepine receptors at the GABA-A ligand-gated chloride channel complex
- Enhances the inhibitory effects of GABA
- Boosts chloride conductance through GABA-regulated channels
- Inhibitory actions in sleep centers may provide sedative hypnotic effects

How Long Until It Works

- Generally takes effect in less than an hour

If It Works

- Improves quality of sleep
- Effects on total wake-time and number of nighttime awakenings may be decreased over time

If It Doesn't Work

- If insomnia does not improve after 7–10 days, it may be a manifestation of a primary psychiatric or physical illness such as obstructive sleep apnea or restless leg syndrome, which requires independent evaluation
- Increase the dose
- Improve sleep hygiene
- Switch to another agent

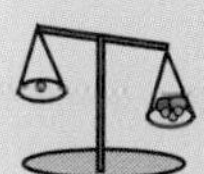

Best Augmenting Combos for Partial Response or Treatment Resistance

- Generally, best to switch to another agent
- Trazodone
- Agents with antihistamine actions (e.g., diphenhydramine, tricyclic antidepressants)

Tests

- In patients with seizure disorders, concomitant medical illness, and/or those with multiple concomitant long-term medications, periodic liver tests and blood counts may be prudent

SIDE EFFECTS

How Drug Causes Side Effects

- Same mechanism for side effects as for therapeutic effects – namely due to excessive actions at benzodiazepine receptors
- Actions at benzodiazepine receptors that carry over to next day can cause daytime sedation, amnesia, and ataxia
- Long-term adaptations in benzodiazepine receptors may explain the development of dependence, tolerance, and withdrawal

Notable Side Effects

✻ Sedation, fatigue, depression
✻ Dizziness, ataxia, slurred speech, weakness
✻ Forgetfulness, confusion
✻ Hyperexcitability, nervousness
- Rare hallucinations, mania
- Rare hypotension
- Hypersalivation, dry mouth
- Rebound insomnia when withdrawing from long-term treatment

Life-Threatening or Dangerous Side Effects

- Respiratory depression, especially when taken with CNS depressants in overdose
- Rare hepatic dysfunction, renal dysfunction, blood dyscrasias

Weight Gain

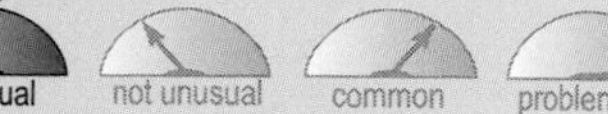

- Reported but not expected

Sedation

unusual not unusual

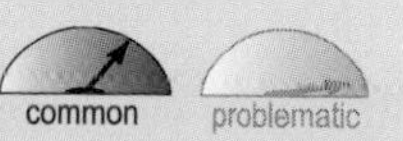

- Many experience and/or can be significant in amount

What to Do About Side Effects

- Wait
- To avoid problems with memory, take estazolam only if planning to have a full night's sleep
- Lower the dose
- Switch to a shorter-acting sedative hypnotic
- Switch to a non-benzodiazepine hypnotic
- Administer flumazenil if side effects are severe or life-threatening

Best Augmenting Agents for Side Effects

- Many side effects cannot be improved with an augmenting agent

DOSING AND USE

Usual Dosage Range

- 1–2 mg/day at bedtime

Dosage Forms

- Tablet 1 mg scored, 2 mg scored

How To Dose

- Initial 1 mg/day at bedtime; increase to 2 mg/day at bedtime if ineffective

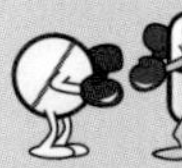

Dosing Tips

- Use lowest possible effective dose and assess need for continued treatment regularly
- Estazolam should generally not be prescribed in quantities greater than a 1-month supply
- Patients with lower body weights may require lower doses
- Risk of dependence may increase with dose and duration of treatment

Overdose

- No death reported in monotherapy; sedation, slurred speech, poor coordination, confusion, coma, respiratory depression

Long-Term Use

- Not generally intended for long-term use
- Evidence of efficacy up to 12 weeks

Habit Forming

- Estazolam is a Schedule IV drug
- Some patients may develop dependence and/or tolerance; risk may be greater with higher doses
- History of drug addiction may increase risk of dependence

How to Stop

- If taken for more than a few weeks, taper to reduce chances of withdrawal effects
- Patients with seizure history may seize upon sudden withdrawal
- Rebound insomnia may occur the first 1–2 nights after stopping
- For patients with severe problems discontinuing a benzodiazepine, dosing may need to be tapered over many months (i.e., reduce dose by 1% every 3 days by crushing tablet and suspending or dissolving in 100 mL of fruit juice and then disposing of 1 mL while drinking the rest; 3–7 days later, dispose of 2 mL, and so on). This is both a form of very slow biological tapering and a form of behavioral desensitization

Pharmacokinetics

- Half-life 10–24 hours
- Inactive metabolites

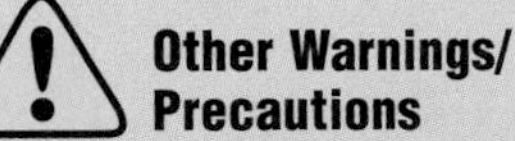

Drug Interactions

- Increased clearance and thus decreased estazolam levels in smokers
- Increased depressive effects when taken with other CNS depressants

Other Warnings/ Precautions

- Insomnia may be a symptom of a primary disorder, rather than a primary disorder itself
- Some patients may exhibit abnormal thinking or behavioral changes similar to those caused by other CNS depressants (i.e., either depressant actions or disinhibiting actions)
- Some depressed patients may experience a worsening of suicidal ideation
- Use only with extreme caution in patients with impaired respiratory function or obstructive sleep apnea
- Estazolam should be administered only at bedtime

Do Not Use
- If patient is pregnant
- If patient has narrow angle-closure glaucoma
- If there is a proven allergy to estazolam or any benzodiazepine

SPECIAL POPULATIONS

Renal Impairment
- Drug should be used with caution

Hepatic Impairment
- Drug should be used with caution

Cardiac Impairment
- Benzodiazepines have been used to treat insomnia associated with acute myocardial infarction

Elderly
- No dose adjustment in healthy patients
- Debilitated patients: recommended initial dose of 0.5 mg/day

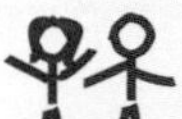

Children and Adolescents
- Safety and efficacy have not been established
- Long-term effects of estazolam in children/adolescents are unknown
- Should generally receive lower doses and be more closely monitored

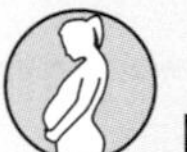

Pregnancy
- Risk Category X [positive evidence of risk to human fetus; contraindicated for use in pregnancy]
- Infants whose mothers received a benzodiazepine late in pregnancy may experience withdrawal effects
- Neonatal flaccidity has been reported in infants whose mothers took a benzodiazepine during pregnancy

Breast Feeding
- Unknown if estazolam is secreted in human breast milk, but all psychotropics assumed to be secreted in breast milk

✻ Recommended either to discontinue drug or bottle feed
- Effects on infant have been observed and include feeding difficulties, sedation, and weight loss

THE ART OF PSYCHOPHARMACOLOGY

Potential Advantages
- Transient insomnia

Potential Disadvantages
- Smokers (may need higher dose)

Primary Target Symptoms
- Time to sleep onset
- Total sleep time
- Nighttime awakenings

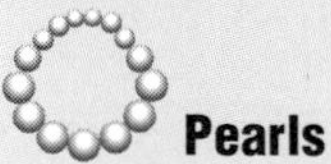

Pearls
- If tolerance develops, it may result in increased anxiety during the day and/or increased wakefulness during the latter part of the night
- Best short-term use is for less than 10 consecutive days, and for less than half of the nights in a month
- Drug holidays may restore drug effectiveness if tolerance develops

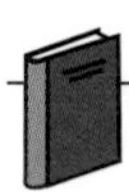

Suggested Reading

Pierce MW, Shu VS. Efficacy of estazolam. The United States clinical experience. Am J Med 1990;88:6S–11S.

Pierce MW, Shu VS, Groves LJ. Safety of estazolam. The United States clinical experience. Am J Med 1990;88:12S–17S.

Vogel GW, Morris D. The effects of estazolam on sleep, performance, and memory: a long-term sleep laboratory study of elderly insomniacs. J Clin Pharmacol 1992; 32:647–51.

THERAPEUTICS

Brands • Lunesta

see index for additional brand names

Generic? No

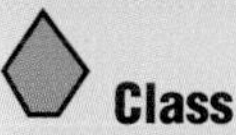

Class

- Non-benzodiazepine hypnotic; alpha 1 isoform selective agonist of GABA-A/benzodiazepine receptors

Commonly Prescribed for

(bold for FDA approved)

- **Insomnia**
- Primary insomnia
- Chronic insomnia
- Transient insomnia
- Insomnia secondary to psychiatric or medical conditions
- Residual insomnia following treatment with antidepressants

How the Drug Works

- May bind selectively to a subtype of the benzodiazepine receptor, the alpha 1 isoform
- May enhance GABA inhibitory actions that provide sedative hypnotic effects more selectively than other actions of GABA
- Boosts chloride conductance through GABA-regulated channels
- Inhibitory actions in sleep centers may provide sedative hypnotic effects

How Long Until It Works

- Generally takes effect in less than an hour

If It Works

- Improves quality of sleep
- Effects on total wake-time and number of nighttime awakenings may be decreased over time

If It Doesn't Work

- If insomnia does not improve after 7–10 days, it may be a manifestation of a primary psychiatric or physical illness such as obstructive sleep apnea or restless leg syndrome, which requires independent evaluation
- Increase the dose
- Improve sleep hygiene
- Switch to another agent

Best Augmenting Combos for Partial Response or Treatment Resistance

- Generally, best to switch to another agent
- Trazodone
- Agents with antihistamine actions (e.g., diphenhydramine, tricyclic antidepressants)

Tests

- None for healthy individuals

SIDE EFFECTS

How Drug Causes Side Effects

- Actions at benzodiazepine receptors that carry over to the next day can cause daytime sedation, amnesia, and ataxia

✻ Chronic studies of eszopiclone suggest lack of notable tolerance or dependence developing over time

Notable Side Effects

✻ Unpleasant taste

- Sedation
- Dizziness
- Dose-dependent amnesia
- Nervousness
- Dry mouth, headache

Life-Threatening or Dangerous Side Effects

- Respiratory depression, especially when taken with other CNS depressants in overdose
- Rare angioedema

Weight Gain

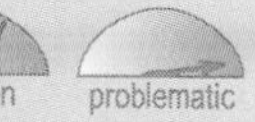

- Reported but not expected

Sedation

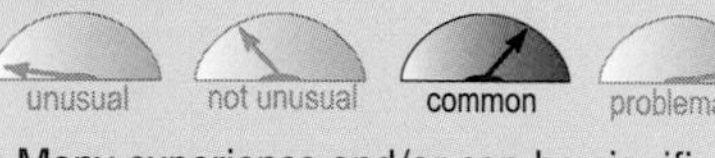

- Many experience and/or can be significant in amount
- Next day carryover sedation following nighttime dosing uncommon

What to Do About Side Effects

- Wait

- To avoid problems with memory, take eszopiclone only if planning to have a full night's sleep
- Lower the dose
- Switch to a shorter-acting sedative hypnotic
- Administer flumazenil if side effects are severe or life-threatening

Best Augmenting Agents for Side Effects

- Many side effects cannot be improved with an augmenting agent

DOSING AND USE

Usual Dosage Range

- 2–3 mg at bedtime

Dosage Forms

- Tablet 1 mg, 2 mg, 3 mg

How To Dose

- No titration, take dose at bedtime

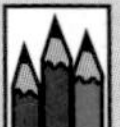

Dosing Tips

- Not restricted to short-term use
- No notable development of tolerance or dependence seen in studies up to 6 months
- Recent study adding eszopiclone to patients with major depression and only a partial response to fluoxetine showed improvement not only in residual insomnia, but in other residual symptoms of depression as well
- Most studies were done with 3 mg dose or less at night, but some patients with insomnia associated with psychiatric disorders may require higher dosing
- However, doses higher than 3 mg may be associated with carryover effects, hallucinations, or other CNS adverse effects
- To avoid problems with memory or carryover sedation, only take eszopiclone if planning to have a full night's sleep
- Most notable side effect may be unpleasant taste
- Other side effects can include sedation, dizziness, dose-dependent amnesia, nervousness, dry mouth, and headache

Overdose

- Few reports of eszopiclone overdose, but probably similar to zopiclone overdose
- Rare fatalities have been reported in zopiclone overdose
- Symptoms associated with zopiclone overdose include clumsiness, mood changes, sedation, weakness, breathing trouble, unconsciousness

Long-Term Use

- No development of tolerance was seen in studies up to 6 months

Habit Forming

- Eszopiclone is a Schedule IV drug
- Some patients could develop dependence and/or tolerance with drugs of this class; risk may be theoretically greater with higher doses
- History of drug addiction may theoretically increase risk of dependence

How to Stop

- Rebound insomnia may occur the first night after stopping
- If taken for more than a few weeks, taper to reduce chances of withdrawal effects

Pharmacokinetics

- Metabolized by CYP450 3A4 and 2E1
- Terminal elimination half-life approximately 6 hours

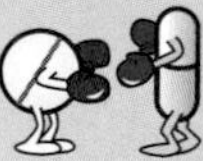

Drug Interactions

- Increased depressive effects when taken with other CNS depressants
- Inhibitors of CYP450 3A4, such as nefazodone and fluvoxamine, could increase plasma levels of eszopiclone
- Inducers of CYP450 3A4, such as rifampicin, could decrease plasma levels of eszopiclone

Other Warnings/ Precautions

- Insomnia may be a symptom of a primary disorder, rather than a primary disorder itself
- Some patients may exhibit abnormal thinking or behavioral changes similar to those caused by other CNS depressants

(i.e., either depressant actions or disinhibiting actions)
- Some depressed patients may experience a worsening of suicidal ideation
- Use only with caution in patients with impaired respiratory function or obstructive sleep apnea
- Eszopiclone should be administered only at bedtime

Do Not Use
- If there is a proven allergy to eszopiclone or zopiclone
- Rare angioedema has occurred with sedative hypnotic use and could potentially cause fatal airway obstruction if it involves the throat, glottis, or larynx; thus if angioedema occurs treatment should be discontinued
- Sleep driving and other complex behaviors, such as eating and preparing food and making phone calls, have been reported in patients taking sedative hypnotics

SPECIAL POPULATIONS

Renal Impairment
- Dose adjustment not generally necessary

Hepatic Impairment
- Dose adjustment not generally recommended for mild-to-moderate hepatic impairment
- For severe impairment, recommended initial dose 1 mg at bedtime; maximum dose 2 mg at bedtime

Cardiac Impairment
- Dosage adjustment may not be necessary

Elderly
- May be more susceptible to adverse effects
- Initial dose 1 mg at bedtime; maximum dose generally 2 mg at bedtime

Children and Adolescents
- Safety and efficacy have not been established
- Long-term effects of eszopiclone in children/adolescents are unknown
- Should generally receive lower doses and be more closely monitored

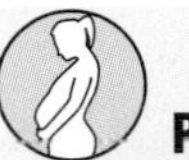

Pregnancy
- Risk Category C [some animal studies show adverse effects; no controlled studies in humans]
- Infants whose mothers took sedative-hypnotics during pregnancy may experience some withdrawal symptoms
- Neonatal flaccidity has been reported in infants whose mothers took sedative hypnotics during pregnancy

Breast Feeding
- Unknown if eszopiclone is secreted in human breast milk, but all psychotropics assumed to be secreted in breast milk
- ✻ Recommended either to discontinue drug or bottle feed

THE ART OF PSYCHOPHARMACOLOGY

Potential Advantages
- Primary insomnia
- Chronic insomnia
- Those who require long-term treatment
- Those with depression whose insomnia does not resolve with antidepressant treatment

Potential Disadvantages
- More expensive than some other sedative hypnotics

Primary Target Symptoms
- Time to sleep onset
- Nighttime awakenings
- Total sleep time

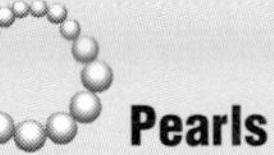

Pearls
- ✻ May be preferred over benzodiazepines because of its rapid onset of action, short duration of effect, and safety profile
- Eszopiclone is the best documented agent to be safe for long-term use, with little or no suggestion of tolerance, dependence, or abuse
- May even be safe to consider in patients with a past history of substance abuse who require treatment with a hypnotic
- May be preferred over benzodiazepine hypnotics, which all cause tolerance, dependence, and abuse as a class

- Not a benzodiazepine itself but binds to the benzodiazepine receptor
- May be a preferred agent in primary insomnia
- Targeting insomnia may prevent the onset of depression and maintain remission after recovery from depression
- Rebound insomnia does not appear to be common

Suggested Reading

Eszopiclone: esopiclone, estorra, S-zopiclone, zopiclone – Sepracor. Drugs R D. 2005;6(2):111–5.

Krystal AD, Walsh JK, Laska E, Caron J, Amato DA, Wessel TC, Roth T. Sustained efficacy of eszopiclone over 6 months of nightly treatment: results of a randomized, double-blind, placebo-controlled study in adults with chronic insomnia. Sleep 2003;26(7):793–9.

Zammit GK, McNabb LJ, Caron J, Amato DA, Roth T. Efficacy and safety of eszopiclone across 6-weeks of treatment for primary insomnia. Curr Med Res Opin 2004;20(12):1979–91.

THERAPEUTICS

Brands
- Romazicon
- Anexate
- Lanexat

see index for additional brand names

Generic? No

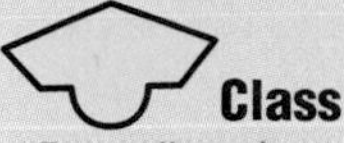

Class
- Benzodiazepine receptor antagonist

Commonly Prescribed for
(bold for FDA approved)
- **Reversal of sedative effects of benzodiazepines after general anesthesia has been induced and/or maintained with benzodiazepines**
- **Reversal of sedative effects of benzodiazepines after sedation has been produced with benzodiazepines for diagnostic and therapeutic procedures**
- **Management of benzodiazepine overdose**
- **Reversal of conscious sedation induced with benzodiazepines (pediatric patients)**

How the Drug Works
- Blocks benzodiazepine receptors at GABA-A ligand-gated chloride channel complex, preventing benzodiazepines from binding there

How Long Until It Works
- Onset of action 1–2 minutes; peak effect 6–10 minutes

If It Works
- ✻ Reverses sedation and psychomotor retardation rapidly, but may not restore memory completely
- ✻ Patients treated for benzodiazepine overdose may experience CNS excitation
- ✻ Patients who receive flumazenil to reverse benzodiazepine effects should be monitored for up to 2 hours for resedation, respiratory depression, or other lingering benzodiazepine effects
- Flumazenil has not been shown to treat hypoventilation due to benzodiazepine treatment

If It Doesn't Work
- Sedation is most likely not due to a benzodiazepine, and treatment with flumazenil should be discontinued and other causes of sedation investigated

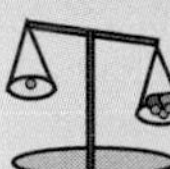

Best Augmenting Combos for Partial Response or Treatment Resistance
- None – flumazenil is basically used as a monotherapy antidote to reverse the actions of benzodiazepines

Tests
- None for healthy individuals

SIDE EFFECTS

How Drug Causes Side Effects
- Blocks benzodiazepine receptors at GABA-A ligand-gated chloride channel complex, preventing benzodiazepines from binding there

Notable Side Effects
- May precipitate benzodiazepine withdrawal in patients dependent upon or tolerant to benzodiazepines
- Dizziness, injection site pain, sweating, headache, blurred vision

Life-Threatening or Dangerous Side Effects
- Seizures
- Death (majority occurred in patients with severe underlying disease or who overdosed with non-benzodiazepines)
- Cardiac dysrhythmia

Weight Gain

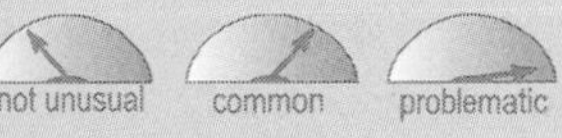

- Reported but not expected

Sedation

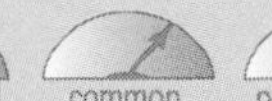
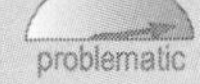

- Reported but not expected
- Patients may experience resedation if the effects of flumazenil wear off before the effects of the benzodiazepine

What to Do About Side Effects
- Monitor patient
- Restrict ambulation because of dizziness, blurred vision, and possibility of resedation

Best Augmenting Agents for Side Effects
- None – augmenting agents are not appropriate to treat side effects associated with flumazenil use

DOSING AND USE

Usual Dosage Range
- 0.4–1 mg generally causes complete antagonism of therapeutic doses of benzodiazepines
- 1–3 mg generally reverses benzodiazepine overdose

Dosage Forms
- Intravenous 0.1 mg/mL – 5 mL multiple-use vial, 10 mL multiple-use vial

How To Dose
- Conscious sedation, general anesthesia: 0.2 mg (2 mL) over 15 seconds; can administer 0.2 mg again after 45 seconds; can administer 0.2 mg each additional 60 seconds; maximum 1 mg
- Benzodiazepine overdose: 0.2 mg over 30 seconds; can administer 0.3 mg over next 30 seconds; can administer 0.5 mg over 30 seconds after 1 minute; maximum 5 mg

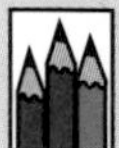

Dosing Tips
- May need to administer follow-up doses to reverse actions of benzodiazepines that have a longer half-life than flumazenil (i.e., longer than 1 hour)

Overdose
- Anxiety, agitation, increased muscle tone, hyperesthesia, convulsions

Long-Term Use
- Not a long-term treatment

Habit Forming
- No

How to Stop
- N/A

Pharmacokinetics
- Terminal half-life 41–79 minutes

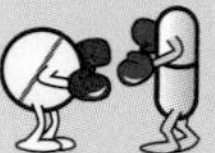

Drug Interactions
- Food increases its clearance

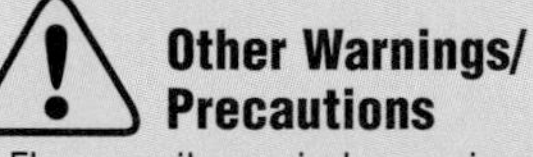

Other Warnings/ Precautions
- Flumazenil may induce seizures, particularly in patients tolerant to or dependent on benzodiazepines, or who have overdosed on cyclic antidepressants, received recent/repeated doses of parenteral benzodiazepines, or have jerking or convulsion during overdose
- Patients dependent on benzodiazepines or receiving benzodiazepines to suppress seizures in cyclic antidepressant overdose should receive the minimally effective dose of flumazenil
- Use with caution in patients with head injury
- Greater risk of resedation if administered to a patient who took a long-acting benzodiazepine or a large dose of a short-acting benzodiazepine
- Flumazenil may induce panic attacks in patients with panic disorder
- Use with caution in cases of mixed overdose because toxic effects of other drugs used in overdose (e.g., convulsions) may appear when the effects of the benzodiazepine are reversed

Do Not Use
- Should not be used until after effects of neuromuscular blockers have been reversed
- If benzodiazepine was prescribed to control a life-threatening condition (e.g., status epilepticus, intracranial pressure)
- If there is a high risk of seizure
- If patient exhibits signs of serious cyclic antidepressant overdose
- If there is a proven allergy to flumazenil or benzodiazepines

SPECIAL POPULATIONS

Renal Impairment
- Dosage adjustment may not be necessary

Hepatic Impairment
- Prolongation of half-life
- Moderate: clearance reduced by half
- Severe: clearance reduced by three-quarters

Cardiac Impairment
- Dosage adjustment may not be necessary

Elderly
- Dosage adjustment may not be necessary

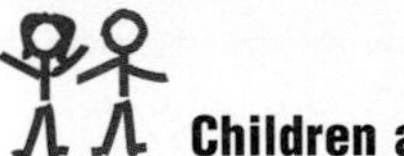

Children and Adolescents
- More variability of pharmacokinetics than in adults
- Safety and efficacy established for reversal of conscious sedation for children over age 1
- Initial 0.01 mg/kg (up to 0.2 mg) over 15 seconds; same dosing pattern as adults; maximum 0.05 mg/kg or 1 mg
- Safety and efficacy for reversal of benzodiazepine overdose, general anesthesia induction or resuscitation of a newborn have not been established, but anecdotal data suggest similar safety and efficacy as for conscious sedation

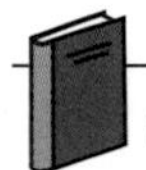

Pregnancy
- Risk Category C [some animal studies show adverse effects; no controlled studies in humans]
- Not recommended to treat the effects of benzodiazepines during labor and delivery because the effects on the infant have not been studied

Breast Feeding
- Unknown if flumazenil is secreted in human breast milk, but all psychotropics assumed to be secreted in breast milk
- If treatment with flumazenil is necessary, it should be administered with caution

THE ART OF PSYCHOPHARMACOLOGY

Potential Advantages
- To reverse a low dose of a short-acting benzodiazepine

Potential Disadvantages
- May be too short-acting

Primary Target Symptoms
- Effects of benzodiazepines
- Sedative effects
- Recall and psychomotor impairments
- Ventilatory depression

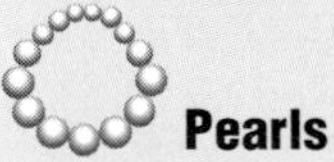

Pearls
- Can precipitate benzodiazepine withdrawal seizures

* Can wear off before the benzodiazepine it is reversing

* Can precipitate anxiety or panic in conscious patients with anxiety disorders

Suggested Reading

Malizia AL, Nutt DJ. The effects of flumazenil in neuropsychiatric disorders. Clin Neuropharmacol 1995;18:215–32.

McCloy RF. Reversal of conscious sedation by flumazenil: current status and future prospects. Acta Anaesthesiol Scand Suppl 1995;108:35–42.

Weinbroum AA, Flaishon R, Sorkine P, Szold O, Rudick V. A risk-benefit assessment of flumazenil in the management of benzodiazepine overdose. Drug Saf 1997; 17:181–96.

Whitwam JG, Amrein R. Pharmacology of flumazenil. Acta Anaesthesiol Scand Suppl 1995;108:3–14.

Whitwam JG. Flumazenil and midazolam in anaesthesia. Acta Anaesthesiol Scand Suppl 1995;108:15–22.

THERAPEUTICS

Brands • Rohypnol

see index for additional brand names

Generic? No

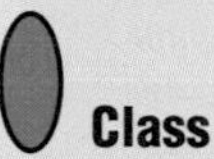

Class

• Benzodiazepine (hypnotic)

Commonly Prescribed for

(bold for FDA approved)

• Short-term treatment of insomnia (severe, disabling)

How the Drug Works

• Binds to benzodiazepine receptors at the GABA-A ligand-gated chloride channel complex
• Enhances the inhibitory effects of GABA
• Boosts chloride conductance through GABA-regulated channels
• Inhibitory actions in sleep centers may provide sedative hypnotic effects

How Long Until It Works

• Generally takes effect in less than an hour

If It Works

• Improves quality of sleep
• Effects on total wake-time and number of nighttime awakenings may be decreased over time

If It Doesn't Work

• If insomnia does not improve after 7–10 days, it may be a manifestation of a primary psychiatric or physical illness such as obstructive sleep apnea or restless leg syndrome, which requires independent evaluation
• Increase the dose
• Improve sleep hygiene
• Switch to another agent

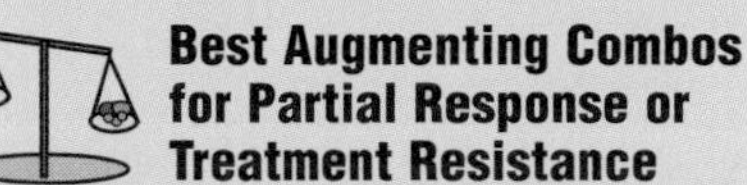

Best Augmenting Combos for Partial Response or Treatment Resistance

• Generally, best to switch to another agent
• Trazodone
• Agents with antihistamine actions (e.g., diphenhydramine, tricyclic antidepressants)

Tests

• In patients with seizure disorders, concomitant medical illness, and/or those with multiple concomitant long-term medications, periodic liver tests and blood counts may be prudent

SIDE EFFECTS

How Drug Causes Side Effects

• Same mechanism for side effects as for therapeutic effects – namely due to excessive actions at benzodiazepine receptors
• Actions at benzodiazepine receptors that carry over to next day can cause daytime sedation, amnesia, and ataxia
• Long-term adaptations in benzodiazepine receptors may explain the development of dependence, tolerance, and withdrawal

Notable Side Effects

* Sedation, fatigue, depression
* Dizziness, ataxia, slurred speech, weakness
* Forgetfulness, confusion
* Hyperexcitability, nervousness
• Rare hallucinations, mania
• Rare hypotension
• Hypersalivation, dry mouth
• Rebound insomnia when withdrawing from long-term treatment

Life-Threatening or Dangerous Side Effects

• Respiratory depression, especially when taken with CNS depressants in overdose
• Rare hepatic dysfunction, renal dysfunction, blood dyscrasias

Weight Gain

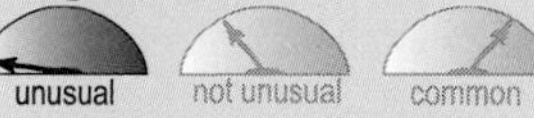

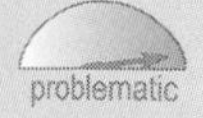

• Reported but not expected

Sedation

unusual not unusual **common** problematic

• Many experience and/or can be significant in amount

What to Do About Side Effects
- Wait
- To avoid problems with memory, only take flunitrazepam if planning to have a full night's sleep
- Lower the dose
- Switch to a shorter-acting sedative hypnotic
- Switch to a non-benzodiazepine hypnotic
- Administer flumazenil if side effects are severe or life-threatening

Best Augmenting Agents for Side Effects
- Many side effects cannot be improved with an augmenting agent

DOSING AND USE

Usual Dosage Range
- 0.5–1 mg/day at bedtime

Dosage Forms
- Tablet 0.5 mg, 1 mg, 2 mg, 4 mg

How To Dose
- Initial 0.5–1 mg/day at bedtime; maximum generally 2 mg/day at bedtime

Dosing Tips
- Use lowest possible effective dose and assess need for continued treatment regularly
- Flunitrazepam should generally not be prescribed in quantities greater than a 1-month supply
- Patients with lower body weights may require lower doses
- Risk of dependence may increase with dose and duration of treatment
- Use doses over 1 mg only in exceptional circumstances
- Patients who request or who require doses over 1 mg may be more likely to have present or past substance abuse
- Flunitrazepam is 10 times more potent than diazepam

Overdose
- Sedation, slurred speech, poor coordination, confusion, coma, respiratory depression

Long-Term Use
- Not generally intended for long-term use
- Use is not recommended to exceed 4 weeks

Habit Forming
- Some patients may develop dependence and/or tolerance; risk may be greater with higher doses
- History of drug addiction may increase risk of dependence
- Currently classified as Schedule III by the World Health Organization
- Currently classified as a Schedule IV drug in the U.S., but not legally available in the U.S.

How to Stop
- If taken for more than a few weeks, taper to reduce chances of withdrawal effects
- Patients with seizure history may seize upon sudden withdrawal
- Rebound insomnia may occur the first 1–2 nights after stopping
- For patients with severe problems discontinuing a benzodiazepine, dosing may need to be tapered over many months (i.e., reduce dose by 1% every 3 days by crushing tablet and suspending or dissolving in 100 mL of fruit juice and then disposing of 1 mL while drinking the rest; 3–7 days later, dispose of 2 mL, and so on). This is both a form of very slow biological tapering and a form of behavioral desensitization

Pharmacokinetics
- Elimination half-life 16–35 hours
- Half-life of active metabolite 23–33 hours

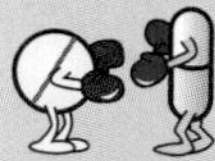

Drug Interactions
- Increased depressive effects when taken with other CNS depressants
- Cisapride may hasten the absorption of flunitrazepam and thus cause a temporary increase in the sedative effects of flunitrazepam

Other Warnings/Precautions
- Insomnia may be a symptom of a primary disorder, rather than a primary disorder itself

- Some patients may exhibit abnormal thinking or behavioural changes similar to those caused by other CNS depressants (i.e., either depressant actions or disinhibiting actions)
- Some depressed patients may experience a worsening of suicidal ideation
- Use only with extreme caution in patients with impaired respiratory function or obstructive sleep apnea
- Flunitrazepam should be administered only at bedtime

Do Not Use

- If patient is pregnant
- If patient has severe chronic hypercapnia, myasthenia gravis, severe respiratory insufficiency, sleep apnea, or severe hepatic insufficiency
- In children
- If patient has narrow angle-closure glaucoma
- If there is a proven allergy to flunitrazepam or any benzodiazepine

SPECIAL POPULATIONS

Renal Impairment

- Drug should be used with caution

Hepatic Impairment

- Dose should be lowered
- Should not be used in patients with severe hepatic insufficiency, as it may precipitate encephalopathy

Cardiac Impairment

- Benzodiazepines have been used to treat insomnia associated with acute myocardial infarction

Elderly

- Initial starting dose 0.5 mg at bedtime; maximum generally 1 mg/day at bedtime
- Paradoxical reactions with restlessness and agitation are more likely to occur in the elderly

Children and Adolescents

- Safety and efficacy have not been established
- Not recommended for use in children or adolescents
- Paradoxical reactions with restlessness and agitation are more likely to occur in children

Pregnancy

- Positive evidence of risk to human fetus; contraindicated for use in pregnancy
- Infants whose mothers received a benzodiazepine late in pregnancy may experience withdrawal effects
- Neonatal flaccidity has been reported in infants whose mothers took a benzodiazepine during pregnancy

Breast Feeding

- Unknown if flunitrazepam is secreted in human breast milk, but all psychotropics assumed to be secreted in breast milk

✻ Recommended either to discontinue drug or bottle feed

- Effects on infant have been observed and include feeding difficulties, sedation, and weight loss

THE ART OF PSYCHOPHARMACOLOGY

Potential Advantages

- For severe, disabling insomnia unresponsive to other sedative hypnotics

Potential Disadvantages

- For those who need treatment for longer than a few weeks
- For those with current or past substance abuse

Primary Target Symptoms

- Time to sleep onset
- Total sleep time
- Nighttime awakenings

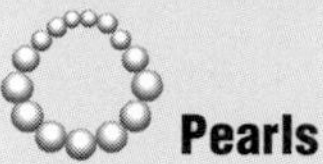

Pearls

✻ Psychiatric symptoms and “paradoxical” reactions may be quite severe with flunitrazepam and may be more frequent than with other benzodiazepines

✻ “Paradoxical” reactions include symptoms such as restlessness, agitation, irritability, aggressiveness, delusions, rage, nightmares, hallucinations, psychosis, inappropriate behavior, and other adverse behavioral effects

- Although legally available in Europe, Mexico, South America, and many other countries, it is not legally available in the U.S.
- Although currently classified as a Schedule IV drug, the U.S. drug enforcement agency is considering reclassifying it as Schedule I
- ✱ Has earned a reputation as a "date rape drug" in which sexual predators have allegedly slipped flunitrazepam into women's drinks to induce sexual relations
- ✱ Flunitrazepam, especially in combination with alcohol, is claimed to reduce the woman's judgment, inhibitions, or physical ability to resist sexual advances, as well as to reduce or eliminate her recall of the events
- ✱ Until 1999 was colorless, but a colorimetric compound is now added that turns the drug blue when added to a liquid, making it obvious that a drink was tampered with
- Illicit use since 1999 has fallen in part due to this additive
- Illicit use has also fallen in the U.S. due to the Drug-Induced Rape Prevention and Punishment act of 1996, making it punishable to commit a violent crime using a controlled substance such as flunitrazepam
- Street names for flunitrazepam, based in part upon its trade name of Rohypnol, manufacturer Roche, and the presence of RO-2 on the surface of the tablets, include "roofies," "ruffies," "roapies," "la roacha," "roach-2," "Mexican valium," "rope," "roache vitamins," and others
- If tolerance develops, it may result in increased anxiety during the day and/or increased wakefulness during the latter part of the night
- Best short-term use is for less than 10 consecutive days, and for less than half of the nights in a month
- Drug holidays may restore drug effectiveness if tolerance develops

Suggested Reading

Simmons MM, Cupp MJ. Use and abuse of flunitrazepam. Ann Pharmacother 1998;32(1):117–9.

Woods JH, Winger G. Abuse liability of flunitrazepam. J Clin Psychopharmacol 1997;17(3 Suppl 2):1S–57S.

THERAPEUTICS

Brands • Prozac • Prozac weekly
• Sarafem

see index for additional brand names

Generic? Yes

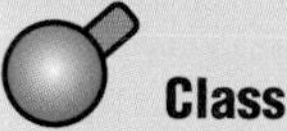

Class

• SSRI (selective serotonin reuptake inhibitor); often classified as an antidepressant, but it is not just an antidepressant

Commonly Prescribed for

(bold for FDA approved)

• **Major depressive disorder**
• **Obsessive-compulsive disorder (OCD)**
• **Premenstrual dysphoric disorder (PMDD)**
• **Bulimia nervosa**
• **Panic disorder**
• **Bipolar depression [in combination with olanzapine (Symbyax)]**
• Social anxiety disorder (social phobia)
• Posttraumatic stress disorder (PTSD)

How the Drug Works

• Boosts neurotransmitter serotonin
• Blocks serotonin reuptake pump (serotonin transporter)
• Desensitizes serotonin receptors, especially serotonin 1A receptors
• Presumably increases serotonergic neurotransmission
✻ Fluoxetine also has antagonist properties at 5HT2C receptors, which could increase norepinephrine and dopamine neurotransmission

How Long Until It Works

✻ Some patients may experience increased energy or activation early after initiation of treatment
• Onset of therapeutic actions usually not immediate, but often delayed 2–4 weeks
• If it is not working within 6–8 weeks, it may require a dosage increase or it may not work at all
• May continue to work for many years to prevent relapse of symptoms

If It Works

• The goal of treatment is complete remission of current symptoms as well as prevention of future relapses
• Treatment most often reduces or even eliminates symptoms, but not a cure since symptoms can recur after medicine stopped
• Continue treatment until all symptoms are gone (remission) or significantly reduced (e.g., OCD, PTSD)
• Once symptoms gone, continue treating for 1 year for the first episode of depression
• For second and subsequent episodes of depression, treatment may need to be indefinite
• For anxiety disorders and bulimia, treatment may also need to be indefinite

If It Doesn't Work

• Many patients have only a partial response where some symptoms are improved but others persist (especially insomnia, fatigue, and problems concentrating in depression)
• Other patients may be nonresponders, sometimes called treatment-resistant or treatment-refractory
• Some patients who have an initial response may relapse even though they continue treatment, sometimes called "poop-out"
• Consider increasing dose, switching to another agent or adding an appropriate augmenting agent
• Consider psychotherapy
• Consider evaluation for another diagnosis or for a comorbid condition (e.g., medical illness, substance abuse, etc.)
• Some patients may experience apparent lack of consistent efficacy due to activation of latent or underlying bipolar disorder, and require antidepressant discontinuation and a switch to a mood stabilizer

Best Augmenting Combos for Partial Response or Treatment Resistance

• Trazodone, especially for insomnia
• Bupropion, mirtazapine, reboxetine, or atomoxetine (add with caution and at lower doses since fluoxetine could theoretically raise atomoxetine levels); use combinations of antidepressants with caution as this may activate bipolar disorder and suicidal ideation

- Modafinil, especially for fatigue, sleepiness, and lack of concentration
- Mood stabilizers or atypical antipsychotics for bipolar depression, psychotic depression, treatment-resistant depression, or treatment-resistant anxiety disorders

✻ Fluoxetine has been specifically studied in combination with olanzapine (olanzapine-fluoxetine combination) with excellent results for bipolar depression, treatment-resistant unipolar depression, and psychotic depression

- Benzodiazepines
- If all else fails for anxiety disorders, consider gabapentin or tiagabine
- Hypnotics for insomnia
- Classically, lithium, buspirone, or thyroid hormone

Tests

- None for healthy individuals

SIDE EFFECTS

How Drug Causes Side Effects

- Theoretically due to increases in serotonin concentrations at serotonin receptors in parts of the brain and body other than those that cause therapeutic actions (e.g., unwanted actions of serotonin in sleep centers causing insomnia, unwanted actions of serotonin in the gut causing diarrhea, etc.)
- Increasing serotonin can cause diminished dopamine release and might contribute to emotional flattening, cognitive slowing, and apathy in some patients
- Most side effects are immediate but often go away with time, in contrast to most therapeutic effects which are delayed and are enhanced over time

✻ Fluoxetine's unique 5HT2C antagonist properties could contribute to agitation, anxiety, and undesirable activation, especially early in dosing

Notable Side Effects

- Sexual dysfunction (men: delayed ejaculation, erectile dysfunction; men and women: decreased sexual desire, anorgasmia)
- Gastrointestinal (decreased appetite, nausea, diarrhea, constipation, dry mouth)
- Mostly central nervous system (insomnia but also sedation, agitation, tremors, headache, dizziness)
- Note: patients with diagnosed or undiagnosed bipolar or psychotic disorders may be more vulnerable to CNS-activating actions of SSRIs
- Autonomic (sweating)
- Bruising and rare bleeding

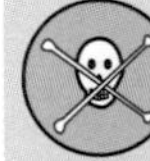

Life-Threatening or Dangerous Side Effects

- Rare seizures
- Rare induction of mania
- Rare activation of suicidal ideation and behavior (suicidality) (short-term studies did not show an increase in the risk of suicidality with antidepressants compared to placebo beyond age 24)

Weight Gain

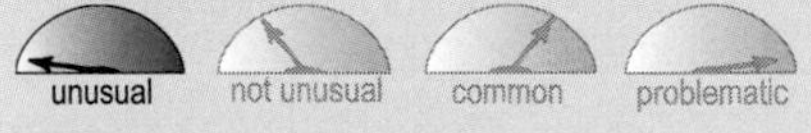

- Reported but not expected
- Possible weight loss, especially short-term

Sedation

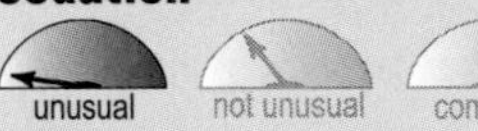

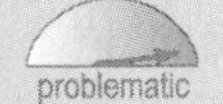

common

- Reported but not expected

What to Do About Side Effects

- Wait
- Wait
- Wait
- If fluoxetine is activating, take in the morning to help reduce insomnia
- Reduce dose to 10 mg, and either stay at this dose if tolerated and effective, or consider increasing again to 20 mg or more if tolerated but not effective at 10 mg
- In a few weeks, switch or add other drugs

Best Augmenting Agents for Side Effects

- Often best to try another SSRI or another antidepressant monotherapy prior to resorting to augmentation strategies to treat side effects
- Trazodone or a hypnotic for insomnia
- Bupropion, sildenafil, vardenafil, or tadalafil for sexual dysfunction
- Bupropion for emotional flattening, cognitive slowing, or apathy

- Mirtazapine for insomnia, agitation, and gastrointestinal side effects
- Benzodiazepines for jitteriness and anxiety, especially at initiation of treatment and especially for anxious patients
- Many side effects are dose-dependent (i.e., they increase as dose increases, or they reemerge until tolerance re-develops)
- Many side effects are time-dependent (i.e., they start immediately upon dosing and upon each dose increase, but go away with time)
- Activation and agitation may represent the induction of a bipolar state, especially a mixed dysphoric bipolar II condition sometimes associated with suicidal ideation, and require the addition of lithium, a mood stabilizer or an atypical antipsychotic, and/or discontinuation of fluoxetine

DOSING AND USE

Usual Dosage Range

- 20–80 mg for depression and anxiety disorders
- 60–80 mg for bulimia

Dosage Forms

- Capsules 10 mg, 20 mg, 40 mg
- Tablet 10 mg
- Liquid 20 mg/5 mL–120 mL bottles
- Weekly capsule 90 mg

How To Dose

- Depression and OCD: Initial dose 20 mg/day in morning, usually wait a few weeks to assess drug effects before increasing dose; maximum dose generally 80 mg/day
- Bulimia: Initial dose 60 mg/day in morning; some patients may need to begin at lower dose and titrate over several days

Dosing Tips

- The long half-lives of fluoxetine and its active metabolites mean that dose changes will not be fully reflected in plasma for several weeks, lengthening titration to final dose and extending withdrawal from treatment
- Give once daily, often in the mornings, but at any time of day tolerated
- Often available in capsules, not tablets, so unable to break capsules in half
- Occasional patients are dosed above 80 mg
- Liquid formulation easiest for doses below 10 mg when used for cases that are very intolerant to fluoxetine or for very slow up and down titration needs

✽ For some patients, weekly dosing with the weekly formulation may enhance compliance

- The more anxious and agitated the patient, the lower the starting dose, the slower the titration, and the more likely the need for a concomitant agent such as trazodone or a benzodiazepine
- If intolerable anxiety, insomnia, agitation, akathisia, or activation occur either upon dosing initiation or discontinuation, consider the possibility of activated bipolar disorder and switch to a mood stabilizer or an atypical antipsychotic

Overdose

- Rarely lethal in monotherapy overdose; respiratory depression especially with alcohol, ataxia, sedation, possible seizures

Long-Term Use

- Safe

Habit Forming

- No

How to Stop

- Taper rarely necessary since fluoxetine tapers itself after immediate discontinuation, due to the long half-life of fluoxetine and its active metabolites

Pharmacokinetics

- Active metabolite (norfluoxetine) has 2 week half-life
- Parent drug has 2–3 day half-life
- Inhibits CYP450 2D6
- Inhibits CYP450 3A4

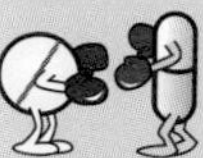

Drug Interactions

- Tramadol increases the risk of seizures in patients taking an antidepressant
- Can increase tricyclic antidepressant levels; use with caution with tricyclic antidepressants or when switching from a TCA to fluoxetine

- Can cause a fatal "serotonin syndrome" when combined with MAO inhibitors, so do not use with MAO inhibitors or for at least 14 days after MAOIs are stopped
- Do not start an MAO inhibitor for at least 5 weeks after discontinuing fluoxetine
- May displace highly protein bound drugs (e.g., warfarin)
- Can rarely cause weakness, hyperreflexia, and incoordination when combined with sumatriptan, or possibly with other triptans, requiring careful monitoring of patient
- Possible increased risk of bleeding, especially when combined with anticoagulants (e.g., warfarin, NSAIDs)
- Via CYP450 2D6 inhibition, could theoretically interfere with the analgesic actions of codeine, and increase the plasma levels of some beta blockers and of atomoxetine
- Via CYP450 2D6 inhibition, fluoxetine could theoretically increase concentrations of thioridazine and cause dangerous cardiac arrhythmias
- May reduce the clearance of diazepam or trazodone, thus increasing their levels
- Via CYP450 3A4 inhibition, may increase the levels of alprazolam, buspirone, and triazolam
- Via CYP450 3A4 inhibition, fluoxetine could theoretically increase concentrations of certain cholesterol lowering HMG CoA reductase inhibitors, especially simvastatin, atorvastatin, and lovastatin, but not pravastatin or fluvastatin, which would increase the risk of rhabdomyolysis; thus, coadministration of fluoxetine with certain HMG CoA reductase inhibitors should proceed with caution
- Via CYP450 3A4 inhibition, fluoxetine could theoretically increase the concentrations of pimozide, and cause QTc prolongation and dangerous cardiac arrhythmias

Other Warnings/ Precautions

✻ Add or initiate other antidepressants with caution for up to 5 weeks after discontinuing fluoxetine
- Use with caution in patients with history of seizure
- Use with caution in patients with bipolar disorder unless treated with concomitant mood-stabilizing agent
- When treating children, carefully weigh the risks and benefits of pharmacological treatment against the risks and benefits of nontreatment with antidepressants and make sure to document this in the patient's chart
- Distribute the brochures provided by the FDA and the drug companies
- Warn patients and their caregivers about the possibility of activating side effects and advise them to report such symptoms immediately
- Monitor patients for activation of suicidal ideation, especially children and adolescents

Do Not Use

- If patient is taking an MAO inhibitor
- If patient is taking thioridazine
- If patient is taking pimozide
- If there is a proven allergy to fluoxetine

SPECIAL POPULATIONS

Renal Impairment

- No dose adjustment
- Not removed by hemodialysis

Hepatic Impairment

- Lower dose or give less frequently, perhaps by half

Cardiac Impairment

- Preliminary research suggests that fluoxetine is safe in these patients
- Treating depression with SSRIs in patients with acute angina or following myocardial infarction may reduce cardiac events and improve survival as well as mood

Elderly

- Some patients may tolerate lower doses better
- Reduction in risk of suicidality with antidepressants compared to placebo in adults age 65 and older

Children and Adolescents

- Carefully weigh the risks and benefits of pharmacological treatment against the risks and benefits of nontreatment with antidepressants and make sure to document this in the patient's chart
- Monitor patients face-to-face regularly, particularly during the first several weeks of treatment
- Use with caution, observing for activation of known or unknown bipolar disorder and/or suicidal ideation, and inform parents or guardian of this risk so they can help observe child or adolescent patients
- Approved for OCD and depression
- Adolescents often receive adult dose, but doses slightly lower for children
- Children taking fluoxetine may have slower growth; long-term effects are unknown

Pregnancy

- Risk Category C [some animal studies show adverse effects; no controlled studies in humans]
- Not generally recommended for use during pregnancy, especially during first trimester
- Nonetheless, continuous treatment during pregnancy may be necessary and has not been proven to be harmful to the fetus
- Current patient registries of children whose mothers took fluoxetine during pregnancy do not show adverse consequences
- At delivery there may be more bleeding in the mother and transient irritability or sedation in the newborn
- Must weigh the risk of treatment (first trimester fetal development, third trimester newborn delivery) to the child against the risk of no treatment (recurrence of depression, maternal health, infant bonding) to the mother and child
- For many patients this may mean continuing treatment during pregnancy
- SSRI use beyond the 20th week of pregnancy may be associated with increased risk of pulmonary hypertension in newborns
- Neonates exposed to SSRIs or SNRIs late in the third trimester have developed complications requiring prolonged hospitalization, respiratory support, and tube feeding; reported symptoms are consistent with either a direct toxic effect of SSRIs and SNRIs or, possibly, a drug discontinuation syndrome, and include respiratory distress, cyanosis, apnea, seizures, temperature instability, feeding difficulty, vomiting, hypoglycemia, hypotonia, hypertonia, hyperreflexia, tremor, jitteriness, irritability, and constant crying

Breast Feeding

- Some drug is found in mother's breast milk
- Trace amounts may be present in nursing children whose mothers are on fluoxetine
- If child becomes irritable or sedated, breast feeding or drug may need to be discontinued
- Immediate postpartum period is a high-risk time for depression, especially in women who have had prior depressive episodes, so drug may need to be reinstituted late in the third trimester or shortly after childbirth to prevent a recurrence during the postpartum period
- Must weigh benefits of breast feeding with risks and benefits of antidepressant treatment versus nontreatment to both the infant and the mother
- For many patients this may mean continuing treatment during breast feeding

THE ART OF PSYCHOPHARMACOLOGY

Potential Advantages

- Patients with atypical depression (hypersomnia, increased appetite)
- Patients with fatigue and low energy
- Patients with comorbid eating and affective disorders
- Generic is less expensive than brand name where available
- Patients for whom weekly administration is desired
- Children with OCD or depression

Potential Disadvantages

- Patients with anorexia
- Initiating treatment in anxious, agitated patients
- Initiating treatment in severe insomnia

Primary Target Symptoms

- Depressed mood
- Energy, motivation, and interest

- Anxiety (eventually, but can actually increase anxiety, especially short-term)
- Sleep disturbance, both insomnia and hypersomnia (eventually, but may actually cause insomnia, especially short-term)

Pearls

✻ May be a first-line choice for atypical depression (e.g., hypersomnia, hyperphagia, low energy, mood reactivity)
- Consider avoiding in agitated insomniacs
- Can cause cognitive and affective "flattening"
- Not as well tolerated as some other SSRIs for panic disorder and other anxiety disorders, especially when dosing is initiated, unless given with co-therapies such as benzodiazepines or trazodone
- Long half-life; even longer lasting active metabolite

✻ Actions at 5HT2C receptors may explain its activating properties

✻ Actions at 5HT2C receptors may explain in part fluoxetine's efficacy in combination with olanzapine for bipolar depression and treatment-resistant depression, since both agents have this property
- For sexual dysfunction, can augment with bupropion, sildenafil, vardenafil, or tadalafil, or switch to a non-SSRI such as bupropion or mirtazapine
- Mood disorders can be associated with eating disorders (especially in adolescent females) and be treated successfully with fluoxetine
- SSRIs may be less effective in women over 50, especially if they are not taking estrogen
- SSRIs may be useful for hot flushes in perimenopausal women
- Some postmenopausal women's depression will respond better to fluoxetine plus estrogen augmentation than to fluoxetine alone
- Nonresponse to fluoxetine in elderly may require consideration of mild cognitive impairment or Alzheimer disease
- SSRIs may not cause as many patients to attain remission of depression as some other classes of antidepressants (e.g., SNRIs)
- A single pill containing both fluoxetine and olanzapine is available for combination treatment of bipolar depression, psychotic depression, and treatment-resistant unipolar depression

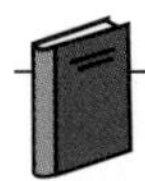

Suggested Reading

Anderson IM. Selective serotonin reuptake inhibitors versus tricyclic antidepressants: a meta-analysis of efficacy and tolerability. Journal of Affective Disorders 2000;58:19–36.

Beasley CM Jr, Ball SG, Nilsson ME, et al. Fluoxetine and adult suicidality revisited: an updated meta-analysis using expanded data sources from placebo-controlled trials. J Clin Psychopharmacol 2007;27(6):682–6.

March JS, Silva S, Petrycki S, et al. The treatment for adolescents with depression study (TADS): long-term effectiveness and safety outcomes. Arch Gen Psychiatry 2007;64(10):1132–43.

Wagstaff AJ, Goa KL. Once-weekly fluoxetine. Drugs 2001;61:2221–8.

FLUPENTHIXOL

THERAPEUTICS

Brands • Depixol

see index for additional brand names

Generic? No

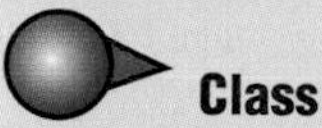

Class

- Conventional antipsychotic (neuroleptic, thioxanthene, dopamine 2 antagonist)

Commonly Prescribed for

(bold for FDA approved)

- Schizophrenia
- Depression (low dose)
- Other psychotic disorders
- Bipolar disorder

How the Drug Works

- Blocks dopamine 2 receptors, reducing positive symptoms of psychosis

How Long Until It Works

- With injection, psychotic symptoms can improve within a few days, but it may take 1–2 weeks for notable improvement
- With oral formulation, psychotic symptoms can improve within 1 week, but it may take several weeks for full effect on behavior

If It Works

- Most often reduces positive symptoms in schizophrenia but does not eliminate them
- Most schizophrenic patients do not have a total remission of symptoms but rather a reduction of symptoms by about a third
- Continue treatment in schizophrenia until reaching a plateau of improvement
- After reaching a satisfactory plateau, continue treatment for at least a year after first episode of psychosis in schizophrenia
- For second and subsequent episodes of psychosis in schizophrenia, treatment may need to be indefinite
- Reduces symptoms of acute psychotic mania but not proven as a mood stabilizer or as an effective maintenance treatment in bipolar disorder
- After reducing acute psychotic symptoms in mania, switch to a mood stabilizer and/or an atypical antipsychotic for mood stabilization and maintenance

If It Doesn't Work

- Consider trying one of the first-line atypical antipsychotics (risperidone, olanzapine, quetiapine, ziprasidone, aripiprazole, paliperidone, amisulpride)
- Consider trying another conventional antipsychotic
- If 2 or more antipsychotic monotherapies do not work, consider clozapine

Best Augmenting Combos for Partial Response or Treatment Resistance

- Augmentation of conventional antipsychotics has not been systematically studied
- Addition of a mood-stabilizing anticonvulsant such as valproate, carbamazepine, or lamotrigine may be helpful in both schizophrenia and bipolar mania
- Augmentation with lithium in bipolar mania may be helpful
- Addition of a benzodiazepine, especially short-term for agitation

Tests

- ✽ Since conventional antipsychotics are frequently associated with weight gain, before starting treatment, weigh all patients and determine if the patient is already overweight (BMI 25.0–29.9) or obese (BMI ≥30)
- Before giving a drug that can cause weight gain to an overweight or obese patient, consider determining whether the patient already has pre-diabetes (fasting plasma glucose 100–25 mg/dL), diabetes (fasting plasma glucose >126 mg/dL), or dyslipidemia (increased total cholesterol, LDL cholesterol and triglycerides; decreased HDL cholesterol), and treat or refer such patients for treatment, including nutrition and weight management, physical activity counseling, smoking cessation, and medical management
- ✽ Monitor weight and BMI during treatment
- ✽ Consider monitoring fasting triglycerides monthly for several months in patients at high risk for metabolic complications and when initiating or switching antipsychotics
- ✽ While giving a drug to a patient who has gained >5% of initial weight, consider evaluating for the presence of pre-diabetes,

diabetes, or dyslipidemia, or consider switching to a different antipsychotic
- Monitoring elevated prolactin levels of dubious clinical benefit

SIDE EFFECTS

How Drug Causes Side Effects

- By blocking dopamine 2 receptors in the striatum, it can cause motor side effects
- By blocking dopamine 2 receptors in the pituitary, it can cause elevations in prolactin
- By blocking dopamine 2 receptors excessively in the mesocortical and mesolimbic dopamine pathways, especially at high doses, it can cause worsening of negative and cognitive symptoms (neuroleptic-induced deficit syndrome)
- Anticholinergic actions may cause sedation, blurred vision, constipation, dry mouth
- Antihistaminic actions may cause sedation, weight gain
- By blocking alpha 1 adrenergic receptors, it can cause dizziness, sedation, and hypotension
- Mechanism of weight gain and any possible increased incidence of diabetes or dyslipidemia with conventional antipsychotics is unknown

Notable Side Effects

✻ Neuroleptic-induced deficit syndrome
✻ Extrapyramidal symptoms (more common at start of treatment), Parkinsonism
✻ Insomnia, restlessness, agitation, sedation
✻ Tardive dyskinesia (risk increases with duration of treatment and with dose)
✻ Galactorrhea, amenorrhea
- Tachycardia
- Weight gain
- Hypomania
- Rare eosinophilia

Life-Threatening or Dangerous Side Effects

- Rare neuroleptic malignant syndrome
- Rare seizures
- Rare jaundice, leucopenia

- Increased risk of death and cerebrovascular events in elderly patients with dementia-related psychosis

Weight Gain

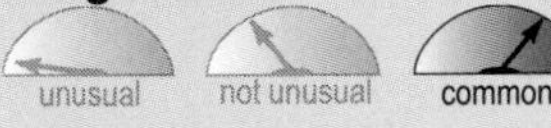

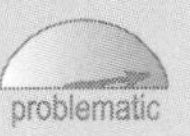

- Many experience and/or can be significant in amount

Sedation

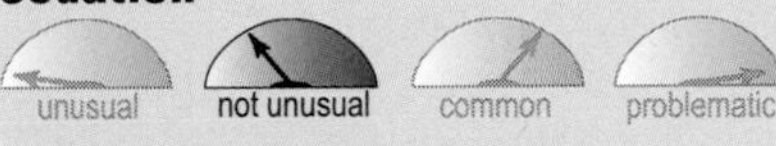

- Occurs in significant minority

What to Do About Side Effects

- Wait
- Wait
- Wait
- For motor symptoms, add an anticholinergic agent
- Reduce the dose
- For sedation, give at night
- Switch to an atypical antipsychotic
- Weight loss, exercise programs, and medical management for high BMIs, diabetes, dyslipidemia

Best Augmenting Agents for Side Effects

- Benztropine or trihexyphenidyl for motor side effects
- Sometimes amantadine can be helpful for motor side effects
- Benzodiazepines may be helpful for akathisia
- Many side effects cannot be improved with an augmenting agent

DOSING AND USE

Usual Dosage Range

- Oral 3–6 mg/day in divided doses
- Intramuscular 40–120 mg every 1–4 weeks

Dosage Forms

- Tablet 0.5 mg, 3 mg
- Injection 20 mg/mL, 100 mg/mL

How To Dose

- Oral: initial 1 mg 3 times a day; increase by 1 mg every 2–3 days; maximum generally 18 mg/day

- Intramuscular: initial dose 20 mg for patients who have not been exposed to long-acting depot antipsychotics, 40 mg for patients who have previously demonstrated tolerance to long-acting depot antipsychotics; after 4–10 days can give additional 20 mg dose; maximum 200 mg every 1–4 weeks

Dosing Tips

- The peak of action for the decanoate is usually 7–10 days, and doses generally have to be administered every 2–3 weeks
- May have more activating effects at low doses, which can sometimes be useful as a second-line, short-term treatment of depression
- Some evidence that flupenthixol may improve anxiety and depression at low doses

Overdose

- Agitation, confusion, sedation, extrapyramidal symptoms, respiratory collapse, circulatory collapse

Long-Term Use

- Safe

Habit Forming

- No

How to Stop

- Slow down-titration of oral formulation (over 6–8 weeks), especially when simultaneously beginning a new antipsychotic while switching (i.e., cross-titration)
- Rapid oral discontinuation may lead to rebound psychosis and worsening of symptoms
- If antiparkinson agents are being used, they should be continued for a few weeks after flupenthixol is discontinued

Pharmacokinetics

- Oral: maximum plasma concentrations within 3–8 hours
- Intramuscular: rate-limiting half-life approximately 8 days with single dose, approximately 17 days with multiple doses

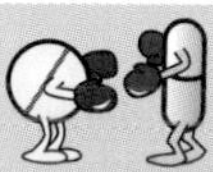

Drug Interactions

- May decrease the effects of levodopa, dopamine agonists
- May increase the effects of antihypertensive drugs except for guanethidine, whose antihypertensive actions flupenthixol may antagonize
- CNS effects may be increased if used with other CNS depressants
- Combined use with epinephrine may lower blood pressure
- Ritonavir may increase plasma levels of flupenthixol
- May increase carbamazepine plasma levels
- Some patients taking a neuroleptic and lithium have developed an encephalopathic syndrome similar to neuroleptic malignant syndrome

Other Warnings/ Precautions

- If signs of neuroleptic malignant syndrome develop, treatment should be immediately discontinued
- Use cautiously in patients with alcohol withdrawal or convulsive disorders because of possible lowering of seizure threshold
- In epileptic patients, dose 10–20 mg every 15 days for intramuscular formulation
- Use with caution if at all in patients with Parkinson's disease, severe arteriosclerosis, or Lewy body dementia
- Possible antiemetic effect of flupenthixol may mask signs of other disorders or overdose; suppression of cough reflex may cause asphyxia
- Avoid extreme heat exposure
- Do not use epinephrine in event of overdose as interaction with some pressor agents may lower blood pressure

Do Not Use

- If patient is taking a large concomitant dose of a sedative hypnotic
- If patient has CNS depression
- If patient is comatose or if there is brain damage
- If there is blood dyscrasia
- In patient has pheochromocytoma
- If patient has liver damage
- If patient has a severe cardiovascular disorder
- If patient has renal insufficiency

- If patient has cerebrovascular insufficiency
- If there is a proven allergy to flupenthixol

SPECIAL POPULATIONS

Renal Impairment
- Oral: recommended to take half or less of usual adult dose
- Intramuscular: recommended dose schedule generally 10–20 mg every 15 days

Hepatic Impairment
- Use with caution
- Oral: recommended to take half or less of usual adult dose

Cardiac Impairment
- Use with caution
- Oral: recommended to take half or less of usual adult dose

Elderly
- Intramuscular: recommended initial dose generally 5 mg; recommended dose schedule generally 10–20 mg every 15 days
- Oral: recommended to take half or less of usual adult dose
- Although conventional antipsychotics are commonly used for behavioral disturbances in dementia, no agent has been approved for treatment of elderly patients with dementia-related psychosis
- Elderly patients with dementia-related psychosis treated with antipsychotics are at an increased risk of death compared to placebo, and also have an increased risk of cerebrovascular events

Children and Adolescents
- Not recommended for use in children

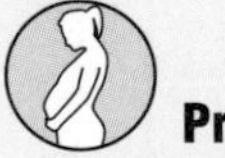

Pregnancy
- Not recommended for use during pregnancy
- Reports of extrapyramidal symptoms, jaundice, hyperreflexia, hyporeflexia in infants whose mothers took a conventional antipsychotic during pregnancy
- Psychotic symptoms may worsen during pregnancy and some form of treatment may be necessary
- Atypical antipsychotics may be preferable to conventional antipsychotics or anticonvulsant mood stabilizers if treatment is required during pregnancy

Breast Feeding
- Some drug is found in mother's breast milk
- * Recommended either to discontinue drug or bottle feed

THE ART OF PSYCHOPHARMACOLOGY

Potential Advantages
- Non-compliant patients

Potential Disadvantages
- Children
- Elderly
- Patients with tardive dyskinesia

Primary Target Symptoms
- Positive symptoms of psychosis
- Negative symptoms of psychosis
- Aggressive symptoms

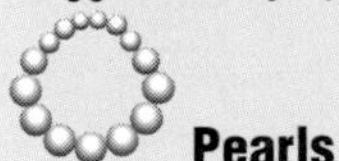

Pearls
- May activate manic patients
- Less sedation and orthostatic hypotension but more extrapyramidal symptoms than some other conventional antipsychotics
- Patients have very similar antipsychotic responses to any conventional antipsychotic, which is different from atypical antipsychotics where antipsychotic responses of individual patients can occasionally vary greatly from one atypical antipsychotic to another
- Patients with inadequate responses to atypical antipsychotics may benefit from a trial of augmentation with a conventional antipsychotic such as flupenthixol or from switching to a conventional antipsychotic such as flupenthixol
- However, long-term polypharmacy with a combination of a conventional antipsychotic such as flupenthixol with an atypical antipsychotic may combine their side effects without clearly augmenting the efficacy of either
- Although a frequent practice by some prescribers, adding 2 conventional antipsychotics together has little rationale and may reduce tolerability without clearly enhancing efficacy

Suggested Reading

Gerlach J. Depot neuroleptics in relapse prevention: advantages and disadvantages. Int Clin Psychopharmacol 1995; 9 Suppl 5:17–20.

Quraishi S, David A. Depot flupenthixol decanoate for schizophrenia or other similar psychotic disorders. Cochrane Database Syst Rev 2000;(2):CD001470.

Soyka M, De Vry J. Flupenthixol as a potential pharmacotreatment of alcohol and cocaine abuse/dependence. Eur Neuropsychopharmacol 2000;10(5):325–32.

THERAPEUTICS

Brands • Prolixin
see index for additional brand names

Generic? Yes

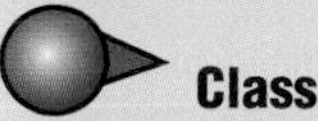

Class
- Conventional antipsychotic (neuroleptic, phenothiazine, dopamine 2 antagonist)

Commonly Prescribed for
(bold for FDA approved)
- **Psychotic disorders**
- Bipolar disorder

How the Drug Works
- Blocks dopamine 2 receptors, reducing positive symptoms of psychosis

How Long Until It Works
- Psychotic symptoms can improve within 1 week, but it may take several weeks for full effect on behavior

If It Works
- Most often reduces positive symptoms in schizophrenia but does not eliminate them
- Most schizophrenic patients do not have a total remission of symptoms but rather a reduction of symptoms by about a third
- Continue treatment in schizophrenia until reaching a plateau of improvement
- After reaching a satisfactory plateau, continue treatment for at least a year after first episode of psychosis in schizophrenia
- For second and subsequent episodes of psychosis in schizophrenia, treatment may need to be indefinite
- Reduces symptoms of acute psychotic mania but not proven as a mood stabilizer or as an effective maintenance treatment in bipolar disorder
- After reducing acute psychotic symptoms in mania, switch to a mood stabilizer and/or an atypical antipsychotic for mood stabilization and maintenance

If It Doesn't Work
- Consider trying one of the first-line atypical antipsychotics (risperidone, olanzapine, quetiapine, ziprasidone, aripiprazole, paliperidone, amisulpride)
- Consider trying another conventional antipsychotic
- If 2 or more antipsychotic monotherapies do not work, consider clozapine

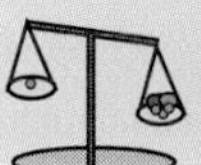

Best Augmenting Combos for Partial Response or Treatment Resistance
- Augmentation of conventional antipsychotics has not been systematically studied
- Addition of a mood-stabilizing anticonvulsant such as valproate, carbamazepine, or lamotrigine may be helpful in both schizophrenia and bipolar mania
- Augmentation with lithium in bipolar mania may be helpful
- Addition of a benzodiazepine, especially short-term for agitation

Tests
✻ Since conventional antipsychotics are frequently associated with weight gain, before starting treatment, weigh all patients and determine if the patient is already overweight (BMI 25.0–29.9) or obese (BMI ≥30)
- Before giving a drug that can cause weight gain to an overweight or obese patient, consider determining whether the patient already has pre-diabetes (fasting plasma glucose 100–25 mg/dL), diabetes (fasting plasma glucose >126 mg/dL), or dyslipidemia (increased total cholesterol, LDL cholesterol and triglycerides; decreased HDL cholesterol), and treat or refer such patients for treatment, including nutrition and weight management, physical activity counseling, smoking cessation, and medical management

✻ Monitor weight and BMI during treatment
✻ Consider monitoring fasting triglycerides monthly for several months in patients at high risk for metabolic complications and when initiating or switching antipsychotics
✻ While giving a drug to a patient who has gained >5% of initial weight, consider evaluating for the presence of pre-diabetes, diabetes, or dyslipidemia, or consider switching to a different antipsychotic
- Should check blood pressure in the elderly before starting and for the first few weeks of treatment

- Monitoring elevated prolactin levels of dubious clinical benefit
- Phenothiazines may cause false-positive phenylketonuria results

SIDE EFFECTS

How Drug Causes Side Effects

- By blocking dopamine 2 receptors in the striatum, it can cause motor side effects
- By blocking dopamine 2 receptors in the pituitary, it can cause elevations in prolactin
- By blocking dopamine 2 receptors excessively in the mesocortical and mesolimbic dopamine pathways, especially at high doses, it can cause worsening of negative and cognitive symptoms (neuroleptic-induced deficit syndrome)
- Anticholinergic actions may cause sedation, blurred vision, constipation, dry mouth
- Antihistaminic actions may cause sedation, weight gain
- By blocking alpha 1 adrenergic receptors, it can cause dizziness, sedation, and hypotension
- Mechanism of weight gain and any possible increased incidence of diabetes or dyslipidemia with conventional antipsychotics is unknown

Notable Side Effects

✽ Neuroleptic-induced deficit syndrome
✽ Akathisia
✽ Priapism
✽ Extrapyramidal symptoms, Parkinsonism, tardive dyskinesia, tardive dystonia
✽ Galactorrhea, amenorrhea
- Dizziness, sedation
- Dry mouth, constipation, urinary retention, blurred vision
- Decreased sweating, depression
- Sexual dysfunction
- Hypotension, tachycardia, syncope
- Weight gain

Life-Threatening or Dangerous Side Effects

- Rare neuroleptic malignant syndrome
- Rare jaundice, agranulocytosis
- Rare seizures
- Increased risk of death and cerebrovascular events in elderly patients with dementia-related psychosis

Weight Gain

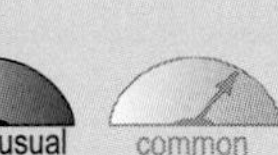

- Occurs in significant minority

Sedation

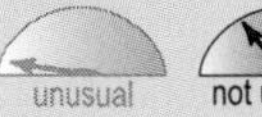
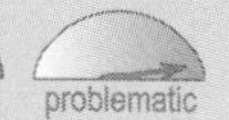

- Occurs in significant minority

What to Do About Side Effects

- Wait
- Wait
- Wait
- For motor symptoms, add an anticholinergic agent
- Reduce the dose
- For sedation, take at night
- Switch to an atypical antipsychotic
- Weight loss, exercise programs, and medical management for high BMIs, diabetes, dyslipidemia

Best Augmenting Agents for Side Effects

- Benztropine or trihexyphenidyl for motor side effects
- Sometimes amantadine can be helpful for motor side effects
- Benzodiazepines may be helpful for akathisia
- Many side effects cannot be improved with an augmenting agent

DOSING AND USE

Usual Dosage Range

- Oral: 1–20 mg/day maintenance
- Intramuscular: generally 1/3 to 1/2 the oral dose
- Decanoate for intramuscular or subcutaneous administration: 12.5 mg/0.5 mL–50 mg/2 mL

Dosage Forms

- Tablet 1 mg, 2.5 mg scored, 5 mg scored, 10 mg scored
- Decanoate for long-acting intramuscular or subcutaneous administration 25 mg/mL
- Injection for acute intramuscular administration 2.5 mg/mL
- Elixir 2.5 mg/5 mL
- Concentrate 5 mg/mL

How To Dose

- Oral: initial 0.5–10 mg/day in divided doses; maximum 40 mg/day
- Intramuscular (short-acting): initial 1.25 mg; 2.5–10 mg/day can be given in divided doses every 6–8 hours; maximum dose generally 10 mg/day
- Decanoate (long-acting): initial 12.5–25 mg (0.5–1 mL); subsequent doses and intervals determined in accordance with the patient's response; generally no more than 50 mg/2 mL given at intervals not longer than 4 weeks

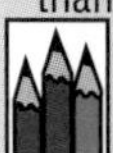

Dosing Tips

- Patients receiving atypical antipsychotics may occasionally require a "top up" of a conventional antipsychotic to control aggression or violent behavior
- Fluphenazine tablets 2.5 mg, 5 mg, and 10 mg contain tartrazine, which can cause allergic reactions, especially in patients sensitive to aspirin
- Oral solution should not be mixed with drinks containing caffeine, tannic acid (tea), or pectinates (apple juice)
- 12.5 mg/0.5 mL every 2 weeks of the long-acting decanoate may be comparable to 10 mg daily of oral fluphenazine
- Onset of action of decanoate at 24–72 hours after injection with significant antipsychotic actions within 48–96 hours

Overdose

- Extrapyramidal symptoms, coma, hypotension, sedation, seizures, respiratory depression

Long-Term Use

- Some side effects may be irreversible (e.g., tardive dyskinesia)

Habit Forming

- No

How to Stop

- Slow down-titration of oral formulation (over 6 to 8 weeks), especially when simultaneously beginning a new antipsychotic while switching (i.e., cross-titration)
- Rapid oral discontinuation may lead to rebound psychosis and worsening of symptoms
- If antiparkinson agents are being used, they should be continued for a few weeks after fluphenazine is discontinued

Pharmacokinetics

- Mean half-life of oral formulation approximately 15 hours
- Mean half-life of intramuscular formulation approximately 6.8–9.6 days

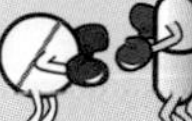

Drug Interactions

- May decrease the effects of levodopa, dopamine agonists
- May increase the effects of antihypertensive drugs except for guanethidine, whose antihypertensive actions fluphenazine may antagonize
- Additive effects may occur if used with CNS depressants
- Additive anticholinergic effects may occur if used with atropine or related compounds
- Alcohol and diuretics may increase the risk of hypotension
- Some patients taking a neuroleptic and lithium have developed an encephalopathic syndrome similar to neuroleptic malignant syndrome
- Combined use with epinephrine may lower blood pressure

Other Warnings/ Precautions

- If signs of neuroleptic malignant syndrome develop, treatment should be immediately discontinued
- Use cautiously in patients with alcohol withdrawal or convulsive disorders because of possible lowering of seizure threshold
- Avoid undue exposure to sunlight
- Use cautiously in patients with respiratory disorders
- Avoid extreme heat exposure
- Antiemetic effect can mask signs of other disorders or overdose
- Do not use epinephrine in event of overdose as interaction with some pressor agents may lower blood pressure
- Use only with caution if at all in Parkinson's disease or Lewy body dementia

Do Not Use

- If patient is in a comatose state or has CNS depression

- If patient is taking cabergoline, pergolide, or metrizamide
- If there is a proven allergy to fluphenazine
- If there is a known sensitivity to any phenothiazine

SPECIAL POPULATIONS

Renal Impairment
- Use with caution; titration should be slower

Hepatic Impairment
- Use with caution; titration should be slower

Cardiac Impairment
- Cardiovascular toxicity can occur, especially orthostatic hypotension

Elderly
- Titration should be slower; lower initial dose (1–2.5 mg/day)
- Elderly patients may be more susceptible to adverse effects
- Although conventional antipsychotics are commonly used for behavioral disturbances in dementia, no agent has been approved for treatment of elderly patients with dementia-related psychosis
- Elderly patients with dementia-related psychosis treated with antipsychotics are at an increased risk of death compared to placebo, and also have an increased risk of cerebrovascular events

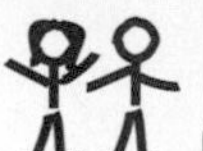

Children and Adolescents
- Safety and efficacy not established
- Decanoate and enanthate injectable formulations are contraindicated in children under age 12
- Generally consider second-line after atypical antipsychotics

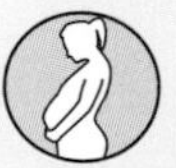

Pregnancy
- Risk Category C [some animal studies show adverse effects; no controlled studies in humans]
- Reports of extrapyramidal symptoms, jaundice, hyperreflexia, hyporeflexia in infants whose mothers took a phenothiazine during pregnancy
- Fluphenazine should be used only during pregnancy if clearly indicated
- Psychotic symptoms may worsen during pregnancy and some form of treatment may be necessary
- Atypical antipsychotics may be preferable to conventional antipsychotics or anticonvulsant mood stabilizers if treatment is required during pregnancy

Breast Feeding
- Some drug is found in mother's breast milk
- Effects on infant have been observed (dystonia, tardive dyskinesia, sedation)
- ✻ Recommended either to discontinue drug or bottle feed

THE ART OF PSYCHOPHARMACOLOGY

Potential Advantages
- Intramuscular formulation for emergency use

Potential Disadvantages
- Patients with tardive dyskinesia
- Children
- Elderly

Primary Target Symptoms
- Positive symptoms of psychosis
- Motor and autonomic hyperactivity
- Violent or aggressive behavior

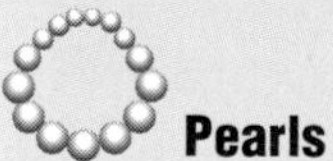

Pearls
- Fluphenazine is a high-potency phenothiazine
- Less risk of sedation and orthostatic hypotension but greater risk of extrapyramidal symptoms than with low-potency phenothiazines
- Conventional antipsychotics are much less expensive than atypical antipsychotics
- Not shown to be effective for behavioral problems in mental retardation
- Patients have very similar antipsychotic responses to any conventional antipsychotic, which is different from atypical antipsychotics where antipsychotic responses of individual patients can occasionally vary greatly from one atypical antipsychotic to another
- Patients with inadequate responses to atypical antipsychotics may benefit from a trial of augmentation with a conventional

antipsychotic such as fluphenazine or from switching to a conventional antipsychotic such as fluphenazine
- However, long-term polypharmacy with a combination of a conventional antipsychotic such as fluphenazine with an atypical antipsychotic may combine their side effects without clearly augmenting the efficacy of either
- Although a frequent practice by some prescribers, adding 2 conventional antipsychotics together has little rationale and may reduce tolerability without clearly enhancing efficacy

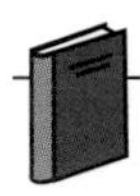

Suggested Reading

Adams CE, Eisenbruch M. Depot fluphenazine for schizophrenia. Cochrane Database Syst Rev 2000;(2):CD000307.

King DJ. Drug treatment of the negative symptoms of schizophrenia. Eur Neuropsychopharmacol 1998;8(1):33–42.

Milton GV, Jann MW. Emergency treatment of psychotic symptoms. Pharmacokinetic considerations for antipsychotic drugs. Clin Pharmacokinet 1995;28(6):494–504.

FLURAZEPAM

THERAPEUTICS

Brands • Dalmane

see index for additional brand names

Generic? Yes

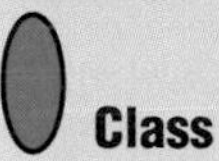

Class

• Benzodiazepine (hypnotic)

Commonly Prescribed for

(bold for FDA approved)

- **Insomnia characterized by difficulty in falling asleep, frequent nocturnal awakenings, and/or early morning awakening**
- **Recurring insomnia or poor sleeping habits**
- **Acute or chronic medical situations requiring restful sleep**

How the Drug Works

- Binds to benzodiazepine receptors at the GABA-A ligand-gated chloride channel complex
- Enhances the inhibitory effects of GABA
- Boosts chloride conductance through GABA-regulated channels
- Inhibitory actions in sleep centers may provide sedative hypnotic effects

How Long Until It Works

- Generally takes effect in less than an hour

If It Works

- Improves quality of sleep
- Effects on total wake-time and number of nighttime awakenings may be decreased over time

If It Doesn't Work

- If insomnia does not improve after 7–10 days, it may be a manifestation of a primary psychiatric or physical illness such as obstructive sleep apnea or restless leg syndrome, which requires independent evaluation
- Increase the dose
- Improve sleep hygiene
- Switch to another agent

Best Augmenting Combos for Partial Response or Treatment Resistance

- Generally, best to switch to another agent
- Trazodone
- Agents with antihistamine actions (e.g., diphenhydramine, tricyclic antidepressants)

Tests

- In patients with seizure disorders, concomitant medical illness, and/or those with multiple concomitant long-term medications, periodic liver tests and blood counts may be prudent

SIDE EFFECTS

How Drug Causes Side Effects

- Same mechanism for side effects as for therapeutic effects – namely due to excessive actions at benzodiazepine receptors
- Actions at benzodiazepine receptors that carry over to the next day can cause daytime sedation, amnesia, and ataxia
- Long-term adaptations in benzodiazepine receptors may explain the development of dependence, tolerance, and withdrawal

Notable Side Effects

- Sedation, fatigue, depression
- Dizziness, ataxia, slurred speech, weakness
- Forgetfulness, confusion
- Hyperexcitability, nervousness
- Rare hallucinations, mania
- Rare hypotension
- Hypersalivation, dry mouth
- Rebound insomnia when withdrawing from long-term treatment

Life-Threatening or Dangerous Side Effects

- Respiratory depression, especially when taken with CNS depressants in overdose
- Rare hepatic dysfunction, renal dysfunction, blood dyscrasias

Weight Gain

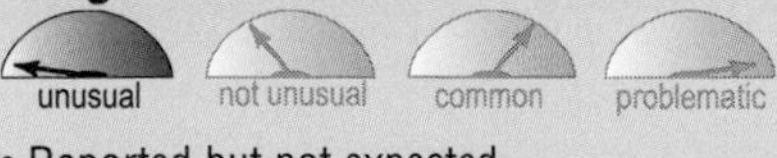

- Reported but not expected

Sedation

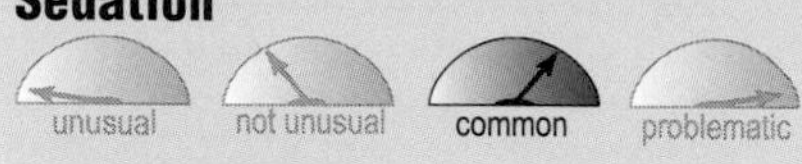

- Many experience and/or can be significant in amount

What to Do About Side Effects

- Wait
- To avoid problems with memory, only take flurazepam if planning to have a full night's sleep
- Lower the dose
- Switch to a shorter-acting sedative hypnotic
- Switch to a non-benzodiazepine hypnotic
- Administer flumazenil if side effects are severe or life-threatening

Best Augmenting Agents for Side Effects

- Many side effects cannot be improved with an augmenting agent

DOSING AND USE

Usual Dosage Range

- 15–30 mg/day at bedtime for 7–10 days

Dosage Forms

- Capsule 15 mg, 30 mg

How To Dose

- 15 mg/day at bedtime; may increase to 30 mg/day at bedtime if ineffective

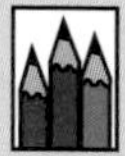

Dosing Tips

✻ Because flurazepam tends to accumulate over time, perhaps not the best hypnotic for chronic nightly use

- Use lowest possible effective dose and assess need for continued treatment regularly
- Flurazepam should generally not be prescribed in quantities greater than a 1-month supply
- Patients with lower body weights may require lower doses
- Risk of dependence may increase with dose and duration of treatment

Overdose

- No death reported in monotherapy; sedation, slurred speech, poor coordination, confusion, coma, respiratory depression

Long-Term Use

- Not generally intended for long-term use

✻ Because of its relatively longer half-life, flurazepam may cause some daytime sedation and/or impaired motor/cognitive function, and may do so progressively over time

Habit Forming

- Flurazepam is a Schedule IV drug
- Some patients may develop dependence and/or tolerance; risk may be greater with higher doses
- History of drug addiction may increase risk of dependence

How to Stop

- If taken for more than a few weeks, taper to reduce chances of withdrawal effects
- Patients with seizure history may seize upon sudden withdrawal
- Rebound insomnia may occur the first 1–2 nights after stopping
- For patients with severe problems discontinuing a benzodiazepine, dosing may need to be tapered over many months (i.e., reduce dose by 1% every 3 days by crushing tablet and suspending or dissolving in 100 mL of fruit juice and then disposing of 1 mL while drinking the rest; 3–7 days later, dispose of 2 mL, and so on). This is both a form of very slow biological tapering and a form of behavioral desensitization

Pharmacokinetics

- Elimination half-life approximately 24–100 hours
- Active metabolites

Drug Interactions

- Cimetidine may decrease flurazepam clearance and thus raise flurazepam levels
- Flurazepam and kava combined use may affect clearance of either drug
- Increased depressive effects when taken with other CNS depressants

Other Warnings/ Precautions

- Insomnia may be a symptom of a primary disorder, rather than a primary disorder itself
- Some patients may exhibit abnormal thinking or behavioral changes similar to those caused by other CNS depressants (i.e., either depressant actions or disinhibiting actions)
- Some depressed patients may experience a worsening of suicidal ideation
- Use only with extreme caution in patients with impaired respiratory function or obstructive sleep apnea
- Flurazepam should be administered only at bedtime

Do Not Use

- If patient is pregnant
- If patient has narrow angle-closure glaucoma
- If there is a proven allergy to flurazepam or any benzodiazepine

SPECIAL POPULATIONS

Renal Impairment

- Recommended dose: 15 mg/day

Hepatic Impairment

- Recommended dose: 15 mg/day

Cardiac Impairment

- Benzodiazepines have been used to treat insomnia associated with acute myocardial infarction

Elderly

- Recommended dose: 15 mg/day

Children and Adolescents

- Safety and efficacy have not been established
- Long-term effects of flurazepam in children/adolescents are unknown
- Should generally receive lower doses and be more closely monitored

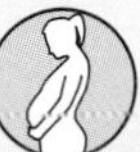

Pregnancy

- Risk Category X [positive evidence of risk to human fetus; contraindicated for use in pregnancy]
- Infants whose mothers received a benzodiazepine late in pregnancy may experience withdrawal effects
- Neonatal flaccidity has been reported in infants whose mothers took a benzodiazepine during pregnancy

Breast Feeding

- Unknown if flurazepam is secreted in human breast milk, but all psychotropics assumed to be secreted in breast milk

✻ Recommended either to discontinue drug or bottle feed

- Effects on infant have been observed and include feeding difficulties, sedation, and weight loss

THE ART OF PSYCHOPHARMACOLOGY

Potential Advantages

- Transient insomnia

Potential Disadvantages

- Chronic nightly insomnia

Primary Target Symptoms

- Time to sleep onset
- Total sleep time
- Nighttime awakenings

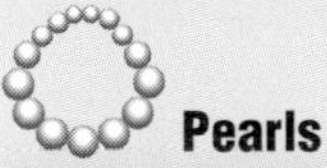

Pearls

✻ Flurazepam has a longer half-life than some other sedative hypnotics, so it may be less likely to cause rebound insomnia on discontinuation

- Flurazepam may not be as effective on the first night as it is on subsequent nights
- Was once one of the most widely used hypnotics

✻ Long-term accumulation of flurazepam and its active metabolites may cause insidious onset of confusion or falls, especially in the elderly

Suggested Reading

Greenblatt DJ. Pharmacology of benzodiazepine hypnotics. J Clin Psychiatry 1992;53 (Suppl):7–13.

Hilbert JM, Battista D. Quazepam and flurazepam: differential pharmacokinetic and pharmacodynamic characteristics. J Clin Psychiatry 1991;52(Suppl):21–6.

Johnson LC, Chernik DA, Sateia MJ. Sleep, performance, and plasma levels in chronic insomniacs during 14-day use of flurazepam and midazolam: an introduction. J Clin Psychopharmacol 1990;10(4 Suppl):5S–9S.

Roth T, Roehrs TA. A review of the safety profiles of benzodiazepine hypnotics. J Clin Psychiatry 1991;52(Suppl):38–41.

FLUVOXAMINE

THERAPEUTICS

Brands • Luvox
• Luvox CR

see index for additional brand names

Generic? Yes (not for fluvoxamine CR)

Class

- SSRI (selective serotonin reuptake inhibitor); often classified as an antidepressant, but it is not just an antidepressant

Commonly Prescribed for

(bold for FDA approved)

- **Obsessive-compulsive disorder (OCD) (fluvoxamine and fluvoxamine CR)**
- **Social anxiety disorder (fluvoxamine CR)**
- Depression
- Panic disorder
- Generalized anxiety disorder (GAD)
- Posttraumatic stress disorder (PTSD)

How the Drug Works

- Boosts neurotransmitter serotonin
- Blocks serotonin reuptake pump (serotonin transporter)
- Desensitizes serotonin receptors, especially serotonin 1A receptors
- Presumably increases serotonergic neurotransmission

✻ Fluvoxamine also has antagonist properties at sigma 1 receptors

How Long Until It Works

✻ Some patients may experience relief of insomnia or anxiety early after initiation of treatment

- Onset of therapeutic actions usually not immediate, but often delayed 2–4 weeks
- If it is not working within 6–8 weeks, it may require a dosage increase or it may not work at all
- May continue to work for many years to prevent relapse of symptoms

If It Works

- The goal of treatment is complete remission of current symptoms as well as prevention of future relapses
- Treatment most often reduces or even eliminates symptoms, but not a cure since symptoms can recur after medicine stopped
- Continue treatment until all symptoms are gone (remission) or significantly reduced (e.g., OCD)
- Once symptoms gone, continue treating for 1 year for the first episode of depression
- For second and subsequent episodes of depression, treatment may need to be indefinite
- Use in anxiety disorders may also need to be indefinite

If It Doesn't Work

- Many patients only have a partial response where some symptoms are improved but others persist (especially insomnia, fatigue, and problems concentrating in depression)
- Other patients may be nonresponders, sometimes called treatment-resistant or treatment-refractory
- Some patients who have an initial response may relapse even though they continue treatment, sometimes called "poop-out"
- Consider increasing dose, switching to another agent or adding an appropriate augmenting agent
- Consider psychotherapy
- Consider evaluation for another diagnosis or for a comorbid condition (e.g., medical illness, substance abuse, etc.)
- Some patients may experience apparent lack of consistent efficacy due to activation of latent or underlying bipolar disorder, and require antidepressant discontinuation and a switch to a mood stabilizer

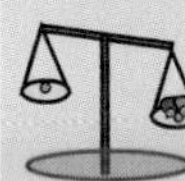

Best Augmenting Combos for Partial Response or Treatment Resistance

- For the expert, consider cautious addition of clomipramine for treatment-resistant OCD
- Trazodone, especially for insomnia
- Bupropion, mirtazapine, reboxetine, or atomoxetine (use combinations of antidepressants with caution as this may activate bipolar disorder and suicidal ideation)
- Modafinil, especially for fatigue, sleepiness, and lack of concentration
- Mood stabilizers or atypical antipsychotics for bipolar depression, psychotic depression, treatment-resistant depression, or treatment-resistant anxiety disorders

- Benzodiazepines
- If all else fails for anxiety disorders, consider gabapentin or tiagabine
- Hypnotics for insomnia
- Classically, lithium, buspirone, or thyroid hormone
- In Europe and Japan, augmentation is more commonly administered for the treatment of depression and anxiety disorders, especially with benzodiazepines and lithium
- In the U.S., augmentation is more commonly administered for the treatment of OCD, especially with atypical antipsychotics, buspirone, or even clomipramine; clomipramine should be added with caution and at low doses as fluvoxamine can alter clomipramine metabolism and raise its levels

Tests

- None for healthy individuals

SIDE EFFECTS

How Drug Causes Side Effects

- Theoretically due to increases in serotonin concentrations at serotonin receptors in parts of the brain and body other than those that cause therapeutic actions (e.g., unwanted actions of serotonin in sleep centers causing insomnia, unwanted actions of serotonin in the gut causing diarrhea, etc.)
- Increasing serotonin can cause diminished dopamine release and might contribute to emotional flattening, cognitive slowing, and apathy in some patients
- Most side effects are immediate but often go away with time, in contrast to most therapeutic effects which are delayed and are enhanced over time

✽ Fluvoxamine's sigma 1 antagonist properties may contribute to sedation and fatigue in some patients

Notable Side Effects

- Sexual dysfunction (men: delayed ejaculation, erectile dysfunction; men and women: decreased sexual desire, anorgasmia)
- Gastrointestinal (decreased appetite, nausea, diarrhea, constipation, dry mouth)
- Mostly central nervous system (insomnia but also sedation, agitation, tremors, headache, dizziness)
- Note: patients with diagnosed or undiagnosed bipolar or psychotic disorders may be more vulnerable to CNS-activating actions of SSRIs
- Autonomic (sweating)
- Bruising and rare bleeding
- Rare hyponatremia

Life-Threatening or Dangerous Side Effects

- Rare seizures
- Rare induction of mania
- Rare activation of suicidal ideation and behavior (suicidality) (short-term studies did not show an increase in the risk of suicidality with antidepressants compared to placebo beyond age 24)

Weight Gain

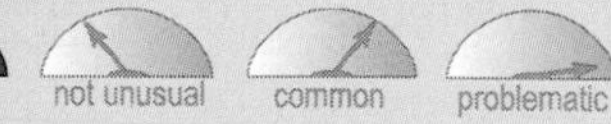

- Reported but not expected
- Patients may actually experience weight loss

Sedation

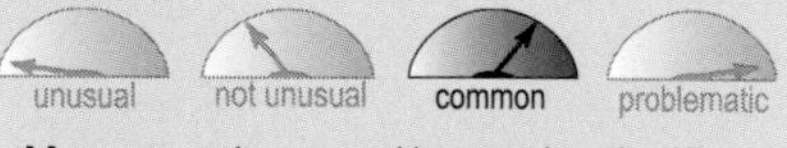

- Many experience and/or can be significant in amount

What to Do About Side Effects

- Wait
- Wait
- Wait
- If fluvoxamine is sedating, take at night to reduce drowsiness
- Reduce dose
- In a few weeks, switch or add other drugs

Best Augmenting Agents for Side Effects

- Often best to try another SSRI or another antidepressant monotherapy prior to resorting to augmentation strategies to treat side effects
- Trazodone or a hypnotic for insomnia
- Bupropion, sildenafil, vardenafil, or tadalafil for sexual dysfunction
- Bupropion for emotional flattening, cognitive slowing, or apathy

- Mirtazapine for insomnia, agitation, and gastrointestinal side effects
- Benzodiazepines for jitteriness and anxiety, especially at initiation of treatment and especially for anxious patients
- Many side effects are dose-dependent (i.e., they increase as dose increases, or they reemerge until tolerance redevelops)
- Many side effects are time-dependent (i.e., they start immediately upon dosing and upon each dose increase, but go away with time)
- Activation and agitation may represent the induction of a bipolar state, especially a mixed dysphoric bipolar II condition sometimes associated with suicidal ideation, and require the addition of lithium, a mood stabilizer or an atypical antipsychotic, and/or discontinuation of fluvoxamine

DOSING AND USE

Usual Dosage Range
- 100–300 mg/day for OCD
- 100–200 mg/day for depression
- 100–300 mg/day for social anxiety disorder

Dosage Forms
- Tablets 25 mg, 50 mg scored, 100 mg scored
- Controlled-release capsules 100 mg, 150 mg

How To Dose
- For immediate-release, initial 50 mg/day; increase by 50 mg/day in 4–7 days; usually wait a few weeks to assess drug effects before increasing dose further, but can increase by 50 mg/day every 4–7 days until desired efficacy is reached; maximum 300 mg/day
- For immediate-release, doses below 100 mg/day usually given as a single dose at bedtime; doses above 100 mg/day can be divided into two doses to enhance tolerability, with the larger dose administered at night, but can also be given as a single dose at bedtime
- For controlled-release, initial 100 mg/day; increase by 50 mg/day each week until desired efficacy is reached; maximum generally 300 mg/day

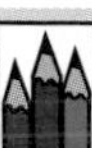

Dosing Tips
- 50-mg and 100-mg tablets are scored, so to save costs, give 25 mg as half of 50 mg tablet, and give 50 mg as half of 100 mg tablet
- To improve tolerability of immediate-release formulation, dosing can either be given once a day, usually all at night, or split either symmetrically or asymmetrically, usually with more of the dose given at night
- Some patients take more than 300 mg/day
- Controlled-release capsules should not be chewed or crushed
- If intolerable anxiety, insomnia, agitation, akathisia, or activation occur either upon dosing initiation or discontinuation, consider the possibility of activated bipolar disorder and switch to a mood stabilizer or an atypical antipsychotic

Overdose
- Rare fatalities have been reported, both in combination with other drugs and alone; sedation, dizziness, vomiting, diarrhea, irregular heartbeat, seizures, coma, breathing difficulty

Long-Term Use
- Safe

Habit Forming
- No

How to Stop
- Taper to avoid withdrawal effects (dizziness, nausea, stomach cramps, sweating, tingling, dysesthesias)
- Many patients tolerate 50% dose reduction for 3 days, then another 50% reduction for 3 days, then discontinuation
- If withdrawal symptoms emerge during discontinuation, raise dose to stop symptoms and then restart withdrawal much more slowly

Pharmacokinetics
- Parent drug has 9–28 hour half-life
- Inhibits CYP450 3A4
- Inhibits CYP450 1A2
- Inhibits CYP450 2C9/2C19

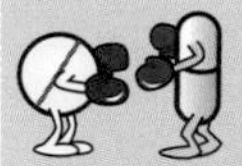

Drug Interactions

- Tramadol increases the risk of seizures in patients taking an antidepressant
- Can increase tricyclic antidepressant levels; use with caution with tricyclic antidepressants
- Can cause a fatal "serotonin syndrome" when combined with MAO inhibitors, so do not use with MAO inhibitors or for at least 14 days after MAOIs are stopped
- Do not start an MAO inhibitor for at least 2 weeks after discontinuing fluvoxamine
- May displace highly protein-bound drugs (e.g., warfarin)
- Can rarely cause weakness, hyperreflexia, and incoordination when combined with sumatriptan or possibly with other triptans, requiring careful monitoring of patient
- Possible increased risk of bleeding, especially when combined with anticoagulants (e.g., warfarin, NSAIDs)
- Via CYP450 1A2 inhibition, fluvoxamine may reduce clearance of theophylline and clozapine, thus raising their levels and requiring their dosing to be lowered
- Fluvoxamine administered with either caffeine or theophylline can thus cause jitteriness, excessive stimulation, or rarely seizures, so concomitant use should proceed cautiously
- Metabolism of fluvoxamine may be enhanced in smokers and thus its levels lowered, requiring higher dosing
- Via CYP450 3A4 inhibition, fluvoxamine may reduce clearance of carbamazepine and benzodiazepines such as alprazolam and triazolam, and thus require dosage reduction
- Via CYP450 3A4 inhibition, fluvoxamine could theoretically increase concentrations of certain cholesterol lowering HMG CoA reductase inhibitors, especially simvastatin, atorvastatin, and lovastatin, but not pravastatin or fluvastatin, which would increase the risk of rhabdomyolysis; thus, coadministration of fluvoxamine with certain HMG CoA reductase inhibitors should proceed with caution
- Via CYP450 3A4 inhibition, fluvoxamine could theoretically increase the concentrations of pimozide, and cause QTc prolongation and dangerous cardiac arrhythmias

Other Warnings/ Precautions

- Add or initiate other antidepressants with caution for up to 2 weeks after discontinuing fluvoxamine
- Use with caution in patients with history of seizure
- Use with caution in patients with bipolar disorder unless treated with concomitant mood-stabilizing agent
- May cause photosensitivity
- When treating children, carefully weigh the risks and benefits of pharmacological treatment against the risks and benefits of nontreatment with antidepressants and make sure to document this in the patient's chart
- Distribute the brochures provided by the FDA and the drug companies
- Warn patients and their caregivers about the possibility of activating side effects and advise them to report such symptoms immediately
- Monitor patients for activation of suicidal ideation, especially children and adolescents

Do Not Use

- If patient is taking an MAO inhibitor
- If patient is taking thioridazine, pimozide, tizanidine, alosetron, or ramelteon
- If there is a proven allergy to fluvoxamine

SPECIAL POPULATIONS

Renal Impairment

- No dose adjustment

Hepatic Impairment

- Lower dose or give less frequently, perhaps by half; use slower titration

Cardiac Impairment

- Preliminary research suggests that fluvoxamine is safe in these patients
- Treating depression with SSRIs in patients with acute angina or following myocardial infarction may reduce cardiac events and improve survival as well as mood

Elderly

- May require lower initial dose and slower titration

- Reduction in risk of suicidality with antidepressants compared to placebo in adults age 65 and older

Children and Adolescents

- Approved for ages 8–17 for OCD
- 8–17: initial 25 mg/day at bedtime; increase by 25 mg/day every 4–7 days; maximum 200 mg/day; doses above 50 mg/day should be divided into 2 doses with the larger dose administered at bedtime
- Preliminary evidence suggests efficacy for other anxiety disorders and depression in children and adolescents
- Carefully weigh the risks and benefits of pharmacological treatment against the risks and benefits of nontreatment with antidepressants and make sure to document this in the patient's chart
- Monitor patients face-to-face regularly, particularly during the first several weeks of treatment
- Use with caution, observing for activation of known or unknown bipolar disorder and/or suicidal ideation, and inform parents or guardians of this risk so they can help observe child or adolescent patients

Pregnancy

- Risk Category C [some animal studies show adverse effects; no controlled studies in humans]
- Not generally recommended for use during pregnancy, especially during first trimester
- Nonetheless, continuous treatment during pregnancy may be necessary and has not been proven to be harmful to the fetus
- At delivery there may be more bleeding in the mother and transient irritability or sedation in the newborn
- Must weigh the risk of treatment (first trimester fetal development, third trimester newborn delivery) to the child against the risk of no treatment (recurrence of depression, maternal health, infant bonding) to the mother and child
- For many patients this may mean continuing treatment during pregnancy
- SSRI use beyond the 20th week of pregnancy may be associated with increased risk of pulmonary hypertension in newborns
- Neonates exposed to SSRIs or SNRIs late in the third trimester have developed complications requiring prolonged hospitalization, respiratory support, and tube feeding; reported symptoms are consistent with either a direct toxic effect of SSRIs and SNRIs or, possibly, a drug discontinuation syndrome, and include respiratory distress, cyanosis, apnea, seizures, temperature instability, feeding difficulty, vomiting, hypoglycemia, hypotonia, hypertonia, hyperreflexia, tremor, jitteriness, irritability, and constant crying

Breast Feeding

- Some drug is found in mother's breast milk
- Trace amounts may be present in nursing children whose mothers are on fluvoxamine
- If child becomes irritable or sedated, breast feeding or drug may need to be discontinued
- Immediate postpartum period is a high-risk time for depression, especially in women who have had prior depressive episodes, so drug may need to be reinstituted late in the third trimester or shortly after childbirth to prevent a recurrence during the postpartum period
- Must weigh benefits of breast feeding with risks and benefits of antidepressant treatment versus nontreatment to both the infant and the mother
- For many patients this may mean continuing treatment during breast feeding

THE ART OF PSYCHOPHARMACOLOGY

Potential Advantages

- Patients with mixed anxiety/depression
- Generic is less expensive than brand name where available

Potential Disadvantages

- Patients with irritable bowel or multiple gastrointestinal complaints
- Can require dose titration and twice daily dosing

Primary Target Symptoms

- Depressed mood
- Anxiety

Pearls

* Often a preferred treatment of anxious depression as well as major depressive disorder comorbid with anxiety disorders
- Some withdrawal effects, especially gastrointestinal effects
- May have lower incidence of sexual dysfunction than other SSRIs
- Preliminary research suggests that fluvoxamine is efficacious in obsessive-compulsive symptoms in schizophrenia when combined with antipsychotics
- Not FDA approved for depression, but used widely for depression in many countries
- CR formulation may be better tolerated than immediate-release formulation, particularly with less sedation
- SSRIs may be less effective in women over 50, especially if they are not taking estrogen
- SSRIs may be useful for hot flushes in perimenopausal women

* Actions at sigma 1 receptors may explain in part fluvoxamine's sometimes rapid onset effects in anxiety disorders and insomnia
* Actions at sigma 1 receptors may explain potential advantages of fluvoxamine for psychotic depression and delusional depression
* For treatment-resistant OCD, consider cautious combination of fluvoxamine and clomipramine by an expert

- Normally, clomipramine (CMI), a potent serotonin reuptake blocker, at steady state is metabolized extensively to its active metabolite desmethyl-clomipramine (de-CMI), a potent noradrenergic reuptake blocker
- Thus, at steady state, plasma drug activity is generally more noradrenergic (with higher de-CMI levels) than serotonergic (with lower parent CMI levels)
- Addition of a CYP450 1A2 inhibitor, fluvoxamine, blocks this conversion and results in higher CMI levels than de-CMI levels
- Thus, addition of the SSRI fluvoxamine to CMI in treatment-resistant OCD can powerfully enhance serotonergic activity, not only due to the inherent serotonergic activity of fluvoxamine, but also due to a favorable pharmacokinetic interaction inhibiting CYP450 1A2 and thus converting CMI's metabolism to a more powerful serotonergic portfolio of parent drug

Suggested Reading

Cheer SM, Figgitt DP. Spotlight on fluvoxamine in anxiety disorders in children and adolescents. CNS Drugs 2002;16:139–44.

Edwards JG, Anderson I. Systematic review and guide to selection of selective serotonin reuptake inhibitors. Drugs 1999;57:507–33.

Figgitt DP, McClellan KJ. Fluvoxamine. An updated review of its use in the management of adults with anxiety disorders. Drugs 2000;60:925–54.

Pigott TA, Seay SM. A review of the efficacy of selective serotonin reuptake inhibitors in obsessive-compulsive disorder. J Clin Psychiatry 1999;60:101–6.

Wares MR. Fluvoxamine: a review of the controlled trials in depression. J Clin Psychiatry 1997;58(suppl 5):15–23.

THERAPEUTICS

Brands • Neurontin

see index for additional brand names

Generic? Not in U.S. or Europe

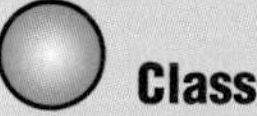

Class

- Anticonvulsant, antineuralgic for chronic pain, alpha 2 delta ligand at voltage-sensitive calcium channels

Commonly Prescribed for

(bold for FDA approved)

- **Partial seizures with or without secondary generalization (adjunctive)**
- **Postherpetic neuralgia**
- Neuropathic pain/chronic pain
- Anxiety (adjunctive)
- Bipolar disorder (adjunctive)

How the Drug Works

- Is a leucine analogue and is transported both into the blood from the gut and also across the blood-brain barrier into the brain from the blood by the system L transport system

✻ Binds to the alpha 2 delta subunit of voltage-sensitive calcium channels

- This closes N and P/Q presynaptic calcium channels, diminishing excessive neuronal activity and neurotransmitter release
- Although structurally related to gamma-aminobutyric acid (GABA), no known direct actions on GABA or its receptors

How Long Until It Works

- Should reduce seizures by 2 weeks
- Should also reduce pain in postherpetic neuralgia by 2 weeks; some patients respond earlier
- May reduce pain in other neuropathic pain syndromes within a few weeks
- If it is not reducing pain within 6–8 weeks, it may require a dosage increase or it may not work at all
- May reduce anxiety in a variety of disorders within a few weeks
- Not yet clear if it has mood-stabilizing effects in bipolar disorder or antineuralgic actions in chronic neuropathic pain, but some patients may respond and if so, would be expected to show clinical effects starting by 2 weeks although it may take several weeks to months to optimize

If It Works

- The goal of treatment is complete remission of symptoms (e.g., seizures)
- The goal of treatment of chronic neuropathic pain is to reduce symptoms as much as possible, especially in combination with other treatments
- Treatment of chronic neuropathic pain most often reduces but does not eliminate symptoms and is not a cure since symptoms usually recur after medicine stopped
- Continue treatment until all symptoms are gone or until improvement is stable and then continue treating indefinitely as long as improvement persists

If It Doesn't Work (for neuropathic pain or bipolar disorder)

✻ May only be effective in a subset of bipolar patients, in some patients who fail to respond to other mood stabilizers, or it may not work at all

- Many patients only have a partial response where some symptoms are improved but others persist or continue to wax and wane without stabilization of pain or mood
- Other patients may be nonresponders, sometimes called treatment-resistant or treatment-refractory
- Consider increasing dose, switching to another agent or adding an appropriate augmenting agent
- Consider biofeedback or hypnosis for pain
- Consider the presence of noncompliance and counsel patient
- Switch to another agent with fewer side effects
- Consider evaluation for another diagnosis or for a comorbid condition (e.g., medical illness, substance abuse, etc.)

Best Augmenting Combos for Partial Response or Treatment Resistance

✻ Gabapentin is itself an augmenting agent to numerous other anticonvulsants in treating epilepsy; and to lithium, atypical antipsychotics and other anticonvulsants in the treatment of bipolar disorder

- For postherpetic neuralgia, gabapentin can decrease concomitant opiate use

* ✻ For neuropathic pain, gabapentin can augment tricyclic antidepressants and SNRIs as well as tiagabine, other anticonvulsants and even opiates if done by experts while carefully monitoring in difficult cases
* For anxiety, gabapentin is a second-line treatment to augment SSRIs, SNRIs, or benzodiazepines

Tests

* None for healthy individuals
* False positive readings with the Ames N-Multistix SG® dipstick test for urinary protein have been reported when gabapentin was administered with other anticonvulsants

SIDE EFFECTS

How Drug Causes Side Effects

* CNS side effects may be due to excessive blockade of voltage-sensitive calcium channels

Notable Side Effects

* ✻ Sedation, dizziness, ataxia, fatigue, nystagmus, tremor
* Vomiting, dyspepsia, diarrhea, dry mouth, constipation, weight gain
* Blurred vision
* Peripheral edema
* Additional effects in children under age 12: hostility, emotional lability, hyperkinesia, thought disorder, weight gain

Life-Threatening or Dangerous Side Effects

* Sudden unexplained deaths have occurred in epilepsy (unknown if related to gabapentin use)
* Rare activation of suicidal ideation and behavior (suicidality)

Weight Gain

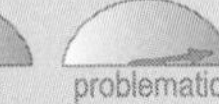

* Occurs in significant minority

Sedation

unusual not unusual common problematic

* Many experience and/or can be significant in amount
* Dose-related; can be problematic at high doses
* Can wear off with time, but may not wear off at high doses

What to Do About Side Effects

* Wait
* Wait
* Wait
* Take more of the dose at night to reduce daytime sedation
* Lower the dose
* Switch to another agent

Best Augmenting Agents for Side Effects

* Many side effects cannot be improved with an augmenting agent

DOSING AND USE

Usual Dosage Range

* 900–1,800 mg/day in 3 divided doses

Dosage Forms

* Capsule 100 mg, 300 mg, 400 mg
* Tablet 600 mg, 800 mg
* Liquid 250 mg/5 mL – 470 mL bottle

How To Dose

* Postherpetic neuralgia: 300 mg on day 1; on day 2 increase to 600 mg in 2 doses; on day 3 increase to 900 mg in 3 doses; maximum dose generally 1,800 mg/day in 3 doses
* Seizures (ages 12 and older): Initial 900 mg/day in 3 doses; recommended dose generally 1800 mg/day in 3 doses; maximum dose generally 3,600 mg/day; time between any 2 doses should usually not exceed 12 hours
* Seizures (under age 13): see Children and Adolescents

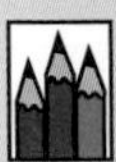

Dosing Tips

* Gabapentin should not be taken until 2 hours after administration of an antacid
* If gabapentin is added to a second anticonvulsant, the titration period should

be at least a week to improve tolerance to sedation
- Some patients need to take gabapentin only twice daily in order to experience adequate symptomatic relief for pain or anxiety
- At the high end of the dosing range, tolerability may be enhanced by splitting dose into more than 3 divided doses
- For intolerable sedation, can give most of the dose at night and less during the day
- To improve slow-wave sleep, may need to take gabapentin only at bedtime

Overdose
- No fatalities; slurred speech, sedation, double vision, diarrhea

Long-Term Use
- Safe

Habit Forming
- No

How to Stop
- Taper over a minimum of 1 week
- Epilepsy patients may seize upon withdrawal, especially if withdrawal is abrupt

✽ Rapid discontinuation may increase the risk of relapse in bipolar disorder
- Discontinuation symptoms uncommon

Pharmacokinetics
- Gabapentin is not metabolized but excreted intact renally
- Not protein bound
- Elimination half-life approximately 5–7 hours

Drug Interactions
- Antacids may reduce the bioavailability of gabapentin, so gabapentin should be administered approximately 2 hours before antacid medication
- Naproxen may increase absorption of gabapentin
- Morphine and hydrocodone may increase plasma AUC (area under the curve) values of gabapentin and thus gabapentin plasma levels over time

Other Warnings/ Precautions
- Depressive effects may be increased by other CNS depressants (alcohol, MAOIs, other anticonvulsants, etc.)
- Dizziness and sedation could increase the chances of accidental injury (falls) in the elderly
- Pancreatic acinar adenocarcinomas have developed in male rats that were given gabapentin, but clinical significance is unknown
- Development of new tumors or worsening of tumors has occurred in humans taking gabapentin; it is unknown whether gabapentin affected the development or worsening of tumors
- Warn patients and their caregivers about the possibility of activation of suicidal ideation and advise them to report such side effects immediately

Do Not Use
- If there is a proven allergy to gabapentin or pregabalin

SPECIAL POPULATIONS

Renal Impairment
- Gabapentin is renally excreted, so the dose may need to be lowered
- Dosing can be adjusted according to creatinine clearance, such that patients with clearance below 16 mL/min should receive 100–300 mg/day in 1 dose, patients with clearance between 16–29 mL/min should receive 200–700 mg/day in 1 dose, and patients with clearance between 30–59 mL/min should receive 400–1,400 mg/day in 2 doses
- Can be removed by hemodialysis; patients receiving hemodialysis may require supplemental doses of gabapentin
- Use in renal impairment has not been studied in children under age 12

Hepatic Impairment
- No available data but not metabolized by the liver and clinical experience suggests normal dosing

Cardiac Impairment
- No specific recommendations

Elderly
- Some patients may tolerate lower doses better
- Elderly patients may be more susceptible to adverse effects

Children and Adolescents
- Approved for use starting at age 3 as adjunct treatment for partial seizures
- Ages 5–12: initial 10–15 mg/kg per day in 3 doses; titrate over 3 days to 25–35 mg/kg per day given in 3 doses; maximum dose generally 50 mg/kg per day; time between any 2 doses should usually not exceed 12 hours
- Ages 3–4: initial 10–15 mg/kg per day in 3 doses; titrate over 3 days to 40 mg/kg per day; maximum dose generally 50 mg/kg per day; time between any 2 doses should usually not exceed 12 hours

Pregnancy
- Risk Category C [some animal studies show adverse effects; no controlled studies in humans]
- Use in women of childbearing potential requires weighing potential benefits to the mother against the risks to the fetus
- Antiepileptic Drug Pregnancy Registry: (888) 233-2334
- Taper drug if discontinuing
- Seizures, even mild seizures, may cause harm to the embryo/fetus

✻ Lack of convincing efficacy for treatment of bipolar disorder or psychosis suggests risk/benefit ratio is in favor of discontinuing gabapentin during pregnancy for these indications

✻ For bipolar patients, gabapentin should generally be discontinued before anticipated pregnancies

✻ For bipolar patients, given the risk of relapse in the postpartum period, mood stabilizer treatment, especially with agents with better evidence of efficacy than gabapentin, should generally be restarted immediately after delivery if patient is unmedicated during pregnancy

✻ Atypical antipsychotics may be preferable to gabapentin if treatment of bipolar disorder is required during pregnancy
- Bipolar symptoms may recur or worsen during pregnancy and some form of treatment may be necessary

Breast Feeding
- Some drug is found in mother's breast milk

✻ Recommended either to discontinue drug or bottle feed
- If drug is continued while breast feeding, infant should be monitored for possible adverse effects
- If infant becomes irritable or sedated, breast feeding or drug may need to be discontinued

✻ Bipolar disorder may recur during the postpartum period, particularly if there is a history of prior postpartum episodes of either depression or psychosis

✻ Relapse rates may be lower in women who receive prophylactic treatment for postpartum episodes of bipolar disorder
- Atypical antipsychotics and anticonvulsants such as valproate may be safer and more effective than gabapentin during the postpartum period when treating a nursing mother with bipolar disorder

THE ART OF PSYCHOPHARMACOLOGY

Potential Advantages
- Chronic neuropathic pain
- Has relatively mild side effect profile
- Has few pharmacokinetic drug interactions
- Treatment-resistant bipolar disorder

Potential Disadvantages
- Usually requires 3 times a day dosing
- Poor documentation of efficacy for many off-label uses, especially bipolar disorder

Primary Target Symptoms
- Seizures
- Pain
- Anxiety

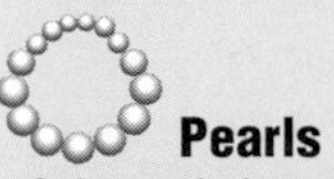

Pearls
- Gabapentin is generally well-tolerated, with only mild adverse effects
- Well-studied in epilepsy and postherpetic neuralgia

* ✻ Most use is off-label
* ✻ Off-label use for first-line treatment of neuropathic pain may be justified
* ✻ Off-label use for second-line treatment of anxiety may be justified
* ✻ Off-label use as an adjunct for bipolar disorder may not be justified
* ✻ Misperceptions about gabapentin's efficacy in bipolar disorder have led to its use in more patients than other agents with proven efficacy, such as lamotrigine
* ✻ Off-label use as an adjunct for schizophrenia may not be justified
* May be useful for some patients in alcohol withdrawal
* ✻ One of the few agents that enhances slow-wave delta sleep, which may be helpful in chronic neuropathic pain syndromes
* ✻ May be a useful adjunct for fibromyalgia
* Drug absorption and clinical efficacy may not necessarily be proportionately increased at high doses, and thus response to high doses may not be consistent

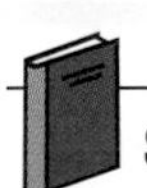

Suggested Reading

Backonja NM. Use of anticonvulsants for treatment of neuropathic pain. Neurology 2002;59(Suppl 2):S14–7.

MacDonald KJ, Young LT. Newer antiepileptic drugs in bipolar disorder. CNS Drugs 2002;16:549–62.

Marson AG, Kadir ZA, Hutton JL, Chadwick DW. Gabapentin for drug-resistant partial epilepsy. Cochrane Database Syst Rev 2000;(2):CD001415.

Rose MA, Kam PC. Gabapentin: pharmacology and its use in pain management. Anaesthesia 2002;57:451–62.

Stahl SM. Anticonvulsants and the relief of chronic pain: pregabalin and gabapentin as alpha(2)delta ligands at voltage-gated calcium channels. J Clin Psychiatry 2004;65:596–7.

Stahl SM. Anticonvulsants as anxiolytics, part 2: Pregabalin and gabapentin as alpha(2)delta ligands at voltage-gated calcium channels. J Clin Psychiatry 2004;65:460–1.

GALANTAMINE

THERAPEUTICS

Brands • Razadyne
• Razadyne ER

see index for additional brand names

Generic? No

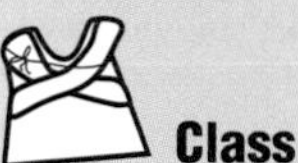

Class

• Cholinesterase inhibitor (acetylcholinesterase inhibitor); also an allosteric nicotinic cholinergic modulator; cognitive enhancer

Commonly Prescribed for

(bold for FDA approved)

• **Alzheimer disease (mild to moderate)**
• Memory disturbances in other dementias
• Memory disturbances in other conditions
• Mild cognitive impairment

How the Drug Works

* Reversibly and competitively inhibits centrally-active acetylcholinesterase (AChE), making more acetylcholine available
• Increased availability of acetylcholine compensates in part for degenerating cholinergic neurons in neocortex that regulate memory
* Modulates nicotinic receptors, which enhances actions of acetylcholine
• Nicotinic modulation may also enhance the actions of other neurotransmitters by increasing the release of dopamine, norepinephrine, serotonin, GABA, and glutamate
• Does not inhibit butyrylcholinesterase
• May release growth factors or interfere with amyloid deposition

How Long Until It Works

• May take up to 6 weeks before any improvement in baseline memory or behavior is evident
• May take months before any stabilization in degenerative course is evident

If It Works

• May improve symptoms and slow progression of disease, but does not reverse the degenerative process

If It Doesn't Work

• Consider adjusting dose, switching to a different cholinesterase inhibitor, or adding an appropriate augmenting agent
• Reconsider diagnosis and rule out other conditions such as depression or a dementia other than Alzheimer disease

Best Augmenting Combos for Partial Response or Treatment Resistance

* Atypical antipsychotics to reduce behavioral disturbances
* Antidepressants if concomitant depression, apathy, or lack of interest
* Memantine for moderate to severe Alzheimer disease
• Divalproex, carbamazepine, or oxcarbazepine for behavioral disturbances
• Not rational to combine with another cholinesterase inhibitor

Tests

• None for healthy individuals

SIDE EFFECTS

How Drug Causes Side Effects

• Peripheral inhibition of acetylcholinesterase can cause gastrointestinal side effects
• Central inhibition of acetylcholinesterase may contribute to nausea, vomiting, weight loss, and sleep disturbances

Notable Side Effects

* Nausea, diarrhea, vomiting, appetite loss, increased gastric acid secretion, weight loss
• Headache, dizziness
• Fatigue, depression

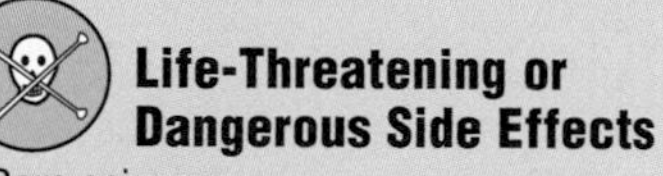

Life-Threatening or Dangerous Side Effects

• Rare seizures
• Rare syncope

Weight Gain

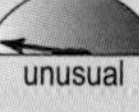

not unusual common

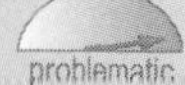

• Reported but not expected
• Some patients may experience weight loss

Sedation

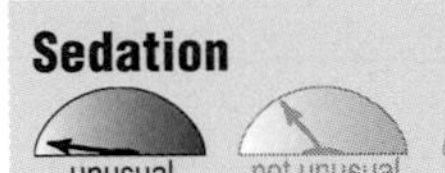

- Reported but not expected

What to Do About Side Effects

- Wait
- Wait
- Wait
- Use slower dose titration
- Consider lowering dose, switching to a different agent or adding an appropriate augmenting agent

Best Augmenting Agents for Side Effects

- Many side effects cannot be improved with an augmenting agent

DOSING AND USE

Usual Dosage Range

- 16–24 mg/day

Dosage Forms

- Tablet 4 mg, 8 mg, 12 mg
- Extended-release capsule 8 mg, 16 mg, 24 mg
- Liquid 4 mg/mL – 100 mL bottle

How To Dose

- Immediate-release: Initial 8 mg twice daily; after 4 weeks may increase dose to 16 mg twice daily; maximum dose generally 32 mg/day
- Extended-release: same titration schedule as immediate-release but dosed once a day in the morning

Dosing Tips

- Gastrointestinal side effects may be reduced if drug is administered with food
- Gastrointestinal side effects may also be reduced if dose is titrated slowly
- Probably best to utilize highest tolerated dose within the usual dosing range

✻ When switching to another cholinesterase inhibitor, probably best to cross-titrate from one to the other to prevent precipitous decline in function if the patient washes out of one drug entirely

Overdose

- Can be lethal; nausea, vomiting, excess salivation, sweating, hypotension, bradycardia, collapse, convulsions, muscle weakness (weakness of respiratory muscles can lead to death)

Long-Term Use

- Drug may lose effectiveness in slowing degenerative course of Alzheimer disease after 6 months
- Can be effective in some patients for several years

Habit Forming

- No

How to Stop

- Taper not necessary
- Discontinuation may lead to notable deterioration in memory and behavior, which may not be restored when drug is restarted or another cholinesterase inhibitor is initiated

Pharmacokinetics

- Terminal elimination half-life approximately 7 hours
- Metabolized by CYP450 2D6 and 3A4

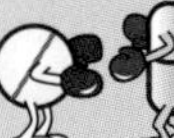

Drug Interactions

- Galantamine may increase the effects of anesthetics and should be discontinued prior to surgery
- Inhibitors of CYP450 2D6 and CYP450 3A4 may inhibit galantamine metabolism and raise galantamine plasma levels
- Galantamine may interact with anticholinergic agents and the combination may decrease the efficacy of both
- Cimetidine may increase bioavailability of galantamine
- May have synergistic effect if administered with cholinomimetics (e.g., bethanechol)
- Bradycardia may occur if combined with beta blockers
- Theoretically, could reduce the efficacy of levodopa in Parkinson's disease
- Not rational to combine with another cholinesterase inhibitor

Other Warnings/ Precautions
- May exacerbate asthma or other pulmonary disease
- Increased gastric acid secretion may increase the risk of ulcers
- Bradycardia or heart block may occur in patients with or without cardiac impairment

Do Not Use
- If there is a proven allergy to galantamine

SPECIAL POPULATIONS

Renal Impairment
- Should be used with caution
- Not recommended for use in patients with severe renal impairment

Hepatic Impairment
- Should be used with caution
- Reduction of clearance may increase with the degree of hepatic impairment
- Not recommended for use in patients with severe hepatic impairment

Cardiac Impairment
- Should be used with caution
- Syncopal episodes have been reported with the use of galantamine

Elderly
- Clearance is reduced in elderly patients

Children and Adolescents
- Safety and efficacy have not been established

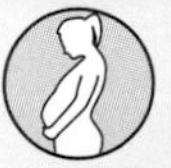

Pregnancy
- Risk Category B [animal studies do not show adverse effects; no controlled studies in humans]

✽ Not recommended for use in pregnant women or in women of childbearing potential

Breast Feeding
- Unknown if galantamine is secreted in human breast milk, but all psychotropics assumed to be secreted in breast milk

✽ Recommended either to discontinue drug or bottle feed
- Galantamine is not recommended for use in nursing women

THE ART OF PSYCHOPHARMACOLOGY

Potential Advantages
- Alzheimer disease with cerebrovascular disease
- Theoretically, nicotinic modulation may provide added therapeutic benefits for memory and behavior in some Alzheimer patients
- Theoretically, nicotinic modulation may also provide efficacy for cognitive disorders other than Alzheimer disease

Potential Disadvantages
- Patients who have difficulty taking a medication twice daily

Primary Target Symptoms
- Memory loss in Alzheimer disease
- Behavioral symptoms in Alzheimer disease
- Memory loss in other dementias

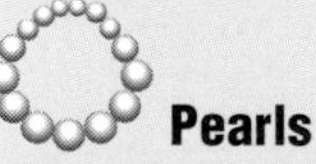

Pearls
- Dramatic reversal of symptoms of Alzheimer disease is not generally seen with cholinesterase inhibitors
- Can lead to therapeutic nihilism among prescribers and lack of an appropriate trial of a cholinesterase inhibitor

✽ Perhaps only 50% of Alzheimer patients are diagnosed, and only 50% of those diagnosed are treated, and only 50% of those treated are given a cholinesterase inhibitor, and then only for 200 days in a disease that lasts 7–10 years
- Must evaluate lack of efficacy and loss of efficacy over months, not weeks

✽ Treats behavioral and psychological symptoms of Alzheimer dementia as well as cognitive symptoms (i.e., especially apathy, disinhibition, delusions, anxiety, cooperation, pacing)
- Patients who complain themselves of memory problems may have depression, whereas patients whose spouses or children complain of the patient's memory problems may have Alzheimer disease

- Treat the patient but ask the caregiver about efficacy
- What you see may depend upon how early you treat
- The first symptoms of Alzheimer disease are generally mood changes; thus, Alzheimer disease may initially be diagnosed as depression
- Women may experience cognitive symptoms in perimenopause as a result of hormonal changes that are not a sign of dementia or Alzheimer disease
- Aggressively treat concomitant symptoms with augmentation (e.g., atypical antipsychotics for agitation, antidepressants for depression)
- If treatment with antidepressants fails to improve apathy and depressed mood in the elderly, it is possible that this represents early Alzheimer disease and a cholinesterase inhibitor like galantamine may be helpful
- What to expect from a cholinesterase inhibitor:
  - Patients do not generally improve dramatically although this can be observed in a significant minority of patients
  - Onset of behavioral problems and nursing home placement can be delayed
  - Functional outcomes, including activities of daily living, can be preserved
  - Caregiver burden and stress can be reduced
- Delay in progression in Alzheimer disease is not evidence of disease-modifying actions of cholinesterase inhibition
- Cholinesterase inhibitors like galantamine depend upon the presence of intact targets for acetylcholine for maximum effectiveness and thus may be most effective in the early stages of Alzheimer disease
- The most prominent side effects of galantamine are gastrointestinal effects, which are usually mild and transient
- For patients with intolerable side effects, generally allow a washout period with resolution of side effects prior to switching to another cholinesterase inhibitor
- Weight loss can be a problem in Alzheimer patients with debilitation and muscle wasting
- Women over 85, particularly with low body weights, may experience more adverse effects
- Use with caution in underweight or frail patients
- Cognitive improvement may be linked to substantial (>65%) inhibition of acetylcholinesterase

✻ Galantamine is a natural product present in daffodils and snowdrops

- New extended-release formulation allows for once daily dosing

✻ Novel dual action uniquely combines acetylcholinesterase inhibition with allosteric nicotine modulation

✻ Novel dual action should theoretically enhance cholinergic actions but incremental clinical benefits have been difficult to demonstrate

✻ Actions at nicotinic receptors enhance not only the release of acetylcholine but also that of other neurotransmitters, which may boost attention and improve behaviors caused by deficiencies in those neurotransmitters in Alzheimer disease

- Some Alzheimer patients who fail to respond to another cholinesterase inhibitor may respond when switched to galantamine
- Some Alzheimer patients who fail to respond to galantamine may respond to another cholinesterase inhibitor
- To prevent potential clinical deterioration, generally switch from long-term treatment with one cholinesterase inhibitor to another without a washout period

✻ Galantamine may slow the progression of mild cognitive impairment to Alzheimer disease

✻ May be useful for dementia with Lewy bodies (DLB, constituted by early loss of attentiveness and visual perception with possible hallucinations, Parkinson-like movement problems, fluctuating cognition such as daytime drowsiness and lethargy, staring into space for long periods, episodes of disorganized speech)

- May decrease delusions, apathy, agitation, and hallucinations in dementia with Lewy bodies

✻ May be useful for vascular dementia (e.g., acute onset with slow stepwise progression that has plateaus, often with gait abnormalities, focal signs, imbalance, and urinary incontinence)

- May be helpful for dementia in Down's syndrome

- Suggestions of utility in some cases of treatment-resistant bipolar disorder
- Theoretically, may be useful for ADHD, but not yet proven
- Theoretically, could be useful in any memory condition characterized by cholinergic deficiency (e.g., some cases of brain injury, cancer chemotherapy-induced cognitive changes, etc.)

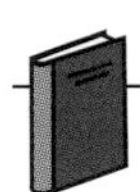

Suggested Reading

Bentue-Ferrer D, Tribut O, Polard E, Allain H. Clinically significant drug interactions with cholinesterase inhibitors: a guide for neurologists. CNS Drugs 2003;17:947–63.

Bonner LT, Peskind ER. Pharmacologic treatments of dementia. Med Clin North Am 2002;86:657–74.

Coyle J, Kershaw P. Galantamine, a cholinesterase inhibitor that allosterically modulates nicotinic receptors: effects on the course of Alzheimer's disease. Biol Psychiatry 2001;49:289–99.

Jones RW. Have cholinergic therapies reached their clinical boundary in Alzheimer's disease? Int J Geriatr Psychiatry 2003;18(Suppl 1): S7–S13.

Olin J, Schneider L. Galantamine for Alzheimer's disease. Cochrane Database Syst Rev 2002;(3):CD001747.

Stahl SM. Cholinesterase inhibitors for Alzheimer's disease. Hosp Pract (Off Ed) 1998;33:131–6.

Stahl SM. The new cholinesterase inhibitors for Alzheimer's disease, part 1. J Clin Psychiatry 2000;61:710–11.

Stahl SM. The new cholinesterase inhibitors for Alzheimer's disease, part 2. J Clin Psychiatry 2000;61:813–14.

THERAPEUTICS

Brands • Intuniv (pending approval)
• Tenex

see index for additional brand names

Generic? Yes (not for guanfacine ER)

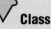

Class

- Centrally acting alpha 2A agonist; antihypertensive

Commonly Prescribed for

(bold for FDA approved)

- **Hypertension**
- Attention deficit hyperactivity disorder (ADHD) in children ages 6–17 (Intuniv, pending approval)
- Oppositional defiant disorder
- Pervasive developmental disorders
- Motor tics
- Tourette's syndrome

How the Drug Works

- For hypertension, stimulates alpha 2A adrenergic receptors in the brain stem, reducing sympathetic outflow from the CNS and decreasing peripheral resistance, renal vascular resistance, heart rate, and blood pressure
- For ADHD, theoretically has central actions on postsynaptic alpha 2A receptors in the prefrontal cortex

How Long Until It Works

- For ADHD, can take a few weeks to see maximum therapeutic benefits
- Blood pressure may be lowered 30–60 minutes after first dose; greatest reduction seen after 2–4 hours
- May take several weeks to control blood pressure adequately

If It Works (for ADHD)

- The goal of treatment of ADHD is reduction of symptoms of inattentiveness, motor hyperactivity, and/or impulsiveness that disrupt social, school, and/or occupational functioning
- Continue treatment until all symptoms are under control or improvement is stable and then continue treatment indefinitely as long as improvement persists
- Reevaluate the need for treatment periodically
- Treatment for ADHD begun in childhood may need to be continued into adolescence and adulthood if continued benefit is documented

If It Doesn't Work (for ADHD)

- Consider adjusting dose or switching to another agent
- Consider behavioral therapy
- Consider the presence of noncompliance and counsel patient and parents
- Consider evaluation for another diagnosis or for a comorbid condition (e.g., bipolar disorder, substance abuse, medical illness, etc.)

Best Augmenting Combos for Partial Response or Treatment Resistance

- Best to attempt another monotherapy prior to augmenting for ADHD
- Possibly combination with stimulants (with caution as benefits of combination poorly documented)
- Combinations for ADHD should be for the expert, while monitoring the patient closely, and when other treatment options have failed
- Chlorthalidone, thyazide-type diuretics, and furosemide for hypertension

Tests

- Blood pressure should be checked regularly during treatment

SIDE EFFECTS

How Drug Causes Side Effects

- Excessive actions on alpha 2A receptors

Notable Side Effects

- Sedation, dizziness
- Dry mouth, constipation
- Fatigue, weakness

Life-Threatening or Dangerous Side Effects

- Sinus bradycardia, hypotension

Weight Gain

- Reported but not expected

Sedation

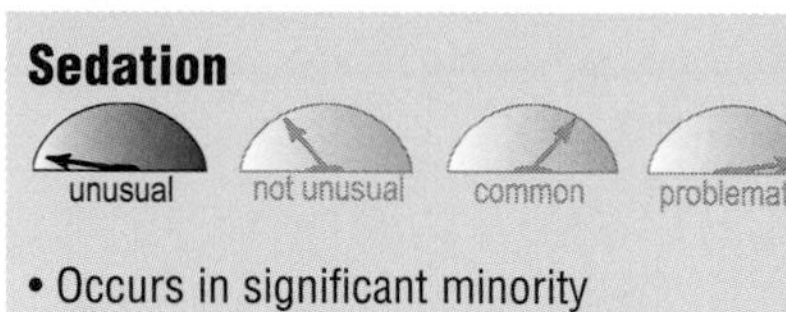

- Occurs in significant minority
- Some patients may not tolerate it
- Can abate with time

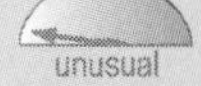
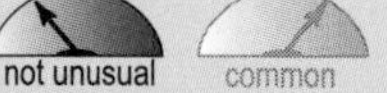

- May be less sedation with controlled-release formulation (pending approval)

What to Do About Side Effects

- Wait
- Adjust dose
- If side effects persist, discontinue use

Best Augmenting Agents for Side Effects

- Dose reduction or switching to another agent may be more effective since most side effects cannot be improved with an augmenting agent

DOSING AND USE

Usual Dosage Range

- Immediate-release: 1–2 mg/day

Dosage Forms

- Immediate-release tablet 1 mg, 2 mg, 3 mg

How To Dose

- Immediate-release: initial 1 mg/day at bedtime; after 3–4 weeks can increase to 2 mg/day

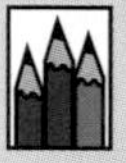

Dosing Tips

- Adverse effects are dose-related and usually transient
- Doses greater than 2 mg/day are associated with increased side effects
- If guanfacine is terminated abruptly, rebound hypertension may occur within 2–4 days
- For hypertension, dose can be raised to 2 mg/day if 1 mg/day is ineffective, but 2 mg may have no more efficacy than 1 mg

Overdose

- Drowsiness, lethargy, bradycardia, hypotension

Long Term Use

- Shown to be safe and effective for treatment of hypertension

Habit Forming

- No

How to Stop

- Taper to avoid rebound effects (nervousness, increased blood pressure)

Pharmacokinetics

- Elimination half-life approximately 17 hours

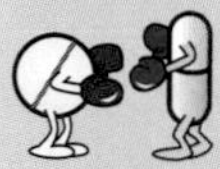

Drug Interactions

- Increased depressive effects when taken with other CNS depressants
- Phenobarbital and phenytoin may reduce plasma concentrations of guanfacine

Other Warnings/Precautions

- Excessive heat (e.g., saunas) may exacerbate some of the side effects, such as dizziness and drowsiness
- Use with caution in patients with severe coronary insufficiency, recent myocardial infarction, cerebrovascular disease, or chronic renal or hepatic failure

Do Not Use

- If there is a proven allergy to guanfacine

SPECIAL POPULATIONS

Renal Impairment

- Patients should receive lower doses

Hepatic Impairment

- Use with caution

Cardiac Impairment

- Use with caution in patients with recent myocardial infarction, severe coronary insufficiency, cerebrovascular disease

Elderly

- Elimination half-life may be longer in elderly patients

- Elderly patients may be more sensitive to sedative effects

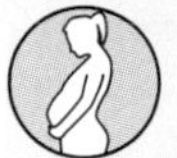

Children and Adolescents

- Safety and efficacy not established in children under age 6
- Some reports of mania and aggressive behavior in ADHD patients taking guanfacine

Pregnancy

- Risk Category B [animal studies do not show adverse effects; no controlled studies in humans]
- Use in women of childbearing potential requires weighing potential benefits to the mother against potential risks to the fetus

Breast Feeding

- Unknown if guanfacine is secreted in human breast milk, but all psychotropics assumed to be secreted in breast milk
- Recommended either to discontinue drug or bottle feed

THE ART OF PSYCHOPHARMACOLOGY

Potential Advantages

- No known abuse potential
- For oppositional behavior associated with ADHD
- Less sedation than clonidine

Potential Disadvantages

- Not well studied in adults with ADHD

Primary Target Symptoms

- Concentration
- Motor hyperactivity
- Oppositional and impulsive behavior
- High blood pressure

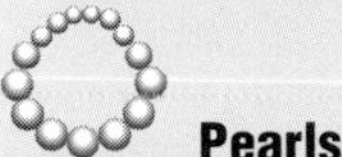

Pearls

- Guanfacine has been shown to be effective in both children and adults, and approval is pending for guanfacine extended-release in children ages 6–17
- Guanfacine can also be used to treat tic disorders, including Tourette's syndrome
- Although both guanfacine and clonidine are alpha 2 adrenergic agonists, guanfacine is relatively selective for alpha 2A receptors, whereas clonidine binds not only alpha 2A, 2B, and 2C receptors but also imidazoline receptors, causing more sedation, hypotension, and side effects than guanfacine
- May be used as monotherapy or in combination with stimulants for the treatment of oppositional behavior in children with or without ADHD

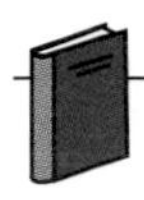

Suggested Reading

Arnsten AF, Scahill L, Findling RL. alpha2-Adrenergic receptor agonists for the treatment of attention-deficit/hyperactivity disorder: emerging concepts from new data. J Child Adolesc Psychopharmacol 2007;17(4):393–406.

Posey DJ, McDouble CJ. Guanfacine and guanfacine extended-release: treatment for ADHD and related disorders. CNS Drug Rev 2007;13(4):465–74.

THERAPEUTICS

Brands • Haldol

see index for additional brand names

Generic? Yes

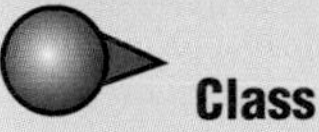

Class

- Conventional antipsychotic (neuroleptic, butyrophenone, dopamine 2 antagonist)

Commonly Prescribed for

(bold for FDA approved)

- **Manifestations of psychotic disorders (oral, immediate-release injection)**
- **Tics and vocal utterances in Tourette's syndrome (oral, immediate-release injection)**
- **Second-line treatment of severe behavior problems in children of combative, explosive hyperexcitability (oral, immediate-release injection)**
- **Second-line short-term treatment of hyperactive children (oral, immediate-release injection)**
- **Treatment of schizophrenic patients who require prolonged parenteral antipsychotic therapy (depot intramuscular decanoate)**
- Bipolar disorder
- Behavioral disturbances in dementias
- Delirium (with lorazepam)

How the Drug Works

- Blocks dopamine 2 receptors, reducing positive symptoms of psychosis and possibly combative, explosive, and hyperactive behaviors
- Blocks dopamine 2 receptors in the nigrostriatal pathway, improving tics and other symptoms in Tourette's syndrome

How Long Until It Works

- Psychotic symptoms can improve within 1 week, but it may take several weeks for full effect on behavior

If It Works

- Most often reduces positive symptoms in schizophrenia but does not eliminate them
- Most schizophrenic patients do not have a total remission of symptoms but rather a reduction of symptoms by about a third
- Continue treatment in schizophrenia until reaching a plateau of improvement
- After reaching a satisfactory plateau, continue treatment for at least a year after first episode of psychosis in schizophrenia
- For second and subsequent episodes of psychosis in schizophrenia, treatment may need to be indefinite
- Reduces symptoms of acute psychotic mania but not proven as a mood stabilizer or as an effective maintenance treatment in bipolar disorder
- After reducing acute psychotic symptoms in mania, switch to a mood stabilizer and/or an atypical antipsychotic for mood stabilization and maintenance

If It Doesn't Work

- Consider trying one of the first-line atypical antipsychotics (risperidone, olanzapine, quetiapine, ziprasidone, aripiprazole, paliperidone, amisulpride)
- Consider trying another conventional antipsychotic
- If 2 or more antipsychotic monotherapies do not work, consider clozapine

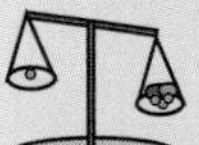

Best Augmenting Combos for Partial Response or Treatment Resistance

- Augmentation of conventional antipsychotics has not been systematically studied
- Addition of a mood-stabilizing anticonvulsant such as valproate, carbamazepine, or lamotrigine may be helpful in both schizophrenia and bipolar mania
- Augmentation with lithium in bipolar mania may be helpful
- Addition of a benzodiazepine, especially short-term for agitation

Tests

* Since conventional antipsychotics are frequently associated with weight gain, before starting treatment, weigh all patients and determine if the patient is already overweight (BMI 25.0–29.9) or obese (BMI ≥30)
- Before giving a drug that can cause weight gain to an overweight or obese patient, consider determining whether the patient already has pre-diabetes (fasting plasma glucose 100–25 mg/dL), diabetes (fasting

plasma glucose >126 mg/dl), or dyslipidemia (increased total cholesterol, LDL cholesterol and triglycerides; decreased HDL cholesterol), and treat or refer such patients for treatment, including nutrition and weight management, physical activity counseling, smoking cessation, and medical management

* ✻ Monitor weight and BMI during treatment
* ✻ Consider monitoring fasting triglycerides monthly for several months in patients at high risk for metabolic complications and when initiating or switching antipsychotics
* ✻ While giving a drug to a patient who has gained >5% of initial weight, consider evaluating for the presence of pre-diabetes, diabetes, or dyslipidemia, or consider switching to a different antipsychotic
* Should check blood pressure in the elderly before starting and for the first few weeks of treatment
* Monitoring elevated prolactin levels of dubious clinical benefit

SIDE EFFECTS

How Drug Causes Side Effects

* By blocking dopamine 2 receptors in the striatum, it can cause motor side effects
* By blocking dopamine 2 receptors in the pituitary, it can cause elevations in prolactin
* By blocking dopamine 2 receptors excessively in the mesocortical and mesolimbic dopamine pathways, especially at high doses, it can cause worsening of negative and cognitive symptoms (neuroleptic-induced deficit syndrome)
* By blocking alpha 1 adrenergic receptors, it can cause dizziness, sedation, and hypotension
* Mechanism of weight gain and any possible increased incidence of diabetes or dyslipidemia with conventional antipsychotics is unknown

Notable Side Effects

* ✻ Neuroleptic-induced deficit syndrome
* ✻ Akathisia
* ✻ Extrapyramidal symptoms, Parkinsonism, tardive dyskinesia, tardive dystonia
* ✻ Galactorrhea, amenorrhea
* Dizziness, sedation
* Dry mouth, constipation, urinary retention, blurred vision
* Decreased sweating
* Hypotension, tachycardia, hypertension
* Weight gain

Life-Threatening or Dangerous Side Effects

* Rare neuroleptic malignant syndrome
* Rare seizures
* Rare jaundice, agranulocytosis, leukopenia
* Increased risk of death and cerebrovascular events in elderly patients with dementia-related psychosis

Weight Gain

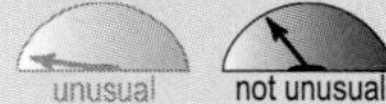

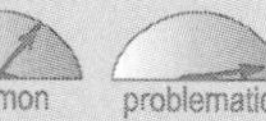

* Occurs in significant minority

Sedation

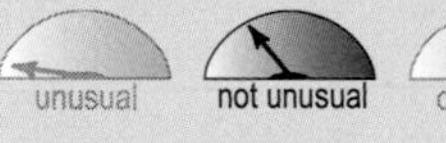

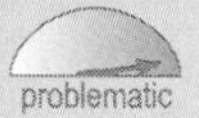

* Sedation is usually transient

What to Do About Side Effects

* Wait
* Wait
* Wait
* For motor symptoms, add an anticholinergic agent
* Reduce the dose
* For sedation, give at night
* Switch to an atypical antipsychotic
* Weight loss, exercise programs, and medical management for high BMIs, diabetes, dyslipidemia

Best Augmenting Agents for Side Effects

* Benztropine or trihexyphenidyl for motor side effects
* Sometimes amantadine can be helpful for motor side effects
* Benzodiazepines may be helpful for akathisia
* Many side effects cannot be improved with an augmenting agent

DOSING AND USE

Usual Dosage Range
- 1–40 mg/day orally
- Immediate-release injection 2–5 mg each dose
- Decanoate injection 10–20 times the previous daily dose of oral antipsychotic

Dosage Forms
- Tablet 0.5 mg scored, 1 mg scored, 2 mg scored, 5 mg scored, 10 mg scored, 20 mg scored
- Concentrate 2 mg/mL
- Solution 1 mg/mL
- Injection 5 mg/mL (immediate-release)
- Decanoate injection 50 mg haloperidol as 70.5 mg/mL haloperidol decanoate, 100 mg haloperidol as 141.04 mg/mL haloperidol decanoate

How To Dose
- Oral: initial 1–15 mg/day; can give once daily or in divided doses at the beginning of treatment during rapid dose escalation; increase as needed; can be dosed up to 100 mg/day; safety not established for doses over 100 mg/day
- Immediate-release injection: initial dose 2–5 mg; subsequent doses may be given as often as every hour; patient should be switched to oral administration as soon as possible
- Decanoate injection: initial dose 10–15 times the previous oral dose for patients maintained on low antipsychotic doses (e.g., up to equivalent of 10 mg/day oral haloperidol); initial dose may be as high as 20 times the previous oral dose for patients maintained on higher antipsychotic doses; maximum dose 100 mg, if higher than 100 mg dose is required the remainder can be administered 3–7 days later; administer total dose every 4 weeks

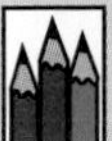

Dosing Tips
- Haloperidol is frequently dosed too high
- Some studies suggest that patients who respond well to low doses of haloperidol (e.g., approximately 2 mg/day) may have efficacy similar to atypical antipsychotics for both positive and negative symptoms of schizophrenia
- Higher doses may actually induce or worsen negative symptoms of schizophrenia
- Low doses, however, may not have beneficial actions on cognitive and affective symptoms in schizophrenia
- One of the only antipsychotics with a depot formulation lasting for up to a month

Overdose
- Fatalities have been reported; extrapyramidal symptoms, hypotension, sedation, respiratory depression, shock-like state

Long-Term Use
- Often used for long-term maintenance
- Some side effects may be irreversible (e.g., tardive dyskinesia)

Habit Forming
- No

How to Stop
- Slow down-titration of oral formulation (over 6–8 weeks), especially when simultaneously beginning a new antipsychotic while switching (i.e., cross-titration)
- Rapid oral discontinuation may lead to rebound psychosis and worsening of symptoms
- If antiparkinson agents are being used, they should be continued for a few weeks after haloperidol is discontinued

Pharmacokinetics
- Decanoate half-life approximately 3 weeks
- Oral half-life approximately 12–38 hours

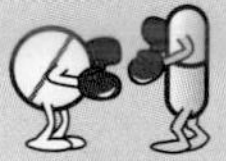

Drug Interactions
- May decrease the effects of levodopa, dopamine agonists
- May increase the effects of antihypertensive drugs except for guanethidine, whose antihypertensive actions haloperidol may antagonize
- Additive effects may occur if used with CNS depressants; dose of other agent should be reduced
- Some pressor agents (e.g., epinephrine) may interact with haloperidol to lower blood pressure

- Haloperidol and anticholinergic agents together may increase intraocular pressure
- Reduces effects of anticoagulants
- Plasma levels of haloperidol may be lowered by rifampin
- Some patients taking haloperidol and lithium have developed an encephalopathic syndrome similar to neuroleptic malignant syndrome
- May enhance effects of antihypertensive drugs

Other Warnings/ Precautions

- If signs of neuroleptic malignant syndrome develop, treatment should be immediately discontinued
- Use with caution in patients with respiratory disorders
- Avoid extreme heat exposure
- If haloperidol is used to treat mania, patients may experience a rapid switch to depression
- Patients with thyrotoxicosis may experience neurotoxicity
- Use only with caution if at all in Parkison's disease on Lewy body dementia
- Higher doses and IV administration may be associated with increased risk of QT prolongation and torsades de pointes; use particular caution if patient has a QT-prolonging condition, underlying cardiac abnormalities, hypothyroidism, familial long-QT syndrome, or is taking a drug known to prolong QT interval

Do Not Use

- If patient is in comatose state or has CNS depression
- If patient has Parkinson's disease
- If there is a proven allergy to haloperidol

SPECIAL POPULATIONS

Renal Impairment

- Use with caution

Hepatic Impairment

- Use with caution

Cardiac Impairment

- Use with caution because of risk of orthostatic hypertension
- Possible increased risk of QT prolongation or torsades de pointes at higher doses or with IV administration

Elderly

- Lower doses should be used and patient should be monitored closely
- Elderly may be more susceptible to respiratory side effects and hypotension
- Although conventional antipsychotics are commonly used for behavioral disturbances in dementia, no agent has been approved for treatment of elderly patients with dementia-related psychosis
- Elderly patients with dementia-related psychosis treated with antipsychotics are at an increased risk of death compared to placebo, and also have an increased risk of cerebrovascular events

Children and Adolescents

- Safety and efficacy have not been established; not intended for use under age 3
- Oral: initial 0.5 mg/day; target dose 0.05–0.15 mg/kg per day for psychotic disorders; 0.05–0.075 mg/kg per day for nonpsychotic disorders
- Generally consider second-line after atypical antipsychotics

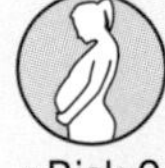

Pregnancy

- Risk Category C [some animal studies show adverse effects; no controlled studies in humans]
- Reports of extrapyramidal symptoms, jaundice, hyperreflexia, hyporeflexia in infants whose mothers took a conventional antipsychotic during pregnancy
- Reports of limb deformity in infants whose mothers took haloperidol during pregnancy
- Haloperidol should generally not be used during the first trimester
- Haloperidol should be used only during pregnancy if clearly needed
- Psychotic symptoms may worsen during pregnancy and some form of treatment may be necessary
- Atypical antipsychotics may be preferable to conventional antipsychotics or anticonvulsant mood stabilizers if treatment is required during pregnancy

Breast Feeding
- Some drug is found in mother's breast milk

* Recommended either to discontinue drug or bottle feed

THE ART OF PSYCHOPHARMACOLOGY

Potential Advantages
- Intramuscular formulation for emergency use
- Depot formulation for noncompliance
- Low-dose responders may have comparable positive and negative symptom efficacy to atypical antipsychotics
- Low-cost, effective treatment

Potential Disadvantages
- Patients with tardive dyskinesia or who wish to avoid tardive dyskinesia and extrapyramidal symptoms
- Vulnerable populations such as children or elderly
- Patients with notable cognitive or mood symptoms

Primary Target Symptoms
- Positive symptoms of psychosis
- Violent or aggressive behavior

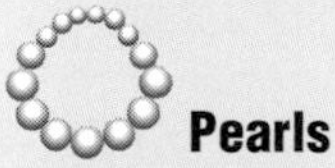

Pearls
- Prior to the introduction of atypical antipsychotics, haloperidol was one of the most preferred antipsychotics
- Haloperidol may still be a useful antipsychotic, especially at low doses for those patients who require management with a conventional antipsychotic or who cannot afford an atypical antipsychotic
- Low doses may not induce negative symptoms, but high doses may
- Not clearly effective for improving cognitive or affective symptoms of schizophrenia
- May be effective for bipolar maintenance, but there may be more tardive dyskinesia when affective disorders are treated with a conventional antipsychotic long-term
- Less sedating than many other conventional antipsychotics, especially "low-potency" phenothiazines
- Haloperidol is often used to treat delirium, generally in combination with lorazepam, with the haloperidol dose 2 times the lorazepam dose
- Haloperidol's long-acting intramuscular formulation lasts up to 4 weeks, whereas some other long-acting intramuscular antipsychotics may last only up to 2 weeks
- Decanoate administration is intended for patients with chronic schizophrenia who have been stabilized on oral antipsychotic medication
- Patients have very similar antipsychotic responses to any conventional antipsychotic, which is different from atypical antipsychotics where antipsychotic responses of individual patients can occasionally vary greatly from one atypical antipsychotic to another
- Conventional antipsychotics are much less expensive than atypical antipsychotics
- Patients receiving atypical antipsychotics may occasionally require a "top up" of a conventional antipsychotic such as haloperidol to control aggression or violent behavior
- Patients with inadequate responses to atypical antipsychotics may benefit from a trial of augmentation with a conventional antipsychotic such as haloperidol or from switching to a conventional antipsychotic such as haloperidol
- However, long-term polypharmacy with a combination of a conventional antipsychotic such as haloperidol with an atypical antipsychotic may combine their side effects without clearly augmenting the efficacy of either
- Although a frequent practice by some prescribers, adding 2 conventional antipsychotics together has little rationale and may reduce tolerability without clearly enhancing efficacy

Suggested Reading

Csernansky JG, Mahmoud R, Brenner R, Risperidone-USA-79 Study Group. A comparison of risperidone and haloperidol for the prevention of relapse in patients with schizophrenia. N Engl J Med 2002;346:16–22.

Davis JM, Chen N, Glick ID. A meta-analysis of the efficacy of second-generation antipsychotics. Arch Gen Psychiatry 2003;60:553–64.

Geddes J, Freemantle N, Harrison P, Bebbington P. Atypical antipsychotics in the treatment of schizophrenia: systematic overview and meta-regression analysis. BMJ 2000;321:1371–6.

Joy CB, Adams CE, Lawrie SM. Haloperidol versus placebo for schizophrenia. Cochrane Database Syst Rev 2001;(2):CD003082.

Kudo S, Ishizaki T. Pharmacokinetics of haloperidol: an update. Clin Pharmacokinet 1999;37:435–56.

Quraishi S ,David A. Depot haloperidol decanoate for schizophrenia. Cochrane Database Syst Rev 2000;(2):CD001361.

THERAPEUTICS

Brands
- Atarax
- Marax
- Vistaril

see index for additional brand names

Generic? Yes

Class
- Antihistamine (anxiolytic, hypnotic, antiemetic)

Commonly Prescribed for
(bold for FDA approved)
- **Anxiety and tension associated with psychoneurosis**
- **Adjunct in organic disease states in which anxiety is manifested**
- **Pruritus due to allergic conditions**
- **Histamine-mediated pruritus**
- **Premedication sedation**
- **Sedation following general anesthesia**
- **Acute disturbance/hysteria (injection)**
- **Anxiety withdrawal symptoms in alcoholics or patients with delirium tremens (injection)**
- **Adjunct in pre/postoperative and pre/postpartum patients to allay anxiety, control emesis, and reduce narcotic dose (injection)**
- **Nausea and vomiting (injection)**
- Insomnia

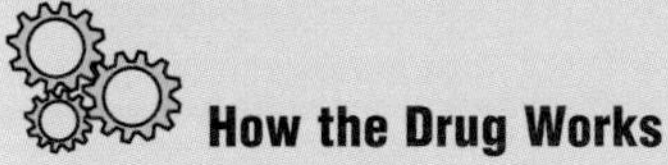

How the Drug Works
- Blocks histamine 1 receptors

How Long Until It Works
- 15–20 minutes (oral administration)
- Some immediate relief with first dosing is common; can take several weeks with daily dosing for maximal therapeutic benefit in chronic conditions

If It Works
- For short-term symptoms of anxiety – after a few weeks, discontinue use or use on an "as-needed" basis
- For chronic anxiety disorders, the goal of treatment is complete remission of symptoms as well as prevention of future relapses
- For chronic anxiety disorders, treatment most often reduces or even eliminates symptoms, but not a cure since symptoms can recur after medicine stopped
- For long-term symptoms of anxiety, consider switching to an SSRI or SNRI for long-term maintenance
- If long-term maintenance is necessary, continue treatment for 6 months after symptoms resolve, and then taper dose slowly
- If symptoms reemerge, consider treatment with an SSRI or SNRI, or consider restarting hydroxyzine

If It Doesn't Work
- Consider switching to another agent or adding an appropriate augmenting agent

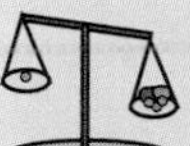

Best Augmenting Combos for Partial Response or Treatment Resistance
- Hydroxyzine can be used as an adjunct to SSRIs or SNRIs in treating anxiety disorders

Tests
- None for healthy individuals
- Hydroxyzine may cause falsely elevated urinary concentrations of 17-hydroxycorticosteroids in certain lab tests (e.g., Porter-Silber reaction, Glenn-Nelson method)

SIDE EFFECTS

How Drug Causes Side Effects
- Blocking histamine 1 receptors can cause sedation

Notable Side Effects
- Dry mouth, sedation, tremor

Life-Threatening or Dangerous Side Effects
- Rare convulsions (generally at high doses)
- Rare cardiac arrest, death (intramuscular formulation combined with CNS depressants)
- Bronchodilation
- Respiratory depression

Weight Gain

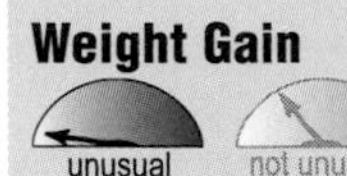
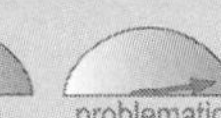

unusual not unusual common problematic

- Reported but not expected

Sedation

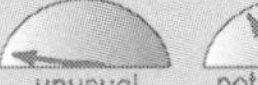
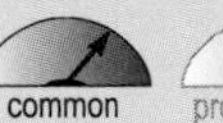

unusual not unusual common problematic

- Many experience and/or can be significant in amount
- Sedation is usually transient

What to Do About Side Effects

- Wait
- Wait
- Wait
- Switch to another agent

Best Augmenting Agents for Side Effects

- Many side effects cannot be improved with an augmenting agent

DOSING AND USE

Usual Dosage Range

- Anxiety: 50–100 mg 4 times a day
- Sedative: 50–100 mg oral, 25–100 mg intramuscular injection
- Pruritus: 75 mg/day divided into 3–4 doses

Dosage Forms

- Tablet 10 mg, 25 mg, 50 mg, 100 mg
- Capsule 25 mg, 50 mg, 100 mg
- Oral Liquid 10 mg/5 mL, 25 mg/5 mL
- Intramuscular 25 mg/mL, 50 mg/mL, 100 mg/2 mL

How To Dose

- Oral dosing does not require titration
- Emergency intramuscular injection: Initial 50–100 mg, repeat every 4–6 hours as needed
- Hydroxyzine intramuscular injection should not be given in the lower or mid-third of the arm and should only be given in the deltoid area if it is well-developed
- In adults, hydroxyzine intramuscular injections may be given in the upper outer quadrant of the buttock or in the mid-lateral thigh

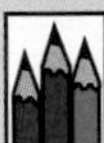

Dosing Tips

- Hydroxyzine may be administered intramuscularly initially, but should be changed to oral administration as soon as possible
- Tolerance usually develops to sedation, allowing higher dosing over time

Overdose

- Sedation, hypotension

Long-Term Use

- Evidence of efficacy for up to 16 weeks

Habit Forming

- No

How to Stop

- Taper generally not necessary

Pharmacokinetics

- Rapidly absorbed from gastrointestinal tract
- Mean elimination half-life approximately 20 hours

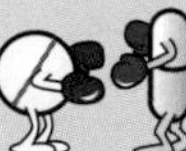

Drug Interactions

- If hydroxyzine is taken in conjunction with another CNS depressant, the dose of the CNS depressant should be reduced by half
- If hydroxyzine is used pre- or post-operatively, the dose of narcotic can be reduced
- If anticholinergic agents are used with hydroxyzine, the anticholinergic effects may be enhanced
- Hydroxyzine may reverse the vasopressor effect of epinephrine; patients requiring a vasopressor agent should use norepinephrine or metaraminol instead

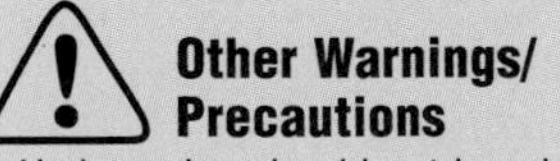

Other Warnings/ Precautions

- Hydroxyzine should not be administered subcutaneously, intra-arterially, or intravenously

Do Not Use

- If patient is in early stages of pregnancy
- If there is a proven allergy to hydroxyzine

SPECIAL POPULATIONS

Renal Impairment
- Dosage adjustment may not be necessary

Hepatic Impairment
- Dosage adjustment may not be necessary

Cardiac Impairment
- Hydroxyzine may be used to treat anxiety associated with cardiac impairment

Elderly
- Some patients may tolerate lower doses better
- Elderly patients may be more sensitive to sedative and anticholinergic effects
- Should be avoided in elderly patients with dementia

Children and Adolescents
- Anxiety, pruritus (6 and older): 50–100 mg/day in divided doses
- Anxiety, pruritus (under 6): 50 mg/day in divided doses
- Sedative: 0.6 mg/kg oral, 0.5 mg/lb intramuscular injection
- Small children should not receive hydroxyzine by intramuscular injection in the periphery of the upper quadrant of the buttock unless absolutely necessary because of risk of damage to the sciatic nerve
- Hyperactive children should be monitored for paradoxical effects

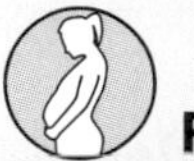

Pregnancy
✻ Hydroxyzine is contraindicated in early pregnancy
- Hydroxyzine intramuscular injection can be used prepartum, reducing narcotic requirements by up to 50%

Breast Feeding
- Unknown if hydroxyzine is secreted in human breast milk, but all psychotropics assumed to be secreted in breast milk

✻ Recommended either to discontinue drug or bottle feed

THE ART OF PSYCHOPHARMACOLOGY

Potential Advantages
- Has multiple formulations, including oral capsules, tablets, and liquid, as well as injectable
- No abuse liability, dependence, or withdrawal

Potential Disadvantages
- Patients with severe anxiety disorders
- Elderly patients
- Dementia patients

Primary Target Symptoms
- Anxiety
- Skeletal muscle tension
- Itching
- Nausea, vomiting

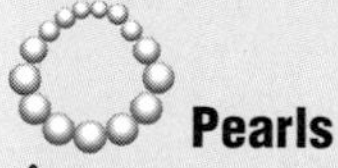

Pearls
✻ A preferred anxiolytic for patients with dermatitis or skin symptoms such as pruritis
- Anxiolytic actions may be proportional to sedating actions
- Hydroxyzine tablets are made with 1,1,1-trichloroethane, which destroys ozone
- Hydroxyzine by intramuscular injection may be used to treat agitation during alcohol withdrawal
- Hydroxyzine may not be as effective as benzodiazepines or newer agents in the management of anxiety

Suggested Reading

Diehn F, Tefferi A. Pruritus in polycythaemia vera: prevalence, laboratory correlates and management. Br J Haematol 2001;115:619–21.

Ferreri M, Hantouche EG. Recent clinical trials of hydroxyzine in generalized anxiety disorder. Acta Psychiatr Scand Suppl 1998;393:102–8.

Paton DM, Webster DR. Clinical pharmacokinetics of H1-receptor antagonists (the antihistamines). Clin Pharmacokinet 1985;10:477–97.

THERAPEUTICS

Brands • Tofranil
see index for additional brand names

Generic? Yes

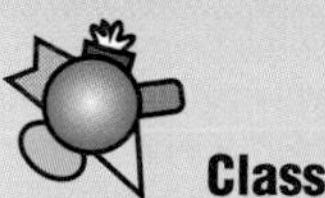

Class

- Tricyclic antidepressant (TCA)
- Serotonin and norepinephrine/noradrenaline reuptake inhibitor

Commonly Prescribed for

(bold for FDA approved)

- **Depression**
- ✱ Enuresis
- Anxiety
- Insomnia
- Neuropathic pain/chronic pain
- Treatment-resistant depression
- Cataplexy syndrome

How the Drug Works

- Boosts neurotransmitters serotonin and norepinephrine/noradrenaline
- Blocks serotonin reuptake pump (serotonin transporter), presumably increasing serotonergic neurotransmission
- Blocks norepinephrine reuptake pump (norepinephrine transporter), presumably increasing noradrenergic neurotransmission
- Presumably desensitizes both serotonin 1A receptors and beta adrenergic receptors
- Since dopamine is inactivated by norepinephrine reuptake in frontal cortex, which largely lacks dopamine transporters, imipramine can increase dopamine neurotransmission in this part of the brain
- May be effective in treating enuresis because of its anticholinergic properties

How Long Until It Works

- May have immediate effects in treating insomnia or anxiety
- Onset of therapeutic actions usually not immediate, but often delayed 2–4 weeks
- If it is not working within 6–8 weeks for depression, it may require a dosage increase or it may not work at all
- May continue to work for many years to prevent relapse of symptoms

If It Works

- The goal of treatment of depression is complete remission of current symptoms as well as prevention of future relapses
- The goal of treatment of chronic neuropathic pain is to reduce symptoms as much as possible, especially in combination with other treatments
- Treatment of depression most often reduces or even eliminates symptoms, but not a cure since symptoms can recur after medicine stopped
- Treatment of chronic neuropathic pain may reduce symptoms, but rarely eliminates them completely, and is not a cure since symptoms can recur after medicine is stopped
- Continue treatment of depression until all symptoms are gone (remission)
- Once symptoms of depression are gone, continue treating for 1 year for the first episode of depression
- For second and subsequent episodes of depression, treatment may need to be indefinite
- Use in anxiety disorders and chronic pain may also need to be indefinite, but long-term treatment is not well studied in these conditions

If It Doesn't Work

- Many depressed patients have only a partial response where some symptoms are improved but others persist (especially insomnia, fatigue, and problems concentrating)
- Other depressed patients may be nonresponders, sometimes called treatment-resistant or treatment-refractory
- Consider increasing dose, switching to another agent or adding an appropriate augmenting agent
- Consider psychotherapy
- Consider evaluation for another diagnosis or for a comorbid condition (e.g., medical illness, substance abuse, etc.)
- Some patients may experience apparent lack of consistent efficacy due to activation of latent or underlying bipolar disorder, and require antidepressant discontinuation and a switch to a mood stabilizer

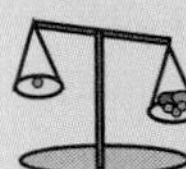

Best Augmenting Combos for Partial Response or Treatment Resistance

- Lithium, buspirone, thyroid hormone (for depression)
- Gabapentin, tiagabine, other anticonvulsants, even opiates if done by experts while monitoring carefully in difficult cases (for chronic pain)

Tests

- None for healthy individuals

✽ Since tricyclic and tetracyclic antidepressants are frequently associated with weight gain, before starting treatment, weigh all patients and determine if the patient is already overweight (BMI 25.0–29.9) or obese (BMI ≥30)

- Before giving a drug that can cause weight gain to an overweight or obese patient, consider determining whether the patient already has pre-diabetes (fasting plasma glucose 100–25 mg/dL), diabetes (fasting plasma glucose >126 mg/dL), or dyslipidemia (increased total cholesterol, LDL cholesterol and triglycerides; decreased HDL cholesterol), and treat or refer such patients for treatment, including nutrition and weight management, physical activity counseling, smoking cessation, and medical management

✽ Monitor weight and BMI during treatment

✽ While giving a drug to a patient who has gained >5% of initial weight, consider evaluating for the presence of pre-diabetes, diabetes, or dyslipidemia, or consider switching to a different antidepressant

- EKGs may be useful for selected patients (e.g., those with personal or family history of QTc prolongation; cardiac arrhythmia; recent myocardial infarction; uncompensated heart failure; or taking agents that prolong QTc interval such as pimozide, thioridazine, selected antiarrhythmics, moxifloxacin, sparfloxacin, etc.)
- Patients at risk for electrolyte disturbances (e.g., patients on diuretic therapy) should have baseline and periodic serum potassium and magnesium measurements

SIDE EFFECTS

How Drug Causes Side Effects

- Anticholinergic activity may explain sedative effects, dry mouth, constipation, and blurred vision
- Sedative effects and weight gain may be due to antihistamine properties
- Blockade of alpha adrenergic 1 receptors may explain dizziness, sedation, and hypotension
- Cardiac arrhythmias and seizures, especially in overdose, may be caused by blockade of ion channels

Notable Side Effects

- Blurred vision, constipation, urinary retention, increased appetite, dry mouth, nausea, diarrhea, heartburn, unusual taste in mouth, weight gain
- Fatigue, weakness, dizziness, sedation, headache, anxiety, nervousness, restlessness
- Sexual dysfunction, sweating

Life-Threatening or Dangerous Side Effects

- Paralytic ileus, hyperthermia (TCAs + anticholinergic agents)
- Lowered seizure threshold and rare seizures
- Orthostatic hypotension, sudden death, arrhythmias, tachycardia
- QTc prolongation
- Hepatic failure, extrapyramidal symptoms
- Increased intraocular pressure, increased psychotic symptoms
- Rare induction of mania
- Rare activation of suicidal ideation and behavior (suicidality) (short-term studies did not show an increase in the risk of suicidality with antidepressants compared to placebo beyond age 24)

Weight Gain

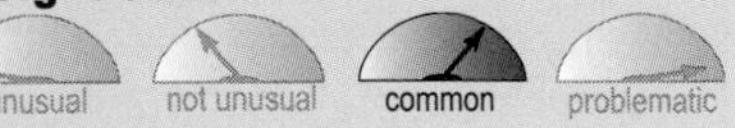

- Many experience and/or can be significant in amount
- Can increase appetite and carbohydrate craving

Sedation

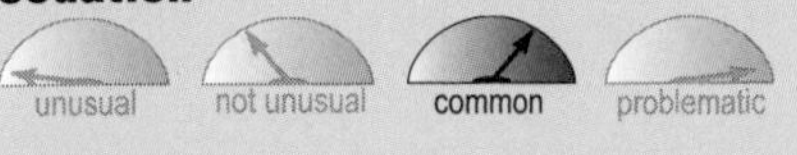

- Many experience and/or can be significant in amount
- Tolerance to sedative effects may develop with long-term use

What To Do About Side Effects

- Wait
- Wait
- Wait
- Lower the dose
- Switch to an SSRI or newer antidepressant

Best Augmenting Agents for Side Effects

- Many side effects cannot be improved with an augmenting agent

DOSING AND USE

Usual Dosage Range

- 50–150 mg/day

Dosage Forms

- Capsule 75 mg, 100 mg, 125 mg, 150 mg
- Tablet 10 mg, 25 mg, 50 mg

How To Dose

- Initial 25 mg/day at bedtime; increase by 25 mg every 3–7 days
- 75–100 mg/day once daily or in divided doses; gradually increase daily dose to achieve desired therapeutic effects; dose at bedtime for daytime sedation and in morning for insomnia; maximum dose 300 mg/day

Dosing Tips

- If given in a single dose, should generally be administered at bedtime because of its sedative properties
- If given in split doses, largest dose should generally be given at bedtime because of its sedative properties
- If patients experience nightmares, split dose and do not give large dose at bedtime
- Patients treated for chronic pain may only require lower doses
- Tofranil-PM(r) (imipramine pamoate) 100- and 125-mg capsules contain the dye tartrazine (FD&C yellow No. 5), which may cause allergic reactions in some patients; this reaction is more likely in patients with sensitivity to aspirin
- If intolerable anxiety, insomnia, agitation, akathisia, or activation occur either upon dosing initiation or discontinuation, consider the possibility of activated bipolar disorder, and switch to a mood stabilizer or an atypical antipsychotic

Overdose

- Death may occur; convulsions, cardiac dysrhythmias, severe hypotension, CNS depression, coma, changes in EKG

Long-Term Use

- Safe

Habit Forming

- No

How to Stop

- Taper to avoid withdrawal effects
- Even with gradual dose reduction some withdrawal symptoms may appear within the first 2 weeks
- Many patients tolerate 50% dose reduction for 3 days, then another 50% reduction for 3 days, then discontinuation
- If withdrawal symptoms emerge during discontinuation, raise dose to stop symptoms and then restart withdrawal much more slowly

Pharmacokinetics

- Substrate for CYP450 2D6 and 1A2
- Metabolized to an active metabolite, desipramine, a predominantly norepinephrine reuptake inhibitor, by demethylation via CYP450 1A2

Drug Interactions

- Tramadol increases the risk of seizures in patients taking TCAs
- Use of TCAs with anticholinergic drugs may result in paralytic ileus or hyperthermia
- Fluoxetine, paroxetine, bupropion, duloxetine, and other CYP450 2D6 inhibitors may increase TCA concentrations
- Fluvoxamine, a CYP450 1A2 inhibitor, can decrease the conversion of imipramine to desmethylimipramine (desipramine) and increase imipramine plasma concentrations
- Cimetidine may increase plasma concentrations of TCAs and cause anticholinergic symptoms

- Phenothiazines or haloperidol may raise TCA blood concentrations
- May alter effects of antihypertensive drugs; may inhibit hypotensive effects of clonidine
- Use with sympathomimetic agents may increase sympathetic activity
- Methylphenidate may inhibit metabolism of TCAs
- Activation and agitation, especially following switching or adding antidepressants, may represent the induction of a bipolar state, especially a mixed dysphoric bipolar II condition sometimes associated with suicidal ideation, and require the addition of lithium, a mood stabilizer or an atypical antipsychotic, and/or discontinuation of imipramine

Other Warnings/ Precautions

- Add or initiate other antidepressants with caution for up to 2 weeks after discontinuing imipramine
- Generally, do not use with MAO inhibitors, including 14 days after MAOIs are stopped; do not start an MAOI until 2 weeks after discontinuing imipramine, but see Pearls
- Use with caution in patients with history of seizure, urinary retention, narrow angle-closure glaucoma, hyperthyroidism
- TCAs can increase QTc interval, especially at toxic doses, which can be attained not only by overdose but also by combining with drugs that inhibit its metabolism via CYP450 2D6, potentially causing torsade de pointes-type arrhythmia or sudden death
- Because TCAs can prolong QTc interval, use with caution in patients who have bradycardia or who are taking drugs that can induce bradycardia (e.g., beta blockers, calcium channel blockers, clonidine, digitalis)
- Because TCAs can prolong QTc interval, use with caution in patients who have hypokalemia and/or hypomagnesemia or who are taking drugs that can induce hypokalemia and/or magnesemia (e.g., diuretics, stimulant laxatives, intravenous amphotericin B, glucocorticoids, tetracosactide)
- When treating children, carefully weigh the risks and benefits of pharmacological treatment against the risks and benefits of nontreatment with antidepressants and make sure to document this in the patient's chart
- Distribute the brochures provided by the FDA and the drug companies
- Warn patients and their caregivers about the possibility of activating side effects and advise them to report such symptoms immediately
- Monitor patients for activation of suicidal ideation, especially children and adolescents

Do Not Use

- If patient is recovering from myocardial infarction
- If patient is taking agents capable of significantly prolonging QTc interval (e.g., pimozide, thioridazine, selected antiarrhythmics, moxifloxacin, sparfloxacin)
- If there is a history of QTc prolongation or cardiac arrhythmia, recent acute myocardial infarction, uncompensated heart failure
- If patient is taking drugs that inhibit TCA metabolism, including CYP450 2D6 inhibitors, except by an expert
- If there is reduced CYP450 2D6 function, such as patients who are poor 2D6 metabolizers, except by an expert and at low doses
- If there is a proven allergy to imipramine, desipramine, or lofepramine

SPECIAL POPULATIONS

Renal Impairment

- Cautious use; may need lower dose

Hepatic Impairment

- Cautious use; may need lower dose

Cardiac Impairment

- TCAs have been reported to cause arrhythmias, prolongation of conduction time, orthostatic hypotension, sinus tachycardia, and heart failure, especially in the diseased heart
- Myocardial infarction and stroke have been reported with TCAs
- TCAs produce QTc prolongation, which may be enhanced by the existence of

bradycardia, hypokalemia, congenital or acquired long QTc interval, which should be evaluated prior to administering imipramine
- Use with caution if treating concomitantly with a medication likely to produce prolonged bradycardia, hypokalemia, slowing of intracardiac conduction, or prolongation of the QTc interval
- Avoid TCAs in patients with a known history of QTc prolongation, recent acute myocardial infarction, and uncompensated heart failure
- TCAs may cause a sustained increase in heart rate in patients with ischemic heart disease and may worsen (decrease) heart rate variability, an independent risk of mortality in cardiac populations
- Since SSRIs may improve (increase) heart rate variability in patients following a myocardial infarct and may improve survival as well as mood in patients with acute angina or following a myocardial infarction, these are more appropriate agents for cardiac population than tricyclic/tetracyclic antidepressants

✻ Risk/benefit ratio may not justify use of TCAs in cardiac impairment

Elderly

- May be more sensitive to anticholinergic, cardiovascular, hypotensive, and sedative effects
- Initial 30–40 mg/day; maximum dose 100 mg/day
- Reduction in risk of suicidality with antidepressants compared to placebo in adults age 65 and older

Children and Adolescents

- Carefully weigh the risks and benefits of pharmacological treatment against the risks and benefits of nontreatment with antidepressants and make sure to document this in the patient's chart
- Monitor patients face-to-face regularly, particularly during the first several weeks of treatment
- Use with caution, observing for activation of known or unknown bipolar disorder and/or suicidal ideation, and inform parents or guardian of this risk so they can help observe child or adolescent patients
- Used age 6 and older for enuresis; age 12 and older for other disorders
- Several studies show lack of efficacy of TCAs for depression
- May be used to treat hyperactive/impulsive behaviors
- Some cases of sudden death have occurred in children taking TCAs
- Adolescents: initial 30–40 mg/day; maximum 100 mg/day
- Children: initial 1.5 mg/kg per day; maximum 5 mg/kg per day
- Functional enuresis: 50 mg/day (age 6–12) or 75 mg/day (over 12)

Pregnancy

- Risk Category D [positive evidence of risk to human fetus; potential benefits may still justify its use during pregnancy]
- Crosses the placenta
- Should be used only if potential benefits outweigh potential risks
- Adverse effects have been reported in infants whose mothers took a TCA (lethargy, withdrawal symptoms, fetal malformations)
- Evaluate for treatment with an antidepressant with a better risk/benefit ratio

Breast Feeding

- Some drug is found in mother's breast milk

✻ Recommended either to discontinue drug or bottle feed

- Immediate postpartum period is a high-risk time for depression, especially in women who have had prior depressive episodes, so drug may need to be reinstituted late in the third trimester or shortly after childbirth to prevent a recurrence during the postpartum period
- Must weigh benefits of breast feeding with risks and benefits of antidepressant treatment versus nontreatment to both the infant and the mother
- For many patients this may mean continuing treatment during breast feeding

THE ART OF PSYCHOPHARMACOLOGY

Potential Advantages

- Patients with insomnia
- Severe or treatment-resistant depression
- Patients with enuresis

Potential Disadvantages

- Pediatric and geriatric patients
- Patients concerned with weight gain
- Cardiac patients

Primary Target Symptoms

- Depressed mood
- Chronic pain

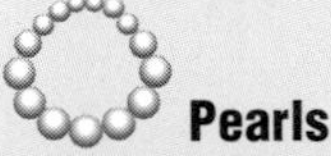

Pearls

- Was once one of the most widely prescribed agents for depression
- * Probably the most preferred TCA for treating enuresis in children
- * Preference of some prescribers for imipramine over other TCAs for the treatment of enuresis is based more upon art and anecdote and empiric clinical experience than comparative clinical trials with other TCAs
- Tricyclic antidepressants are no longer generally considered a first-line treatment option for depression because of their side effect profile
- TCAs may aggravate psychotic symptoms
- Alcohol should be avoided because of additive CNS effects
- Underweight patients may be more susceptible to adverse cardiovascular effects
- Children, patients with inadequate hydration, and patients with cardiac disease may be more susceptible to TCA-induced cardiotoxicity than healthy adults
- For the expert only: although generally prohibited, a heroic but potentially dangerous treatment for severely treatment-resistant patients is to give a tricyclic/tetracyclic antidepressant other than clomipramine simultaneously with an MAO inhibitor for patients who fail to respond to numerous other antidepressants
- If this option is elected, start the MAOI with the tricyclic/tetracyclic antidepressant simultaneously at low doses after appropriate drug washout, then alternately increase doses of these agents every few days to a week as tolerated
- Although very strict dietary and concomitant drug restrictions must be observed to prevent hypertensive crises and serotonin syndrome, the most common side effects of MAOI/tricyclic or tetracyclic combinations may be weight gain and orthostatic hypotension
- Patients on TCAs should be aware that they may experience symptoms such as photosensitivity or blue-green urine
- SSRIs may be more effective than TCAs in women, and TCAs may be more effective than SSRIs in men
- Since tricyclic/tetracyclic antidepressants are substrates for CYP450 2D6, and 7% of the population (especially Caucasians) may have a genetic variant leading to reduced activity of 2D6, such patients may not safely tolerate normal doses of tricyclic/tetracyclic antidepressants and may require dose reduction
- Phenotypic testing may be necessary to detect this genetic variant prior to dosing with a tricyclic/tetracyclic antidepressant, especially in vulnerable populations such as children, elderly, cardiac populations, and those on concomitant medications
- Patients who seem to have extraordinarily severe side effects at normal or low doses may have this phenotypic CYP450 2D6 variant and require low doses or switching to another antidepressant not metabolized by 2D6

Suggested Reading

Anderson IM. Meta-analytical studies on new antidepressants. Br Med Bull 2001; 57:161–178.

Anderson IM. Selective serotonin reuptake inhibitors versus tricyclic antidepressants: a meta-analysis of efficacy and tolerability. J Aff Disorders 2000;58:19–36.

Preskorn SH. Comparison of the tolerability of bupropion, fluoxetine, imipramine, nefazodone, paroxetine, sertraline, and venlafaxine. J Clin Psychiatry 1995;56(Suppl 6):12–21.

Workman EA, Short DD. Atypical antidepressants versus imipramine in the treatment of major depression: a meta-analysis. J Clin Psychiatry 1993;54:5–12.

THERAPEUTICS

Brands • Marplan

see index for additional brand names

Generic? Not in U.S.

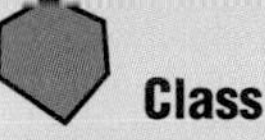

Class

- Monoamine oxidase inhibitor (MAOI)

Commonly Prescribed for

(bold for FDA approved)

- **Depression**
- Treatment-resistant depression
- Treatment-resistant panic disorder
- Treatment-resistant social anxiety disorder

How the Drug Works

- Irreversibly blocks monoamine oxidase (MAO) from breaking down norepinephrine, serotonin, and dopamine
- This presumably boosts noradrenergic, serotonergic, and dopaminergic neurotransmission

How Long Until It Works

- Onset of therapeutic actions usually not immediate, but often delayed 2–4 weeks
- If it is not working within 6–8 weeks, it may require a dosage increase or it may not work at all
- May continue to work for many years to prevent relapse of symptoms

If It Works

- The goal of treatment is complete remission of current symptoms as well as prevention of future relapses
- Treatment most often reduces or even eliminates symptoms, but not a cure since symptoms can recur after medicine stopped
- Continue treatment until all symptoms are gone (remission)
- Once symptoms gone, continue treating for 1 year for the first episode of depression
- For second and subsequent episodes of depression, treatment may need to be indefinite
- Use in anxiety disorders may also need to be indefinite

If It Doesn't Work

- Many patients only have a partial response where some symptoms are improved but others persist (especially insomnia, fatigue, and problems concentrating)
- Other patients may be nonresponders, sometimes called treatment-resistant or treatment-refractory
- Some patients who have an initial response may relapse even though they continue treatment, sometimes called "poop-out"
- Consider increasing dose, switching to another agent or adding an appropriate augmenting agent
- Consider psychotherapy
- Consider evaluation for another diagnosis or for a comorbid condition (e.g., medical illness, substance abuse, etc.)
- Some patients may experience apparent lack of consistent efficacy due to activation of latent or underlying bipolar disorder, and require antidepressant discontinuation and a switch to a mood stabilizer

Best Augmenting Combos for Partial Response or Treatment Resistance

✻ Augmentation of MAOIs has not been systematically studied, and this is something for the expert, to be done with caution and with careful monitoring

✻ A stimulant such as d-amphetamine or methylphenidate (with caution; may activate bipolar disorder and suicidal ideation; may elevate blood pressure)

- Lithium
- Mood-stabilizing anticonvulsants
- Atypical antipsychotics (with special caution for those agents with monoamine reuptake blocking properties, such as ziprasidone and zotepine)

Tests

- Patients should be monitored for changes in blood pressure
- Patients receiving high doses or long-term treatment should have hepatic function evaluated periodically

✻ Since MAO inhibitors are frequently associated with weight gain, before starting treatment, weigh all patients and determine if the patient is already overweight (BMI 25.0–29.9) or obese (BMI ≥30)

- Before giving a drug that can cause weight gain to an overweight or obese patient, consider determining whether the patient already has pre-diabetes (fasting plasma glucose 100–25 mg/dL), diabetes (fasting plasma glucose >126 mg/dL), or dyslipidemia (increased total cholesterol, LDL cholesterol and triglycerides; decreased HDL cholesterol), and treat or refer such patients for treatment, including nutrition and weight management, physical activity counseling, smoking cessation, and medical management

✻ Monitor weight and BMI during treatment

✻ While giving a drug to a patient who has gained >5% of initial weight, consider evaluating for the presence of pre-diabetes, diabetes, or dyslipidemia, or consider switching to a different antidepressant

SIDE EFFECTS

How Drug Causes Side Effects

- Theoretically due to increases in monoamines in parts of the brain and body and at receptors other than those that cause therapeutic actions (e.g., unwanted actions of serotonin in sleep centers causing insomnia, unwanted actions of norepinephrine on vascular smooth muscle causing hypertension, etc.)
- Side effects are generally immediate, but immediate side effects often disappear in time

Notable Side Effects

- Dizziness, sedation, headache, sleep disturbances, fatigue, weakness, tremor, movement problems, blurred vision, increased sweating
- Constipation, dry mouth, nausea, change in appetite, weight gain
- Sexual dysfunction
- Orthostatic hypotension (dose-related); syncope may develop at high doses

Life-Threatening or Dangerous Side Effects

- Hypertensive crisis (especially when MAOIs are used with certain tyramine-containing foods or prohibited drugs)
- Induction of mania
- Rare activation of suicidal ideation and behavior (suicidality) (short-term studies did not show an increase in the risk of suicidality with antidepressants compared to placebo beyond age 24)
- Seizures
- Hepatotoxicity

Weight Gain

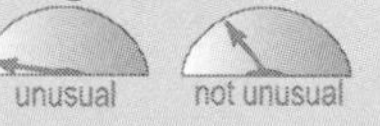

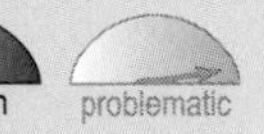

- Many experience and/or can be significant in amount

Sedation

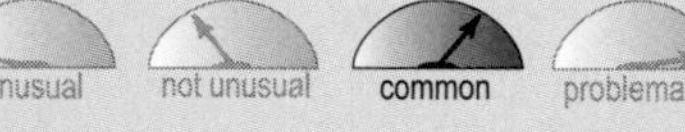

- Many experience and/or can be significant in amount
- Can also cause activation

What To Do About Side Effects

- Wait
- Wait
- Wait
- Lower the dose
- Take at night if daytime sedation
- Switch after appropriate washout to an SSRI or newer antidepressant

Best Augmenting Agents for Side Effects

- Trazodone (with caution) for insomnia
- Benzodiazepines for insomnia

✻ Single oral or sublingual dose of a calcium channel blocker (e.g., nifedipine) for urgent treatment of hypertension due to drug interaction or dietary tyramine

- Many side effects cannot be improved with an augmenting agent

DOSING AND USE

Usual Dosage Range

- 40–60 mg/day

Dosage Forms

- Tablet 10 mg

How To Dose

- Initial 10 mg twice a day; increase by 10 mg/day every 2–4 days; dosed 2–4 times/day; maximum dose 60 mg/day

Dosing Tips

- Orthostatic hypotension, especially at high doses, may require splitting into 3 or 4 daily doses
- Patients receiving high doses may need to be evaluated periodically for effects on the liver
- Little evidence to support efficacy of isocarboxazid at doses below 30 mg/day

Overdose

- Dizziness, sedation, ataxia, headache, insomnia, restlessness, anxiety, irritability; cardiovascular effects, confusion, respiratory depression, or coma may also occur

Long-Term Use

- May require periodic evaluation of hepatic function
- MAOIs may lose some efficacy long-term

Habit Forming

- Some patients have developed dependence to MAOIs

How to Stop

- Generally no need to taper, as drug wears off slowly over 2–3 weeks

Pharmacokinetics

- Clinical duration of action may be up to 21 days due to irreversible enzyme inhibition

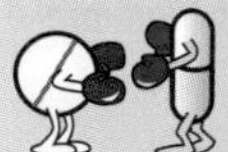

Drug Interactions

- Tramadol may increase the risk of seizures in patients taking an MAO inhibitor
- Can cause a fatal "serotonin syndrome" when combined with drugs that block serotonin reuptake (e.g., SSRIs, SNRIs, sibutramine, tramadol, etc.), so do not use with a serotonin reuptake inhibitor or for up to 5 weeks after stopping the serotonin reuptake inhibitor
- Hypertensive crisis with headache, intracranial bleeding, and death may result from combining MAO inhibitors with sympathomimetic drugs (e.g., amphetamines, methylphenidate, cocaine, dopamine, epinephrine, norepinephrine, and related compounds methyldopa, levodopa, *L*-tryptophan, *L*-tyrosine, and phenylalanine)
- Excitation, seizures, delirium, hyperpyrexia, circulatory collapse, coma, and death may result from combining MAO inhibitors with mepiridine or dextromethorphan
- Do not combine with another MAO inhibitor, alcohol, buspirone, bupropion, or guanethidine
- Adverse drug reactions can results from combining MAO inhibitors with tricyclic/tetracyclic antidepressants and related compounds, including carbamazepine, cyclobenzaprine, and mirtazapine, and should be avoided except by experts to treat difficult cases (see Pearls)
- MAO inhibitors in combination with spinal anesthesia may cause combined hypotensive effects
- Combination of MAOIs and CNS depressants may enhance sedation and hypotension

Other Warnings/ Precautions

- Use requires low tyramine diet
- Patients taking MAO inhibitors should avoid high-protein food that has undergone protein breakdown by aging, fermentation, pickling, smoking, or bacterial contamination
- Patients taking MAO inhibitors should avoid cheeses (especially aged varieties), pickled herring, beer, wine, liver, yeast extract, dry sausage, hard salami, pepperoni, Lebanon bologna, pods of broad beans (fava beans), yogurt, and excessive use of caffeine and chocolate
- Patient and prescriber must be vigilant to potential interactions with any drug, including antihypertensives and over-the-counter cough/cold preparations
- Over-the-counter medications to avoid include cough and cold preparations, including those containing dextromethorphan, nasal decongestants (tablets, drops, or spray), hay-fever medications, sinus medications, asthma inhalant medications, anti-appetite medications, weight reducing preparations, "pep" pills

- Use cautiously in patients receiving reserpine, anesthetics, disulfiram, metrizamide, anticholinergic agents
- Isocarboxazid is not recommended for use in patients who cannot be monitored closely
- When treating children, carefully weigh the risks and benefits of pharmacological treatment against the risks and benefits of nontreatment with antidepressants and make sure to document this in the patient's chart
- Distribute the brochures provided by the FDA and the drug companies
- Warn patients and their caregivers about the possibility of activating side effects and advise them to report such symptoms immediately
- Monitor patients for activation of suicidal ideation, especially children and adolescents

Do Not Use

- If patient is taking meperidine (pethidine)
- If patient is taking a sympathomimetic agent or taking guanethidine
- If patient is taking another MAOI
- If patient is taking any agent that can inhibit serotonin reuptake (e.g., SSRIs, sibutramine, tramadol, milnacipran, duloxetine, venlafaxine, clomipramine, etc.)
- If patient is taking diuretics, dextromethorphan, buspirone, bupropion
- If patient has pheochromocytoma
- If patient has cardiovascular or cerebrovascular disease
- If patient has frequent or severe headaches
- If patient is undergoing elective surgery and requires general anesthesia
- If patient has a history of liver disease or abnormal liver function tests
- If patient is taking a prohibited drug
- If patient is not compliant with a low-tyramine diet
- If there is a proven allergy to isocarboxazid

SPECIAL POPULATIONS

Renal Impairment

- Use with caution – drug may accumulate in plasma
- May require lower than usual adult dose

Hepatic Impairment

- Not for use in hepatic impairment

Cardiac Impairment

- Contraindicated in patients with congestive heart failure or hypertension
- Any other cardiac impairment may require lower than usual adult dose
- Patients with angina pectoris or coronary artery disease should limit their exertion

Elderly

- Initial dose lower than usual adult dose
- Elderly patients may have greater sensitivity to adverse effects
- Reduction in risk of suicidality with antidepressants compared to placebo in adults age 65 and older

Children and Adolescents

- Not recommended for use in children under age 16
- Carefully weigh the risks and benefits of pharmacological treatment against the risks and benefits of nontreatment with antidepressants and make sure to document this in the patient's chart
- Distribute the brochures provided by the FDA and the drug companies
- Warn patients and their caregivers about the possibility of activating side effects and advise them to report such symptoms immediately
- Use with caution, observing for activation of known or unknown bipolar disorder and/or suicidal ideation, and inform parents or guardian of this risk so they can help observe child or adolescent patients

Pregnancy

- Risk Category C [some animal studies show adverse effects; no controlled studies in humans]
- Not generally recommended for use during pregnancy, especially during first trimester
- Should evaluate patient for treatment with an antidepressant with a better risk/benefit ratio

Breast Feeding

- Some drug is found in mother's breast milk
- Immediate postpartum period is a high-risk time for depression, especially in women

who have had prior depressive episodes, so drug may need to be reinstituted late in the third trimester or shortly after childbirth to prevent a recurrence during the postpartum period
- Should evaluate patient for treatment with an antidepressant with a better risk/benefit ratio

THE ART OF PSYCHOPHARMACOLOGY

Potential Advantages
- Atypical depression
- Severe depression
- Treatment-resistant depression or anxiety disorders

Potential Disadvantages
- Requires compliance to dietary restrictions, concomitant drug restrictions
- Patients with cardiac problems or hypertension
- Multiple daily doses

Primary Target Symptoms
- Depressed mood
- Somatic symptoms
- Sleep and eating disturbances
- Psychomotor retardation
- Morbid preoccupation

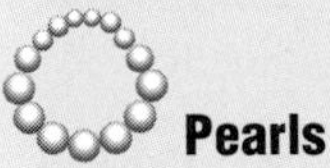

Pearls
- MAOIs are generally reserved for second-line use after SSRIs, SNRIs, and combinations of newer antidepressants have failed
- Despite little utilization, some patients respond to isocarboxazid who do not respond to other antidepressants including other MAOIs
- Patient should be advised not to take any prescription or over-the-counter drugs without consulting their doctor because of possible drug interactions with the MAOI
- Headache is often the first symptom of hypertensive crisis
- Foods generally to avoid as they are usually high in tyramine content: dry sausage, pickled herring, liver, broad bean pods, sauerkraut, cheese, yogurt, alcoholic beverages, nonalcoholic beer and wine, chocolate, caffeine, meat, and fish
- The rigid dietary restrictions may reduce compliance
- Mood disorders can be associated with eating disorders (especially in adolescent females), and isocarboxazid can be used to treat both depression and bulimia
- MAOIs are a viable second-line treatment option in depression, but are not frequently used

✻ Myths about the danger of dietary tyramine can be exaggerated, but prohibitions against concomitant drugs often not followed closely enough
- Orthostatic hypotension, insomnia, and sexual dysfunction are often the most troublesome common side effects

✻ MAOIs should be for the expert, especially if combining with agents of potential risk (e.g., stimulants, trazodone, TCAs)

✻ MAOIs should not be neglected as therapeutic agents for the treatment-resistant
- Although generally prohibited, a heroic but potentially dangerous treatment for severely treatment-resistant patients is for an expert to give a tricyclic/tetracyclic antidepressant other than clomipramine simultaneously with an MAO inhibitor for patients who fail to respond to numerous other antidepressants
- Use of MAOIs with clomipramine is always prohibited because of the risk of serotonin syndrome and death
- Amoxapine may be the preferred trycyclic/tetracyclic antidepressant to combine with an MAOI in heroic cases due to its theoretically protective 5HT2A antagonist properties
- If this option is elected, start the MAOI with the tricyclic/tetracyclic antidepressant simultaneously at low doses after appropriate drug washout, then alternately increase doses of these agents every few days to a week as tolerated
- Although very strict dietary and concomitant drug restrictions must be observed to prevent hypertensive crises and serotonin syndrome, the most common side effects of MAOI and tricyclic/tetracyclic combinations may be weight gain and orthostatic hypotension

Suggested Reading

Kennedy SH. Continuation and maintenance treatments in major depression: the neglected role of monoamine oxidase inhibitors. J Psychiatry Neurosci 1997;22:127–31.

Lippman SB, Nash K. Monoamine oxidase inhibitor update. Potential adverse food and drug interactions. Drug Saf 1990;5:195–204.

Larsen JK, Rafaelsen OJ. Long-term treatment of depression with isocarboxazide. Acta Psychiatr Scand 1980;62(5):456–63.

THERAPEUTICS

Brands • Lamictal
• Labileno
• Lamictin

see index for additional brand names

Generic? Yes

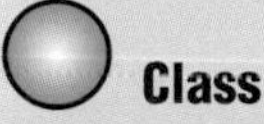

Class

• Anticonvulsant, mood stabilizer, voltage-sensitive sodium channel antagonist

Commonly Prescribed for

(bold for FDA approved)

• **Maintenance treatment of bipolar I disorder**
• **Partial seizures (adjunctive; adults and children over age 2)**
• **Generalized seizures of Lennox-Gastaut syndrome (adjunctive; adults and children over age 2)**
• **Conversion to monotherapy in adults with partial seizures who are receiving treatment with carbamazepine, phenytoin, phenobarbital, primidone, or valproate**
• Bipolar depression
• Bipolar mania (adjunctive and second-line)
• Psychosis, schizophrenia (adjunctive)
• Neuropathic pain/chronic pain
• Major depressive disorder (adjunctive)
• Other seizure types and as initial monotherapy for epilepsy

How the Drug Works

❋ Acts as a use-dependent blocker of voltage-sensitive sodium channels
❋ Interacts with the open channel conformation of voltage-sensitive sodium channels
❋ Interacts at a specific site of the alpha pore-forming subunit of voltage-sensitive sodium channels
• Inhibits release of glutamate and asparate

How Long Until It Works

• May take several weeks to improve bipolar depression
• May take several weeks to months to optimize an effect on mood stabilization
• Can reduce seizures by 2 weeks, but may take several weeks to months to reduce seizures

If It Works

• The goal of treatment is complete remission of symptoms (e.g., seizures, depression, pain)
• Continue treatment until all symptoms are gone or until improvement is stable and then continue treating indefinitely as long as improvement persists
• Continue treatment indefinitely to avoid recurrence of mania, depression, and/or seizures
• Treatment of chronic neuropathic pain may reduce but does not eliminate pain symptoms and is not a cure since pain usually recurs after medicine stopped

If It Doesn't Work (for bipolar disorder)

❋ Many patients only have a partial response where some symptoms are improved but others persist or continue to wax and wane without stabilization of mood
• Other patients may be nonresponders, sometimes called treatment-resistant or treatment-refractory
• Consider increasing dose, switching to another agent or adding an appropriate augmenting agent
• Consider adding psychotherapy
• Consider biofeedback or hypnosis for pain
• Consider the presence of noncompliance and counsel patient
• Switch to another mood stabilizer with fewer side effects
• Consider evaluation for another diagnosis or for a comorbid condition (e.g., medical illness, substance abuse, etc.)

Best Augmenting Combos for Partial Response or Treatment Resistance (for bipolar disorder)

• Lithium
• Atypical antipsychotics (especially risperidone, olanzapine, quetiapine, ziprasidone, and aripiprazole)
❋ Valproate (with caution and at half dose of lamotrigine in the presence of valproate, because valproate can double lamotrigine levels)
❋ Antidepressants (with caution because

antidepressants can destabilize mood in some patients, including induction of rapid cycling or suicidal ideation; in particular consider bupropion; also SSRIs, SNRIs, others; generally avoid TCAs, MAOIs)

Tests

- None required
- The value of monitoring plasma concentrations of lamotrigine has not been established
- Because lamotrigine binds to melanin-containing tissues, ophthalmological checks may be considered

SIDE EFFECTS

How Drug Causes Side Effects

- CNS side effects theoretically due to excessive actions at voltage-sensitive sodium channels
- Rash hypothetically an allergic reaction

Notable Side Effects

✻ Benign rash (approximately 10%)

- Sedation, blurred or double vision, dizziness, ataxia, headache, tremor, insomnia, poor coordination, fatigue
- Nausea, vomiting, dyspepsia, abdominal pain, constipation, rhinitis
- Additional effects in pediatric patients with epilepsy: infection, pharyngitis, asthenia

Life-Threatening or Dangerous Side Effects

✻ Rare serious rash (risk may be greater in pediatric patients but still rare)

- Rare multi-organ failure associated with Stevens Johnson syndrome, toxic epidermal necrolysis or drug hypersensitivity syndrome
- Rare blood dyscrasias
- Rare sudden unexplained deaths have occurred in epilepsy (unknown if related to lamotrigine use)
- Withdrawal seizures upon abrupt withdrawal
- Rare activation of suicidal ideation and behavior (suicidality)

Weight Gain

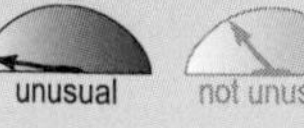

- Reported but not expected

Sedation

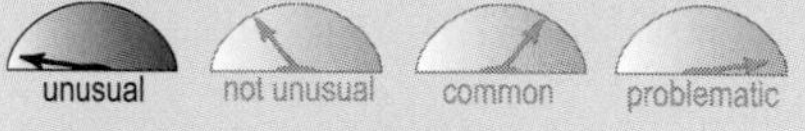

- Reported but not expected
- Dose-related
- Can wear off with time

What To Do About Side Effects

- Wait
- Take at night to reduce daytime sedation
- Divide dosing to twice daily

✻ If patient develops signs of a rash with benign characteristics (i.e., a rash that peaks within days, settles in 10–14 days, is spotty, nonconfluent, nontender, has no systemic features, and laboratory tests are normal):

- Reduce lamotrigine dose or stop dosage increase
- Warn patient to stop drug and contact physician if rash worsens or new symptoms emerge
- Prescribe antihistamine and/or topical corticosteroid for pruritis
- Monitor patient closely

✻ If patient develops signs of a rash with serious characteristics (i.e., a rash that is confluent and widespread, or purpuric or tender; with any prominent involvement of neck or upper trunk; any involvement of eyes, lips, mouth, etc.; any associated fever, malaise, pharyngitis, anorexia, or lymphadenopathy; abnormal laboratory tests for complete blood count, liver function, urea, creatinine):

- Stop lamotrigine (and valproate if administered)
- Monitor and investigate organ involvement (hepatic, renal, hematologic)
- Patient may require hospitalization
- Monitor patient very closely

Best Augmenting Agents for Side Effects

- Antihistamines and/or topical corticosteroid for rash, pruritis
- Many side effects cannot be improved with an augmenting agent

DOSING AND USE

Usual Dosage Range

- Monotherapy for bipolar disorder: 100–200 mg/day
- Adjunctive treatment for bipolar disorder: 100 mg/day in combination with valproate; 400 mg/day in combination with enzyme-inducing antiepileptic drugs such as carbamazepine, phenobarbital, phenytoin, and primidone
- Monotherapy for seizures in patients over age 12: 300–500 mg/day in 2 doses
- Adjunctive treatment for seizures in patients over age 12: 100–400 mg/day for regimens containing valproate; 100–200 mg/day for valproate alone; 300–500 mg/day in 2 doses for regimens not containing valproate
- Patients ages 2–12 with epilepsy are dosed based on body weight and concomitant medications

Dosage Forms

- Tablet 25 mg scored, 100 mg scored, 150 mg scored, 200 mg scored
- Chewable tablet 2 mg, 5 mg, 25 mg

How To Dose

✲ Bipolar disorder (monotherapy, see chart): for the first 2 weeks administer 25 mg/day; at week 3 increase to 50 mg/day; at week 5 increase to 100 mg/day; at week 6 increase to 200 mg/day; maximum dose generally 200 mg/day

✲ Bipolar disorder (adjunct to valproate): for the first 2 weeks administer 25 mg every other day; at week 3 increase to 25 mg/day; at week 5 increase to 50 mg/day; at week 6 increase to 100 mg/day; maximum dose generally 100 mg/day

- Bipolar disorder (adjunct to enzyme-inducing antiepileptic drugs): for the first 2 weeks administer 50 mg/day; at week 3 increase to 100 mg/day in divided doses; starting at week 5 increase by 100 mg/day each week; maximum dose generally 400 mg/day in divided doses
- When lamotrigine is added to epilepsy treatment that includes valproate (ages 12 and older): for the first 2 weeks administer 25 mg every other day; at week 3 increase to 25 mg/day; every 1–2 weeks can increase by 25–50 mg/day; usual maintenance dose 100–400 mg/day in 1–2 doses or 100–200 mg/day if lamotrigine is added to valproate alone
- When lamotrigine is added to epilepsy treatment that includes carbamazepine, phenytoin, phenobarbital, or primidone (without valproate) (ages 12 and older): for the first 2 weeks administer 50 mg/day; at week 3 increase to 100 mg/day in 2 doses; every 1–2 weeks can increase by 100 mg/day; usual maintenance dose 300–500 mg/day in 2 doses

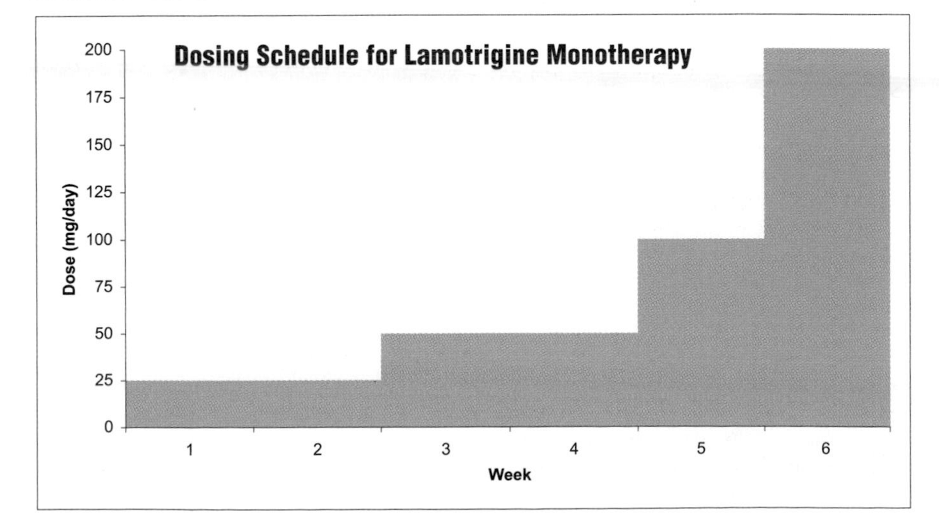

- When converting from a single enzyme-inducing antiepileptic drug to lamotrigine monotherapy for epilepsy: titrate as described above to 500 mg/day in 2 doses while maintaining dose of previous medication; decrease first drug in 20% decrements each week over the next 4 weeks
- When converting from valproate to lamotrigine monotherapy for epilepsy: titrate as described above to 200 mg/day while maintaining dose of valproate, then gradually increase lamotrigine up to 500 mg/day while gradually discontinuing valproate
- Seizures (under age 12): see Children and Adolescents

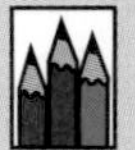

Dosing Tips

✻ Very slow dose titration may reduce the incidence of skin rash
- Therefore, dose should not be titrated faster than recommended because of possible risk of increased side effects, including rash
- If patient stops taking lamotrigine for 5 days or more it may be necessary to restart the drug with the initial dose titration, as rashes have been reported on reexposure
- Advise patient to avoid new medications, foods, or products during the first 3 months of lamotrigine treatment in order to decrease the risk of unrelated rash; patient should also not start lamotrigine within 2 weeks of a viral infection, rash, or vaccination

✻ If lamotrigine is added to patients taking valproate, remember that valproate inhibits lamotrigine metabolism and therefore titration rate and ultimate dose of lamotrigine should be reduced by 50% to reduce the risk of rash

✻ Thus, if concomitant valproate is discontinued after lamotrigine dose is stabilized, then the lamotrigine dose should be cautiously doubled over at least 2 weeks in equal increments each week following discontinuation of valproate
- Also, if concomitant enzyme-inducing antiepileptic drugs such as carbamazepine, phenobarbital, phenytoin, and primidone are discontinued after lamotrigine dose is stabilized, then the lamotrigine dose should be maintained for 1 week following discontinuation of the other drug and then reduced by half over 2 weeks in equal decrements each week
- Since oral contraceptives and pregnancy can decrease lamotrigine levels, adjustments to the maintenance dose of lamotrigine are recommended in women taking, starting, or stopping oral contraceptives, becoming pregnant, or after delivery
- Chewable dispersible tablets should only be administered as whole tablets; dose should be rounded down to the nearest whole tablet
- Chewable dispersible tablets can be dispersed by adding the tablet to liquid (enough to cover the drug); after approximately 1 minute the solution should be stirred and then consumed immediately in its entirety

Overdose

- Some fatalities have occurred; ataxia, nystagmus, seizures, coma, intraventricular conduction delay

Long-Term Use

- Safe

Habit Forming

- No

How to Stop

- Taper over at least 2 weeks

✻ Rapid discontinuation can increase the risk of relapse in bipolar disorder
- Patients with epilepsy may seize upon withdrawal, especially if withdrawal is abrupt
- Discontinuation symptoms uncommon

Pharmacokinetics

- Elimination half-life in healthy volunteers approximately 33 hours after a single dose of lamotrigine
- Elimination half-life in patients receiving concomitant valproate treatment approximately 59 hours after a single dose of lamotrigine
- Elimination half-life in patients receiving concomitant enzyme-inducing antiepileptic drugs (such as carbamazepine, phenobarbital, phenytoin, and primidone)

approximately 14 hours after a single dose of lamotrigine
- Metabolized in the liver through glucorunidation but not through the CYP450 enzyme system
- Inactive metabolite
- Renally excreted
- Lamotrigine inhibits dihydrofolate reductase and may therefore reduce folate concentrations
- Rapidly and completely absorbed; bioavailability not affected by food

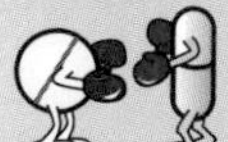

Drug Interactions

✻ Valproate increases plasma concentrations and half-life of lamotrigine, requiring lower doses of lamotrigine (half or less)
✻ Use of lamotrigine with valproate may be associated with an increased incidence of rash
- Enzyme-inducing antiepileptic drugs (e.g., carbamazepine, phenobarbital, phenytoin, primidone) may increase the clearance of lamotrigine and lower its plasma levels
- Oral contraceptives may decrease plasma levels of lamotrigine
- No likely pharmacokinetic interactions of lamotrigine with lithium, oxcarbazepine, atypical antipsychotics, or antidepressants

Other Warnings/ Precautions

✻ Life-threatening rashes have developed in association with lamotrigine use; lamotrigine should generally be discontinued at the first sign of serious rash
✻ Risk of rash may be increased with higher doses, faster dose escalation, concomitant use of valproate, or in children under age 12
- Patient should be instructed to report any symptoms of hypersensitivity immediately (fever; flu-like symptoms; rash; blisters on skin or in eyes, mouth, ears, nose, or genital areas; swelling of eyelids, conjunctivitis, lymphadenopathy)
- Depressive effects may be increased by other CNS depressants (alcohol, MAOIs, other anticonvulsants, etc.)
- A small number of people may experience a worsening of seizures
- May cause photosensitivity
- Lamotrigine binds to tissue that contains melanin, so for long-term treatment ophthalmological checks may be considered
- Warn patients and their caregivers about the possibility of activation of suicidal ideation and advise them to report such side effects immediately

Do Not Use

- If there is a proven allergy to lamotrigine

SPECIAL POPULATIONS

Renal Impairment

- Lamotrigine is renally excreted, so the maintenance dose may need to be lowered
- Can be removed by hemodialysis; patients receiving hemodialysis may require supplemental doses of lamotrigine

Hepatic Impairment

- Dose may need to be reduced and titration may need to be slower, perhaps by 50% in patients with moderate impairment and 75% in patients with severe impairment

Cardiac Impairment

- Clinical experience is limited
- Drug should be used with caution

Elderly

- Some patients may tolerate lower doses better
- Elderly patients may be more susceptible to adverse effects

Children and Adolescents

- Ages 2 and older: approved as add-on for Lennox-Gastaut syndrome
- Ages 2 and older: approved as add-on for partial seizures
- No other use of lamotrigine is approved for patients under 16 years of age

✻ Risk of rash is increased in pediatric patients, especially in children under 12 and in children taking valproate
- When lamotrigine is added to treatment that includes valproate (ages 2–12): for the first 2 weeks administer 0.15 mg/kg per day in 1–2 doses rounded down to the nearest whole tablet; at week 3 increase to

0.3 mg/kg per day in 1–2 doses rounded down to the nearest whole tablet; every 1–2 weeks can increase by 0.3 mg/kg per day rounded down to the nearest whole tablet; usual maintenance dose 1–5 mg/kg per day in 1–2 doses (maximum generally 200 mg/day) or 1–3 mg/kg per day in 1–2 doses if lamotrigine is added to valproate alone
- When lamotrigine is added to treatment with carbamazepine, phenytoin, phenobarbital, or primidone (without valproate) (ages 2–12): for the first 2 weeks administer 0.6 mg/kg per day in 2 doses rounded down to the nearest whole tablet; at week 3 increase to 1.2 mg/kg per day in 2 doses rounded down to the nearest whole tablet; every 1–2 weeks can increase by 1.2 mg/kg per day rounded down to the nearest whole tablet; usual maintenance dose 5–15 mg/kg per day in 2 doses (maximum dose generally 400 mg per day)
- Clearance of lamotrigine may be influenced by weight, such that patients weighing less than 30 kg may require an increase of up to 50% for maintenance doses

Pregnancy
- Risk Category C [some animal studies show adverse effects; no controlled studies in humans]
- Use in women of childbearing potential requires weighing potential benefits to the mother against the risks to the fetus
- Pregnancy registry data show increased risk of isolated cleft palate or cleft lip deformity with first trimester exposure
- ✻ If treatment with lamotrigine is continued, plasma concentrations of lamotrigine may be reduced during pregnancy, possibly requiring increased doses with dose reduction following delivery
- Pregnancy exposure registry for lamotrigine: (800) 336-2176
- Taper drug if discontinuing
- Seizures, even mild seizures, may cause harm to the embryo/fetus
- Recurrent bipolar illness during pregnancy can be quite disruptive
- ✻ For bipolar patients, lamotrigine should generally be discontinued before anticipated pregnancies
- ✻ For bipolar patients in whom treatment is discontinued, given the risk of relapse in the postpartum period, lamotrigine should generally be restarted immediately after delivery
- ✻ Atypical antipsychotics may be preferable to lithium or anticonvulsants such as lamotrigine if treatment of bipolar disorder is required during pregnancy, but lamotrigine may be preferable to other anticonvulsants such as valproate if anticonvulsant treatment is required during pregnancy
- Bipolar symptoms may recur or worsen during pregnancy and some form of treatment may be necessary

Breast Feeding
- Some drug is found in mother's breast milk
- ✻ Generally recommended either to discontinue drug or bottle feed
- If drug is continued while breast feeding, infant should be monitored for possible adverse effects
- If infant shows signs of irritability or sedation, drug may need to be discontinued
- ✻ Bipolar disorder may recur during the postpartum period, particularly if there is a history of prior postpartum episodes of either depression or psychosis
- ✻ Relapse rates may be lower in women who receive prophylactic treatment for postpartum episodes of bipolar disorder
- Atypical antipsychotics and anticonvulsants such as valproate may be preferable to lithium or lamotrigine during the postpartum period when breast feeding

THE ART OF PSYCHOPHARMACOLOGY

Potential Advantages
- Depressive stages of bipolar disorder (bipolar depression)
- To prevent recurrences of both depression and mania in bipolar disorder

Potential Disadvantages
- May not be as effective in the manic stage of bipolar disorder

Primary Target Symptoms
- Incidence of seizures

- Unstable mood, especially depression, in bipolar disorder
- Pain

Pearls

- ✻ Lamotrigine is a first-line treatment option that may be best for patients with bipolar depression
- ✻ Seems to be more effective in treating depressive episodes than manic episodes in bipolar disorder (treats from below better than it treats from above)
- ✻ Seems to be effective in preventing both manic relapses as well as depressive relapses (stabilizes both from above and from below) although it may be even better for preventing depressive relapses than for preventing manic relapses
- ✻ Despite convincing evidence of efficacy in bipolar disorder, is often used less frequently than anticonvulsants without convincing evidence of efficacy in bipolar disorder (e.g., gabapentin or topiramate)
- ✻ Low levels of use may be based upon exaggerated fears of skin rashes or lack of knowledge about how to manage skin rashes if they occur
- ✻ May actually be one of the best tolerated mood stabilizers with little weight gain or sedation
- Actual risk of serious skin rash may be comparable to agents erroneously considered "safer" including carbamazepine, phenytoin, phenobarbital, and zonisamide
- Rashes are common even in placebo-treated patients in clinical trials of bipolar patients (5–10%) due to non-drug related causes including eczema, irritant, and allergic contact dermatitis, such as poison ivy and insect bite reactions
- ✻ To manage rashes in bipolar patients receiving lamotrigine, realize that rashes that occur within the first 5 days or after 8–12 weeks of treatment are rarely drug-related, and learn the clinical distinctions between a benign rash and a serious rash (see What to Do About Side Effects above)
- Rash, including serious rash, appears riskiest in younger children, in those who are receiving concomitant valproate, and/or in those receiving rapid lamotrigine titration and/or high dosing
- Risk of serious rash is less than 1% and has been declining since slower titration, lower dosing, adjustments to use of concomitant valproate administration, and limitations on use in children under 12 have been implemented
- Incidence of serious rash is very low (approaching zero) in recent studies of bipolar patients
- Benign rashes related to lamotrigine may affect up to 10% of patients and resolve rapidly with drug discontinuation
- ✻ Given the limited treatment options for bipolar depression, patients with benign rashes can even be rechallenged with lamotrigine 5–12 mg/day with very slow titration after risk/benefit analysis if they are informed, reliable, closely monitored, and warned to stop lamotrigine and contact their physician if signs of hypersensitivity occur
- Only a third of bipolar patients experience adequate relief with a monotherapy, so most patients need multiple medications for best control
- Lamotrigine is useful in combination with atypical antipsychotics and/or lithium for acute mania
- Usefulness for bipolar disorder in combination with anticonvulsants other than valproate is not well demonstrated; such combinations can be expensive and are possibly ineffective or even irrational
- May be useful as an adjunct to atypical antipsychotics for rapid onset of action in schizophrenia
- May be useful as an adjunct to antidepressants in major depressive disorder
- Early studies suggest possible utility for patients with neuropathic pain such as diabetic peripheral neuropathy, HIV-associated neuropathy, and other pain conditions including migraine

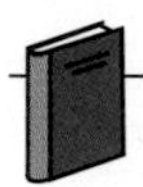

Suggested Reading

Calabrese JR, Bowden CL, Sachs GS, et al. A double-blind placebo-controlled study of lamotrigine monotherapy in outpatients with bipolar I depression. J Clin Psych 1999;60:79–88.

Calabrese JR, Sullivan JR, Bowden CL, Suppes T, Goldberg JF, Sachs GS, Shelton MD, Goodwin FK, Frye MA, Kusumakar V. Rash in multicenter trials of lamotrigine in mood disorders: clinical relevance and management. J Clin Psychiatry 2002;63:1012–19.

Culy CR, Goa KL. Lamotrigine. A review of its use in childhood epilepsy. Paediatr Drugs 2000; 2: 299–330.

Cunningham M, Tennis P, and the International Lamotrigine Pregnancy Registry Scientific Advisory Committee. Lamotrigine and the risk of malformations in pregnancy. Neurology 2005;64:955–60.

Green B. Lamotrigine in mood disorders. Curr Med Res Opin 2003;19:272–7.

Goodwin GM, Bowden CL, Calabrese JR et al. A pooled analysis of 2 placebo-controlled 18-month trials of lamotrigine and lithium maintenance treatment in bipolar I disorder. J Clin Psychiatry 2004;65:432–41.

LEVETIRACETAM

THERAPEUTICS

Brands • Keppra
• Keppra XR

see index for additional brand names

Generic? No

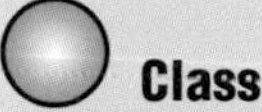

Class

• Anticonvulsant, synaptic vesicle protein SV2A modulator

Commonly Prescribed for

(bold for FDA approved)

• **Adjunct therapy for partial seizures in epilepsy (ages 4 and older)**
• **Adjunct therapy for myoclonic seizures in juvenile myoclonic epilepsy (ages 12 and older)**
• **Adjunct therapy for primary generalized tonic-clonic seizures in idiopathic generalized epilepsy (ages 6 and older)**
• Neuropathic pain/chronic pain
• Mania

How the Drug Works

* Binds to synaptic vesicle protein SV2A, which is involved in synaptic vesicle exocytosis
• Opposes the activity of negative modulators of GABA- and glycine-gated currents and partially inhibits N-type calcium currents in neuronal cells

How Long Until It Works

• Should reduce seizures by 2 weeks
• Not yet clear if it has mood-stabilizing effects in bipolar disorder or antineuralgic actions in chronic neuropathic pain, but some patients may respond and if so, would be expected to show clinical effects starting by 2 weeks although it may take several weeks to months to optimize clinical effects

If It Works

• The goal of treatment is complete remission of symptoms (e.g., seizures, mania, pain)
• The goal of treatment of chronic neuropathic pain is to reduce symptoms as much as possible, especially in combination with other treatments
• Treatment of chronic neuropathic pain most often reduces but does not eliminate symptoms and is not a cure since symptoms usually recur after medicine stopped
• Continue treatment until all symptoms are gone or until mood is stable and then continue treating indefinitely as long as improvement persists
• Continue treatment indefinitely to avoid recurrence of seizures, mania, and pain

If It Doesn't Work (for bipolar disorder or neuropathic pain)

* May be effective only in a subset of bipolar patients, in some patients who fail to respond to other mood stabilizers, or it may not work at all
• Many patients have only a partial response where some symptoms are improved but others persist or continue to wax and wane without stabilization of pain or mood
• Other patients may be nonresponders, sometimes called treatment-resistant or treatment-refractory
• Consider increasing dose or switching to another agent with better demonstrated efficacy in bipolar disorder or neuropathic pain

Best Augmenting Combos for Partial Response or Treatment Resistance

• Levetiracetam is itself a second-line augmenting agent to numerous other anticonvulsants, lithium, and atypical antipsychotics for bipolar disorder and to gabapentin, tiagabine, other anticonvulsants, SNRIs, and tricyclic antidepressants for neuropathic pain

Tests

• None for healthy individuals

SIDE FFECTS

How Drug Causes Side Effects

• CNS side effects may be due to excessive actions on SV2A synaptic vesicle proteins or to actions on various voltage-sensitive ion channels

Notable Side Effects

- ✻ Sedation, dizziness, ataxia, asthenia
- Hematologic abnormalities (decrease in red blood cell count and hemoglobin)

Life-Threatening or Dangerous Side Effects

- Activation of suicidal ideation and acts (rare)
- Changes in behavior (aggression, agitation, anxiety, hostility)
- Rare activation of suicidal ideation and behavior (suicidality)

Weight Gain

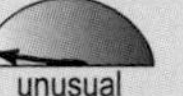
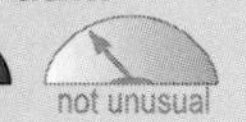

unusual | not unusual | common | problematic

- Reported but not expected

Sedation

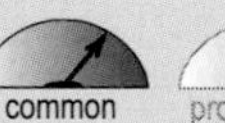

unusual | not unusual | common | problematic

- Many experience and/or can be significant in amount

What To Do About Side Effects

- Wait
- Wait
- Wait
- Take more of the dose at night to reduce daytime sedation
- Lower the dose
- Switch to another agent

Best Augmenting Agents for Side Effects

- Many side effects cannot be improved with an augmenting agent

DOSING AND USE

Usual Dosage Range

- 1,000–3,000 mg/day

Dosage Forms

- Tablet 250 mg, 500 mg, 750 mg
- Extended-release tablet 500 mg
- Oral solution 100 mg/mL

How To Dose

- Initial 1,000 mg/day in 1 (extended-release) or 2 (immediate-release) doses; after 2 weeks can increase by 1,000 mg/day every 2 weeks; maximum dose generally 3,000 mg/day

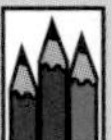

Dosing Tips

- For intolerable sedation, can give most of the dose at night and less during the day
- Some patients may tolerate and respond to doses greater than 3,000 mg/day

Overdose

- No fatalities; sedation, agitation, aggression, respiratory depression, coma

Long-Term Use

- Safe

Habit Forming

- No

How to Stop

- Taper
- Epilepsy patients may seize upon withdrawal, especially if withdrawal is abrupt
- ✻ Rapid discontinuation can increase the risk of relapse in bipolar disorder
- Discontinuation symptoms uncommon

Pharmacokinetics

- Elimination half-life approximately 6–8 hours
- Inactive metabolites
- Not metabolized by CYP450 enzymes
- Does not inhibit/induce CYP450 enzymes
- Renally excreted

Drug Interactions

- Because levetiracetam is not metabolized by CYP450 enzymes and does not inhibit or induce CYP450 enzymes, it is unlikely to have significant pharmacokinetic drug interactions

Other Warnings/ Precautions

- Depressive effects may be increased by other CNS depressants (alcohol, MAOIs, other anticonvulsants, etc.)
- Warn patients and their caregivers about the possibility of activation of suicidal ideation and advise them to report such side effects immediately

- Monitor patients for behavioral symptoms (aggression, agitation, anger, anxiety, apathy, depression, hostility, irritability) as well as for possible psychotic symptoms or suicidality

Do Not Use

- If there is a proven allergy to levetiracetam

SPECIAL PPULATIONS

Renal Impairment

- Recommended dose for patients with mild impairment may be between 500 mg and 1,500 mg twice a day
- Recommended dose for patients with moderate impairment may be between 250 mg and 750 mg twice a day
- Recommended dose for patients with severe impairment may be between 250 mg and 500 mg twice a day
- Patients on dialysis may require doses between 500 mg and 1,000 mg once a day, with a supplemental dose of 250–500 mg following dialysis

Hepatic Impairment

- Dose adjustment usually not necessary

Cardiac Impairment

- No specific recommendations

Elderly

- Some patients may tolerate lower doses better
- Elderly patients may be more susceptible to adverse effects

Children and Adolescents

- Safety and efficacy not established under age 16
- Children may require higher doses than adults; dosing should be adjusted according to weight

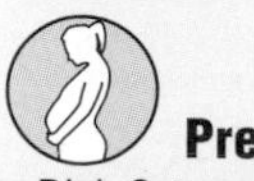

Pregnancy

- Risk Category C [some animal studies show adverse effects; no controlled studies in humans]
- Use in women of childbearing potential requires weighing potential benefits to the mother against the risks to the fetus
- Antiepileptic Drug Pregnancy Registry: (888) 233-2334
- Taper drug if discontinuing
- Seizures, even mild seizures, may cause harm to the embryo/fetus
- Lack of convincing efficacy for treatment of bipolar disorder or chronic neuropathic pain suggests risk/benefit ratio is in favor of discontinuing levetiracetam during pregnancy for these indications
- * For bipolar patients, given the risk of relapse in the postpartum period, mood stabilizer treatment, especially with agents with better evidence of efficacy than levetiracetam, should generally be restarted immediately after delivery if patient is unmedicated during pregnancy
- * For bipolar patients, levetiracetam should generally be discontinued before anticipated pregnancies
- * Atypical antipsychotics may be preferable to levetiracetam if treatment of bipolar disorder is required during pregnancy
- Bipolar symptoms may recur or worsen during pregnancy and some form of treatment may be necessary

Breast Feeding

- Some drug is found in mother's breast milk
- * Recommended either to discontinue drug or bottle feed
- If drug is continued while breast feeding, infant should be monitored for possible adverse effects
- If infant becomes irritable or sedated, breast feeding or drug may need to be discontinued
- * Bipolar disorder may recur during the postpartum period, particularly if there is a history of prior postpartum episodes of either depression or psychosis
- * Relapse rates may be lower in women who receive prophylactic treatment for postpartum episodes of bipolar disorder
- Atypical antipsychotics and anticonvulsants such as valproate may be safer than levetiracetam during the postpartum period when breast feeding

THE ART OF PSYCHOPHARMACOLOGY

Potential Advantages
- Patients on concomitant drugs (lack of drug interactions)
- Treatment-refractory bipolar disorder
- Treatment-refractory neuropathic pain

Potential Disadvantages
- Patients noncompliant with twice daily dosing
- Efficacy for bipolar disorder or neuropathic pain not well documented

Primary Target Symptoms
- Seizures
- Pain
- Mania

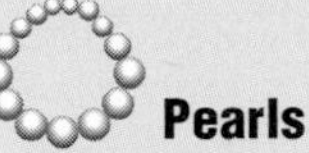

Pearls
- Well studied in epilepsy

✱ Off-label use second-line and as an augmenting agent may be justified for bipolar disorder and neuropathic pain unresponsive to other treatments

✱ Unique mechanism of action suggests utility where other anticonvulsants fail to work

✱ Unique mechanism of action as modulator of synaptic vesicle release suggests theoretical utility for clinical conditions that are hypothetically linked to excessively activated neuronal circuits, such as anxiety disorders and neuropathic pain as well as epilepsy

Suggested Reading

Ben-Menachem E. Levetiracetam: treatment in epilepsy. Expert Opin Pharmacother 2003;4(11):2079–88.

French J. Use of levetiracetam in special populations. Epilepsia 2001;42 Suppl 4:40–3.

Leppik IE. Three new drugs for epilepsy: levetiracetam, oxcarbazepine, and zonisamide. J Child Neurol 2002;17 Suppl 1:S53–7.

Lynch BA, Lambeng N, Nocka K, Kensel-Hammes P, Bajjalieh SM, Matagne A, Fuks B.. The synaptic vesicle protein SV2A is the binding site for the antiepileptic drug levetiracetam. Proc Natl Acad Sci USA 2004;101:9861–6.

Pinto A, Sander JW. Levetiracetam: a new therapeutic option for refractory epilepsy. Int J Clin Pract 2003;57(7):616–21.

THERAPEUTICS

Brands • Vyvanse
see index for additional brand names

Generic? No

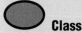

Class
- Stimulant

Commonly Prescribed for
(bold for FDA approved)
- **Attention deficit hyperactivity disorder (ADHD) in children ages 6–12 and in adults**
- Narcolepsy
- Treatment-resistant depression

How the Drug Works
* Lisdexamfetamine is a prodrug of dextroamphetamine and is thus not active until after it has been absorbed by the intestinal tract and converted to dextroamphetamine (active component) and l-lysine
* Once converted to dextroamphetamine, it increases norepinephrine and especially dopamine actions by blocking their reuptake and facilitating their release
- Enhancement of dopamine and norepinephrine in certain brain regions (e.g., dorsolateral prefrontal cortex) may improve attention, concentration, executive dysfunction, and wakefulness
- Enhancement of dopamine actions in other brain regions (e.g., basal ganglia) may improve hyperactivity
- Enhancement of dopamine and norepinephrine in yet other brain regions (e.g., medial prefrontal cortex, hypothalamus) may improve depression, fatigue, and sleepiness

How Long Until It Works
- Some immediate effects can be seen with first dosing
- Can take several weeks to attain maximum therapeutic benefit

If It Works (for ADHD)
- The goal of treatment of ADHD is reduction of symptoms of inattentiveness, motor hyperactivity, and/or impulsiveness that disrupt social, school and/or occupational functioning
- Continue treatment until all symptoms are under control or improvement is stable and then continue treatment indefinitely as long as improvement persists
- Reevaluate the need for treatment periodically
- Treatment for ADHD begun in childhood may need to be continued into adolescence and adulthood if continued benefit is documented

If It Doesn't Work (for ADHD)
- Consider adjusting dose or switching to another formulation of d-amphetamine or to another agent
- Consider behavioral therapy
- Consider the presence of noncompliance and counsel patients and parents
- Consider evaluation for another diagnosis or for a comorbid condition (e.g., bipolar disorder, substance abuse, medical illness, etc.)
* Some ADHD patients and some depressed patients may experience lack of consistent efficacy due to activation of latent or underlying bipolar disorder, and require either augmenting with a mood stabilizer or switching to a mood stabilizer

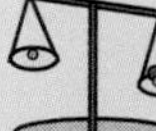

Best Augmenting Combos for Partial Response or Treatment Resistance
* Best to attempt other monotherapies prior to augmenting
- For the expert, can combine with modafinil or atomoxetine for ADHD
- For the expert, can occasionally combine with atypical antipsychotics in highly treatment-resistant cases of bipolar disorder or ADHD
- For the expert, can combine with antidepressants to boost antidepressant efficacy in highly treatment-resistant cases of depression while carefully monitoring patient

Tests
- Blood pressure should be monitored regularly
- In children, monitor weight and height

SIDE EFFECTS

How Drug Causes Side Effects
- Increases in norepinephrine especially peripherally can cause autonomic side effects, including tremor, tachycardia, hypertension, and cardiac arrhythmias
- Increases in norepinephrine and dopamine centrally can cause CNS side effects such as insomnia, agitation, psychosis, and substance abuse

Notable Side Effects
✻ Insomnia, headache, exacerbation of tics, nervousness, irritability, overstimulation, tremor, dizziness

✻ Anorexia, nausea, dry mouth, constipation, diarrhea, weight loss
- Can temporarily slow normal growth in children (controversial)
- Sexual dysfunction long-term (impotence, libido changes), but can also improve sexual dysfunction short-term

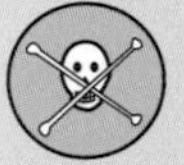

Life-Threatening or Dangerous Side Effects
- Psychotic episodes
- Seizures
- Palpitations, tachycardia, hypertension
- Rare activation of hypomania, mania, or suicidal ideation (controversial)
- Cardiovascular adverse effects, sudden death in patients with preexisting cardiac structural abnormalities

Weight Gain

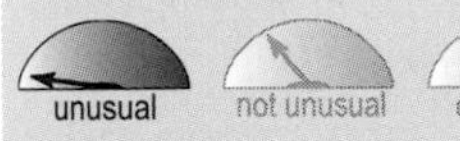

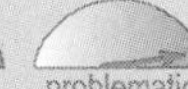

- Reported but not expected
- Some patients may experience weight loss

Sedation

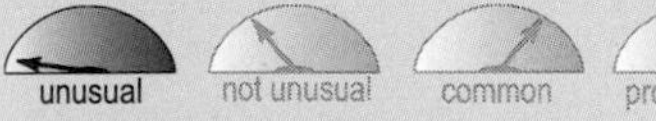

- Reported but not expected
- Activation much more common than sedation

What To Do About Side Effects
- Wait
- Adjust dose
- Switch to another long-acting stimulant
- Switch to another agent
- For insomnia, avoid dosing in afternoon/evening

Best Augmenting Agents for Side Effects
- Beta-blockers for peripheral autonomic side effects
- Dose reduction or switching to another agent may be more effective since most side effects cannot be improved with an augmenting agent

DOSING AND USE

Usual Dosage Range
- 30 mg/day

Dosage Forms
- Capsule 20 mg, 30 mg, 40 mg, 50 mg, 60 mg, 70 mg

How To Dose
- Initial 30 mg/day in the morning; can increase by 10–20 mg each week; maximum dose generally 70 mg

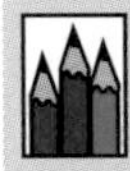

Dosing Tips
- 10–12 hour duration of clinical action
- Capsules can either be taken whole or they can be opened and the contents dissolved in water
- When taken in water, the entire solution should be consumed immediately
- Dose of a single capsule should not be divided

* Once daily dosing can be an important practical element in stimulant utilization, eliminating the hassle and pragmatic difficulties of lunchtime dosing at school, including storage problems, potential diversion, and the need for a medical professional to supervise dosing away from home
- Avoid dosing after the morning because of the risk of insomnia

✻ May be possible to dose only during the school week for some ADHD patients

✻ May be able to give drug holidays over the summer in order to reassess therapeutic utility and effects on growth

suppression as well as to assess any other side effects and the need to reinstitute stimulant treatment for the next school term
- Can be taken with or without food

Overdose
- Rarely fatal; panic, hyperreflexia, rhabdomyolysis, rapid respiration, confusion, coma, hallucination, convulsion, arrhythmia, change in blood pressure, circulatory collapse

Long Term Use
- Can be used long-term for ADHD when ongoing monitoring documents continued efficacy
- Dependence and/or abuse may develop
- Tolerance to therapeutic effects may develop in some patients
- Long-term stimulant use may be associated with growth suppression in children (controversial)
- Periodic monitoring of weight, blood pressure, CBC, platelet counts, and liver function may be prudent

Habit Forming
- Schedule II drug
- Patients may develop tolerance, psychological dependence
- Theoretically less abuse potential than other stimulants when taken as directed because it is inactive until it reaches the gut and thus has delayed time to onset as well as long duration of action

How to Stop
- Taper to avoid withdrawal effects
- Withdrawal following chronic therapeutic use may unmask symptoms of the underlying disorder and may require follow-up and reinstitution of treatment
- Careful supervision is required during withdrawal from abuse use since severe depression may occur

Pharmacokinetics
- 1 hour to maximum concentration of lisdexamfetamine, 3.5 hours to maximum concentration of dextroamphetamine
- Duration of clinical action 10–12 hours

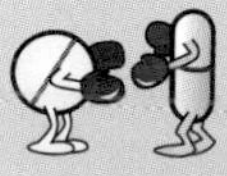

Drug Interactions
- May affect blood pressure and should be used cautiously with agents used to control blood pressure
- Gastrointestinal acidifying agents (guanethidine, reserpine, glutamic acid, ascorbic acid, fruit juices, etc.) and urinary acidifying agents (ammonium chloride, sodium phosphate, etc.) lower amphetamine plasma levels, so such agents can be useful to administer after an overdose but may also lower therapeutic efficacy of amphetamines
- Gastrointestinal alkalinizing agents (sodium bicarbonate, etc.) and urinary alkalinizing agents (acetazolamide, some thiazides) increase amphetamine plasma levels and potentiate amphetamine's actions
- Desipramine and protryptiline can cause striking and sustained increases in brain concentrations of d-amphetamine and may also add to d-amphetamine's cardiovascular effects
- Theoretically, other agents with norepinephrine reuptake blocking properties, such as venlafaxine, duloxetine, atomoxetine, milnacipran, and reboxetine, could also add to amphetamine's CNS and cardiovascular effects
- Amphetamines may counteract the sedative effects of antihistamines
- Haloperidol, chlorpromazine, and lithium may inhibit stimulatory effects of amphetamine
- Theoretically, atypical antipsychotics should also inhibit stimulatory effects of amphetamines
- Theoretically, amphetamines could inhibit the antipsychotic actions of antipsychotics
- Theoretically, amphetamines could inhibit the mood-stabilizing actions of atypical antipsychotics in some patients
- Combinations of amphetamines with mood stabilizers (lithium, anticonvulsants, atypical antipsychotics) is generally something for experts only, when monitoring patients closely and when other options fail
- Absorption of amphetamines is delayed by phenobarbital, phenytoin, ethosuximide
- Amphetamines inhibit adrenergic blockers and enhance adrenergic effects of norepinephrine

- Amphetamines may antagonize hypotensive effects of Veratrum alkaloids and other antihypertensives
- Amphetamines increase the analgesic effects of meperidine
- Amphetamines contribute to excessive CNS stimulation if used with large doses of propoxyphene
- Amphetamines can raise plasma corticosteroid levels
- MAOIs slow absorption of amphetamines and thus potentiate their actions, which can cause headache, hypertension, and rarely hypertensive crisis and malignant hyperthermia, sometimes with fatal results
- Use with MAOIs, including within 14 days of MAOI use, is not advised, but this can sometimes be considered by experts who monitor depressed patients closely when other treatment options for depression fail

Other Warnings/ Precautions

- Use with caution in patients with any degree of hypertension, hyperthyroidism, or history of drug abuse
- Children who are not growing or gaining weight should stop treatment, at least temporarily
- May worsen motor and phonic tics
- May worsen symptoms of thought disorder and behavior disturbance in psychotic patients
- Stimulants have a high potential for abuse and must be used with caution in anyone with a current or past history of substance abuse or alcoholism or in emotionally unstable patients
- Administration of stimulants for prolonged periods of time should be avoided whenever possible or done only with close monitoring, as it may lead to marked tolerance and drug dependence, including psychological dependence with varying degrees of abnormal behavior
- Particular attention should be paid to the possibility of subjects obtaining stimulants for nontherapeutic use or distribution to others and the drugs should in general be prescribed sparingly with documentation of appropriate use
- Unusual dosing has been associated with sudden death in children with structural cardiac abnormalities
- Not an appropriate first-line treatment for depression or for normal fatigue
- May lower the seizure threshold
- Emergence or worsening of activation and agitation may represent the induction of a bipolar state, especially a mixed dysphoric bipolar II condition sometimes associated with suicidal ideation, and require the addition of a mood stabilizer and/or discontinuation of lisdexamfetamine

Do Not Use

- If patient has extreme anxiety or agitation
- If patient has motor tics or Tourette's syndrome or if there is a family history of Tourette's, unless administered by an expert in cases when the potential benefits for ADHD outweigh the risks of worsening tics
- Should generally not be administered with an MAOI, including within 14 days of MAOI use, except in heroic circumstances and by an expert
- If patient has arteriosclerosis, cardiovascular disease, or severe hypertension
- If patient has glaucoma
- If patient has structural cardiac abnormalities
- If patient has hyperthyroidism
- If there is a proven allergy to any sympathomimetic agent

SPECIAL POPULATIONS

Renal Impairment

- No dose adjustment necessary

Hepatic Impairment

- Use with caution

Cardiac Impairment

- Use with caution, particularly in patients with recent myocardial infarction or other conditions that could be negatively affected by increased blood pressure
- Do not use in patients with structural cardiac abnormalities

Elderly

- Some patients may tolerate lower doses better

Children and Adolescents

- Safety and efficacy not established in children under age 6
- Use in young children should be reserved for the expert
- d-amphetamine may worsen symptoms of behavioral disturbance and thought disorder in psychotic children
- d-amphetamine has acute effects on growth hormone; long-term effects are unknown but weight and height should be monitored during long-term treatment
- American Heart Association recommends EKG prior to initiating stimulant treatment in children, although not all experts agree

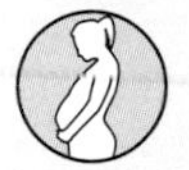

Pregnancy

- Risk Category C [some animal studies show adverse effects; no controlled studies in humans]
- There is a greater risk of premature birth and low birth weight in infants whose mothers take d-amphetamine during pregnancy
- Infants whose mothers take d-amphetamine during pregnancy may experience withdrawal symptoms
- Use in women of childbearing potential requires weighing potential benefits to the mother against potential risks to the fetus

* For ADHD patients, lisdexamfetamine should generally be discontinued before anticipated pregnancies

Breast Feeding

- Some drug is found in mother's breast milk

* Recommended either to discontinue drug or bottle feed

- If infant shows signs of irritability, drug may need to be discontinued

THE ART OF PSYCHOPHARMACOLOGY

Potential Advantages

- Although restricted as a Schedule II controlled substance like other stimulants, as a prodrug lisdexamfetamine may have less propensity for abuse, intoxication, or dependence than other stimulants
- May be particularly useful in adult patients without prior diagnosis and treatment of ADHD as a child to prevent abuse and diversion since lisdexamfetamine may be less abusable than other stimulants

Potential Disadvantages

- Patients with current or past substance abuse
- Patients with current or past bipolar disorder or psychosis

Primary Target Symptoms

- Concentration, attention span
- Motor hyperactivity
- Impulsiveness
- Physical and mental fatigue
- Daytime sleepiness
- Depression

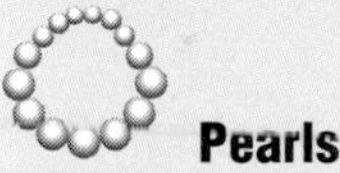

Pearls

- May be useful for treatment of depressive symptoms in medically ill elderly patients
- May be useful for treatment of post-stroke depression
- A classical augmentation strategy for treatment-refractory depression
- Specifically, may be useful for treatment of cognitive dysfunction and fatigue as residual symptoms of major depressive disorder unresponsive to multiple prior treatments
- May also be useful for the treatment of cognitive impairment, depressive symptoms, and severe fatigue in patients with HIV infection and in cancer patients
- Can be used to potentiate opioid analgesia and reduce sedation, particularly in end-of-life management
- Some patients respond to or tolerate lisdexamfetamine better than methylphenidate or amphetamine and vice versa

* Despite warnings, can be a useful adjunct to MAOIs for heroic treatment of highly refractory mood disorders when monitored with vigilance

* Can reverse sexual dysfunction caused by psychiatric illness and by some drugs such as SSRIs, including decreased libido, erectile dysfunction, delayed ejaculation, and anorgasmia

- Atypical antipsychotics may be useful in treating stimulant or psychotic consequences of overdose

- Half-life and duration of clinical action tend to be shorter in younger children
- Drug abuse may actually be lower in ADHD adolescents treated with stimulants than in ADHD adolescents who are not treated

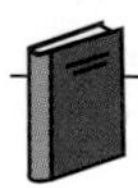

Suggested Reading

Biederman J, Boellner SW, Childress A, et al. Lisdexamfetamine dimesylate and mixed amphetamine salts extended-release in children with ADHD: a double-blind, placebo-controlled, crossover analog classroom study. Biol Psychiatry 2007;62(9):970-6.

Biederman J, Krishnan S, Zhang Y, McGough JJ, Findling RL. Efficacy and tolerability of lisdexamfetamine dimesylate (NRP-104) in children with attention-deficit/hyperactivity disorder: a phase III, multicenter, randomized, double-blind, forced-dose, parallel-group study. Clin Ther 2007;29(3):450-63.

THERAPEUTICS

Brands
- Eskalith
- Eskalith CR
- Lithobid slow-release tablets
- Lithostat tablets
- Lithium carbonate tablets
- Lithium citrate syrup

see index for additional brand names

Generic? Yes

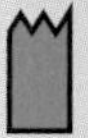

Class
- Mood stabilizer

Commonly Prescribed for
(bold for FDA approved)
- **Manic episodes of manic-depressive illness**
- **Maintenance treatment for manic-depressive patients with a history of mania**
- Bipolar depression
- Major depressive disorder (adjunctive)
- Vascular headache
- Neutropenia

How the Drug Works
- Unknown and complex
- Alters sodium transport across cell membranes in nerve and muscle cells
- Alters metabolism of neurotransmitters including catecholamines and serotonin
- ✻ May alter intracellular signaling through actions on second messenger systems
- Specifically, inhibits inositol monophosphatase, possibly affecting neurotransmission via phosphatidyl inositol second messenger system
- Also reduces protein kinase C activity, possibly affecting genomic expression associated with neurotransmission
- Increases cytoprotective proteins, activates signaling cascade utilized by endogenous growth factors, and increases gray matter content, possibly by activating neurogenesis and enhancing trophic actions that maintain synapses

How Long Until It Works
- 1–3 weeks

If It Works
- The goal of treatment is complete remission of symptoms (i.e., mania and/or depression)
- Continue treatment until all symptoms are gone or until improvement is stable and then continue treating indefinitely as long as improvement persists
- Continue treatment indefinitely to avoid recurrence of mania or depression

If It Doesn't Work
- ✻ Many patients have only a partial response where some symptoms are improved but others persist or continue to wax and wane without stabilization of mood
- Other patients may be nonresponders, sometimes called treatment-resistant or treatment-refractory
- Consider checking plasma drug level, increasing dose, switching to another agent, or adding an appropriate augmenting agent
- Consider adding psychotherapy
- Consider the presence of noncompliance and counsel patient
- Switch to another mood stabilizer with fewer side effects
- Consider evaluation for another diagnosis or for a comorbid condition (e.g., medical illness, substance abuse, etc.)

Best Augmenting Combos for Partial Response or Treatment Resistance
- Valproate
- Atypical antipsychotics (especially risperidone, olanzapine, quetiapine, ziprasidone, and aripiprazole)
- Lamotrigine
- ✻ Antidepressants (with caution because antidepressants can destabilize mood in some patients, including induction of rapid cycling or suicidal ideation; in particular consider bupropion; also SSRIs, SNRIs, others; generally avoid TCAs, MAOIs)

Tests
- ✻ Before initiating treatment, kidney function tests (including creatinine and urine specific gravity) and thyroid function tests; electrocardiogram for patients over 50
- Repeat kidney function tests 1–2 times/year

✽ Frequent tests to monitor trough lithium plasma levels (should generally be between 1.0 and 1.5 mEq/L for acute treatment, 0.6 and 1.2 mEq/L for chronic treatment)
✽ Since lithium is frequently associated with weight gain, before starting treatment, weigh all patients and determine if the patient is already overweight (BMI 25.0–29.9) or obese (BMI ≥30)
- Before giving a drug that can cause weight gain to an overweight or obese patient, consider determining whether the patient already has pre-diabetes (fasting plasma glucose 100–25 mg/dL), diabetes (fasting plasma glucose >126 mg/dL), or dyslipidemia (increased total cholesterol, LDL cholesterol and triglycerides; decreased HDL cholesterol), and treat or refer such patients for treatment, including nutrition and weight management, physical activity counseling, smoking cessation, and medical management

✽ Monitor weight and BMI during treatment
✽ While giving a drug to a patient who has gained >5% of initial weight, consider evaluating for the presence of pre-diabetes, diabetes, or dyslipidemia, or consider switching to a different agent

SIDE EFFECTS

How Drug Causes Side Effects

- Unknown and complex
- CNS side effects theoretically due to excessive actions at the same or similar sites that mediate its therapeutic actions
- Some renal side effects theoretically due to lithium's actions on ion transport

Notable Side Effects

✽ Ataxia, dysarthria, delirium, tremor, memory problems
✽ Polyuria, polydipsia (nephrogenic diabetes insipidus)
✽ Diarrhea, nausea
✽ Weight gain
- Euthyroid goiter or hypothyroid goiter, possibly with increased TSH and reduced thyroxine levels
- Acne, rash, alopecia
- Leukocytosis
- Side effects are typically dose-related

Life-Threatening or Dangerous Side Effects

- Lithium toxicity
- Renal impairment (interstitial nephritis)
- Nephrogenic diabetes insipidus
- Arrhythmia, cardiovascular changes, sick sinus syndrome, bradycardia, hypotension
- T wave flattening and inversion
- Rare pseudotumor cerebri
- Rare seizures

Weight Gain

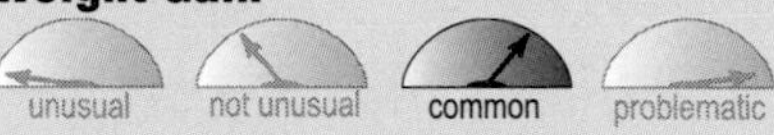

- Many experience and/or can be significant in amount
- Can become a health problem in some
- May be associated with increased appetite

Sedation

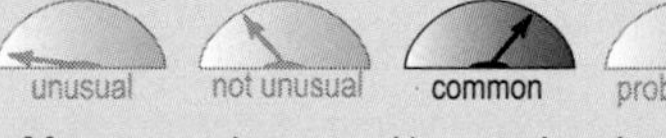

- Many experience and/or can be significant in amount
- May wear off with time

What To Do About Side Effects

- Wait
- Wait
- Wait
- Lower the dose

✽ Take entire dose at night as long as efficacy persists all day long with this administration
✽ Change to a different lithium preparation (e.g., controlled-release)
✽ Reduce dosing from 3 times/day to 2 times/day
- If signs of lithium toxicity occur, discontinue immediately
- For stomach upset, take with food
- For tremor, avoid caffeine
- Switch to another agent

Best Augmenting Agents for Side Effects

✽ Propranolol 20–30 mg 2–3 times/day may reduce tremor
- For the expert, cautious addition of a diuretic (e.g., chlorothiazide 50 mg/day) while reducing lithium dose by 50% and monitoring plasma lithium levels may

reduce polydipsia and polyuria that does not go away with time alone
- Many side effects cannot be improved with an augmenting agent

DOSING AND USE

Usual Dosage Range
- 1,800 mg/day in divided doses (acute)
- 900–1,200 mg/day in divided doses (maintenance)
- Liquid: 10 mL three times/day (acute mania); 5 mL 3–4 times/day (long-term)

Dosage Forms
- Tablet 300 mg (slow-release), 450 mg (controlled-release)
- Capsule 150 mg, 300 mg, 600 mg
- Liquid 8 mEq/5 mL

How To Dose
- Start 300 mg 2–3 times/day and adjust dosage upward as indicated by plasma lithium levels

Dosing Tips
✻ Sustained-release formulation may reduce gastric irritation, lower peak lithium plasma levels, and diminish peak dose side effects (i.e., side effects occurring 1–2 hours after each dose of standard lithium carbonate may be improved by sustained-release formulation)
- Lithium sulfate and other dosage strengths for lithium are available in Europe
- Check therapeutic blood levels as "trough" levels about 12 hours after the last dose
- After stabilization, some patients may do best with a once daily dose at night
- Responses in acute mania may take 7–14 days even with adequate plasma lithium levels

✻ Some patients apparently respond to doses as low as 300 mg twice a day, even with plasma lithium levels below 0.5 mEq/L
- Use the lowest dose of lithium associated with adequate therapeutic response
- Lower doses and lower plasma lithium levels (<0.6 mEq/L) are often adequate and advisable in the elderly

✻ Rapid discontinuation increases the risk of relapse and possibly suicide, so lithium may need to be tapered slowly over 3 months if it is to be discontinued after long-term maintenance

Overdose
- Fatalities have occurred; tremor, dysarthria, delirium, coma, seizures, autonomic instability

Long-Term Use
- Indicated for long-term prevention of relapse
- May cause reduced kidney function
- Requires regular therapeutic monitoring of lithium levels as well as of kidney function and thyroid function

Habit Forming
- No

How to Stop
- Taper gradually over 3 months to avoid relapse
- Rapid discontinuation increases the risk of relapse, and possibly suicide
- Discontinuation symptoms uncommon

Pharmacokinetics
- Half life 18–30 hours

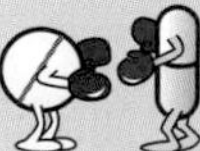

Drug Interactions
✻ Nonsteroidal anti-inflammatory agents, including ibuprofen and selective COX-2 inhibitors (cyclooxygenase 2), can increase plasma lithium concentrations; add with caution to patients stabilized on lithium

✻ Diuretics, especially thiazides, can increase plasma lithium concentrations; add with caution to patients stabilized on lithium
- Angiotensin-converting enzyme inhibitors can increase plasma lithium concentrations; add with caution to patients stabilized on lithium
- Metronidazole can lead to lithium toxicity through decreased renal clearance
- Acetazolamide, alkalizing agents, xanthine preparations, and urea may lower lithium plasma concentrations
- Methyldopa, carbamazepine, and phenytoin may interact with lithium to increase its toxicity

- Use lithium cautiously with calcium channel blockers, which may also increase lithium toxicity
- Use of lithium with an SSRI may raise risk of dizziness, confusion, diarrhea, agitation, tremor
- Some patients taking haloperidol and lithium have developed an encephalopathic syndrome similar to neuroleptic malignant syndrome
- Lithium may prolong effects of neuromuscular blocking agents
- No likely pharmacokinetic interactions of lithium with mood-stabilizing anticonvulsants or atypical antipsychotics

Other Warnings/ Precautions

* Toxic levels are near therapeutic levels; signs of toxicity include tremor, ataxia, diarrhea, vomiting, sedation
- Monitor for dehydration; lower dose if patient exhibits signs of infection, excessive sweating, diarrhea
- Closely monitor patients with thyroid disorders

Do Not Use

- If patient has severe kidney disease
- If patient has severe cardiovascular disease
- If patient has severe dehydration
- If patient has sodium depletion
- If there is a proven allergy to lithium

SPECIAL POPULATIONS

Renal Impairment

- Not recommended for use in patients with severe impairment

Hepatic Impairment

- No special indications

Cardiac Impairment

- Not recommended for use in patients with severe impairment

Elderly

- Likely that elderly patients will require lower doses to achieve therapeutic serum levels
- Elderly patients may be more sensitive to adverse effects

* Neurotoxicity, including delirium and other mental status changes, may occur even at therapeutic doses in elderly and organically compromised patients
- Lower doses and lower plasma lithium levels (<0.6 mEg/L) are often adequate and advisable in the elderly

Children and Adolescents

- Safety and efficacy not established in children under age 12
- Use only with caution
- Younger children tend to have more frequent and severe side effects
- Children should be monitored more frequently

Pregnancy

- Risk Category D [positive evidence of risk to human fetus; potential benefits may still justify its use during pregnancy]

* Evidence of increased risk of major birth defects (perhaps 2–3 times the general population), but probably lower than with some other mood stabilizers (e.g., valproate)
- Evidence of increase in cardiac anomalies (especially Ebstein's anomaly) in infants whose mothers took lithium during pregnancy
- Lithium administration during delivery may be associated with hypotonia in the infant
- Use in women of childbearing potential requires weighing potential benefits to the mother against the risks to the fetus
- Taper drug if discontinuing

* For bipolar patients, lithium should generally be discontinued before anticipated pregnancies
- Recurrent bipolar illness during pregnancy can be quite disruptive

* For bipolar patients, given the risk of relapse in the postpartum period, lithium should generally be restarted immediately after delivery, but this generally means no breast feeding
* Atypical antipsychotics may be preferable to lithium or anticonvulsants if treatment of bipolar disorder is required during pregnancy

- Bipolar symptoms may recur or worsen during pregnancy and some form of treatment may be necessary

Breast Feeding

- Some drug is found in mother's breast milk, possibly at full therapeutic levels since lithium is soluble in breast milk
- ✽ Recommended either to discontinue drug or bottle feed
- ✽ Bipolar disorder may recur during the postpartum period, particularly if there is a history of prior postpartum episodes of either depression or psychosis
- ✽ Relapse rates may be lower in women who receive prophylactic treatment for postpartum episodes of bipolar disorder
- Atypical antipsychotics and anticonvulsants such as valproate may be safer than lithium during the postpartum period when breast feeding

THE ART OF PSYCHOPHARMACOLOGY

Potential Advantages

- Euphoric mania
- Treatment-resistant depression
- Reduces suicide risk
- Works well in combination with atypical antipsychotics and/or mood-stabilizing anticonvulsants such as valproate

Potential Disadvantages

- Dysphoric mania
- Mixed mania, rapid-cycling mania
- Depressed phase of bipolar disorder
- Patients unable to tolerate weight gain, sedation, gastrointestinal effects, renal effects, and other side effects
- Requires blood monitoring

Primary Target Symptoms

- Unstable mood
- Mania

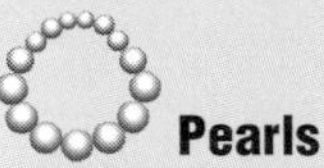

Pearls

- ✽ Lithium was the original mood stabilizer and is still a first-line treatment option but may be underutilized since it is an older agent and is less promoted for use in bipolar disorder than newer agents
- ✽ May be best for euphoric mania; patients with rapid-cycling and mixed state types of bipolar disorder generally do less well on lithium
- ✽ Seems to be more effective in treating manic episodes than depressive episodes in bipolar disorder (treats from above better than it treats from below)
- ✽ May also be more effective in preventing manic relapses than in preventing depressive episodes (stabilizes from above better than it stabilizes from below)
- ✽ May decrease suicide and suicide attempts not only in bipolar I disorder but also in bipolar II disorder and in unipolar depression
- ✽ Due to its narrow therapeutic index, lithium's toxic side effects occur at doses close to its therapeutic effects
- Close therapeutic monitoring of plasma drug levels is required during lithium treatment; lithium is the first psychiatric drug that required blood level monitoring
- Probably less effective than atypical antipsychotics for severe, excited, disturbed, hyperactive, or psychotic patients with mania
- Due to delayed onset of action, lithium monotherapy may not be the first choice in acute mania, but rather may be used as an adjunct to atypical antipsychotics, benzodiazepines, and/or valproate loading
- After acute symptoms of mania are controlled, some patients can be maintained on lithium monotherapy
- However, only a third of bipolar patients experience adequate relief with a monotherapy, so most patients need multiple medications for best control
- Lithium is not a convincing augmentation agent to atypical antipsychotics for the treatment of schizophrenia
- Lithium is one of the most useful adjunctive agents to augment antidepressants for treatment-resistant unipolar depression
- Lithium may be useful for a number of patients with episodic, recurrent symptoms with or without affective illness, including episodic rage, anger or violence, and self-destructive behavior; such symptoms may be associated with psychotic or nonpsychotic illnesses, personality disorders, organic disorders, or mental retardation

- Lithium is better tolerated during acute manic phases than when manic symptoms have abated
- Adverse effects generally increase in incidence and severity as lithium serum levels increase
- Although not recommended for use in patients with severe renal or cardiovascular disease, dehydration, or sodium depletion, lithium can be administered cautiously in a hospital setting to such patients, with lithium serum levels determined daily
- Lithium-induced weight gain may be more common in women than in men

Suggested Reading

Delva NJ, Hawken ER. Preventing lithium intoxication. Guide for physicians. Can Fam Physician 2001;47:1595–600.

Goodwin FK. Rationale for using lithium in combination with other mood stabilizers in the management of bipolar disorder. J Clin Psychiatry 2003;64(Suppl 5):18–24.

Goodwin GM, Bowden CL, Calabrese JR, et al. A pooled analysis of 2 placebo-controlled 18-month trials of lamotrigine and lithium maintenance treatment in bipolar I disorder. J Clin Psychiatry 2004;65:432–41.

Maj M. The effect of lithium in bipolar disorder: a review of recent research evidence. Bipolar Disord 2003;5:180–8.

Tueth MJ, Murphy TK, Evans DL. Special considerations: use of lithium in children, adolescents, and elderly populations. J Clin Psychiatry 1998;59 (Suppl 6):66–73.

THERAPEUTICS

Brands
- Deprimyl
- Gamanil

see index for additional brand names

Generic? Yes

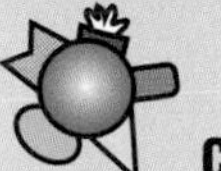

Class
- Tricyclic antidepressant (TCA)
- Predominantly a norepinephrine/noradrenaline reuptake inhibitor

Commonly Prescribed for
(bold for FDA approved)
- Major depressive disorder
- Anxiety
- Insomnia
- Neuropathic pain/chronic pain
- Treatment-resistant depression

How the Drug Works
- Boosts neurotransmitter norepinephrine/noradrenaline
- Blocks norepinephrine reuptake pump (norepinephrine transporter), presumably increasing noradrenergic neurotransmission
- Since dopamine is inactivated by norepinephrine reuptake in frontal cortex, which largely lacks dopamine transporters, lofepramine can increase dopamine neurotransmission in this part of the brain
- A more potent inhibitor of norepinephrine reuptake pump than serotonin reuptake pump (serotonin transporter)
- At high doses may also boost neurotransmitter serotonin and presumably increase serotonergic neurotransmission

How Long Until It Works
- May have immediate effects in treating insomnia or anxiety
- Onset of therapeutic actions usually not immediate, but often delayed 2–4 weeks
- If it is not working within 6–8 weeks for depression, it may require a dosage increase or it may not work at all
- May continue to work for many years to prevent relapse of symptoms

If It Works
- The goal of treatment of depression is complete remission of current symptoms as well as prevention of future relapses
- The goal of treatment of chronic neuropathic pain is to reduce symptoms as much as possible, especially in combination with other treatments
- Treatment of depression most often reduces or even eliminates symptoms, but not a cure since symptoms can recur after medicine stopped
- Treatment of chronic neuropathic pain may reduce symptoms, but rarely eliminates them completely, and is not a cure since symptoms can recur after medicine is stopped
- Continue treatment of depression until all symptoms are gone (remission)
- Once symptoms of depression are gone, continue treating for 1 year for the first episode of depression
- For second and subsequent episodes of depression, treatment may need to be indefinite
- Use in anxiety disorders and chronic pain may also need to be indefinite, but long-term treatment is not well studied in these conditions

If It Doesn't Work
- Many depressed patients only have a partial response where some symptoms are improved but others persist (especially insomnia, fatigue, and problems concentrating)
- Other depressed patients may be nonresponders, sometimes called treatment-resistant or treatment-refractory
- Consider increasing dose, switching to another agent or adding an appropriate augmenting agent
- Consider psychotherapy
- Consider evaluation for another diagnosis or for a comorbid condition (e.g, medical illness, substance abuse, etc.)
- Some patients may experience apparent lack of consistent efficacy due to activation of latent or underlying bipolar disorder, and require antidepressant discontinuation and a switch to a mood stabilizer

Best Augmenting Combos for Partial Response or Treatment Resistance

- Lithium, buspirone, thyroid hormone (for depression)
- Gabapentin, tiagabine, other anticonvulsants, even opiates if done by experts while monitoring carefully in difficult cases (for chronic pain)

Tests

- None for healthy individuals
- ✻ Since tricyclic and tetracyclic antidepressants are frequently associated with weight gain, before starting treatment, weigh all patients and determine if the patient is already overweight (BMI 25.0–29.9) or obese (BMI ≥30)
- Before giving a drug that can cause weight gain to an overweight or obese patient, consider determining whether the patient already has pre-diabetes (fasting plasma glucose 100–25 mg/dL), diabetes (fasting plasma glucose >126 mg/dL), or dyslipidemia (increased total cholesterol, LDL cholesterol and triglycerides; decreased HDL cholesterol), and treat or refer such patients for treatment, including nutrition and weight management, physical activity counseling, smoking cessation, and medical management
- ✻ Monitor weight and BMI during treatment
- ✻ While giving a drug to a patient who has gained >5% of initial weight, consider evaluating for the presence of pre-diabetes, diabetes, or dyslipidemia, or consider switching to a different antidepressant
- EKGs may be useful for selected patients (e.g., those with personal or family history of QTc prolongation; cardiac arrhythmia; recent myocardial infarction; uncompensated heart failure; or taking agents that prolong QTc interval such as pimozide, thioridazine, selected antiarrhythmics, moxifloxacin, sparfloxacin, etc.)
- Patients at risk for electrolyte disturbances (e.g., patients on diuretic therapy) should have baseline and periodic serum potassium and magnesium measurements

SIDE EFFECTS

How Drug Causes Side Effects

- Anticholinergic activity may explain sedative effects, dry mouth, constipation, and blurred vision
- Sedative effects and weight gain may be due to antihistamine properties
- Blockade of alpha adrenergic 1 receptors may explain dizziness, sedation, and hypotension
- Cardiac arrhythmias and seizures, especially in overdose, may be caused by blockade of ion channels

Notable Side Effects

- Blurred vision, constipation, urinary retention, increased appetite, dry mouth, nausea, diarrhea, heartburn, unusual taste in mouth, weight gain
- Fatigue, weakness, dizziness, sedation, headache, anxiety, nervousness, restlessness
- Sexual dysfunction, sweating

Life-Threatening or Dangerous Side Effects

- Paralytic ileus, hyperthermia (TCAs + anticholinergic agents)
- Lowered seizure threshold and rare seizures
- Orthostatic hypotension, sudden death, arrhythmias, tachycardia
- QTc prolongation
- Hepatic failure, extrapyramidal symptoms
- Increased intraocular pressure
- Rare induction of mania
- Rare activation of suicidal ideation and behavior (suicidality) (short-term studies did not show an increase in the risk of suicidality with antidepressants compared to placebo beyond age 24)

Weight Gain

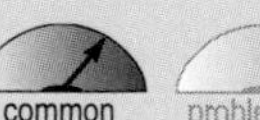

- Many experience and/or can be significant in amount
- Can increase appetite and carbohydrate craving

Sedation

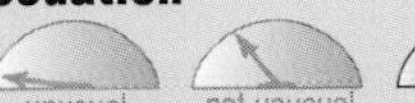

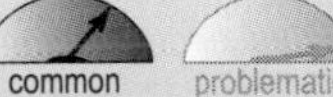

- Many experience and/or can be significant in amount
- Tolerance to sedative effect may develop with long-term use

What To Do About Side Effects

- Wait
- Wait
- Wait
- Lower the dose
- Switch to an SSRI or newer antidepressant

Best Augmenting Agents for Side Effects

- Many side effects cannot be improved with an augmenting agent

DOSING AND USE

Usual Dosage Range

- 140–210 mg/day

Dosage Forms

- Tablet 70 mg multiscored
- Liquid 70 mg/5mL

How To Dose

- Initial 70 mg/day once daily or in divided doses; gradually increase daily dose to achieve desired therapeutic effects; dose at bedtime for daytime sedation and in morning for insomnia; maximum dose 280 mg/day for inpatients, 210 mg/day for outpatients

Dosing Tips

- If given in a single dose, should generally be administered at bedtime because of its sedative properties
- If given in split doses, largest dose should generally be given at bedtime because of its sedative properties
- If patients experience nightmares, split dose and do not give large dose at bedtime
- Unusual dose compared to most TCAs
- Patients treated for chronic pain may only require lower doses
- If intolerable anxiety, insomnia, agitation, akathisia, or activation occur either upon dosing initiation or discontinuation, consider the possibility of activated bipolar disorder, and switch to a mood stabilizer or an atypical antipsychotic

Overdose

- Death may occur; convulsions, cardiac dysrhythmias, severe hypotension, CNS depression, coma, changes in EKG

Long-Term Use

- Safe

Habit Forming

- No

How to Stop

- Taper to avoid withdrawal effects
- Even with gradual dose reduction some withdrawal symptoms may appear within the first 2 weeks
- Many patients tolerate 50% dose reduction for 3 days, then another 50% reduction for 3 days, then discontinuation
- If withdrawal symptoms emerge during discontinuation, raise dose to stop symptoms and then restart withdrawal much more slowly

Pharmacokinetics

- Substrate for CYP450 2D6
- Half-life of parent compound approximately 1.5–6 hours

* Major metabolite is the antidepressant desipramine, with a half-life of approximately 24 hours

Drug Interactions

- Tramadol increases the risk of seizures in patients taking TCAs
- Use of TCAs with anticholinergic drugs may result in paralytic ileus or hyperthermia
- Fluoxetine, paroxetine, bupropion, duloxetine, and other CYP450 2D6 inhibitors may increase TCA concentrations
- Cimetidine may increase plasma concentrations of TCAs and cause anticholinergic symptoms
- Phenothiazines or haloperidol may raise TCA blood concentrations

- May alter effects of antihypertensive drugs; may inhibit hypotensive effects of clonidine
- Use with sympathomimetic agents may increase sympathetic activity
- Methylphenidate may inhibit metabolism of TCAs
- Activation and agitation, especially following switching or adding antidepressants, may represent the induction of a bipolar state, especially a mixed dysphoric bipolar II condition sometimes associated with suicidal ideation, and require the addition of lithium, a mood stabilizer or an atypical antipsychotic, and/or discontinuation of lofepramine

Other Warnings/ Precautions

- Add or initiate other antidepressants with caution for up to 2 weeks after discontinuing lofepramine
- Generally, do not use with MAO inhibitors, including 14 days after MAOIs are stopped; do not start an MAOI until 2 weeks after discontinuing lofepramine, but see Pearls
- Use with caution in patients with history of seizure, urinary retention, narrow angle-closure glaucoma, hyperthyroidism
- TCAs can increase QTc interval, especially at toxic doses, which can be attained not only by overdose but also by combining with drugs that inhibit its metabolism via CYP450 2D6, potentially causing torsade de pointes-type arrhythmia or sudden death
- Because TCAs can prolong QTc interval, use with caution in patients who have bradycardia or who are taking drugs that can induce bradycardia (e.g., beta blockers, calcium channel blockers, clonidine, digitalis)
- Because TCAs can prolong QTc interval, use with caution in patients who have hypokalemia and/or hypomagnesemia or who are taking drugs that can induce hypokalemia and/or magnesemia (e.g., diuretics, stimulant laxatives, intravenous amphotericin B, glucocorticoids, tetracosactide)
- When treating children, carefully weigh the risks and benefits of pharmacological treatment against the risks and benefits of nontreatment with antidepressants and make sure to document this in the patient's chart
- Distribute the brochures provided by the FDA and the drug companies
- Warn patients and their caregivers about the possibility of activating side effects and advise them to report such symptoms immediately
- Monitor patients for activation of suicidal ideation, especially children and adolescents

Do Not Use

- If patient is recovering from myocardial infarction
- If patient is taking agents capable of significantly prolonging QTc interval (e.g., pimozide, thioridazine, selected antiarrhythmics, moxifloxacin, sparfloxacin)
- If there is a history of QTc prolongation or cardiac arrhythmia, recent acute myocardial infarction, uncompensated heart failure
- If patient is taking drugs that inhibit TCA metabolism, including CYP450 2D6 inhibitors, except by an expert
- If there is reduced CYP450 2D6 function, such as patients who are poor 2D6 metabolizers, except by an expert and at low doses
- If there is a proven allergy to lofepramine, desipramine, or imipramine

SPECIAL POPULATIONS

Renal Impairment

- Use with caution

Hepatic Impairment

- Use with caution

Cardiac Impairment

- TCAs have been reported to cause arrhythmias, prolongation of conduction time, orthostatic hypotension, sinus tachycardia, and heart failure, especially in the diseased heart
- Myocardial infarction and stroke have been reported with TCAs
- TCAs produce QTc prolongation, which may be enhanced by the existence of bradycardia, hypokalemia, congenital or acquired long QTc interval, which should

be evaluated prior to administering lofepramine
- Use with caution if treating concomitantly with a medication likely to produce prolonged bradycardia, hypokalemia, slowing of intracardiac conduction, or prolongation of the QTc interval
- Avoid TCAs in patients with a known history of QTc prolongation, recent acute myocardial infarction, and uncompensated heart failure
- TCAs may cause a sustained increase in heart rate in patients with ischemic heart disease and may worsen (decrease) heart rate variability, an independent risk of mortality in cardiac populations
- Since SSRIs may improve (increase) heart rate variability in patients following a myocardial infarct and may improve survival as well as mood in patients with acute angina or following a myocardial infarction, these are more appropriate agents for cardiac population than tricyclic/tetracyclic antidepressants

❋ Risk/benefit ratio may not justify use of TCAs in cardiac impairment

Elderly

- May be more sensitive to anticholinergic, cardiovascular, hypotensive, and sedative effects
- Reduction in risk of suicidality with antidepressants compared to placebo in adults age 65 and older

Children and Adolescents

- Carefully weigh the risks and benefits of pharmacological treatment against the risks and benefits of nontreatment with antidepressants and make sure to document this in the patient's chart
- Monitor patients face-to-face regularly, particularly during the first several weeks of treatment
- Use with caution, observing for activation of known or unknown bipolar disorder and/or suicidal ideation, and inform parents or guardian of this risk so they can help observe child or adolescent patients
- Not recommended for use under age 18
- Several studies show lack of efficacy of TCAs for depression
- May be used to treat enuresis or hyperactive/impulsive behaviors
- Some cases of sudden death have occurred in children taking TCAs

Pregnancy

- Risk Category C [some animal studies show adverse effects; no controlled studies in humans]
- Crosses the placenta
- Adverse effects have been reported in infants whose mothers took a TCA (lethargy, withdrawal symptoms, fetal malformations)
- Not generally recommended for use during pregnancy, especially during first trimester
- Must weigh the risk of treatment (first trimester fetal development, third trimester newborn delivery) to the child against the risk of no treatment (recurrence of depression, maternal health, infant bonding) to the mother and child
- For many patients this may mean continuing treatment during pregnancy

Breast Feeding

- Some drug is found in mother's breast milk

❋ Recommended either to discontinue drug or bottle feed

- Immediate postpartum period is a high-risk time for depression, especially in women who have had prior depressive episodes, so drug may need to be reinstituted late in the third trimester or shortly after childbirth to prevent a recurrence during the postpartum period
- Must weigh benefits of breast feeding with risks and benefits of antidepressant treatment versus nontreatment to both the infant and the mother
- For many patients this may mean continuing treatment during breast feeding

THE ART OF PSYCHOPHARMACOLOGY

Potential Advantages

- Patients with insomnia
- Severe or treatment-resistant depression
- Anxious depression

Potential Disadvantages

- Pediatric and geriatric patients

- Patients concerned with weight gain
- Cardiac patients

Primary Target Symptoms

- Depressed mood

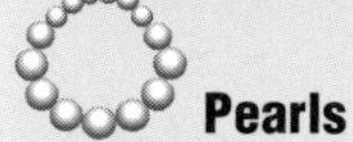

Pearls

- Tricyclic antidepressants are often a first-line treatment option for chronic pain
- Tricyclic antidepressants are no longer generally considered a first-line option for depression because of their side effect profile
- Tricyclic antidepressants continue to be useful for severe or treatment-resistant depression
- Noradrenergic reuptake inhibitors such as lofepramine can be used as a second-line treatment for smoking cessation, cocaine dependence, and attention deficit disorder

✻ Lofepramine is a short-acting prodrug of the TCA desipramine

✻ Fewer anticholinergic side effects, particularly sedation, than some other tricyclics

- Once a popular TCA in the U.K., but not widely marketed throughout the world
- TCAs may aggravate psychotic symptoms
- Alcohol should be avoided because of additive CNS effects
- Underweight patients may be more susceptible to adverse cardiovascular effects
- Children, patients with inadequate hydration, and patients with cardiac disease may be more susceptible to TCA-induced cardiotoxicity than healthy adults
- For the expert only: although generally prohibited, a heroic treatment (but potentially dangerous) for severely treatment-resistant patients is to give a tricyclic/tetracyclic antidepressant other than clomipramine simultaneously with an MAO inhibitor for patients who fail to respond to numerous other antidepressants
- If this option is elected, start the MAOI with the tricyclic/tetracyclic antidepressant simultaneously at low doses after appropriate drug washout, then alternately increase doses of these agents every few days to a week as tolerated
- Although very strict dietary and concomitant drug restrictions must be observed to prevent hypertensive crises and serotonin syndrome, the most common side effects of MAOI/tricyclic or tetracyclic combinations may be weight gain and orthostatic hypotension
- Patients on TCAs should be aware that they may experience symptoms such as photosensitivity or blue-green urine
- SSRIs may be more effective than TCAs in women, and TCAs may be more effective than SSRIs in men
- Since tricyclic/tetracyclic antidepressants are substrates for CYP450 2D6, and 7% of the population (especially Caucasians) may have a genetic variant leading to reduced activity of 2D6, such patients may not safely tolerate normal doses of tricyclic/tetracyclic antidepressants and may require dose reduction
- Phenotypic testing may be necessary to detect this genetic variant prior to dosing with a tricyclic/tetracyclic antidepressant, especially in vulnerable populations such as children, elderly, cardiac populations, and those on concomitant medications
- Patients who seem to have extraordinarily severe side effects at normal or low doses may have this phenotypic CYP450 2D6 variant and require low doses or switching to another antidepressant not metabolized by 2D6

Suggested Reading

Anderson IM. Meta-analytical studies on new antidepressants. Br Med Bull 2001;57:161–78.

Anderson IM. Selective serotonin reuptake inhibitors versus tricyclic antidepressants: a meta-analysis of efficacy and tolerability. J Aff Disorders 2000;58:19–36.

Kerihuel JC, Dreyfus JF. Meta-analyses of the efficacy and tolerability of the tricyclic antidepressant lofepramine. J Int Med Res 1991;19:183–201.

Lancaster SG, Gonzales JP. Lofepramine. A review of its pharmacodynamic and pharmacokinetic properties, and therapeutic efficacy in depressive illness. Drugs. 1989; 37:123–40.

LOFLAZEPATE

THERAPEUTICS

Brands • Meilax

see index for additional brand names

Generic? No

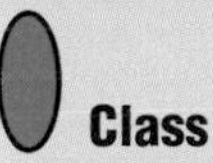

Class

- Benzodiazepine (anxiolytic)

Commonly Prescribed for

(bold for FDA approved)

- Anxiety, tension, depression, or sleep disorder in patients with neurosis
- Anxiety, tension, depression, or sleep disorder in patients with psychosomatic disease

How the Drug Works

- Binds to benzodiazepine receptors at the GABA-A ligand-gated chloride channel complex
- Enhances the inhibitory effects of GABA
- Boosts chloride conductance through GABA-regulated channels
- Inhibits neuronal activity presumably in amygdala-centered fear circuits to provide therapeutic benefits in anxiety disorders

How Long Until It Works

- Some immediate relief with first dosing is common; can take several weeks with daily dosing for maximal therapeutic benefit

If It Works

- For short-term symptoms of anxiety – after a few weeks, discontinue use or use on an "as-needed" basis
- For chronic anxiety disorders, the goal of treatment is complete remission of symptoms as well as prevention of future relapses
- For chronic anxiety disorders, treatment most often reduces or even eliminates symptoms, but not a cure since symptoms can recur after medicine stopped
- For long-term symptoms of anxiety, consider switching to an SSRI or SNRI for long-term maintenance
- If long-term maintenance with a benzodiazepine is necessary, continue treatment for 6 months after symptoms resolve, and then taper dose slowly
- If symptoms reemerge, consider treatment with an SSRI or SNRI, or consider restarting the benzodiazepine; sometimes benzodiazepines have to be used in combination with SSRIs or SNRIs for best results

If It Doesn't Work

- Consider switching to another agent or adding an appropriate augmenting agent
- Consider psychotherapy, especially cognitive behavioral psychotherapy
- Consider presence of concomitant substance abuse
- Consider presence of loflazepate abuse
- Consider another diagnosis, such as a comorbid medical condition

Best Augmenting Combos for Partial Response or Treatment Resistance

- Benzodiazepines are frequently used as augmenting agents for antipsychotics and mood stabilizers in the treatment of psychotic and bipolar disorders
- Benzodiazepines are frequently used as augmenting agents for SSRIs and SNRIs in the treatment of anxiety disorders
- Not generally rational to combine with other benzodiazepines
- Caution if using as an anxiolytic concomitantly with other sedative hypnotics for sleep

Tests

- In patients with seizure disorders, concomitant medical illness, and/or those with multiple concomitant long-term medications, periodic liver tests and blood counts may be prudent

SIDE EFFECTS

How Drug Causes Side Effects

- Same mechanism for side effects as for therapeutic effects – namely due to excessive actions at benzodiazepine receptors
- Long-term adaptations in benzodiazepine receptors may explain the development of dependence, tolerance, and withdrawal
- Side effects are generally immediate, but immediate side effects often disappear in time

Notable Side Effects

- ✻ Sedation, fatigue, depression
- ✻ Dizziness, ataxia, slurred speech, weakness
- ✻ Forgetfulness, confusion
- ✻ Hyperexcitability, nervousness
- Rare hallucinations, mania
- Rare hypotension
- Hypersalivation, dry mouth

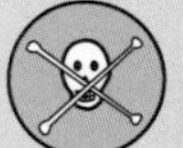

Life-Threatening or Dangerous Side Effects

- Respiratory depression, especially when taken with CNS depressants in overdose
- Rare hepatic dysfunction, renal dysfunction, blood dyscrasias

Weight Gain

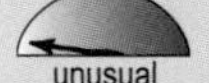

not unusual
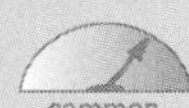

problematic

- Reported but not expected

Sedation

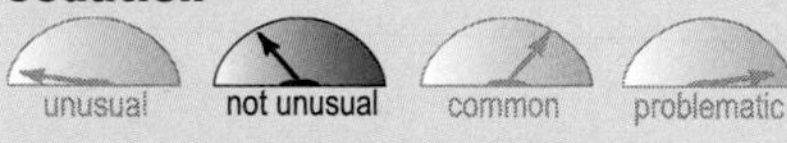

- Occurs in significant minority
- Especially at initiation of treatment or when dose increases
- Tolerance often develops over time

What To Do About Side Effects

- Wait
- Wait
- Wait
- Lower the dose
- Take largest dose at bedtime to avoid sedative effects during the day
- Switch to another agent
- Administer flumazenil if side effects are severe or life-threatening

Best Augmenting Agents for Side Effects

- Many side effects cannot be improved with an augmenting agent

DOSING AND USE

Usual Dosage Range

- 1 mg once or twice a day

Dosage Forms

- Tablet 1 mg, 2 mg

How To Dose

- Start at 1 mg, increase to 1 mg twice/day or 2 mg once a day in a few days if necessary

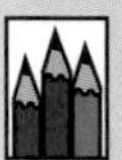

Dosing Tips

- ✻ Because of its long half-life, patients who require chronic treatment may need dose reduction after a few weeks due to drug accumulation
- ✻ Because of its long half-life, once daily dosing is the most frequent dosing generally necessary
- ✻ Because of its long half-life, some patients may have sustained benefits even if dosing is intermittently skipped on some days
- Use lowest possible effective dose for the shortest possible period of time (a benzodiazepine-sparing strategy)
- Assess need for continued treatment regularly
- Risk of dependence may increase with dose and duration of treatment
- For interdose symptoms of anxiety, can either increase dose or maintain same total daily dose but divide into more frequent doses
- Can also use an as-needed occasional "top up" dose for interdose anxiety
- Because panic disorder can require doses higher than 2 mg/day, the risk of dependence may be greater in these patients
- Some severely ill patients may require more than 2 mg/day
- Frequency of dosing in practice is often greater than predicted from half-life, as duration of biological activity is often shorter than pharmacokinetic terminal half-life, which is why once daily dosing is usually the favored option despite the long half-life

Overdose

- Sedation, confusion, poor coordination, diminished reflexes, coma

Long-Term Use

- Risk of dependence, particularly for treatment periods longer than 12 weeks and especially in patients with past or current polysubstance abuse

Habit Forming
- Patients may develop dependence and/or tolerance with long-term use

How to Stop
- Patients with history of seizures may seize upon withdrawal, especially if withdrawal is abrupt
- Taper by 0.5 mg every 3–7 days to reduce chances of withdrawal effects
- For difficult to taper cases, consider reducing dose much more slowly after reaching 3 mg/day, perhaps by as little as 0.25 mg every 7–10 days or slower
- For other patients with severe problems discontinuing a benzodiazepine, dosing may need to be tapered over many months (i.e., reduce dose by 1% every 3 days by crushing tablet and suspending or dissolving in 100 mL of fruit juice and then disposing of 1 mL while drinking the rest; 3–7 days later, dispose of 2 mL, and so on). This is both a form of very slow biological tapering and a form of behavioral desensitization
- Be sure to differentiate reemergence of symptoms requiring reinstitution of treatment from withdrawal symptoms
- Benzodiazepine-dependent anxiety patients and insulin-dependent diabetics are not addicted to their medications. When benzodiazepine-dependent patients stop their medication, disease symptoms can reemerge, disease symptoms can worsen (rebound), and/or withdrawal symptoms can emerge

Pharmacokinetics
- Elimination half-life approximately 122 hours (ultra-long half-life)

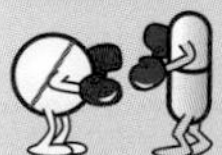

Drug Interactions
- Increased depressive effects when taken with other CNS depressants
- Cimetidine raises loflazepate plasma levels
- Rapid dose reduction or discontinuation of loflazepate during concomitant use with tetracyclic antidepressants such as maprotiline may result in convulsive seizures, possibly due to the loss of anticonvulsant actions that suppress the proconvulsant actions of tetracyclic antidepressants

Other Warnings/ Precautions
- Dosage changes should be made in collaboration with prescriber
- Use with caution in patients with pulmonary disease; rare reports of death after initiation of benzodiazepines in patients with severe pulmonary impairment
- History of drug or alcohol abuse often creates greater risk for dependency
- Hypomania and mania have occurred in depressed patients taking loflazepate
- Use only with extreme caution if patient has obstructive sleep apnea
- Some depressed patients may experience a worsening of suicidal ideation
- Some patients may exhibit abnormal thinking or behavioral changes similar to those caused by other CNS depressants (i.e., either depressant actions or disinhibiting actions)

Do Not Use
- If patient has narrow angle-closure glaucoma
- If patient has myasthenia gravis
- If there is a proven allergy to loflazepate or any benzodiazepine

SPECIAL POPULATIONS

Renal Impairment
- Drug should be used with caution

Hepatic Impairment
- Drug should be used with caution

Cardiac Impairment
- Benzodiazepines have been used to treat anxiety associated with acute myocardial infarction

Elderly
- Drug should be used with caution
- Should begin with lower starting dose

Children and Adolescents
- Safety and efficacy have not been established
- Benzodiazepines are often used in children and adolescents, especially short-term and at the lower end of the dosing scale

- Long-term effects of loflazepate in children/adolescents are unknown
- Should generally receive lower doses and be more closely monitored

Pregnancy

- Possible increased risk of birth defects when benzodiazepines taken during pregnancy
- Because of the potential risks, loflazepate is not generally recommended as treatment for anxiety during pregnancy, especially during the first trimester
- Drug should be tapered if discontinued
- Infants whose mothers received a benzodiazepine late in pregnancy may experience withdrawal effects
- Neonatal flaccidity has been reported in infants whose mothers took a benzodiazepine during pregnancy
- Seizures, even mild seizures, may cause harm to the embryo/fetus

Breast Feeding

- Some drug is found in mother's breast milk
- ✱ Recommended either to discontinue drug or bottle feed
- Effects on infant have been observed and include feeding difficulties, sedation, and weight loss

THE ART OF PSYCHOPHARMACOLOGY

Potential Advantages

- Patients who have interdose anxiety on shorter-acting benzodiazepines
- Patients who wish to take drug only once daily
- Patients who occasionally forget to take their dose

Potential Disadvantages

- Drug may accumulate in long-term users and require dosage reduction

Primary Target Symptoms

- Anxiety
- Tension

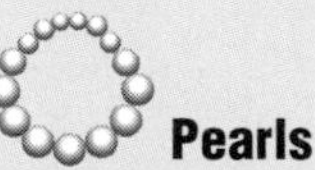

Pearls

- ✱ Is the only "ultra-long half-life" benzodiazepine with a half-life much longer than 24 hours
- ✱ Less interdose anxiety than other benzodiazepines
- ✱ Long half-life could theoretically reduce abuse and withdrawal symptoms
- Is a very useful adjunct to SSRIs and SNRIs in the treatment of numerous anxiety disorders
- Not effective for treating psychosis as a monotherapy, but can be used as an adjunct to antipsychotics
- Not effective for treating bipolar disorder as a monotherapy, but can be used as an adjunct to mood stabilizers and antipsychotics
- May both cause depression and treat depression in different patients
- Risk of seizure is greatest during the first 3 days after discontinuation of loflazepate, especially in those with prior seizures, head injuries or withdrawal from drugs of abuse
- Clinical duration of action may be shorter than plasma half-life, leading to dosing more frequently than 2–3 times daily in some patients
- When using to treat insomnia, remember that insomnia may be a symptom of some other primary disorder itself, and thus warrant evaluation for comorbid psychiatric and/or medical conditions

Suggested Reading

Ba BB, Iliadis A, Cano JP. Pharmacokinetic modeling of ethyl loflazepate (Victan) and its main active metabolites. Ann Biomed Eng 1989;17(6):633–46.

Chambon JP, Perio A, Demarne H, Hallot A, Dantzer R, Roncucci R, Biziere K. Ethyl loflazepate: a prodrug from the benzodiazepine series designed to dissociate anxiolytic and sedative activities. Arzneimittelforschung 1985;35(10):1573–7.

Murasaki M, Mori A, Noguchi T, Hada Y, Hasegawa K, Jinbo S, Kamijima K. Comparison of therapeutic efficacy of neuroses between CM6912 (ethyl loflazepate) and diazepam in a double-blind trial. Prog Neuropsychopharmacol Biol Psychiatry 1989;13(1–2):145–54.

THERAPEUTICS

Brands • Ativan

see index for additional brand names

Generic? Yes

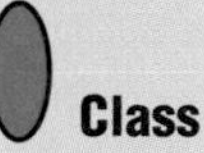

Class

- Benzodiazepine (anxiolytic, anticonvulsant)

Commonly Prescribed for

(bold for FDA approved)

- **Anxiety disorder (oral)**
- **Anxiety associated with depressive symptoms (oral)**
- **Initial treatment of status epilepticus (injection)**
- **Preanesthetic (injection)**
- Insomnia
- Muscle spasm
- Alcohol withdrawal psychosis
- Headache
- Panic disorder
- Acute mania (adjunctive)
- Acute psychosis (adjunctive)
- Delirium (with haloperidol)

How the Drug Works

- Binds to benzodiazepine receptors at the GABA-A ligand-gated chloride channel complex
- Enhances the inhibitory effects of GABA
- Boosts chloride conductance through GABA-regulated channels
- Inhibits neuronal activity presumably in amygdala-centered fear circuits to provide therapeutic benefits in anxiety disorders
- Inhibitory actions in cerebral cortex may provide therapeutic benefits in seizure disorders

How Long Until It Works

- Some immediate relief with first dosing is common; can take several weeks for maximal therapeutic benefit with daily dosing

If It Works

- For short-term symptoms of anxiety – after a few weeks, discontinue use or use on an "as-needed" basis
- For chronic anxiety disorders, the goal of treatment is complete remission of symptoms as well as prevention of future relapses
- For chronic anxiety disorders, treatment most often reduces or even eliminates symptoms, but not a cure since symptoms can recur after medicine stopped
- For long-term symptoms of anxiety, consider switching to an SSRI or SNRI for long-term maintenance
- If long-term maintenance with a benzodiazepine is necessary, continue treatment for 6 months after symptoms resolve, and then taper dose slowly
- If symptoms reemerge, consider treatment with an SSRI or SNRI, or consider restarting the benzodiazepine; sometimes benzodiazepines have to be used in combination with SSRIs or SNRIs for best results

If It Doesn't Work

- Consider switching to another agent or adding an appropriate augmenting agent
- Consider psychotherapy, especially cognitive behavioral psychotherapy
- Consider presence of concomitant substance abuse
- Consider presence of lorazepam abuse
- Consider another diagnosis such as a comorbid medical condition

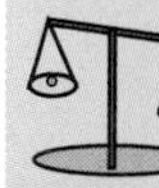

Best Augmenting Combos for Partial Response or Treatment Resistance

- Benzodiazepines are frequently used as augmenting agents for antipsychotics and mood stabilizers in the treatment of psychotic and bipolar disorders
- Benzodiazepines are frequently used as augmenting agents for SSRIs and SNRIs in the treatment of anxiety disorders
- Not generally rational to combine with other benzodiazepines
- Caution if using as an anxiolytic concomitantly with other sedative hypnotics for sleep

Tests

- In patients with seizure disorders, concomitant medical illness, and/or those with multiple concomitant long-term medications, periodic liver tests and blood counts may be prudent

SIDE EFFECTS

How Drug Causes Side Effects

- Same mechanism for side effects as for therapeutic effects – namely due to excessive actions at benzodiazepine receptors
- Long-term adaptations in benzodiazepine receptors may explain the development of dependence, tolerance, and withdrawal
- Side effects are generally immediate, but immediate side effects often disappear in time

Notable Side Effects

✻ Sedation, fatigue, depression
✻ Dizziness, ataxia, slurred speech, weakness
✻ Forgetfulness, confusion
✻ Hyperexcitability, nervousness
✻ Pain at injection site
- Rare hallucinations, mania
- Rare hypotension
- Hypersalivation, dry mouth

Life-Threatening or Dangerous Side Effects

- Respiratory depression, especially when taken with CNS depressants in overdose
- Rare hepatic dysfunction, renal dysfunction, blood dyscrasias

Weight Gain

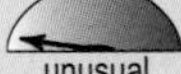

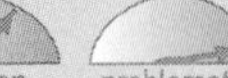

- Reported but not expected

Sedation

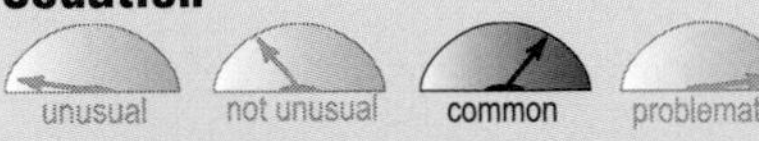

- Many experience and/or can be significant in amount
- Especially at initiation of treatment or when dose increases
- Tolerance often develops over time

What To Do About Side Effects

- Wait
- Wait
- Wait
- Lower the dose
- Take largest dose at bedtime to avoid sedative effects during the day
- Switch to another agent
- Administer flumazenil if side effects are severe or life-threatening

Best Augmenting Agents for Side Effects

- Many side effects cannot be improved with an augmenting agent

DOSING AND USE

Usual Dosage Range

- Oral: 2–6 mg/day in divided doses, largest dose at bedtime
- Injection: 4 mg administered slowly

Dosage Forms

- Tablet 0.5 mg, 1 mg, 2 mg
- Liquid 0.5 mg/5 mL, 2 mg/mL
- Injection 1 mg/0.5 mL, 2 mg/mL, 4 mg/mL

How To Dose

- Oral: Initial 2–3 mg/day in 2–3 doses; increase as needed, starting with evening dose; maximum generally 10 mg/day
- Injection: Initial 4 mg administered slowly; after 10–5 minutes may administer again
- Take liquid formulation with water, soda, applesauce, or pudding

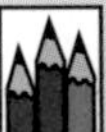

Dosing Tips

✻ One of the few benzodiazepines available in an oral liquid formulation
✻ One of the few benzodiazepines available in an injectable formulation
- Lorazepam injection is intended for acute use; patients who require long-term treatment should be switched to the oral formulation
- Use lowest possible effective dose for the shortest possible period of time (a benzodiazepine-sparing strategy)
- Assess need for continued treatment regularly
- Risk of dependence may increase with dose and duration of treatment
- For interdose symptoms of anxiety, can either increase dose or maintain same total daily dose but divide into more frequent doses
- Can also use an as-needed occasional "top up" dose for interdose anxiety

- Because panic disorder can require doses higher than 6 mg/day, the risk of dependence may be greater in these patients
- Some severely ill patients may require 10 mg/day or more
- Frequency of dosing in practice is often greater than predicted from half-life, as duration of biological activity is often shorter than pharmacokinetic terminal half-life

Overdose
- Fatalities can occur; hypotension, tiredness, ataxia, confusion, coma

Long-Term Use
- Evidence of efficacy up to 16 weeks
- Risk of dependence, particularly for treatment periods longer than 12 weeks and especially in patients with past or current polysubstance abuse

Habit Forming
- Lorazepam is a Schedule IV drug
- Patients may develop dependence and/or tolerance with long-term use

How to Stop
- Patients with history of seizure may seize upon withdrawal, especially if withdrawal is abrupt
- Taper by 0.5 mg every 3 days to reduce chances of withdrawal effects
- For difficult to taper cases, consider reducing dose much more slowly once reaching 3 mg/day, perhaps by as little as 0.25 mg per week or less
- For other patients with severe problems discontinuing a benzodiazepine, dosing may need to be tapered over many months (i.e., reduce dose by 1% every 3 days by crushing tablet and suspending or dissolving in 100 mL of fruit juice and then disposing of 1 mL while drinking the rest; 3–7 days later, dispose of 2 mL, and so on). This is both a form of very slow biological tapering and a form of behavioral desensitization
- Be sure to differentiate reemergence of symptoms requiring reinstitution of treatment from withdrawal symptoms
- Benzodiazepine-dependent anxiety patients and insulin-dependent diabetics are not addicted to their medications. When benzodiazepine-dependent patients stop their medication, disease symptoms can reemerge, disease symptoms can worsen (rebound), and/or withdrawal symptoms can emerge

Pharmacokinetics
- Elimination half-life 10–20 hours
- No active metabolites

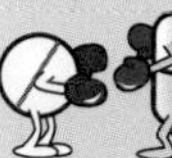

Drug Interactions
- Increased depressive effects when taken with other CNS depressants
- Valproate and probenecid may reduce clearance and raise plasma concentrations of lorazepam
- Oral contraceptives may increase clearance and lower plasma concentrations of lorazepam
- Flumazenil (used to reverse the effects of benzodiazepines) may precipitate seizures and should not be used in patients treated for seizure disorders with lorazepam

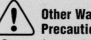

Other Warnings/ Precautions
- Dosage changes should be made in collaboration with prescriber
- Use with caution in patients with pulmonary disease; rare reports of death after initiation of benzodiazepines in patients with severe pulmonary impairment
- History of drug or alcohol abuse often creates greater risk for dependency
- Use oral formulation only with extreme caution if patient has obstructive sleep apnea; injection is contraindicated in patients with sleep apnea
- Some depressed patients may experience a worsening of suicidal ideation
- Some patients may exhibit abnormal thinking or behavioral changes similar to those caused by other CNS depressants (i.e., either depressant actions or disinhibiting actions)

Do Not Use
- If patient has narrow angle-closure glaucoma
- If patient has sleep apnea (injection)
- Must not be given intra-arterially because it may cause arteriospasm and result in gangrene

- If there is a proven allergy to lorazepam or any benzodiazepine

SPECIAL POPULATIONS

Renal Impairment
- 1–2 mg/day in 2–3 doses

Hepatic Impairment
- 1–2 mg/day in 2–3 doses
- Because of its short half-life and inactive metabolites, lorazepam may be a preferred benzodiazepine in some patients with liver disease

Cardiac Impairment
- Benzodiazepines have been used to treat anxiety associated with acute myocardial infarction
- Lorazepam may be used as an adjunct to control drug-induced cardiovascular emergencies

Elderly
- 1–2 mg/day in 2–3 doses
- May be more sensitive to sedative or respiratory effects

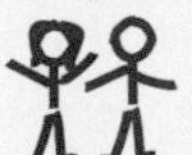

Children and Adolescents
- Oral: safety and efficacy not established in children under age 12
- Injection: safety and efficacy not established in children under age 18
- Long-term effects of lorazepam in children/adolescents are unknown
- Should generally receive lower doses and be more closely monitored

Pregnancy
- Risk Category D [positive evidence of risk to human fetus; potential benefits may still justify its use]
- Possible increased risk of birth defects when benzodiazepines taken during pregnancy
- Because of the potential risks, lorazepam is not generally recommended as treatment for anxiety during pregnancy, especially during the first trimester
- Drug should be tapered if discontinued
- Infants whose mothers received a benzodiazepine late in pregnancy may experience withdrawal effects
- Neonatal flaccidity has been reported in infants whose mothers took a benzodiazepine during pregnancy
- Seizures, even mild seizures, may cause harm to the embryo/fetus

Breast Feeding
- Some drug is found in mother's breast milk
- ✻ Recommended either to discontinue drug or bottle feed
- Effects on infant have been observed and include feeding difficulties, sedation, and weight loss

THE ART OF PSYCHOPHARMACOLOGY

Potential Advantages
- Rapid onset of action
- Availability of oral liquid as well as injectable dosage formulations

Potential Disadvantages
- Euphoria may lead to abuse
- Abuse especially risky in past or present substance abusers
- Possibly more sedation than some other benzodiazepines commonly used to treat anxiety

Primary Target Symptoms
- Panic attacks
- Anxiety
- Muscle spasms
- Incidence of seizures (adjunct)

Pearls
- ✻ One of the most popular and useful benzodiazepines for treatment of agitation associated with psychosis, bipolar disorder, and other disorders, especially in the inpatient setting; this is due in part to useful sedative properties and flexibility of administration with oral tablets, oral liquid, or injectable formulations, which is often useful in treating uncooperative patients
- Is a very useful adjunct to SSRIs and SNRIs in the treatment of numerous anxiety disorders

- Not effective for treating psychosis as a monotherapy, but can be used as an adjunct to antipsychotics
- Not effective for treating bipolar disorder as a monotherapy, but can be used as an adjunct to mood stabilizers and antipsychotics
- Because of its short half-life and inactive metabolites, lorazepam may be preferred over some benzodiazepines for patients with liver disease
- ❋ Lorazepam may be preferred over other benzodiazepines for the treatment of delirium
- When treating delirium, lorazepam is often combined with haloperidol, with the haloperidol dose 2 times the lorazepam dose
- ❋ Lorazepam is often used to induce pre-operative anterograde amnesia to assist in anesthesiology
- May both cause depression and treat depression in different patients
- Clinical duration of action may be shorter than plasma half-life, leading to dosing more frequently than 2–3 times daily in some patients
- When using to treat insomnia, remember that insomnia may be a symptom of some other primary disorder itself, and thus warrant evaluation for comorbid psychiatric and/or medical conditions

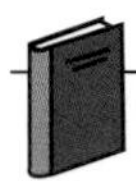

Suggested Reading

Bonnet MH, Arand DL. The use of lorazepam TID for chronic insomnia. Int Clin Psychopharmacol 1999;14:81–9.

Greenblatt DJ. Clinical pharmacokinetics of oxazepam and lorazepam. Clin Pharmacokinet 1981;6:89–105.

Starreveld E, Starreveld AA. Status epilepticus. Current concepts and management. Can Fam Physician 2000;46:1817–23.

Wagner BK, O'Hara DA, Hammond JS. Drugs for amnesia in the ICU. Am J Crit Care 1997; 6:192–201.

THERAPEUTICS

Brands • Loxitane

see index for additional brand names

Generic? Yes

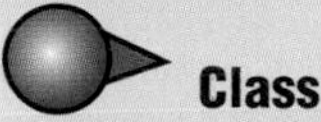

Class

- Conventional antipsychotic (neuroleptic, dopamine 2 antagonist, serotonin dopamine antagonist)

Commonly Prescribed for

(bold for FDA approved)

- **Schizophrenia**
- Other psychotic disorders
- Bipolar disorder

How the Drug Works

- Blocks dopamine 2 receptors, reducing positive symptoms of psychosis

✽ Although classified as a conventional antipsychotic, loxapine is a potent serotonin 2A antagonist

- Serotonin 2A antagonist properties might be relevant at low doses, but generally are overwhelmed by high dosing

How Long Until It Works

- Psychotic symptoms can improve within 1 week, but it may take several weeks for full effect on behavior

If It Works

- Most often reduces positive symptoms in schizophrenia but does not eliminate them
- Most schizophrenic patients do not have a total remission of symptoms but rather a reduction of symptoms by about a third
- Continue treatment in schizophrenia until reaching a plateau of improvement
- After reaching a satisfactory plateau, continue treatment for at least a year after first episode of psychosis in schizophrenia
- For second and subsequent episodes of psychosis in schizophrenia, treatment may need to be indefinite
- Reduces symptoms of acute psychotic mania but not proven as a mood stabilizer or as an effective maintenance treatment in bipolar disorder
- After reducing acute psychotic symptoms in mania, switch to a mood stabilizer and/or an atypical antipsychotic for mood stabilization and maintenance

If It Doesn't Work

- Consider trying one of the first-line atypical antipsychotics (risperidone, olanzapine, quetiapine, ziprasidone, aripiprazole, paliperidone, amisulpride)
- Consider trying another conventional antipsychotic
- If 2 or more antipsychotic monotherapies do not work, consider clozapine

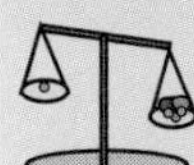

Best Augmenting Combos for Partial Response or Treatment Resistance

- Augmentation of conventional antipsychotics has not been systematically studied
- Addition of a mood stabilizing anticonvulsant such as valproate, carbamazepine, or lamotrigine may be helpful in both schizophrenia and bipolar mania
- Augmentation with lithium in bipolar mania may be helpful
- Addition of a benzodiazepine, especially short-term for agitation

Tests

✽ Since conventional antipsychotics are frequently associated with weight gain, before starting treatment, weigh all patients and determine if the patient is already overweight (BMI 25.0–29.9) or obese (BMI ≥30)

- Before giving a drug that can cause weight gain to an overweight or obese patient, consider determining whether the patient already has pre-diabetes (fasting plasma glucose 100–25 mg/dL), diabetes (fasting plasma glucose >126 mg/dL), or dyslipidemia (increased total cholesterol, LDL cholesterol and triglycerides; decreased HDL cholesterol), and treat or refer such patients for treatment, including nutrition and weight management, physical activity counseling, smoking cessation, and medical management

✽ Monitor weight and BMI during treatment

✽ Consider monitoring fasting triglycerides monthly for several months in patients at high risk for metabolic complications and when initiating or switching antipsychotics

❋ While giving a drug to a patient who has gained >5% of initial weight, consider evaluating for the presence of pre-diabetes, diabetes, or dyslipidemia, or consider switching to a different antipsychotic
- Should check blood pressure in the elderly before starting and for the first few weeks of treatment
- Monitoring elevated prolactin levels of dubious clinical benefit

SIDE EFFECTS

How Drug Causes Side Effects
- By blocking dopamine 2 receptors in the striatum, it can cause motor side effects
- By blocking dopamine 2 receptors in the pituitary, it can cause elevations in prolactin
- By blocking dopamine 2 receptors excessively in the mesocortical and mesolimbic dopamine pathways, especially at high doses, it can cause worsening of negative and cognitive symptoms (neuroleptic-induced deficit syndrome)
- Anticholinergic actions may cause sedation, blurred vision, constipation, dry mouth
- Antihistaminic actions may cause sedation, weight gain
- By blocking alpha 1 adrenergic receptors, it can cause dizziness, sedation, and hypotension
- Mechanism of weight gain and any possible increased incidence of diabetes or dyslipidemia with conventional antipsychotics is unknown

Notable Side Effects
❋ Neuroleptic-induced deficit syndrome
❋ Akathisia
❋ Extrapyramidal symptoms, Parkinsonism, tardive dyskinesia
❋ Galactorrhea, amenorrhea
- Sedation
- Dry mouth, constipation, vision disturbance, urninary retention
- Hypotension, tachycardia

Life-Threatening or Dangerous Side Effects
- Rare neuroleptic malignant syndrome
- Rare agranulocytosis
- Rare hepatocellular injury
- Rare seizures
- Increased risk of death and cerebrovascular events in elderly patients with dementia-related psychosis

Weight Gain
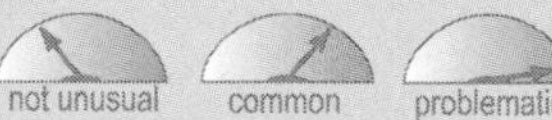

- Reported but not expected

Sedation
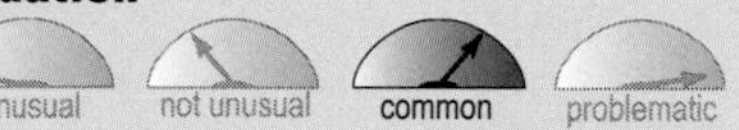

- Many experience and/or can be significant in amount
- Sedation is usually transient
- Sedation is usually dose-dependent and may not be experienced at low doses where loxapine may function as an atypical antipsychotic (e.g., <50 mg/day; especially 5–25 mg/day)

What To Do About Side Effects
- Wait
- Wait
- Wait
- For motor symptoms, add an anticholinergic agent
- Reduce the dose
- For sedation, give at night
- Switch to an atypical antipsychotic
- Weight loss, exercise programs, and medical management for high BMIs, diabetes, dyslipidemia

Best Augmenting Agents for Side Effects
- Benztropine or trihexyphenidyl for motor side effects
- Sometimes amantadine can be helpful for motor side effects
- Benzodiazepines may be helpful for akathisia
- Many side effects cannot be improved with an augmenting agent

DOSING AND USE

Usual Dosage Range
- 60–100 mg/day in divided doses

Dosage Forms

- Capsule 6.8 mg loxapine succinate equivalent to 5 mg loxapine, 13.6 mg loxapine succinate equivalent to 10 mg loxapine, 34.0 mg loxapine succinate equivalent to 25 mg loxapine, 68.1 mg loxapine succinate equivalent to 50 mg loxapine
- Oral liquid 25 mg/mL
- Injection 50 mg/mL

How To Dose

- Initial 20 mg/day in 2 doses; titrate over 7–10 days to 60–100 mg/day in 2–4 doses; maximum generally 250 mg/day
- Take liquid formulation in orange or grapefruit juice

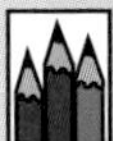

Dosing Tips

- Has conventional antipsychotic properties at originally recommended doses (i.e., starting at 10 mg twice a day, maintenance 60–100 mg/day, maximum 250 mg/day given in 2 divided doses)
- ✻ Binding studies, PET studies, and anecdotal clinical observations suggest that loxapine may be atypical at lower doses (perhaps 5–30 mg/day) but further studies needed
- Anecdotal evidence that many patients can be maintained at 20–60 mg/day as monotherapy
- To augment partial responders to an atypical antipsychotic, consider doses of loxapine as low as 5–60 mg/day, but use full doses if necessary
- No formal studies, but some patients may do well on once-daily dosing, especially at night, rather than twice-daily dosing
- Available as 5 mg and 10 mg capsules for low dose use and as 25 mg and 50 mg capsules for routine use
- Available as a liquid dosage formulation
- Available for acute intramuscular administration (50 mg/mL)
- Intramuscular loxapine may have faster onset of action and superior efficacy for agitated/excited and aggressive behavior in some patients than intramuscular haloperidol
- In the acute situation, give 25–50 mg intramuscularly (0.5–1.0 mL of 50 mg/mL solution) with onset of action within 60 minutes
- When initiating therapy with an atypical antipsychotic in an acute situation, consider short-term intramuscular loxapine to "lead in" to orally administered atypical; e.g., initiate oral dosing of an atypical antipsychotic with 25–50 mg loxapine 2–3 times a day intramuscularly to achieve antipsychotic effects without extrapyramidal symptoms and sedation
- When using loxapine to "top-up" previously stabilized patients now decompensating, may use loxapine as single 25–50 mg doses as needed intramuscularly or as oral liquid or tablets
- Patients receiving atypical antipsychotics may occasionally require a "top up" of a conventional antipsychotic to control aggression or violent behavior

Overdose

- Deaths have occurred; extrapyramidal symptoms, CNS depression, cardiovascular effects, hypotension, seizures, respiratory depression, renal failure, coma

Long-Term Use

- Some side effects may be irreversible (e.g., tardive dyskinesia)

Habit Forming

- No

How to Stop

- Slow down-titration of oral formulation (over 6–8 weeks), especially when simultaneously beginning a new antipsychotic while switching (i.e., cross-titration)
- Rapid oral discontinuation may lead to rebound psychosis and worsening of symptoms
- If antiparkinson agents are being used, they should be continued for a few weeks after loxapine is discontinued

Pharmacokinetics

- Half-life approximately 4 hours for oral formulation
- Half-life approximately 12 hours for intramuscular formulation
- Multiple active metabolites with longer half-lives than parent drug
- ✻ *N*-desmethyl loxapine is amoxapine, an antidepressant

- 8-hydroxyloxapine and 7-hydroxyloxapine are also serotonin-dopamine antagonists
- 8-hydroxyamoxapine and 7-hydroxyamoxapine are also serotonin-dopamine antagonists

Drug Interactions

- Respiratory depression may occur when loxapine is combined with lorazepam
- Additive effects may occur if used with CNS depressants
- May decrease the effects of levodopa, dopamine agonists
- Some patients taking a neuroleptic and lithium have developed an encephalopathic syndrome similar to neuroleptic malignant syndrome
- Combined use with epinephrine may lower blood pressure
- May increase the effects of antihypertensive drugs except for guanethidine, whose antihypertensive actions loxapine may antagonize

Other Warnings/ Precautions

- If signs of neuroleptic malignant syndrome develop, treatment should be immediately discontinued
- Use cautiously in patients with alcohol withdrawal or convulsive disorders because of possible lowering of seizure threshold
- Antiemetic effect can mask signs of other disorders or overdose
- Do not use epinephrine in event of overdose, as interaction with some pressor agents may lower blood pressure
- Use cautiously in patients with glaucoma, urinary retention
- Observe for signs of ocular toxicity (pigmentary retinopathy, lenticular pigmentation)
- Avoid extreme heat exposure
- Use only with caution if at all in Parkinson's disease or Lewy body dementia

Do Not Use

- If patient is in a comatose state or has CNS depression
- If there is a proven allergy to loxapine
- If there is a known sensitivity to any dibenzoxazepine

SPECIAL POPULATIONS

Renal Impairment

- Use with caution

Hepatic Impairment

- Use with caution

Cardiac Impairment

- Use with caution

Elderly

- Some patients may tolerate lower doses better
- Although conventional antipsychotics are commonly used for behavioral disturbances in dementia, no agent has been approved for treatment of elderly patients with dementia-related psychosis
- Elderly patients with dementia-related psychosis treated with antipsychotics are at an increased risk ofdeath compared to placebo, and also have an increased risk of cerebrovascular events

Children and Adolescents

- Safety and efficacy not established
- Generally, consider second-line after atypical antipsychotics

Pregnancy

- Renal papillary abnormalities have been seen in rats during pregnancy
- No studies in pregnant women
- Psychotic symptoms may worsen during pregnancy and some form of treatment may be necessary
- Atypical antipsychotics may be preferable to conventional antipsychotics or anticonvulsant mood stabilizers if treatment is required during pregnancy

Breast Feeding

- Unknown if loxapine is secreted in human breast milk, but all psychotropics assumed to be secreted in breast milk

* Recommended either to discontinue drug or bottle feed

THE ART OF PSYCHOPHARMACOLOGY

Potential Advantages

- Intramuscular formulation for emergency use

Potential Disadvantages

- Patients with tardive dyskinesia

Primary Target Symptoms

- Positive symptoms of psychosis
- Motor and autonomic hyperactivity
- Violent or aggressive behavior

Pearls

✻ Recently discovered to be a serotonin dopamine antagonist (binding studies and PET scans)

✻ Active metabolites are also serotonin dopamine antagonists with longer half-lives than parent drug, thus possibly allowing once-daily treatment

✻ One active metabolite is an antidepressant (amoxapine, also known as *N*-desmethyl-loxapine)

- Theoretically, loxapine should have antidepressant actions, especially at high doses, but no controlled studies
- Theoretically, loxapine may have advantages for short-term use in some patients with psychotic depression
- Developed as a conventional antipsychotic; i.e., reduces positive symptoms, but causes extrapyramidal symptoms and prolactin elevations
- Lower extrapyramidal symptoms than haloperidol in some studies, but not fixed dose studies and no low dose studies

✻ Causes less weight gain than other antipsychotics, both atypical and conventional, and may even be associated with weight loss

- No formal studies of negative symptoms, but some studies show superiority to conventional antipsychotics for emotional withdrawal and social competence
- Best use may be as low-cost augmentation agent to atypical antipsychotics

✻ Enhances efficacy in clozapine partial responders when given concomitantly with clozapine

- For previously stabilized patients with "breakthrough" agitation or incipient decompensation, "top-up" the atypical antipsychotic with as-needed intramuscular or oral single doses of loxapine
- Patients have very similar antipsychotic responses to any conventional antipsychotic, which is different from atypical antipsychotics where antipsychotic responses of individual patients can occasionally vary greatly from one atypical antipsychotic to another
- Patients with inadequate responses to atypical antipsychotics may benefit from a trial of augmentation with a conventional antipsychotic such as loxapine or from switching to a conventional antipsychotic such as loxapine
- However, long-term polypharmacy with a combination of a conventional antipsychotic such as loxapine with an atypical antipsychotic may combine their side effects without clearly augmenting the efficacy of either
- Although a frequent practice by some prescribers, adding 2 conventional antipsychotics together has little rationale and may reduce tolerability without clearly enhancing efficacy

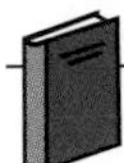

Suggested Reading

Fenton M, Murphy B, Wood J, Bagnall A, Chue P, Leitner M. Loxapine for schizophrenia. Cochrane Database Syst Rev 2000;(2):CD001943.

Heel RC, Brogden RN, Speight TM, Avery GS. Loxapine: a review of its pharmacological properties and therapeutic efficacy as an antipsychotic agent. Drugs 1978;15(3):198–217.

Zisook S, Click MA Jr. Evaluations of loxapine succinate in the ambulatory treatment of acute schizophrenic episodes. Int Pharmacopsychiatry 1980;15(6):365–78.

THERAPEUTICS

Brands • Ludiomil

see index for additional brand names

Generic? Yes

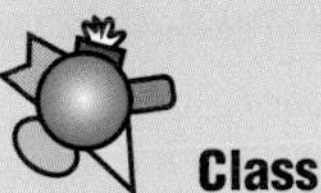

Class

- Tricyclic antidepressant (TCA), sometimes classified as a tetracyclic antidepressant (tetra)
- Predominantly a norepinephrine/ noradrenaline reuptake inhibitor

Commonly Prescribed for

(bold for FDA approved)

- **Depression**
- Anxiety
- Insomnia
- Neuropathic pain/chronic pain
- Treatment-resistant depression

How the Drug Works

- Boosts neurotransmitter norepinephrine/noradrenaline
- Blocks norepinephrine reuptake pump (norepinephrine transporter), presumably increasing noradrenergic neurotransmission
- Since dopamine is inactivated by norepinephrine reuptake in frontal cortex, which largely lacks dopamine transporters, maprotiline can thus increase dopamine neurotransmission in this part of the brain
- A more potent inhibitor of norepinephrine reuptake pump than serotonin reuptake pump (serotonin transporter)
- At high doses may also boost neurotransmitter serotonin and presumably increase serotonergic neurotransmission

How Long Until It Works

- Onset of therapeutic actions usually not immediate, but often delayed 2–4 weeks
- If it is not working within 6–8 weeks for depression, it may require a dosage increase or it may not work at all
- May continue to work for many years to prevent relapse of symptoms

If It Works

- The goal of treatment of depression is complete remission of current symptoms as well as prevention of future relapses
- The goal of treatment of chronic neuropathic pain is to reduce symptoms as much as possible, especially in combination with other treatments
- Treatment of depression most often reduces or even eliminates symptoms, but not a cure since symptoms can recur after medicine is stopped
- Treatment of chronic neuropathic pain may reduce symptoms, but rarely eliminates them completely, and is not a cure since symptoms can recur after medicine stopped
- Continue treatment of depression until all symptoms are gone (remission)
- Once symptoms of depression are gone, continue treating for 1 year for the first episode of depression
- For second and subsequent episodes of depression, treatment may need to be indefinite
- Use in anxiety disorders and chronic pain may also need to be indefinite, but long-term treatment is not well-studied in these conditions

If It Doesn't Work

- Many depressed patients have only a partial response where some symptoms are improved but others persist (especially insomnia, fatigue, and problems concentrating)
- Other depressed patients may be nonresponders, sometimes called treatment-resistant or treatment-refractory
- Consider increasing dose, switching to another agent or adding an appropriate augmenting agent
- Consider psychotherapy
- Consider evaluation for another diagnosis or for a comorbid condition (e.g., medical illness, substance abuse, etc.)
- Some patients may experience apparent lack of consistent efficacy due to activation of latent or underlying bipolar disorder, and require antidepressant discontinuation and a switch to a mood stabilizer

Best Augmenting Combos for Partial Response or Treatment Resistance

- Lithium, buspirone, thyroid hormone (for depression)
- Gabapentin, tiagabine, other anticonvulsants, even opiates if done by experts while monitoring carefully in difficult cases (for chronic pain)

Tests

- None for healthy individuals

✻ Since tricyclic and tetracyclic antidepressants are frequently associated with weight gain, before starting treatment, weigh all patients and determine if the patient is already overweight (BMI 25.0–29.9) or obese (BMI ≥30)

- Before giving a drug that can cause weight gain to an overweight or obese patient, consider determining whether the patient already has pre-diabetes (fasting plasma glucose 100–25 mg/dL), diabetes (fasting plasma glucose >126 mg/dL), or dyslipidemia (increased total cholesterol, LDL cholesterol and triglycerides; decreased HDL cholesterol), and treat or refer such patients for treatment, including nutrition and weight management, physical activity counseling, smoking cessation, and medical management

✻ Monitor weight and BMI during treatment

✻ While giving a drug to a patient who has gained >5% of initial weight, consider evaluating for the presence of pre-diabetes, diabetes, or dyslipidemia, or consider switching to a different antidepressant

- EKGs may be useful for selected patients (e.g., those with personal or family history of QTc prolongation; cardiac arrhythmia; recent myocardial infarction; uncompensated heart failure; or taking agents that prolong QTc interval such as pimozide, thioridazine, selected antiarrhythmics, moxifloxacin, sparfloxacin, etc.)
- Patients at risk for electrolyte disturbances (e.g., patients on diuretic therapy) should have baseline and periodic serum potassium and magnesium measurements

SIDE EFFECTS

How Drug Causes Side Effects

- Anticholinergic activity may explain sedative effects, dry mouth, constipation, and blurred vision
- Sedative effects and weight gain may be due to antihistamine properties
- Blockade of alpha adrenergic 1 receptors may explain dizziness, sedation, and hypotension
- Cardiac arrhythmias and seizures, especially in overdose, may be caused by blockade of ion channels

Notable Side Effects

- Blurred vision, constipation, urinary retention, increased appetite, dry mouth, nausea, diarrhea, heartburn, unusual taste in mouth, weight gain
- Fatigue, weakness, dizziness, sedation, headache, anxiety, nervousness, restlessness
- Sexual dysfunction (impotence, change in libido)
- Sweating, rash, itching

Life-Threatening or Dangerous Side Effects

- Paralytic ileus, hyperthermia (TCAs/ tetracylics + anticholinergic agents)
- Lowered seizure threshold and rare seizures
- Orthostatic hypotension, sudden death, arrhythmias, tachycardia
- QTc prolongation
- Hepatic failure, extrapyramidal symptoms
- Increased intraocular pressure
- Rare induction of mania
- Rare activation of suicidal ideation and behavior (suicidality) (short-term studies did not show an increase in the risk of suicidality with antidepressants compared to placebo beyond age 24)

Weight Gain

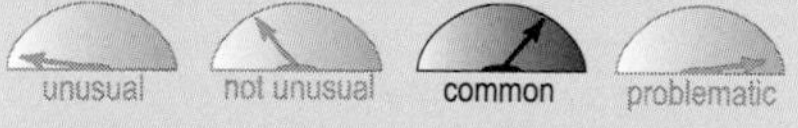

- Many experience and/or can be significant in amount
- Can increase appetite and carbohydrate craving

Sedation

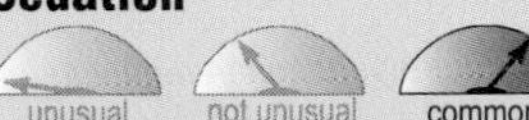

- Many experience and/or can be significant in amount
- Tolerance to sedative effect may develop with long-term use

What To Do About Side Effects

- Wait
- Wait
- Wait
- Lower the dose
- Switch to an SSRI or newer antidepressant

Best Augmenting Agents for Side Effects

- Many side effects cannot be improved with an augmenting agent

DOSING AND USE

Usual Dosage Range

- 75–150 mg/day (for depression)
- 50–150 mg/day (for chronic pain)

Dosage Forms

- Tablet 25 mg, 50 mg, 75 mg

How To Dose

- Initial 25 mg/day at bedtime; increase by 25 mg every 3–7 days
- 75 mg/day; after 2 weeks increase dose gradually by 25 mg/day; maximum dose generally 225 mg/day

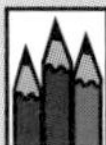

Dosing Tips

- If given in a single dose, should generally be administered at bedtime because of its sedative properties
- If given in split doses, largest dose should generally be given at bedtime because of its sedative properties
- If patients experience nightmares, split dose and do not give large dose at bedtime
- Patients treated for chronic pain may only require lower doses

✻ Risk of seizures increases with dose, especially with maprotiline above 200 mg/day

- If intolerable anxiety, insomnia, agitation, akathisia, or activation occur either upon dosing initiation or discontinuation, consider the possibility of activated bipolar disorder, and switch to a mood stabilizer or an atypical antipsychotic

Overdose

- Death may occur; convulsions, cardiac dysrhythmias, severe hypotension, CNS depression, coma, changes in EKG

Long-Term Use

- Safe

Habit Forming

- No

How to Stop

- Taper to avoid withdrawal effects
- Even with gradual dose reduction some withdrawal symptoms may appear within the first 2 weeks
- Many patients tolerate 50% dose reduction for 3 days, then another 50% reduction for 3 days, then discontinuation
- If withdrawal symptoms emerge during discontinuation, raise dose to stop symptoms and then restart withdrawal much more slowly

Pharmacokinetics

- Substrate for CYP450 2D6
- Mean half-life approximately 51 hours
- Peak plasma concentration 8–24 hours

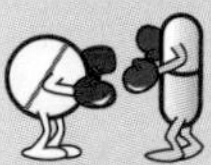

Drug Interactions

- Tramadol increases the risk of seizures in patients taking TCAs
- Use of TCAs/tetracyclics with anticholinergic drugs may result in paralytic ileus or hyperthermia
- Fluoxetine, paroxetine, bupropion, duloxetine, and other CYP450 2D6 inhibitors may increase TCA/tetracyclic concentrations
- Cimetidine may increase plasma concentrations of TCAs/tetracyclics and cause anticholinergic symptoms
- Phenothiazines or haloperidol may raise TCA/tetracyclic blood concentrations
- May alter effects of antihypertensive drugs; may inhibit hypotensive effects of clonidine

- Use with sympathomimetic agents may increase sympathetic activity
- Methylphenidate may inhibit metabolism of TCAs/tetracyclics
- Activation and agitation, especially following switching or adding antidepressants, may represent the induction of a bipolar state, especially a mixed dysphoric bipolar II condition sometimes associated with suicidal ideation, and require the addition of lithium, a mood stabilizer or an atypical antipsychotic, and/or discontinuation of maprotiline

Other Warnings/ Precautions

- Add or initiate other antidepressants with caution for up to 2 weeks after discontinuing maprotiline
- Generally, do not use with MAO inhibitors, including 14 days after MAOIs are stopped; do not start an MAOI until 2 weeks after discontinuing maprotiline, but see Pearls
- Use with caution in patients with history of seizures, urinary retention, narrow angle-closure glaucoma, hyperthyroidism
- TCAs/tetracyclics can increase QTc interval, especially at toxic doses, which can be attained not only by overdose but also by combining with drugs that inhibit TCA/ tetracyclic metabolism via CYP450 2D6, potentially causing torsade de pointes-type arrhythmia or sudden death
- Because TCAs/tetracyclics can prolong QTc interval, use with caution in patients who have bradycardia or who are taking drugs that can induce bradycardia (e.g., beta blockers, calcium channel blockers, clonidine, digitalis)
- Because TCAs/tetracyclics can prolong QTc interval, use with caution in patients who have hypokalemia and/or hypomagnesemia or who are taking drugs that can induce hypokalemia and/or magnesemia (e.g., diuretics, stimulant laxatives, intravenous amphotericin B, glucocorticoids, tetracosactide)
- When treating children, carefully weigh the risks and benefits of pharmacological treatment against the risks and benefits of nontreatment with antidepressants and make sure to document this in the patient's chart
- Distribute the brochures provided by the FDA and the drug companies
- Warn patients and their caregivers about the possibility of activating side effects and advise them to report such symptoms immediately
- Monitor patients for activation of suicidal ideation, especially children and adolescents

Do Not Use

- If patient is recovering from myocardial infarction
- If patient is taking agents capable of significantly prolonging QTc interval (e.g., pimozide, thioridazine, selected antiarrhythmics, moxifloxacin, sparfloxacin)
- If there is a history of QTc prolongation or cardiac arrhythmia, recent acute myocardial infarction, uncompensated heart failure
- If patient is taking drugs that inhibit TCA/tetracyclic metabolism, including CYP450 2D6 inhibitors, except by an expert
- If there is reduced CYP450 2D6 function, such as patients who are poor 2D6 metabolizers, except by an expert and at low doses
- If there is a proven allergy to maprotiline

SPECIAL POPULATIONS

Renal Impairment

- Use with caution

Hepatic Impairment

- Use with caution

Cardiac Impairment

- TCAs/tetracyclics have been reported to cause arrhythmias, prolongation of conduction time, orthostatic hypotension, sinus tachycardia, and heart failure, especially in the diseased heart
- Myocardial infarction and stroke have been reported with TCAs/tetracyclics
- TCAs/tetracyclics produce QTc prolongation, which may be enhanced by the existence of bradycardia, hypokalemia, congenital or acquired long QTc interval, which should be evaluated prior to administering maprotiline

- Use with caution if treating concomitantly with a medication likely to produce prolonged bradycardia, hypokalemia, slowing of intracardiac conduction, or prolongation of the QTc interval
- Avoid TCAs/tetracyclics in patients with a known history of QTc prolongation, recent acute myocardial infarction, and uncompensated heart failure
- TCAs/tetracyclics may cause a sustained increase in heart rate in patients with ischemic heart disease and may worsen (decrease) heart rate variability, an independent risk of mortality in cardiac populations
- Since SSRIs may improve (increase) heart rate variability in patients following a myocardial infarct and may improve survival as well as mood in patients with acute angina or following a myocardial infarction, these are more appropriate agents for cardiac population than tricyclic/tetracyclic antidepressants

✻ Risk/benefit ratio may not justify use of TCAs/tetracyclics in cardiac impairment

Elderly

- May be more sensitive to anticholinergic, cardiovascular, hypotensive, and sedative effects
- Usual dose generally 50–75 mg/day
- Reduction in risk of suicidality with antidepressants compared to placebo in adults age 65 and older

Children and Adolescents

- Carefully weigh the risks and benefits of pharmacological treatment against the risks and benefits of nontreatment with antidepressants and make sure to document this in the patient's chart
- Monitor patients face-to-face regularly, particularly during the first several weeks of treatment
- Use with caution, observing for activation of known or unknown bipolar disorder and/or suicidal ideation, and inform parents or guardian of this risk so they can help observe child or adolescent patients
- Not recommended for use under age 18
- Several studies show lack of efficacy of TCAs/tetracyclics for depression
- May be used to treat enuresis or hyperactive/impulsive behaviors
- Maximum dose for children and adolescents is 75 mg/day

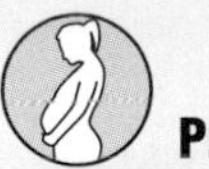

Pregnancy

- Risk Category B [animal studies do not show adverse effects; no controlled studies in humans]
- Adverse effects have been reported in infants whose mothers took a TCA/tetracyclic (lethargy, withdrawal symptoms, fetal malformations)
- Must weigh the risk of treatment (first trimester fetal development, third trimester newborn delivery) to the child against the risk of no treatment (recurrence of depression, maternal health, infant bonding) to the mother and child
- For many patients this may mean continuing treatment during pregnancy

Breast Feeding

- Some drug is found in mother's breast milk

✻ Recommended either to discontinue drug or bottle feed

- Immediate postpartum period is a high-risk time for depression, especially in women who have had prior depressive episodes, so drug may need to be reinstituted late in the third trimester or shortly after childbirth to prevent a recurrence during the postpartum period
- Must weigh benefits of breast feeding with risks and benefits of antidepressant treatment versus nontreatment to both the infant and the mother
- For many patients this may mean continuing treatment during breast feeding

THE ART OF PSYCHOPHARMACOLOGY

Potential Advantages

- Patients with insomnia
- Severe or treatment-resistant depression

Potential Disadvantages

- Pediatric and geriatric patients
- Patients concerned with weight gain
- Cardiac patients
- Patients with seizure disorders

Primary Target Symptoms

- Depressed mood
- Chronic pain

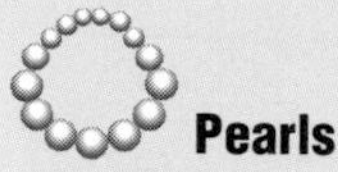

Pearls

- Tricyclic/tetracyclic antidepressants are often a first-line treatment option for chronic pain
- Tricyclic/tetracyclic antidepressants are no longer generally considered a first-line treatment option for depression because of their side effect profile
- Tricyclic/tetracyclic antidepressants continue to be useful for severe or treatment-resistant depression
- ✻ May have somewhat increased risk of seizures compared to some other TCAs, especially at higher doses
- TCAs/tetracyclics may aggravate psychotic symptoms
- Alcohol should be avoided because of additive CNS effects
- Underweight patients may be more susceptible to adverse cardiovascular effects
- Children, patients with inadequate hydration, and patients with cardiac disease may be more susceptible to TCA/tetracyclic-induced cardiotoxicity than healthy adults
- For the expert only: a heroic treatment (but potentially dangerous) for severely treatment-resistant patients is to give simultaneously with monoamine oxidase inhibitors for patients who fail to respond to numerous other antidepressants
- If this option is elected, start the MAOI with the tricyclic/tetracyclic antidepressant simultaneously at low doses after appropriate drug washout, then alternately increase doses of these agents every few days to a week as tolerated
- Although very strict dietary and concomitant drug restrictions must be observed to prevent hypertensive crises and serotonin syndrome, the most common side effects of MAOI/ tricyclic or tetracyclic combinations may be weight gain and orthostatic hypotension
- Patients on tricyclics/tetracyclics should be aware that they may experience symptoms such as photosensitivity or blue-green urine
- SSRIs may be more effective than TCAs/tetracyclics in women, and TCAs/tetracyclics may be more effective than SSRIs in men
- ✻ May have a more rapid onset of action than some other TCAs/tetracyclics
- Since tricyclic/tetracyclic antidepressants are substrates for CYP450 2D6, and 7% of the population (especially Caucasians) may have a genetic variant leading to reduced activity of 2D6, such patients may not safely tolerate normal doses of tricyclic/tetracyclic antidepressants and may require dose reduction
- Phenotypic testing may be necessary to detect this genetic variant prior to dosing with a tricyclic/tetracyclic antidepressant, especially in vulnerable populations such as children, elderly, cardiac populations, and those on concomitant medications
- Patients who seem to have extraordinarily severe side effects at normal or low doses may have this phenotypic CYP450 2D6 variant and require low doses or switching to another antidepressant not metabolized by 2D6

Suggested Reading

Anderson IM. Meta-analytical studies on new antidepressants. Br Med Bull 2001;57:161–78.

Anderson IM. Selective serotonin reuptake inhibitors versus tricyclic antidepressants: a meta-analysis of efficacy and tolerability. J Aff Disorders 2000;58:19–36.

Kane JM, Lieberman J. The efficacy of amoxapine, maprotiline, and trazodone in comparison to imipramine and amitriptyline: a review of the literature. Psychopharmacol Bull 1984;20:240–9.

THERAPEUTICS

Brands • Namenda

see index for additional brand names

Generic? No

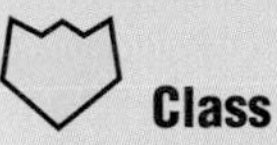

Class

- NMDA receptor antagonist; *N*-methyl-D-aspartate (NMDA) subtype of glutamate receptor antagonist; cognitive enhancer

Commonly Prescribed for

(bold for FDA approved)

- **Alzheimer disease (moderate to severe)**
- Alzheimer disease (mild to moderate)
- Memory disorders in other conditions
- Mild cognitive impairment
- Chronic pain

How the Drug Works

- ✻ Is a low to moderate affinity noncompetitive (open-channel) NMDA receptor antagonist, which binds preferentially to the NMDA receptor-operated cation channels
- Presumably interferes with the postulated persistent activation of NMDA receptors by excessive glutamate release in Alzheimer disease

How Long Until It Works

- Memory improvement is not expected and it may take months before any stabilization in degenerative course is evident

If It Works

- May slow progression of disease, but does not reverse the degenerative process

If It Doesn't Work

- Consider adjusting dose, switching to a cholinesterase inhibitor or adding a cholinesterase inhibitor
- Reconsider diagnosis and rule out other conditions such as depression or a dementia other than Alzheimer disease

Best Augmenting Combos for Partial Response or Treatment Resistance

- ✻ Atypical antipsychotics to reduce behavioral disturbances
- ✻ Antidepressants if concomitant depression, apathy, or lack of interest
- ✻ May be combined with cholinesterase inhibitors
- Divalproex, carbamazepine, or oxcarbazepine for behavioral disturbances

Tests

- None for healthy individuals

SIDE EFFECTS

How Drug Causes Side Effects

- Presumably due to excessive actions at NMDA receptors

Notable Side Effects

- Dizziness, headache
- Constipation

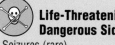

Life-Threatening or Dangerous Side Effects

- Seizures (rare)

Weight Gain

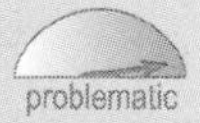

unusual | not unusual | common | problematic

- Reported but not expected

Sedation

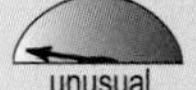
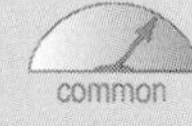
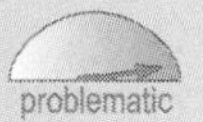

unusual | not unusual | common | problematic

- Reported but not expected
- Fatigue may occur

What to Do About Side Effects

- Wait
- Wait
- Wait
- Consider lowering dose or switching to a different agent

Best Augmenting Agents for Side Effects

- Many side effects cannot be improved with an augmenting agent

DOSING AND USE

Usual Dosage Range

- 10 mg twice daily

Dosage Forms
- Tablet 5 mg, 10 mg
- Oral solution 2 mg/mL

How To Dose
- Initial 5 mg/day; can increase by 5 mg each week; doses over 5 mg should be divided; maximum dose 10 mg twice daily

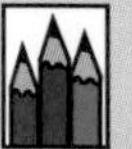

Dosing Tips
* Despite very long half-life, is generally dosed twice daily, although some data suggest once daily is safe and tolerable
- Both the patient and the patient's caregiver should be instructed on how to dose memantine since patients themselves have moderate to severe dementia and may require assistance
* Memantine is unlikely to affect pharmacokinetics of acetylcholinesterase inhibitors
- Absorption not affected by food

Overdose
- No fatalities have been reported; restlessness, psychosis, visual hallucinations, sedation, stupor, loss of consciousness

Long-Term Use
- Drug may lose effectiveness in slowing degenerative course of Alzheimer disease after 6 months

Habit Forming
- No

How to Stop
- No known withdrawal symptoms
- Theoretically, discontinuation could lead to notable deterioration in memory and behavior which may not be restored when drug is restarted or a cholinesterase inhibitor is initiated

Pharmacokinetics
- Little metabolism; mostly excreted unchanged in the urine
- Terminal elimination half-life approximately 60–80 hours
- Minimal inhibition of CYP450 enzymes

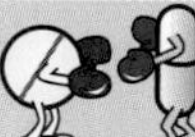

Drug Interactions
- No interactions with drugs metabolized by CYP450 enzymes
- Drugs that raise the urine pH (e.g., carbonic anhydrase inhibitors, sodium bicarbonate) may reduce elimination of memantine and raise plasma levels of memantine
* No interactions with cholinesterase inhibitors

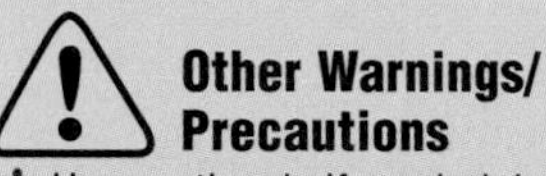

Other Warnings/ Precautions
* Use cautiously if coadministering with other NMDA antagonists such as amantadine, ketamine, and dextromethorphan

Do Not Use
- If there is a proven allergy to memantine

SPECIAL POPULATIONS

Renal Impairment
- Use with caution; dose may need to be reduced
- Not recommended for use in severe renal impairment

Hepatic Impairment
- Not likely to require dosage adjustment

Cardiac Impairment
- Not likely to require dosage adjustment

Elderly
- Pharmacokinetics similar to younger adults

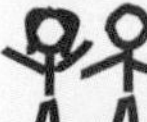

Children and Adolescents
- Memantine use has not been studied in children or adolescents

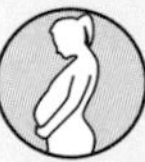

Pregnancy
- Risk Category B [animal studies do not show adverse effects; no controlled studies in humans]
* Not recommended for use in pregnant women or women of childbearing potential

Breast Feeding

- Unknown if memantine is secreted in human breast milk, but all psychotropics assumed to be secreted in breast milk
- ✽ Recommended either to discontinue drug or bottle feed
- Memantine is not recommended for use in nursing women

THE ART OF PSYCHOPHARMACOLOGY

Potential Advantages

- In patients with more advanced Alzheimer disease

Potential Disadvantages

- Unproven to be effective in mild to moderate Alzheimer disease
- Patients who have difficulty taking a medication twice daily

Primary Target Symptoms

- Memory loss in Alzheimer disease
- Behavioral symptoms in Alzheimer disease
- Memory loss in other dementias

Pearls

- ✽ One of only two drugs indicated for moderate to severe Alzheimer disease
- Recently approved in the U.S. but available for many years in other countries (e.g., Germany)
- ✽ Memantine's actions are somewhat like the natural inhibition of NMDA receptors by magnesium, and thus memantine is a sort of "artificial magnesium"
- Theoretically, NMDA antagonism of memantine is strong enough to block chronic low-level overexcitation of glutamate receptors associated with Alzheimer disease, but not strong enough to interfere with periodic high level utilization of glutamate for plasticity, learning, and memory
- Structurally related to the antiparkinsonian and anti-influenza agent amantadine, which is also a weak NMDA antagonist
- ✽ Memantine is well-tolerated with a low incidence of adverse effects
- Antagonist actions at 5HT3 receptors have unknown clinical consequences but may contribute to low incidence of gastrointestinal side effects
- Treat the patient but ask the caregiver about efficacy
- Delay in progression of Alzheimer disease is not evidence of disease-modifying actions of NMDA antagonism
- May or may not be effective in vascular dementia
- Under investigation for dementia associated with HIV/AIDS
- May or may not be effective in chronic neuropathic pain
- ✽ Theoretically, could be useful for any condition characterized by moderate over-activation of NMDA glutamate receptors (possibly neurodegenerative conditions or even bipolar disorder, anxiety disorders, or chronic neuropathic pain), but this is not proven

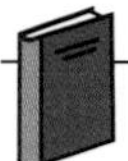

Suggested Reading

Areosa SA, Sherriff F. Memantine for dementia. Cochrane Database Syst Rev 2003;(3):CD003154.

Doggrell S. Is memantine a breakthrough in the treatment of moderate-to-severe Alzheimer's disease? Expert Opin Pharmacother 2003;4:1857–60.

Mobius HJ. Memantine: update on the current evidence. Int J Geriatr Psychiatry 2003;18(Suppl 1):S47–54.

Tariot PN, Federoff HJ. Current treatment for Alzheimer disease and future prospects. Alzheimer Dis Assoc Disord 2003;17 Suppl 4: S105–13.

THERAPEUTICS

Brands • Serentil
• Lidanil

see index for additional brand names

Generic? Yes

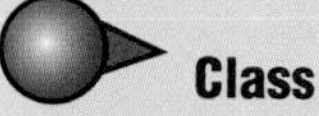

Class

• Conventional antipsychotic (neuroleptic, phenothiazine, dopamine 2 antagonist)

Commonly Prescribed for

(bold for FDA approved)

• **Management of schizophrenic patients who fail to respond adequately to treatment with other antipsychotic drugs**

How the Drug Works

• Blocks dopamine 2 receptors, reducing positive symptoms of psychosis

How Long Until It Works

• Psychotic symptoms can improve within 1 week, but it may take several weeks for full effect on behavior

If It Works

• Is a second-line treatment option

* Should evaluate for switching to an antipsychotic with a better risk/benefit ratio

If It Doesn't Work

• Consider trying one of the first-line atypical antipsychotics (risperidone, olanzapine, quetiapine, ziprasidone, aripiprazole, paliperidone, amisulpride)

• Consider trying another conventional antipsychotic

• If 2 or more antipsychotic monotherapies do not work, consider clozapine

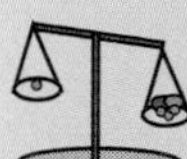

Best Augmenting Combos for Partial Response or Treatment Resistance

• Augmentation of mesoridazine has not been systematically studied and can be dangerous, especially with drugs that can prolong QTc interval

Tests

* Baseline EKG and serum potassium levels should be determined

* Periodic evaluation of EKG and serum potassium levels

• Serum magnesium levels may also need to be monitored

* Since conventional antipsychotics are frequently associated with weight gain, before starting treatment, weigh all patients and determine if the patient is already overweight (BMI 25.0–29.9) or obese (BMI ≥30)

• Before giving a drug that can cause weight gain to an overweight or obese patient, consider determining whether the patient already has pre-diabetes (fasting plasma glucose 100–25 mg/dL), diabetes (fasting plasma glucose >126 mg/dL), or dyslipidemia (increased total cholesterol, LDL cholesterol and triglycerides; decreased HDL cholesterol), and treat or refer such patients for treatment, including nutrition and weight management, physical activity counseling, smoking cessation, and medical management

* Monitor weight and BMI during treatment

* Consider monitoring fasting triglycerides monthly for several months in patients at high risk for metabolic complications and when initiating or switching antipsychotics

* While giving a drug to a patient who has gained >5% of initial weight, consider evaluating for the presence of pre-diabetes, diabetes, or dyslipidemia, or consider switching to a different antipsychotic

• Should check blood pressure in the elderly before starting and for the first few weeks of treatment

• Monitoring elevated prolactin levels of dubious clinical benefit

• Phenothiazines may cause false-positive phenylketonuria results

SIDE EFFECTS

How Drug Causes Side Effects

• By blocking dopamine 2 receptors in the striatum, it can cause motor side effects

• By blocking dopamine 2 receptors in the pituitary, it can cause elevations in prolactin

• By blocking dopamine 2 receptors excessively in the mesocortical and mesolimbic dopamine pathways, especially at high doses, it can cause worsening of

negative and cognitive symptoms (neuroleptic-induced deficit syndrome)
- Anticholinergic actions may cause sedation, blurred vision, constipation, dry mouth
- Antihistaminic actions may cause sedation, weight gain
- By blocking alpha 1 adrenergic receptors, it can cause dizziness, sedation, and hypotension
- Mechanism of weight gain and any possible increased incidence of diabetes or dyslipidemia with conventional antipsychotics is unknown

✻ Mechanism of potentially dangerous QTc prolongation may be related to actions at ion channels

Notable Side Effects

✻ Neuroleptic-induced deficit syndrome
✻ Akathisia
✻ Priapism
✻ Extrapyramidal symptoms, Parkinsonism, tardive dyskinesia
✻ Galactorrhea, amenorrhea
✻ Pigmentary retinopathy at high doses
- Dizziness, sedation
- Dry mouth, constipation, blurred vision
- Decreased sweating
- Sexual dysfunction
- Hypotension
- Weight gain

Life-Threatening or Dangerous Side Effects

- Rare neuroleptic malignant syndrome
- Rare jaundice, agranulocytosis
- Rare seizures

✻ Dose-dependent QTc prolongation
- Ventricular arrhythmias and sudden death
- Increased risk of death and cerebrovascular events in elderly patients with dementia-related psychosis

Weight Gain

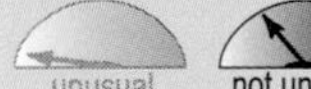

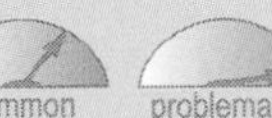

common problematic

- Occurs in significant minority

Sedation

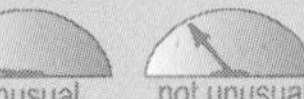

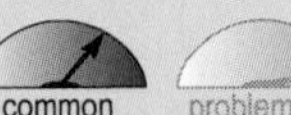

common problematic

- Many experience and/or can be significant in amount
- Sedation is usually transient

What to Do About Side Effects

- Wait
- Wait
- Wait
- For motor symptoms, add an anticholinergic agent
- Reduce the dose
- For sedation, give at night
- Switch to an atypical antipsychotic
- Weight loss, exercise programs, and medical management for high BMIs, diabetes, dyslipidemia

Best Augmenting Agents for Side Effects

- Augmentation of mesoridazine has not been systematically studied and can be dangerous

DOSING AND USE

Usual Dosage Range

- Oral: 100–400 mg/day
- Injection: 25–200 mg/day

Dosage Forms

- Tablet 10 mg, 25 mg, 50 mg, 100 mg
- Ampul 25 mg/mL, 1 mL
- Concentrate 25 mg/mL

How To Dose

- Oral: initial 50 mg 3 times a day; increase dose cautiously as needed
- Injection: initial 25 mg; repeat after 30–60 minutes if needed
- Take liquid formulation in water, orange juice, or grapefruit juice

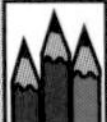

Dosing Tips

✻ The effects of mesoridazine on the QTc interval are dose-dependent, so start low and go slow while carefully monitoring QTc interval

Overdose

- Deaths have occurred; sedation, confusion, agitation, respiratory depression, cardiac disturbances, coma

Long-Term Use
- Some side effects may be irreversible (e.g., tardive dyskinesia)

Habit Forming
- No

How to Stop
- Slow down-titration of oral formulation (over 6–8 weeks), especially when simultaneously beginning a new antipsychotic while switching (i.e., cross-titration)
- Rapid oral discontinuation may lead to rebound psychosis and worsening of symptoms
- If antiparkinson agents are being used, they should be continued for a few weeks after mesoridazine is discontinued

Pharmacokinetics
- Half-life approximately 2–9 hours

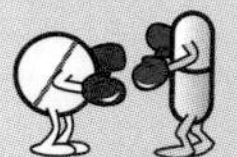

Drug Interactions
- May decrease the effects of levodopa, dopamine agonists
- May increase the effects of antihypertensive drugs
- May enhance QTc prolongation of other drugs capable of prolonging QTc interval
- Additive effects may occur if used with CNS depressants
- Respiratory depression or respiratory arrest may occur if mesoridazine is used with a barbiturate
- Some patients taking a neuroleptic and lithium have developed an encephalopathic syndrome similar to neuroleptic malignant syndrome
- Combined use with epinephrine may lower blood pressure

Other Warnings/ Precautions
- If signs of neuroleptic malignant syndrome develop, treatment should be immediately discontinued
- Use with caution in patients with respiratory disorders, glaucoma, or urinary retention
- Use cautiously in patients with alcohol withdrawal or convulsive disorders because of possible lowering of seizure threshold
- Use with caution if at all in Parkinson's disease or Lewy body dementia
- Avoid extreme heat exposure
- Antiemetic effect can mask signs of other disorders or overdose
- Do not use epinephrine in event of overdose as interaction with some pressor agents may lower blood pressure
- Because mesoridazine may dose-dependently prolong QTc interval, use with caution in patients who have bradycardia or who are taking drugs that can induce bradycardia (e.g., beta blockers, calcium channel blockers, clonidine, digitalis)
- Because mesoridazine may dose-dependently prolong QTc interval, use with caution in patients who have hypokalemia and/or hypomagnesemia or who are taking drugs that can induce hypokalemia and/or magnesemia (e.g., diuretics, stimulant laxatives, intravenous amphotericin B, glucocorticoids, tetracosactide)
- Mesoridazine can increase the QTc interval, potentially causing torsades de pointes-type arrhythmia or sudden death

Do Not Use
- If there is a history of QTc prolongation or cardiac arrhythmia, recent acute myocardial infarction, uncompensated heart failure
- ✻ If QTc interval greater than 450 msec or if taking an agent capable of prolonging the QTc interval
- If patient is in a comatose state or has CNS depression
- If there is a proven allergy to mesoridazine
- If there is a known sensitivity to any phenothiazine

SPECIAL POPULATIONS

Renal Impairment
- Use with caution

Hepatic Impairment
- Use with caution

Cardiac Impairment
- Mesoridazine produces a dose-dependent prolongation of QTc interval, which may be enhanced by the existence of bradycardia,

hypokalemia, congenital or acquired long QTc interval, which should be evaluated prior to administering mesoridazine
- Use with caution if treating concomitantly with a medication likely to produce prolonged bradycardia, hypokalemia, slowing of intracardiac conduction, or prolongation of the QTc interval
- Avoid mesoridazine in patients with a known history of QTc prolongation, recent acute myocardial infarction, and uncompensated heart failure

✲ Risk/benefit ratio may not justify use in cardiac impairment

Elderly
- Lower doses should be used and patient should be monitored closely
- Although conventional antipsychotics are commonly used for behavioral disturbances in dementia, no agent has been approved for treatment of elderly patients with dementia-related psychosis
- Elderly patients with dementia-related psychosis treated with antipsychotics are at an increased risk of death compared to placebo, and also have an increased risk of cerebrovascular events

Children and Adolescents
- Safety and efficacy not established

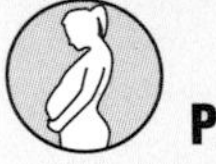

Pregnancy
- Risk Category C [some animal studies show adverse effects; no controlled studies in humans]
- Reports of extrapyramidal symptoms, jaundice, hyperreflexia, hyporeflexia in infants whose mothers took a phenothiazine during pregnancy
- Psychotic symptoms may worsen during pregnancy and some form of treatment may be necessary
- Atypical antipsychotics may be preferable to conventional antipsychotics or anticonvulsant mood stabilizers if treatment is required during pregnancy
- Mesoridazine should generally not be used during the first trimester
- Should evaluate for an antipsychotic with a better risk/benefit ratio if treatment is required during pregnancy

Breast Feeding
- Some drug is found in mother's breast milk
- Effects on infant have been observed (dystonia, tardive dyskinesia, sedation)

✲ Recommended either to discontinue drug or bottle feed

THE ART OF PSYCHOPHARMACOLOGY

Potential Advantages
- Only for patients who respond to this agent and not other antipsychotics

Potential Disadvantages
- Vulnerable populations such as children or elderly
- Patients on other drugs

Primary Target Symptoms
- Positive symptoms of psychosis in patients who fail to respond to treatment with other antipsychotics
- Motor and autonomic hyperactivity in patients who fail to respond to treatment with other antipsychotics
- Violent or aggressive behavior in patients who fail to respond to treatment with other antipsychotics

Pearls

✲ Generally, the benefits of mesoridazine do not outweigh its risks for most patients

✲ Because of its effects on the QTc interval, mesoridazine is not intended for use unless other options (at least 2 antipsychotics) have failed

- Mesoridazine has not been systematically studied in treatment-refractory schizophrenia
- Conventional antipsychotics are much less expensive than atypical antipsychotics

Suggested Reading

Frankenburg FR. Choices in antipsychotic therapy in schizophrenia. Harv Rev Psychiatry 1999;6:241–9.

Gardos G, Tecce JJ, Hartmann E, Bowers P, Cole JO. Treatment with mesoridazine and thioridazine in chronic schizophrenia: II. Potential predictors of drug response. Compr Psychiatry 1978;19:527–32.

Gershon S, Sakalis G, Bowers PA. Mesoridazine–a pharmacodynamic and pharmacokinetic profile. J Clin Psychiatry 1981;42:463–9.

METHYLPHENIDATE (D)

THERAPEUTICS

Brands
- Focalin
- Focalin XR

see index for additional brand names

Generic? Yes

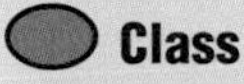 **Class**
- Stimulant

Commonly Prescribed for
(bold for FDA approved)
- **Attention deficit hyperactivity disorder (ADHD) in children ages 6–17 (Focalin, Focalin XR) and in adults (Focalin XR)**
- Narcolepsy
- Treatment-resistant depression

How the Drug Works
✻ Increases norepinephrine and especially dopamine actions by blocking their reuptake
- Enhancement of dopamine and norepinephrine actions in certain brain regions (e.g., dorsolateral prefrontal cortex) may improve attention, concentration, executive function, and wakefulness
- Enhancement of dopamine actions in other brain regions (e.g., basal ganglia) may improve hyperactivity
- Enhancement of dopamine and norepinephrine in yet other brain regions (e.g., medial prefrontal cortex, hypothalamus) may improve depression, fatigue, and sleepiness

How Long Until It Works
- Some immediate effects can be seen with first dosing
- Can take several weeks to attain maximum therapeutic benefit

If It Works (for ADHD)
- The goal of treatment of ADHD is reduction of symptoms of inattentiveness, motor hyperactivity, and/or impulsiveness that disrupt social, school, and/or occupational functioning
- Continue treatment until all symptoms are under control or improvement is stable and then continue treatment indefinitely as long as improvement persists
- Reevaluate the need for treatment periodically
- Treatment for ADHD begun in childhood may need to be continued into adolescence and adulthood if continued benefit is documented

If It Doesn't Work (for ADHD)
- Consider adjusting dose or switching to a formulation of d,l-methylphenidate or to another agent
- Consider behavioral therapy
- Consider the presence of noncompliance and counsel patient and parents
- Consider evaluation for another diagnosis or for a comorbid condition (e.g., bipolar disorder, substance abuse, medical illness, etc.)

✻ Some ADHD patients and some depressed patients may experience lack of consistent efficacy due to activation of latent or underlying bipolar disorder, and require either augmenting with a mood stabilizer or switching to a mood stabilizer

Best Augmenting Combos for Partial Response or Treatment Resistance
✻ Best to attempt other monotherapies prior to augmenting
- For the expert, can combine immediate-release formulation of d-methylphenidate with a sustained-release formulation of d-methylphenidate for ADHD
- For the expert, can combine with modafinil or atomoxetine for ADHD
- For the expert, can occasionally combine with atypical antipsychotics in highly treatment-resistant cases of bipolar disorder or ADHD
- For the expert, can combine with antidepressants to boost antidepressant efficacy in highly treatment-resistant cases of depression while carefully monitoring patient

Tests
- Blood pressure should be monitored regularly
- In children, monitor weight and height
- Periodic complete blood cell and platelet counts may be considered during prolonged therapy (rare leukopenia and/or anemia)

SIDE EFFECTS

How Drug Causes Side Effects

- Increases in norepinephrine peripherally can cause autonomic side effects, including tremor, tachycardia, hypertension, and cardiac arrhythmias
- Increases in norepinephrine and dopamine centrally can cause CNS side effects such as insomnia, agitation, psychosis, and substance abuse

Notable Side Effects

✱ Insomnia, headache, exacerbation of tics, nervousness, irritability, overstimulation, tremor, dizziness
- Anorexia, nausea, abdominal pain, weight loss
- Can temporarily slow normal growth in children (controversial)
- Blurred vision

Life-Threatening or Dangerous Side Effects

- Psychotic episodes, especially with parenteral abuse
- Seizures
- Palpitations, tachycardia, hypertension
- Rare neuroleptic malignant syndrome
- Rare activation of hypomania, mania, or suicidal ideation (controversial)
- Cardiovascular adverse effects, sudden death in patients with preexisting cardiac structural abnormalities

Weight Gain

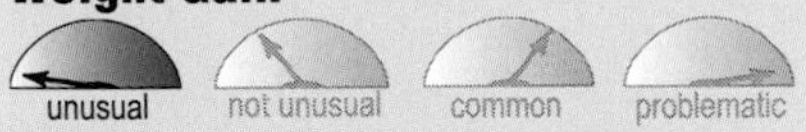

- Reported but not expected
- Some patients may experience weight loss

Sedation

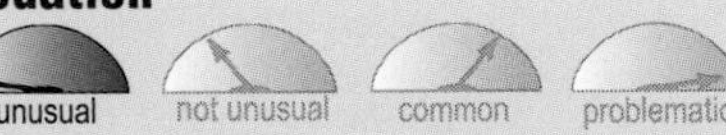

- Reported but not expected
- Activation much more common than sedation

What to Do About Side Effects

- Wait
- Adjust dose
- Switch to a formulation of d,l-methylphenidate
- Switch to another agent
- For insomnia, avoid dosing in afternoon/evening

Best Augmenting Agents for Side Effects

- Betablockers for peripheral autonomic side effects
- Dose reduction or switching to another agent may be more effective since most side effects cannot be improved with an augmenting agent

DOSING AND USE

Usual Dosage Range

- 2.5–10 mg twice per day

Dosage Forms

- Tablet 2.5 mg, 5 mg, 10 mg
- Extended-release capsule 5 mg, 10 mg, 20 mg

How To Dose

- Immediate-release: for patients who are not taking racemic d,l-methylphenidate, initial 2.5 mg twice per day in 4-hour intervals; may adjust dose in weekly intervals by 2.5–5 mg/day; maximum dose generally 10 mg twice per day
- Immediate-release: for patients currently taking racemic d,l-methylphenidate, initial dose should be half the current dose of racemic d,l-methylphenidate; maximum dose generally 10 mg twice per day
- Extended-release: for children, same titration schedule as immediate-release but dosed once in the morning
- Extended-release: for adults not taking racemic d,l-methylphenidate, initial 10 mg/day in the morning; may adjust dose in weekly intervals by 10 mg/day; maximum dose generally 20 mg/day

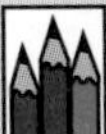

Dosing Tips

✱ Immediate-release d-methylphenidate has the same onset of action and duration of action as immediate-release racemic d,l-methylphenidate (i.e., 2–4 hours) but at half the dose
- Extended-release d-methylphenidate contains half the dose as immediate-

release beads and half as delayed-release beads, so the dose is released in 2 pulses
- Although d-methylphenidate is generally considered to be twice as potent as racemic d,l-methylphenidate, some studies suggest that the d-isomer is actually more than twice as effective as racemic d,l-methylphenidate
- Side effects are generally dose-related
- Off-label uses are dosed the same as for ADHD

✻ May be possible to dose only during the school week for some ADHD patients

✻ May be able to give drug holidays over the summer in order to reassess therapeutic utility and effects on growth and to allow catch-up from any growth suppression as well as to assess any other side effects and the need to reinstitute stimulant treatment for the next school term

- Avoid dosing late in the day because of the risk of insomnia
- Taking with food may delay peak actions for 2–3 hours

Overdose

- Vomiting, tremor, coma, convulsion, hyperreflexia, euphoria, confusion, hallucination, tachycardia, flushing, palpitations, sweating, hyperpyrexia, hypertension, arrhythmia, mydriasis, agitation, delirium, headache

Long-Term Use

- Often used long-term for ADHD when ongoing monitoring documents continued efficacy
- Dependence and/or abuse may develop
- Tolerance to therapeutic effects may develop in some patients
- Long-term stimulant use may be associated with growth suppression in children (controversial)
- Periodic monitoring of weight, blood pressure, CBC, platelet counts, and liver function may be prudent

Habit Forming

- High abuse potential, Schedule II drug
- Patients may develop tolerance, psychological dependence

How to Stop

- Taper to avoid withdrawal effects
- Withdrawal following chronic therapeutic use may unmask symptoms of the underlying disorder and may require follow-up and reinstitution of treatment
- Careful supervision is required during withdrawal from abusive use since severe depression may occur

Pharmacokinetics

- d-*threo*-enantiomer of racemic d,l-methylphenidate
- Mean plasma elimination half-life approximately 2.2 hours (same as d,l-methylphenidate)
- Does not inhibit CYP450 enzymes

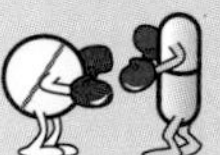

Drug Interactions

- May affect blood pressure and should be used cautiously with agents used to control blood pressure
- May inhibit metabolism of SSRIs, anticonvulsants (phenobarbital, phenytoin, primidone), tricyclic antidepressants, and coumarin anticoagulants, requiring downward dosage adjustments of these drugs
- Serious adverse effects may occur if combined with clonidine (controversial)
- Use with MAOIs, including within 14 days of MAOI use, is not advised, but this can sometimes be considered by experts who monitor depressed patients closely when other treatment options for depression fail
- CNS and cardiovascular actions of d-methylphenidate could theoretically be enhanced by combination with agents that block norepinephrine reuptake, such as the tricyclic antidepressants desipramine or protriptyline, venlafaxine, duloxetine, atomoxetine, milnacipran, and reboxetine
- Theoretically, antipsychotics should inhibit the stimulatory effects of d-methylphenidate
- Theoretically, d-methylphenidate could inhibit the antipsychotic actions of antipsychotics
- Theoretically, d-methylphenidate could inhibit the mood-stabilizing actions of atypical antipsychotics in some patients
- Combinations of d-methylphenidate with mood-stabilizers (lithium, anticonvulsants, atypical antipsychotics) is generally something for experts only, when

monitoring patients closely and when other options fail

Other Warnings/ Precautions

- Use with caution in patients with any degree of hypertension, hyperthyroidism, or history of drug abuse
- Children who are not growing or gaining weight should stop treatment, at least temporarily
- May worsen motor and phonic tics
- May worsen symptoms of thought disorder and behavioral disturbance in psychotic patients
- Stimulants have a high potential for abuse and must be used with caution in anyone with a current or past history of substance abuse or alcoholism or in emotionally unstable patients
- Administration of stimulants for prolonged periods of time should be avoided whenever possible or done only with close monitoring, as it may lead to marked tolerance and drug dependence, including psychological dependence with varying degrees of abnormal behavior
- Particular attention should be paid to the possibility of subjects obtaining stimulants for nontherapeutic use or distribution to others and the drugs should in general be prescribed sparingly with documentation of appropriate use
- Unusual dosing has been associated with sudden death in children with structural cardiac abnormalities
- Not an appropriate first-line treatment for depression or for normal fatigue
- May lower the seizure threshold
- Emergence or worsening of activation and agitation may represent the induction of a bipolar state, especially a mixed dysphoric bipolar II condition sometimes associated with suicidal ideation, and require the addition of a mood stabilizer and/or discontinuation of d-methylphenidate

Do Not Use

- If patient has extreme anxiety or agitation
- If patient has motor tics or Tourette's syndrome or if there is a family history of Tourette's, unless administered by an expert in cases when the potential benefits for ADHD outweigh the risks of worsening tics
- Should generally not be administered with an MAOI, including within 14 days of MAOI use, except in heroic circumstances and by an expert
- If patient has glaucoma
- If patient has structural cardiac abnormalities
- If there is a proven allergy to methylphenidate

SPECIAL POPULATIONS

Renal Impairment

- No dose adjustment necessary

Hepatic Impairment

- No dose adjustment necessary

Cardiac Impairment

- Use with caution, particularly in patients with recent myocardial infarction or other conditions that could be negatively affected by increased blood pressure
- Do not use in patients with structural cardiac abnormalities

Elderly

- Some patients may tolerate lower doses better

Children and Adolescents

- Safety and efficacy not established in children under age 6
- Use in young children should be reserved for the expert
- Methylphenidate has acute effects on growth hormone; long-term effects are unknown but weight and height should be monitored during long-term treatment
- American Heart Association recommends EKG prior to initiating stimulant treatment in children, although not all experts agree

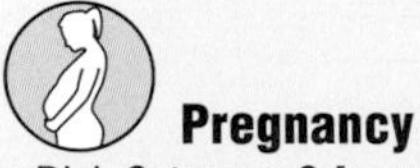

Pregnancy

- Risk Category C [some animal studies show adverse effects; no controlled studies in humans]

- Infants whose mothers took methylphenidate during pregnancy may experience withdrawal symptoms
- Use in women of childbearing potential requires weighing potential benefits to the mother against potential risks to the fetus

✻ For ADHD patients, methylphenidate should generally be discontinued before anticipated pregnancies

Breast Feeding

- Unknown if methylphenidate is secreted in human breast milk, but all psychotropics assumed to be secreted in breast milk

✻ Recommended either to discontinue drug or bottle feed

- If infant shows signs of irritability, drug may need to be discontinued

THE ART OF PSYCHOPHARMACOLOGY

Potential Advantages

- The active d enantiomer of methylphenidate may be slightly more than twice as efficacious as racemic d,l-methylphenidate

Potential Disadvantages

- Patients with current or past substance abuse, bipolar disorder, or psychosis

Primary Target Symptoms

- Concentration, attention span
- Motor hyperactivity
- Impulsiveness
- Physical and mental fatigue
- Daytime sleepiness
- Depression

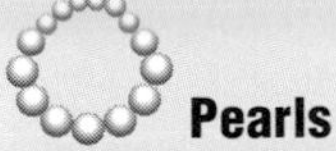

Pearls

- May be useful for treatment of depressive symptoms in medically ill elderly patients
- May be useful for treatment of post-stroke depression
- A classical augmentation strategy for treatment-refractory depression
- Specifically, may be useful for treatment of cognitive dysfunction and fatigue as residual symptoms of major depressive disorder unresponsive to multiple prior treatments
- May also be useful for the treatment of cognitive impairment, depressive symptoms, and severe fatigue in patients with HIV infection and in cancer patients
- Can be used to potentiate opioid analgesia and reduce sedation, particularly in end-of-life management
- Atypical antipsychotics may be useful in treating stimulant or psychotic consequences of overdose
- Some patients respond to or tolerate methylphenidate better than amphetamine, and vice versa
- Taking with food may delay peak actions of immediate-release d-methylphenidate for 2–3 hours
- Half-life and duration of clinical action tend to be shorter in younger children
- Drug abuse may actually be lower in ADHD adolescents treated with stimulants than in ADHD adolescents who are not treated
- New extended-release formulation is truly a once daily dose
- Extended-release capsule can be sprinkled over applesauce for patients unable to swallow the capsule
- Some patients may benefit from an occasional addition of an immediate-release dose of d-methylphenidate to the daily base dose of extended-release d-methylphenidate

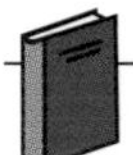

Suggested Reading

Dexmethylphenidate—Novartis/Celgene. Focalin, D-MPH, D-methylphenidate hydrochloride, D-methylphenidate, dexmethylphenidate, dexmethylphenidate hydrochloride. Drugs R D 2002;3(4):279–82.

Keating GM, Figgitt DP. Dexmethylphenidate. Drugs 2002;62(13):1899–904.

THERAPEUTICS

Brands
- Concerta
- Metadate CD
- Ritalin
- Ritalin LA
- Daytrana

see index for additional brand names

Generic? Yes (for immediate-release methylphenidate)

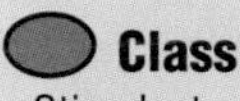

Class
- Stimulant

Commonly Prescribed for
(bold for FDA approved)
- **Attention deficit hyperactivity disorder (ADHD) in children and adults (approved ages vary based on formulation)**
- **Narcolepsy (Metadate ER, Methylin ER, Ritalin, Ritalin SR)**
- Treatment-resistant depression

How the Drug Works
* Increases norepinephrine and especially dopamine actions by blocking their reuptake
- Enhancement of dopamine and norepinephrine actions in certain brain regions (e.g., dorsolateral prefrontal cortex) may improve attention, concentration, executive function, and wakefulness
- Enhancement of dopamine actions in other brain regions (e.g., basal ganglia) may improve hyperactivity
- Enhancement of dopamine and norepinephrine in yet other brain regions (e.g., medial prefrontal cortex, hypothalamus) may improve depression, fatigue, and sleepiness

How Long Until It Works
- Some immediate effects can be seen with first dosing
- Can take several weeks to attain maximum therapeutic benefit

If It Works (for ADHD)
- The goal of treatment of ADHD is reduction of symptoms of inattentiveness, motor hyperactivity, and/or impulsiveness that disrupt social, school, and/or occupational functioning
- Continue treatment until all symptoms are under control or improvement is stable and then continue treatment indefinitely as long as improvement persists
- Reevaluate the need for treatment periodically
- Treatment for ADHD begun in childhood may need to be continued into adolescence and adulthood if continued benefit is documented

If It Doesn't Work (for ADHD)
- Consider adjusting dose or switching to another formulation of d,l-methylphenidate or to another agent
- Consider behavioral therapy
- Consider the presence of noncompliance and counsel patient and parents
- Consider evaluation for another diagnosis or for a comorbid condition (e.g., bipolar disorder, substance abuse, medical illness, etc.)

* Some ADHD patients and some depressed patients may experience lack of consistent efficacy due to activation of latent or underlying bipolar disorder, and require either augmenting with a mood stabilizer or switching to a mood stabilizer

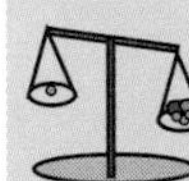

Best Augmenting Combos for Partial Response or Treatment Resistance
* Best to attempt other monotherapies prior to augmenting
- For the expert, can combine immediate-release formulation with a sustained-release formulation of d,l-methylphenidate for ADHD
- For the expert, can combine with modafinil or atomoxetine for ADHD
- For the expert, can occasionally combine with atypical antipsychotics in highly treatment-resistant cases of bipolar disorder or ADHD
- For the expert, can combine with antidepressants to boost antidepressant efficacy in highly treatment-resistant cases of depression while carefully monitoring patient

Tests
- Blood pressure should be monitored regularly

- In children, monitor weight and height
- Periodic complete blood cell and platelet counts may be considered during prolonged therapy (rare leukopenia and/or anemia)

SIDE EFFECTS

How Drug Causes Side Effects

- Increases in norepinephrine peripherally can cause autonomic side effects, including tremor, tachycardia, hypertension, and cardiac arrhythmias
- Increases in norepinephrine and dopamine centrally can cause CNS side effects such as insomnia, agitation, psychosis, and substance abuse

Notable Side Effects

✽ Insomnia, headache, exacerbation of tics, nervousness, irritability, overstimulation, tremor, dizziness
- Anorexia, nausea, abdominal pain, weight loss
- Can temporarily slow normal growth in children (controversial)
- Blurred vision
- Transdermal: application site reactions, including contact sensitization (erythema, edema, papules, vesicles)

Life-Threatening or Dangerous Side Effects

- Psychotic episodes, especially with parenteral abuse
- Seizures
- Palpitations, tachycardia, hypertension
- Rare neuroleptic malignant syndrome
- Rare activation of hypomania, mania, or suicidal ideation (controversial)
- Cardiovascular adverse effects, sudden death in patients with preexisting cardiac structural abnormalities

Weight Gain

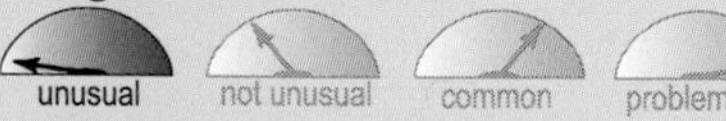

- Reported but not expected
- Some patients may experience weight loss

Sedation

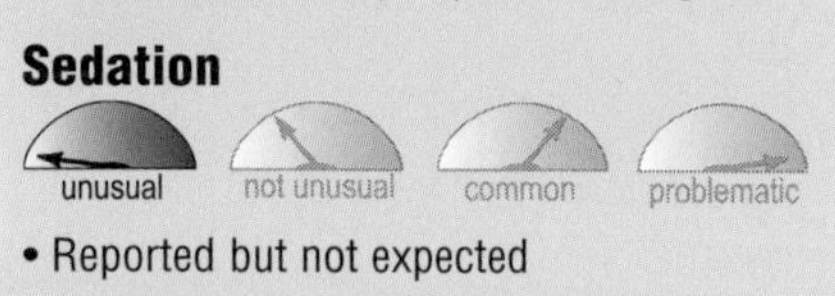

- Reported but not expected
- Activation much more common than sedation

What to Do About Side Effects

- Wait
- Adjust dose
- Switch to another formulation of d,l-methylphenidate
- Switch to another agent
- For insomnia, avoid dosing in afternoon/evening

Best Augmenting Agents for Side Effects

- Betablockers for peripheral autonomic side effects
- Dose reduction or switching to another agent may be more effective since most side effects cannot be improved with an augmenting agent

DOSING AND USE

Usual Dosage Range

- ADHD (oral): up to 2 mg/kg per day in children 6 years and older, with a maximum daily dose of 60 mg/day; in adults usually 20–30 mg/day, but may use up to 40–60 mg/day
- ADHD (transdermal): 10–30 mg/9 hours
- Narcolepsy: 20–60 mg/day in 2–3 divided doses

Dosage Forms

- Immediate-release tablets 5 mg, 10 mg, 20 mg (Ritalin, Methylin, generic methylphenidate)
- Immediate-release chewable tablets 2.5 mg, 5 mg, 10 mg
- Oral solution 5 mg/mL, 10 mg/5 mL
- Older sustained-release tablets 10 mg, 20 mg (Metadate ER, Methylin ER); 20 mg (Ritalin SR)

✽ Newer sustained-release capsules 20 mg, 30 mg, 40 mg (Ritalin LA); 10 mg, 20 mg, 30 mg (Metadate CD)

✽ Newer sustained-release tablets 18 mg, 27 mg, 36 mg, 54 mg (Concerta)
- Transdermal patch 27 mg/12.5 cm^2 (10 mg/9 hours), 41.3 mg/18.75 cm^2 (15 mg/9 hours), 55 mg/25 cm^2 (20 mg/9 hours), 82.5 mg/37.5 cm^2 (30 mg/9 hours)

How To Dose

- Immediate-release Ritalin, Methylin, and generic methylphenidate (2–4 hour duration of action)
  - ADHD: initial 5 mg in morning, 5 mg at lunch; can increase by 5–10 mg each week; maximum dose generally 60 mg/day
  - Narcolepsy: give each dose 30–45 minutes before meals; maximum dose generally 60 mg/day
- Older extended-release Ritalin SR, Methylin SR, and Metadate ER
  - These formulations have a duration of action of approximately 4–6 hours; therefore, these formulations may be used in place of immediate-release formulations when the 4–6 hour dosage of these sustained-release formulations corresponds to the titrated 4–6 hour dosage of the immediate-release formulation
  - Average dose is 20–30 mg/day, usually in 2 divided doses
- ✻ Newer sustained-release formulations for ADHD
  - Concerta (up to 12 hours duration of action): initial 18 mg/day in morning; can increase by 18 mg each week; maximum dose generally 72 mg/day
  - Ritalin LA and Metadate CD (up to 8 hours duration of action): initial 20 mg once daily; dosage may be adjusted in weekly 10-mg increments to a maximum of 60 mg/day taken in the morning
- ✻ Transdermal formulation for ADHD
  - Initial 10 mg/9 hours; can increase by 5 mg/9 hours every week; maximum dose generally 30 mg/9 hours
  - Patch should be applied 2 hours before effect is needed and should be worn for 9 hours
  - Patients should follow the same titration schedule when they are naive to methylphenidate or are switching from another formulation
- oral formulations

Dosing Tips

- Clinical duration of action often differs from pharmacokinetic half-life
- Taking oral formulations with food may delay peak actions for 2–3 hours
- ✻ Immediate-release formulations (Ritalin, Methylin, generic methylphenidate) have 2–4 hour durations of clinical action
- ✻ Older sustained-release formulations such as Methylin ER, Ritalin SR, Metadate ER, and generic methylphenidate sustained-release all have approximately 4–6 hour durations of clinical action, which for most patients is generally not long enough for once daily dosing in the morning and thus generally requires lunchtime dosing at school
- ✻ The newer sustained-release Metadate CD has an early peak and an 8-hour duration of action
- ✻ The newer sustained-release Ritalin LA also has an early peak and an 8-hour duration of action, with 2 pulses (immediate and after 4 hours)
- ✻ The newer sustained-release Concerta trilayer tablet has longest duration of action (12 hours)
- Sustained-release formulations (especially Concerta, Metadate CD, and Ritalin LA) should not be chewed but rather should only be swallowed whole
- ✻ All 3 newer sustained-release formulations have a sufficiently long duration of clinical action to eliminate the need for a lunchtime dosing if taken in the morning
- ✻ This innovation can be an important practical element in stimulant utilization, eliminating the hassle and pragmatic difficulties of lunchtime dosing at school, including storage problems, potential diversion, and the need for a medical professional to supervise dosing away from home
- Off-label uses are dosed the same as for ADHD
- ✻ May be possible to dose only during the school week for some ADHD patients
- ✻ May be able to give drug holidays over the summer in order to reassess therapeutic utility and effects on growth and to allow catch-up from any growth suppression as well as to assess any other side effects and the need to reinstitute stimulant treatment for the next school term
- Avoid dosing late in the day because of the risk of insomnia

- Concerta tablet does not change shape in the GI tract and generally should not be used in patients with gastrointestinal narrowing because of the risk of intestinal obstruction
- Side effects are generally dose-related
- Transdermal patch should be applied to dry, intact skin on the hip
- New application site should be selected for each day; only one patch should be applied at a time; patches should not be cut
- Avoid touching the exposed (sticky) side of the patch, and after application, wash hands with soap and water; do not touch eyes until after hands have been washed
- Heat can increase the amount of methylphenidate absorbed from the transdermal patch, so patients should avoid exposing the application site to external source of direct heat (e.g., heating pads, prolonged direct sunlight)
- If a patch comes off a new patch may be applied at a different site; total daily wear time should remain 9 hours regardless of number of patches used
- Early removal of transdermal patch can be useful to terminate drug action when desired

Overdose

- Vomiting, tremor, coma, convulsion, hyperreflexia, euphoria, confusion, hallucination, tachycardia, flushing, palpitations, sweating, hyperprexia, hypertension, arrhythmia, mydriasis

Long-Term Use

- Often used long-term for ADHD when ongoing monitoring documents continued efficacy
- Dependence and/or abuse may develop
- Tolerance to therapeutic effects may develop in some patients
- Long-term stimulant use may be associated with growth suppression in children (controversial)
- Periodic monitoring of weight, blood pressure, CBC, platelet counts, and liver function may be prudent

Habit Forming

- High abuse potential, Schedule II drug
- Patients may develop tolerance, psychological dependence

How to Stop

- Taper to avoid withdrawal effects
- Withdrawal following chronic therapeutic use may unmask symptoms of the underlying disorder and may require follow-up and reinstitution of treatment
- Careful supervision is required during withdrawal from abusive use since severe depression may occur

Pharmacokinetics

- Average half-life in adults is 3.5 hours (1.3–7.7 hours)
- Average half-life in children is 2.5 hours (1.5–5 hours)
- First-pass metabolism is not extensive with transdermal dosing, thus resulting in notably higher exposure to methylphenidate and lower exposure to metabolites as compared to oral dosing

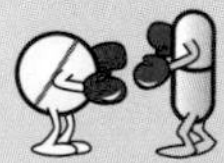

Drug Interactions

- May affect blood pressure and should be used cautiously with agents used to control blood pressure
- May inhibit metabolism of SSRIs, anticonvulsants (phenobarbital, phenytoin, primidone), tricyclic antidepressants, and coumarin anticoagulants, requiring downward dosage adjustments of these drugs
- Serious adverse effects may occur if combined with clonidine (controversial)
- Use with MAOIs, including within 14 days of MAOI use, is not advised, but this can sometimes be considered by experts who monitor depressed patients closely when other treatment options for depression fail
- CNS and cardiovascular actions of d,l-methylphenidate could theoretically be enhanced by combination with agents that block norepinephrine reuptake, such as the tricyclic antidepressants desipramine or protriptyline, venlafaxine, duloxetine, atomoxetine, milnacipran, and reboxetine
- Theoretically, antipsychotics should inhibit the stimulatory effects of d,l-methylphenidate
- Theoretically, d,l-methylphenidate could inhibit the antipsychotic actions of antipsychotics
- Theoretically, d,l-methylphenidate could inhibit the mood-stabilizing actions of atypical antipsychotics in some patients

- Combination of d,l-methylphenidate with mood stabilizers (lithium, anticonvulsants, atypical antipsychotics) is generally something for experts only, when monitoring patients closely and when other options fail

Other Warnings/ Precautions

- Use with caution in patients with any degree of hypertension, hyperthyroidism, or history of drug abuse
- Children who are not growing or gaining weight should stop treatment, at least temporarily
- May worsen motor and phonic tics
- May worsen symptoms of thought disorder and behavioral disturbance in psychotic patients
- Stimulants have a high potential for abuse and must be used with caution in anyone with a current or past history of substance abuse or alcoholism or in emotionally unstable patients
- Administration of stimulants for prolonged periods of time should be avoided whenever possible or done only with close monitoring, as it may lead to marked tolerance and drug dependence, including psychological dependence with varying degrees of abnormal behavior
- Particular attention should be paid to the possibility of subjects obtaining stimulants for nontherapeutic use or distribution to others and the drugs should in general be prescribed sparingly with documentation of appropriate use
- Unusual dosing has been associated with sudden death in children with structural cardiac abnormalities
- Not an appropriate first-line treatment for depression or for normal fatigue
- May lower the seizure threshold
- Emergence or worsening of activation and agitation may represent the induction of a bipolar state, especially a mixed dysphoric bipolar II condition sometimes associated with suicidal ideation, and require the addition of a mood stabilizer and/or discontinuation of d,l-methylphenidate

Do Not Use

- If patient has extreme anxiety or agitation
- If patient has motor tics or Tourette's syndrome or if there is a family history of Tourette's, unless administered by an expert in cases when the potential benefits for ADHD outweigh the risks of worsening tics
- Should generally not be administered with an MAOI, including within 14 days of MAOI use, except in heroic circumstances and by an expert
- If patient has glaucoma
- If patient has structural cardiac abnormalities
- If there is a proven allergy to methylphenidate

SPECIAL POPULATIONS

Renal Impairment

- No dose adjustment necessary

Hepatic Impairment

- No dose adjustment necessary

Cardiac Impairment

- Use with caution, particularly in patients with recent myocardial infarction or other conditions that could be negatively affected by increased blood pressure
- Do not use in patients with structural cardiac abnormalities

Elderly

- Some patients may tolerate lower doses better

Children and Adolescents

- Safety and efficacy not established in children under age 6
- Use in young children should be reserved for the expert
- Methylphenidate has acute effects on growth hormone; long-term effects are unknown but weight and height should be monitored during long-term treatment
- American Heart Association recommends EKG prior to initiating stimulant treatment in children, although not all experts agree

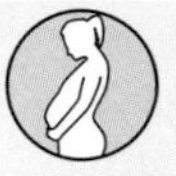

Pregnancy

- Risk Category C [some animal studies show adverse effects; no controlled studies in humans]
- Infants whose mothers took methylphenidate during pregnancy may experience withdrawal symptoms
- Use in women of childbearing potential requires weighing potential benefits to the mother against potential risks to the fetus

✽ For ADHD patients, methylphenidate should generally be discontinued before anticipated pregnancies

Breast Feeding

- Unknown if methylphenidate is secreted in human breast milk, but all psychotropics assumed to be secreted in breast milk

✽ Recommended either to discontinue drug or bottle feed

- If infant shows signs of irritability, drug may need to be discontinued

THE ART OF PSYCHOPHARMACOLOGY

Potential Advantages

- Established long-term efficacy as a first-line treatment for ADHD
- Multiple options for drug delivery, peak actions, and duration of action

Potential Disadvantages

- Patients with current or past substance abuse
- Patients with current or past bipolar disorder or psychosis

Primary Target Symptoms

- Concentration, attention span
- Motor hyperactivity
- Impulsiveness
- Physical and mental fatigue
- Daytime sleepiness
- Depression

Pearls

✽ May be useful for treatment of depressive symptoms in medically ill elderly patients

✽ May be useful for treatment of post-stroke depression

✽ A classical augmentation strategy for treatment-refractory depression

✽ Specifically, may be useful for treatment of cognitive dysfunction and fatigue as residual symptoms of major depressive disorder unresponsive to multiple prior treatments

✽ May also be useful for the treatment of cognitive impairment, depressive symptoms, and severe fatigue in patients with HIV infection and in cancer patients

- Can be used to potentiate opioid analgesia and reduce sedation, particularly in end-of-life management
- Atypical antipsychotics may be useful in treating stimulant or psychotic consequences of overdose
- Some patients respond to or tolerate methylphenidate better than amphetamine and vice versa
- Taking with food may delay peak actions of oral formulations for 2–3 hours
- Half-life and duration of clinical action tend to be shorter in younger children
- Drug abuse may actually be lower in ADHD adolescents treated with stimulants than in ADHD adolescents who are not treated
- Older sustained-release technologies for methylphenidate were not significant advances over immediate-release methylphenidate because they did not eliminate the need for lunchtime dosing or allow once daily administration

✽ Newer sustained-release technologies are truly once a day dosing systems

✽ Metadate CD and Ritalin LA are somewhat similar to each other, both with an early peak and duration of action of about 8 hours

✽ Concerta has less of an early peak but a longer duration of action (up to 12 hours)

✽ Concerta trilayer tablet consists of 3 compartments (2 containing drug, 1 a "push" compartment) and an orifice at the head of the first drug compartment; water fills the push compartment and gradually pushes drug up and out of the tablet through the orifice

✽ Concerta may be preferable for those ADHD patients who work in the evening or do homework up to 12 hours after morning dosing

✽ Metadate CD and Ritalin LA may be preferable for those ADHD patients who

lose their appetite for dinner or have insomnia with Concerta
- Some patients may benefit from an occasional addition of 5–10 mg of immediate-release methylphenidate to their daily base of sustained release methylphenidate
- Transdermal formulation may confer lower abuse potential than oral formulations
- Transdermal formulation may enhance adherence to treatment compared to some oral formulations because it allows once daily application with all day efficacy, has a smoother absorption curve, and allows for daily customization of treatment (i.e., it can be removed early if desired)
- On the other hand, transdermal formulation has slower onset than oral formulations, requires a specific removal time, can cause skin sensitization, can be large depending on dose, and may lead to reduced efficacy if removed prematurely

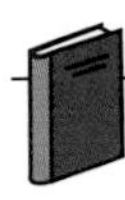

Suggested Reading

Challman TD, Lipsky JJ. Methylphenidate: its pharmacology and uses. Mayo Clin Proc 2000;75:711–21.

Kimko HC, Cross JT, Abemethy DR. Pharmacokinetics and clinical effectiveness of methylphenidate. Clin Pharmacokinet 1999;37:457–70.

Wolraich ML, Greenhill LL, Pelham W, Swanson J, Wilens T, Palumbo D, Atkins M, McBurnett K, Bukstein O, August G. Randomized, controlled trial of oros methylphenidate once a day in children with attention-deficit/hyperactivity disorder. Pediatrics 2001;108:883–92.

THERAPEUTICS

Brands • Versed

see index for additional brand names

Generic? No

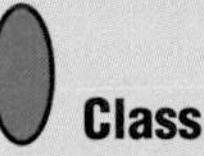

Class

- Benzodiazepine (hypnotic)

Commonly Prescribed for

(bold for FDA approved)

- **Sedation in pediatric patients**
- **Sedation (adjunct to anesthesia)**
- **Preoperative anxiolytic**
- **Drug-induced amnesia**

How the Drug Works

- Binds to benzodiazepine receptors at the GABA-A ligand-gated chloride channel complex
- Enhances the inhibitory effects of GABA
- Boosts chloride conductance through GABA-regulated channels
- Inhibitory actions in sleep centers may provide sedative hypnotic effects

How Long Until It Works

- Intravenous injection: onset 3–5 minutes
- Intramuscular injection: onset 15 minutes, peak 30–60 minutes

If It Works

- Patients generally recover 2–6 hours after awakening

If It Doesn't Work

- Increase the dose
- Switch to another agent

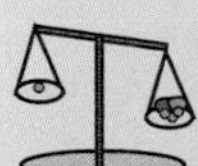

Best Augmenting Combos for Partial Response or Treatment Resistance

- Augmenting agents have not been adequately studied

Tests

- None for healthy individuals

SIDE EFFECTS

How Drug Causes Side Effects

- Actions at benzodiazepine receptors that carry over to next day can cause daytime sedation, amnesia, and ataxia

Notable Side Effects

- Oversedation, impaired recall, agitation, involuntary movements, headache
- Nausea, vomiting
- Hiccups, fluctuation in vital signs, irritation/pain at site of injection
- Hypotension

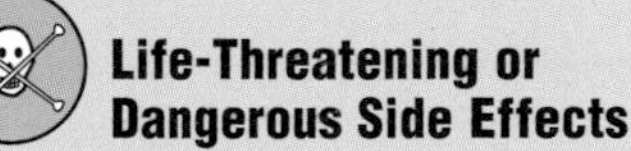

Life-Threatening or Dangerous Side Effects

- Respiratory depression, apnea, respiratory arrest
- Cardiac arrest

Weight Gain

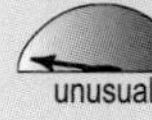

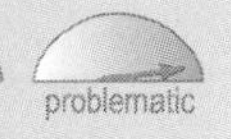

- Reported but not expected

Sedation

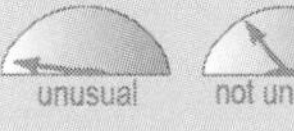

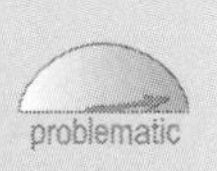

- Many experience and/or can be significant in amount

What to Do About Side Effects

- Wait
- Switch to another agent
- Administer flumazenil if side effects are severe or life-threatening

Best Augmenting Agents for Side Effects

- Many side effects cannot be improved with an augmenting agent

DOSING AND USE

Usual Dosage Range

- Intravenous (adults): 1–2.5 mg
- Liquid (age 16 and under): 0.25–1.0 mg/kg

Dosage Forms

- Intravenous: 5 mg/mL – 1 mL vial, 2 mL vial, 5 mL vial, 10 mL vial
- Liquid: 2 mg/mL – 118 mL bottle

How To Dose

- Liquid single dose: 0.25–1.0 mg/kg; maximum dose generally 20 mg
- Intravenous (adults): administer over 2 minutes; monitor patient over the next 2 or more minutes to determine effects; allow 3–5 minutes between administrations; maximum 2.5 mg within 2 minutes

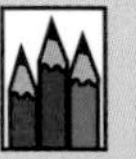

Dosing Tips

- Better to underdose, observe for effects, and then prudently raise dose while monitoring carefully

Overdose

- Sedation, confusion, poor coordination, respiratory depression, coma

Long-Term Use

- Not generally intended for long-term use

Habit Forming

- Some patients may develop dependence and/or tolerance; risk may be greater with higher doses
- History of drug addiction may increase risk of dependence

How to Stop

- If administration was prolonged, do not stop abruptly

Pharmacokinetics

- Elimination half-life 1.8–6.4 hours
- Active metabolite

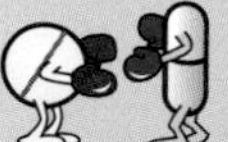

Drug Interactions

- If CNS depressants are used concomitantly, midazolam dose should be reduced by half or more
- Increased depressive effects when taken with other CNS depressants
- Drugs that inhibit CYP450 3A4, such as nefazodone and fluvoxamine, may reduce midazolam clearance and thus raise midazolam levels
- Midazolam decreases the minimum alveolar concentration of halothane needed for general anesthesia

Other Warnings/ Precautions

- Midazolam should be used only in an environment in which the patient can be closely monitored (e.g., hospital) because of the risk of respiratory depression and respiratory arrest
- Sedated pediatric patients should be monitored throughout the procedure
- Patients with chronic obstructive pulmonary disease should receive lower doses
- Use with caution in patients with impaired respiratory function

Do Not Use

- If patient has narrow angle-closure glaucoma
- If there is a proven allergy to midazolam or any benzodiazepine

SPECIAL POPULATIONS

Renal Impairment

- May have longer elimination half-life, prolonging time to recovery

Hepatic Impairment

- Longer elimination half-life; clearance is reduced

Cardiac Impairment

- Longer elimination half-life; clearance is reduced

Elderly

- Longer elimination half-life; clearance is reduced
- Intravenous: 1–3.5 mg; maximum 1.5 mg within 2 minutes

Children and Adolescents

- In most pediatric populations, pharmacokinetic properties are similar to those in adults
- Seriously ill neonates have reduced clearance and longer elimination half-life
- Hypotension has occurred in neonates given midazolam and fentanyl
- Intravenous dose: dependent on age, weight, route, procedure

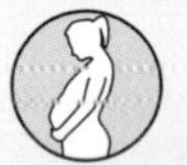

Pregnancy

- Risk Category D [positive evidence of risk to human fetus; potential benefits may still justify its use during pregnancy]
- Midazolam crosses the placenta
- Neonatal flaccidity has been reported in infants whose mother took a benzodiazepine during pregnancy

Breast Feeding

- Some drug is found in mother's breast milk
- Effects on infant have been observed and include feeding difficulties, sedation, and weight loss
- Midazolam can be used to relieve postoperative pain after cesarean section

THE ART OF PSYCHOPHARMACOLOGY

Potential Advantages

- Fast onset
- Parenteral dosage forms

Potential Disadvantages

- Can be oversedating

Primary Target Symptoms

- Anxiety

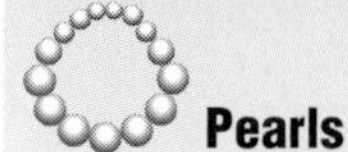

Pearls

- Recovery (e.g., ability to stand/walk) generally takes 2–6 hours after wakening
- Half-life may be longer in obese patients
- Patients with premenstrual syndrome may be less sensitive to midazolam than healthy women throughout the cycle
- Midazolam clearance may be reduced in postmenopausal women compared to premenopausal women

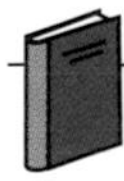

Suggested Reading

Blumer JL. Clinical pharmacology of midazolam in infants and children. Clin Pharmacokinet 1998;35:37–47.

Fountain NB, Adams RE. Midazolam treatment of acute and refractory status epilepticus. Clin Neuropharmacol 1999;22:261–7.

Shafer A. Complications of sedation with midazolam in the intensive care unit and a comparison with other sedative regimens. Crit Care Med 1998;26:947–56.

Yuan R, Flockhart DA, Balian JD. Pharmacokinetic and pharmacodynamic consequences of metabolism-based drug interactions with alprazolam, midazolam, and triazolam. J Clin Pharmacol 1999;39:1109–25.

THERAPEUTICS

Brands
- Toledomin
- Ixel
- Savella

see index for additional brand names

Generic? No

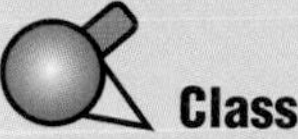

Class

- SNRI (dual serotonin and norepinephrine reuptake inhibitor); antidepressant; chronic pain treatment

Commonly Prescribed for

(bold for FDA approved)

- **Fibromyalgia**
- Major depressive disorder
- Neuropathic pain/chronic pain

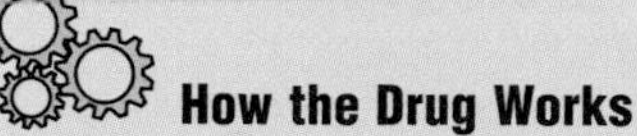

How the Drug Works

- Boosts neurotransmitters serotonin, norepinephrine/noradrenaline, and dopamine
- Blocks serotonin reuptake pump (serotonin transporter), presumably increasing serotonergic neurotransmission
- Blocks norepinephrine reuptake pump (norepinephrine transporter), presumably increasing noradrenergic neurotransmission
- Presumably desensitizes both serotonin 1A receptors and beta adrenergic receptors

* Weak noncompetitive NMDA-receptor antagonist (high doses), which may contribute to actions in chronic pain

- Since dopamine is inactivated by norepinephrine reuptake in frontal cortex, which largely lacks dopamine transporters, milnacipran can increase dopamine neurotransmission in this part of the brain

How Long Until It Works

- Onset of therapeutic actions usually not immediate, but often delayed 2–4 weeks
- If it is not working within 6–8 weeks, it may require a dosage increase or it may not work at all
- May continue to work for many years to prevent relapse of symptoms in depression

If It Works

- The goal of treatment of depression is complete remission of current symptoms as well as prevention of future relapses
- The goal of treatment of fibromyalgia and chronic neuropathic pain is to reduce symptoms as much as possible, especially in combination with other treatments
- Treatment of depression most often reduces or even eliminates symptoms, but is not a cure since symptoms can recur after medicine stopped
- Treatment of fibromyalgia and chronic neuropathic pain may reduce symptoms, but rarely eliminates them completely, and is not a cure since symptoms can recur after medicine is stopped
- Continue treatment of depression until all symptoms are gone (remission)
- Once symptoms of depression are gone, continue treating for 1 year for the first episode of depression
- For second and subsequent episodes of depression, treatment may need to be indefinite
- Use in fibromyalgia and chronic neuropathic pain may also need to be indefinite, but long-term treatment is not well-studied in these conditions

If It Doesn't Work

- Many depressed patients have only a partial response where some symptoms are improved but others persist (especially insomnia, fatigue, and problems concentrating)
- Other depressed patients may be nonresponders, sometimes called treatment-resistant or treatment-refractory
- Some depressed patients who have an initial response may relapse even though they continue treatment, sometimes called "poop-out"
- Consider increasing dose, switching to another agent or adding an appropriate augmenting agent
- Consider psychotherapy
- Consider evaluation for another diagnosis or for a comorbid condition (e.g., medical illness, substance abuse, etc.)
- Some patients may experience apparent lack of consistent efficacy due to activation of latent or underlying bipolar disorder, and require antidepressant discontinuation and switch to a mood stabilizer

Best Augmenting Combos for Partial Response or Treatment Resistance

- Augmentation experience is limited compared to other antidepressants
- Benzodiazepines can reduce insomnia and anxiety
- Adding other agents to milnacipran for treating depression could follow the same practice for augmenting SSRIs or other SNRIs if done by experts while monitoring carefully in difficult cases
- Although no controlled studies and little clinical experience, adding other agents for treating fibromyalgia and chronic neuropathic pain could theoretically include gabapentin, tiagabine, other anticonvulsants, or even opiates if done by experts while monitoring carefully in difficult cases
- Mirtazapine, bupropion, reboxetine, atomoxetine (use combinations of antidepressants with caution as this may activate bipolar disorder and suicidal ideation)
- Modafinil, especially for fatigue, sleepiness, and lack of concentration
- Mood stabilizers or atypical antipsychotics for bipolar depression, psychotic depression or treatment-resistant depression
- Hypnotics or trazodone for insomnia
- Classically, lithium, buspirone, or thyroid hormone

Tests

- Check blood pressure before initiating treatment and regularly during treatment

SIDE EFFECTS

How Drug Causes Side Effects

- Theoretically due to increases in serotonin and norepinephrine concentrations at receptors in parts of the brain and body other than those that cause therapeutic actions (e.g., unwanted actions of serotonin in sleep centers causing insomnia, unwanted actions of norepinephrine on acetylcholine release causing urinary retention or constipation)
- Most side effects are immediate but often go away with time

Notable Side Effects

- Most side effects increase with higher doses, at least transiently
- Headache, nervousness, insomnia, sedation
- Nausea, diarrhea, decreased appetite
- Sexual dysfunction (abnormal ejaculation/orgasm, impotence)
- Asthenia, sweating
- SIADH (syndrome of inappropriate antidiuretic hormone secretion)
- Dose-dependent increased blood pressure
- Dry mouth, constipation
- Dysuria, urological complaints, urinary hesitancy, urinary retention
- Increase in heart rate
- Palpitations

Life-Threatening or Dangerous Side Effects

- Rare induction of mania
- Rare activation of suicidal ideation and behavior (suicidality) (short-term studies did not show an increase in the risk of suicidality with antidepressants compared to placebo beyond age 24)
- Rare seizures

Weight Gain

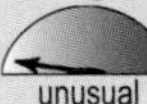
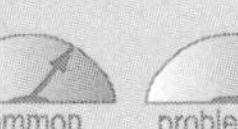

unusual | not unusual | common | problematic

- Reported but not expected

Sedation

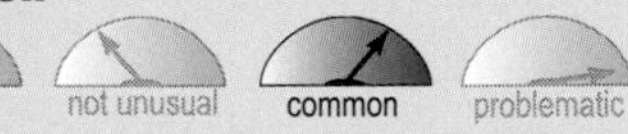

unusual | not unusual | common | problematic

- Many experience and/or can be significant in amount

What to Do About Side Effects

- Wait
- Wait
- Wait
- Lower the dose
- In a few weeks, switch or add other drugs

Best Augmenting Agents for Side Effects

❊ For urinary hesitancy, give an alpha 1 blocker such as tamsulosin or naftopidil
- Often best to try another antidepressant monotherapy prior to resorting to augmentation strategies to treat side effects
- Trazodone or a hypnotic for insomnia

- Bupropion, sildenafil, vardenafil, or tadalafil for sexual dysfunction
- Benzodiazepines for anxiety, agitation
- Mirtazapine for insomnia, agitation, and gastrointestinal side effects
- Many side effects are dose dependent (i.e., they increase as dose increases, or they reemerge until tolerance redevelops)
- Many side effects are time-dependent (i.e., they start immediately upon dosing and upon each dose increase, but go away with time)
- Activation and agitation may represent the induction of a bipolar state, especially a mixed dysphoric bipolar II condition sometimes associated with suicidal ideation, and require the addition of lithium, a mood stabilizer or an atypical antipsychotic, and/or discontinuation of milnacipran

DOSING AND USE

Usual Dosage Range

- 30–200 mg/day in 2 doses

Dosage Forms

- Capsule 25 mg, 50 mg (France, other European countries, and worldwide markets)
- Capsule 15 mg, 25 mg, 50 mg (Japan)
- Tablet 12.5 mg, 25 mg, 50 mg, 100 mg

How To Dose

- Should be administered in 2 divided doses
- Initial 12.5 mg once daily; increase to 25 mg/day in 2 divided doses on day 2; increase to 50 mg/day in 2 divided doses on day 4; increase to 100 mg/day in 2 divided doses on day 7; maximum dose generally 200 mg/day

Dosing Tips

- Preferred dose for fibromyalgia may be 100 mg twice daily
- Higher doses usually well tolerated in fibromyalgia patients

✻ Once daily dosing has far less consistent efficacy, so only give as twice daily

- Higher doses (>200 mg/day) not consistently effective in all studies of depression
- Nevertheless, some patients respond better to higher doses (200–300 mg/day) than to lower doses
- Different doses in different countries
- Different doses in different indications and different populations
- Preferred dose for depression may be 50 mg twice daily to 100 mg twice daily in France
- Preferred dose for depression in the elderly may be 15 mg twice daily to 25 mg twice daily in Japan
- Preferred dosing for depression in other adults may be 25 mg twice daily to 50 mg twice daily in Japan

✻ Thus, clinicians must be aware that titration of twice daily dosing across a 10-fold range (30 mg–300 mg total daily dose) can optimize milnacipran's efficacy in broad clinical use

- Patients with agitation or anxiety may require slower titration to optimize tolerability
- No pharmacokinetic drug interactions (not an inhibitor of CYP450 2D6 or 3A4)
- As milnacipran is a more potent norepinephrine reuptake inhibitor than a serotonin reuptake inhibitor, some patients may require dosing at the higher end of the dosing range to obtain robust dual SNRI actions
- At high doses, NMDA glutamate antagonist actions may be a factor

Overdose

- Vomiting, hypertension, sedation, tachycardia
- The emetic effect of high doses of milnacipran may reduce the risk of serious adverse effects

Long-Term Use

- Safe

Habit Forming

- No

How to Stop

- Taper is prudent, but usually not necessary

Pharmacokinetics

- Half-life 8 hours
- No active metabolite

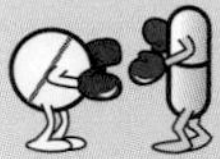

Drug Interactions

- Tramadol increases the risk of seizures in patients taking an antidepressant
- Can cause a fatal "serotonin syndrome" when combined with MAO inhibitors, so do not use with MAO inhibitors or for at least 14 days after MAOIs are stopped
- Do not start an MAO inhibitor for at least 2 weeks after discontinuing milnacipran
- Possible increased risk of bleeding, especially when combined with anticoagulants (e.g., warfarin, NSAIDs)
- Switching from or addition of other norepinephrine reuptake inhibitors should be done with caution, as the additive pro-noradrenergic effects may enhance therapeutic actions in depression, but also enhance noradrenergically mediated side effects
- Few known adverse pharmacokinetic drug interactions

Other Warnings/ Precautions

- Use with caution in patients with history of seizures
- Use with caution in patients with bipolar disorder unless treated with concomitant mood-stabilizing agent
- Can cause mild elevations in ALT/AST, so avoid use with alcohol or in cases of chronic liver disease
- When treating children, carefully weigh the risks and benefits of pharmacological treatment against the risks and benefits of nontreatment with antidepressants and make sure to document this in the patient's chart
- Distribute the brochures provided by the FDA and the drug companies
- Warn patients and their caregivers about the possibility of activating side effects and advise them to report such symptoms immediately
- Monitor patients for activation of suicidal ideation, especially children and adolescents

Do Not Use

- If patient has uncontrolled narrow angle-closure glaucoma
- If patient is taking an MAO inhibitor
- If there is a proven allergy to milnacipran

SPECIAL POPULATIONS

Renal Impairment

- Use caution for moderate impairment
- For severe impairment, 50 mg/day; can increase to 100 mg/day if needed

Hepatic Impairment

- No dose adjustment necessary
- Not recommended for us in chronic liver disease

Cardiac Impairment

- Drug should be used with caution

Elderly

- Some patients may tolerate lower doses better
- Reduction in risk of suicidality with antidepressants compared to placebo in adults age 65 and older

Children and Adolescents

- Carefully weigh the risks and benefits of pharmacological treatment against the risks and benefits of nontreatment with antidepressants and make sure to document this in the patient's chart
- Monitor patients face-to-face regularly, particularly during the first several weeks of treatment
- Use with caution, observing for activation of known or unknown bipolar disorder and/or suicidal ideation, and inform parents or guardians of this risk so they can help observe child or adolescent patients
- Not well-studied

Pregnancy

- Risk Category C [some animal studies show adverse effects; no controlled studies in humans]
- Not generally recommended for use during pregnancy, especially during first trimester
- Nonetheless, continuous treatment during pregnancy may be necessary and has not been proven to be harmful to the fetus
- Must weigh the risk of treatment (first trimester fetal development, third trimester newborn delivery) to the child against the risk of no treatment (recurrence of depression, maternal health, infant bonding) to the mother and child

- For many patients this may mean continuing treatment during pregnancy
- Neonates exposed to SSRIs or SNRIs late in the third trimester have developed complications requiring prolonged hospitalization, respiratory support, and tube feeding; reported symptoms are consistent with either a direct toxic effect of SSRIs and SNRIs or, possibly, a drug discontinuation syndrome, and include respiratory distress, cyanosis, apnea, seizures, temperature instability, feeding difficulty, vomiting, hypoglycemia, hypotonia, hypertonia, hyperreflexia, tremor, jitteriness, irritability, and constant crying

Breast Feeding

- Unknown if milnacipran is secreted in human breast milk, but all psychotropics assumed to be secreted in breast milk
- Immediate postpartum period is a high-risk time for depression, especially in women who have had prior depressive episodes, so drug may need to be reinstituted late in the third trimester or shortly after childbirth to prevent a recurrence during the postpartum period
- Must weigh benefits of breast feeding with risks and benefits of antidepressant treatment versus nontreatment to both the infant and the mother
- For many patients, this may mean continuing treatment during breast feeding

THE ART OF PSYCHOPHARMACOLOGY

Potential Advantages

- Fibromyalgia, chronic pain syndrome
- Patients with retarded depression
- Patients with hypersomnia
- Patients with atypical depression
- Patients with depression may have higher remission rates on SNRIs than on SSRIs
- Depressed patients with somatic symptoms, fatigue, and pain

Potential Disadvantages

- Patients with urologic disorders, prostate disorders
- Patients with borderline or uncontrolled hypertension
- Patients with agitation and anxiety (short-term)

Primary Target Symptoms

- Pain
- Physical symptoms
- Depressed mood
- Energy, motivation, and interest
- Sleep disturbance

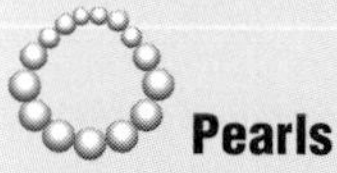

Pearls

- Approved in the United States for use in pain and fibromyalgia
- Not studied in stress urinary incontinence
- Not well studied in ADHD or anxiety disorders, but may be effective

✻ Has greater potency for norepinephrine reuptake blockade than for serotonin reuptake blockade, but this is of unclear clinical significance as a differentiating feature from other SNRIs, although it might contribute to its therapeutic activity in fibromyalgia and chronic pain

✻ Onset of action in fibromyalgia may be somewhat faster than depression (i.e., 2 weeks rather than 2–8 weeks)

- Therapeutic actions in fibromyalgia are partial, with symptom reduction but not necessarily remission of painful symptoms in many patients

✻ Potent noradrenergic actions may account for possibly higher incidence of sweating and urinary hesitancy than other SNRIs

- Urinary hesitancy more common in men than women and in older men than in younger men
- Alpha 1 antagonists such as tamsulosin or naftopidil can reverse urinary hesitancy or retention
- Alpha 1 antagonists given prophylactically may prevent urinary hesitancy or retention in patients at higher risk, such as elderly men with borderline urine flow
- May be better tolerated than tricyclic or tetracyclic antidepressants in the treatment of fibromyalgia or other chronic pain syndromes
- No pharmacokinetic interactions or elevations in plasma drug levels of tricyclic or tetracyclic antidepressants when adding or switching to or from milnacipran

Suggested Reading

Bisserbe JC. Clinical utility of milnacipran in comparison with other antidepressants. Int Clin Psychopharmacol 2002;17 Suppl 1:S43–50.

Leo RJ, Brooks VL. Clinical potential of milnacipran, a serotonin and norepinephrine reuptake inhibitor, in pain. Curr Opin Investig Drugs 2006;7(7):637–42.

Puozzo C, Panconi E, Deprez D. Pharmacology and pharmacokinetics of milnacipran. Int Clin Psychopharmacol 2002;17 Suppl 1:S25–35.

THERAPEUTICS

Brands • Remeron

see index for additional brand names

Generic? Yes

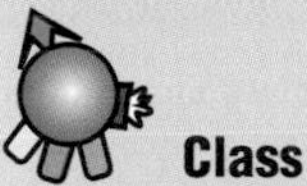

Class

- Alpha 2 antagonist; NaSSA (noradrenaline and specific serotonergic agent); dual serotonin and norepinephrine agent; antidepressant

Commonly Prescribed for

(bold for FDA approved)

- **Major depressive disorder**
- Panic disorder
- Generalized anxiety disorder
- Posttraumatic stress disorder

How the Drug Works

- Boosts neurotransmitters serotonin and norepinephrine/noradrenaline
- Blocks alpha 2 adrenergic presynaptic receptor, thereby increasing norepinephrine neurotransmission
- Blocks alpha 2 adrenergic presynaptic receptor on serotonin neurons (heteroreceptors), thereby increasing serotonin neurotransmission
- This is a novel mechanism independent of norepinephrine and serotonin reuptake blockade
- Blocks 5HT2A, 5HT2C, and 5HT3 serotonin receptors
- Blocks H1 histamine receptors

How Long Until It Works

✻ Actions on insomnia and anxiety can start shortly after initiation of dosing

- Onset of therapeutic actions in depression, however, is usually not immediate, but often delayed 2–4 weeks
- If it is not working within 6–8 weeks for depression, it may require a dosage increase or it may not work at all
- May continue to work for many years to prevent relapse of symptoms

If It Works

- The goal of treatment is complete remission of current symptoms as well as prevention of future relapses
- Treatment most often reduces or even eliminates symptoms, but not a cure since symptoms can recur after medicine stopped
- Continue treatment until all symptoms are gone (remission)
- Once symptoms gone, continue treating for 1 year for the first episode of depression
- For second and subsequent episodes of depression, treatment may need to be indefinite
- Use in anxiety disorders may also need to be indefinite

If It Doesn't Work

- Many patients only have a partial response where some symptoms are improved but others persist (especially insomnia, fatigue, and problems concentrating)
- Other patients may be nonresponders, sometimes called treatment-resistant or treatment-refractory
- Consider increasing dose, switching to another agent or adding an appropriate augmenting agent
- Consider psychotherapy
- Consider evaluation for another diagnosis or for a comorbid condition (e.g., medical illness, substance abuse, etc.)
- Some patients may experience apparent lack of consistent efficacy due to activation of latent or underlying bipolar disorder, and require antidepressant discontinuation and a switch to a mood stabilizer

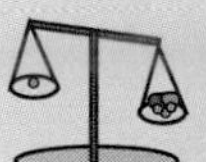

Best Augmenting Combos for Partial Response or Treatment Resistance

- SSRIs, bupropion, reboxetine, atomoxetine (use combinations of antidepressants with caution as this may activate bipolar disorder and suicidal ideation)

✻ Venlafaxine ("California rocket fuel"; a potentially powerful dual serotonin and norepinephrine combination, but observe for activation of bipolar disorder and suicidal ideation)

- Modafinil, especially for fatigue, sleepiness, and lack of concentration
- Mood stabilizers or atypical antipsychotics for bipolar depression, psychotic

depression, or treatment-resistant depression
- Benzodiazepines
- Hypnotics or trazodone for insomnia

Tests
- None for healthy individuals
- May need liver function tests for those with hepatic abnormalities before initiating treatment
- May need to monitor blood count during treatment for those with blood dyscrasias, leucopenia, or granulocytopenia
- Since some antidepressants such as mirtazapine can be associated with significant weight gain, before starting treatment, weigh all patients and determine if the patient is already overweight (BMI >25.0–29.9) or obese (BMI>30)
- Before giving a drug that can cause weight gain to an overweight or obese patient, consider determining whether the patient already has pre-diabetes (fasting plasma glucose 100–25 mg/dL), diabetes (fasting plasma glucose >126 mg/dL), or dyslipidemia (increased total cholesterol, LDL cholesterol and triglycerides; decreased HDL cholesterol), and treat or refer such patients for treatment, including nutrition and weight management, physical activity counseling, smoking cessation, and medical management

✻ Monitor weight and BMI during treatment

✻ While giving a drug to a patient who has gained >5% of initial weight, consider evaluating for the presence of pre-diabetes, diabetes, or dyslipidemia, or consider switching to a different antipsychotic

SIDE EFFECTS

How Drug Causes Side Effects
- Most side effects are immediate but often go away with time

✻ Histamine 1 receptor antagonism may explain sedative effects

✻ Histamine 1 receptor antagonism plus 5HT2C antagonism may explain some aspects of weight gain

Notable Side Effects
- Dry mouth, constipation, increased appetite, weight gain
- Sedation, dizziness, abnormal dreams, confusion
- Flu-like symptoms (may indicate low white blood cell or granulocyte count)
- Change in urinary function
- Hypotension

Life-Threatening or Dangerous Side Effects
- Rare seizures
- Rare induction of mania
- Rare activation of suicidal ideation and behavior (suicidality) (short-term studies did not show an increase in the risk of suicidality with antidepressants compared to placebo beyond age 24)

Weight Gain

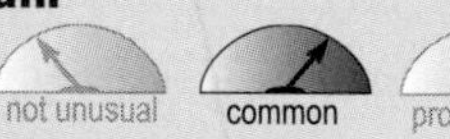

- Many experience and/or can be significant in amount

Sedation

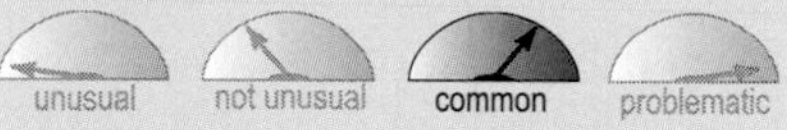

- Many experience and/or can be significant in amount

What to Do About Side Effects
- Wait
- Wait
- Wait
- Switch to another drug

Best Augmenting Agents for Side Effects
- Often best to try another antidepressant monotherapy prior to resorting to augmentation strategies to treat side effects
- Many side effects are dose-dependent (i.e., they increase as dose increases, or they reemerge until tolerance redevelops)
- Many side effects are time-dependent (i.e., they start immediately upon dosing and upon each dose increase, but go away with time)
- Trazodone or a hypnotic for insomnia
- Many side effects cannot be improved with an augmenting agent
- Activation and agitation may represent the induction of a bipolar state, especially a

mixed dysphoric bipolar II condition sometimes associated with suicidal ideation, and require the addition of lithium, a mood stabilizer or an atypical antipsychotic, and/or discontinuation of mirtazapine

DOSING AND USE

Usual Dosage Range

- 15–45 mg at night

Dosage Forms

- Tablet 15 mg scored, 30 mg scored, 45 mg
- SolTab disintegrating tablet 15 mg, 30 mg, 45 mg

How To Dose

- Initial 15 mg/day in the evening; increase every 1–2 weeks until desired efficacy is reached; maximum generally 45 mg/day

Dosing Tips

- Sedation may not worsen as dose increases

✻ Breaking a 15-mg tablet in half and administering 7.5 mg dose may actually increase sedation

- Some patients require more than 45 mg daily, including up to 90 mg in difficult patients who tolerate these doses
- If intolerable anxiety, insomnia, agitation, akathisia, or activation occur either upon dosing initiation or discontinuation, consider the possibility of activated bipolar disorder and switch to a mood stabilizer or an atypical antipsychotic

Overdose

- Rarely lethal; all fatalities have involved other medications; symptoms include sedation, disorientation, memory impairment, rapid heartbeat

Long-Term Use

- Safe

Habit Forming

- Not expected

How to Stop

- Taper is prudent to avoid withdrawal effects, but tolerance, dependence, and withdrawal effects not reliably reported

Pharmacokinetics

- Half-life 20–40 hours

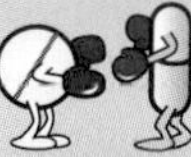

Drug Interactions

- Tramadol increases the risk of seizures in patients taking an antidepressant
- No significant pharmacokinetic drug interactions
- Can cause a fatal "serotonin syndrome" when combined with MAO inhibitors, so do not use with MAO inhibitors or for at least 14 days after MAOIs are stopped
- Do not start an MAO inhibitor for at least 2 weeks after discontinuing mirtazapine

Other Warnings/ Precautions

- Drug may lower white blood cell count (rare; may not be increased compared to other antidepressants but controlled studies lacking; not a common problem reported in post-marketing surveillance)
- Drug may increase cholesterol
- May cause photosensitivity
- Avoid alcohol, which may increase sedation and cognitive and motor effects
- Use with caution in patients with history of seizures
- Use with caution in patients with bipolar disorder unless treated with concomitant mood-stabilizing agent
- When treating children, carefully weigh the risks and benefits of pharmacological treatment against the risks and benefits of nontreatment with antidepressants and make sure to document this in the patient's chart
- Distribute the brochures provided by the FDA and the drug companies
- Warn patients and their caregivers about the possibility of activating side effects and advise them to report such symptoms immediately
- Monitor patients for activation of suicidal ideation, especially children and adolescents

Do Not Use

- If patient is taking an MAO inhibitor
- If there is a proven allergy to mirtazapine

SPECIAL POPULATIONS

Renal Impairment

- Drug should be used with caution

Hepatic Impairment

- Drug should be used with caution
- May require lower dose

Cardiac Impairment

- Drug should be used with caution
- The potential risk of hypotension should be considered

Elderly

- Some patients may tolerate lower doses better
- Reduction in risk of suicidality with antidepressants compared to placebo in adults age 65 and older

Children and Adolescents

- Carefully weigh the risks and benefits of pharmacological treatment against the risks and benefits of nontreatment with antidepressants and make sure to document this in the patient's chart
- Monitor patients face-to-face regularly, particularly during the first several weeks of treatment
- Use with caution, observing for activation of known or unknown bipolar disorder and/or suicidal ideation, and inform parents or guardian of this risk so they can help observe child or adolescent patients
- Safety and efficacy have not been established

Pregnancy

- Risk Category C [some animal studies show adverse effects; no controlled studies in humans]
- Not generally recommended for use during pregnancy, especially during first trimester
- Must weigh the risk of treatment (first trimester fetal development, third trimester newborn delivery) to the child against the risk of no treatment (recurrence of depression, maternal health, infant bonding) to the mother and child
- For many patients this may mean continuing treatment during pregnancy

Breast Feeding

- Unknown if mirtazapine is secreted in human breast milk, but all psychotropics assumed to be secreted in breast milk
- If child becomes irritable or sedated, breast feeding or drug may need to be discontinued
- Immediate postpartum period is a high-risk time for depression, especially in women who have had prior depressive episodes, so drug may need to be reinstituted late in the third trimester or shortly after childbirth to prevent a recurrence during the postpartum period
- Must weigh benefits of breast feeding with risks and benefits of antidepressant treatment versus nontreatment to both the infant and the mother
- For many patients, this may mean continuing treatment during breast feeding

THE ART OF PSYCHOPHARMACOLOGY

Potential Advantages

- Patients particularly concerned about sexual side effects
- Patients with symptoms of anxiety
- Patients on concomitant medications
- As an augmenting agent to boost the efficacy of other antidepressants

Potential Disadvantages

- Patients particularly concerned about gaining weight
- Patients with low energy

Primary Target Symptoms

- Depressed mood
- Sleep disturbance
- Anxiety

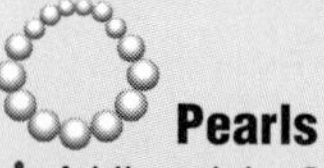

Pearls

- ✻ Adding alpha 2 antagonism to agents that block serotonin and/or norepinephrine reuptake may be synergistic for severe depression
- Adding mirtazapine to venlafaxine or SSRIs may reverse drug-induced anxiety and insomnia
- Adding mirtazapine's 5HT3 antagonism to venlafaxine or SSRIs may reverse drug-induced nausea, diarrhea, stomach cramps, and gastrointestinal side effects

- SSRIs, venlafaxine, bupropion, phentermine, or stimulants may mitigate mirtazapine-induced weight gain
- If weight gain has not occurred by week 6 of treatment, it is less likely for there to be significant weight gain
- Has been demonstrated to have an earlier onset of action than SSRIs

✻ Does not affect the CYP450 system, and so may be preferable in patients requiring concomitant medications

- Preliminary evidence suggests efficacy as an augmenting agent to haloperidol in treating negative symptoms of schizophrenia
- Anecdotal reports of efficacy in recurrent brief depression
- Weight gain as a result of mirtazapine treatment is more likely in women than in men, and before menopause rather than after

✻ May cause sexual dysfunction only infrequently

- Patients can have carryover sedation and intoxicated-like feeling if particularly sensitive to sedative side effects when initiating dosing
- Rarely, patients may complain of visual "trails" or after-images on mirtazapine

Suggested Reading

Anttila SA, Leinonen EV. A review of the pharmacological and clinical profile of mirtazapine. CNS Drug Rev 2001;7(3):249–64.

Benkert O, Muller M, Szegedi A. An overview of the clinical efficacy of mirtazapine. Hum Psychopharmacol 2002;17 Suppl 1:S23–6.

Falkai P. Mirtazapine: other indications. J Clin Psychiatry 1999;60(Suppl 17):36–40.

Fawcett J, Barkin RL. A meta-analysis of eight randomized, double-blind, controlled clinical trials of mirtazapine for the treatment of patients with major depression and symptoms of anxiety. J Clin Psychiatry 1998; 59:123–27.

Masand PS, Gupta S. Long-term side effects of newer-generation antidepressants: SSRIS, venlafaxine, nefazodone, bupropion, and mirtazapine. Ann Clin Psychiatry 2002; 14:175–82.

MOCLOBEMIDE

THERAPEUTICS

Brands
- Aurorix
- Arima
- Manerix

see index for additional brand names

Generic? No

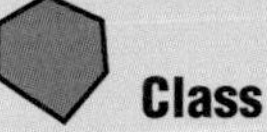

Class
- Reversible inhibitor of monoamine oxidase A (MAO-A) (RIMA)

Commonly Prescribed for
(bold for FDA approved)
- Depression
- Social anxiety disorder

How the Drug Works
- Reversibly blocks MAO-A from breaking down norepinephrine, dopamine, and serotonin
- This presumably boosts noradrenergic, serotonergic, and dopaminergic neurotransmission
- MAO-A inhibition predominates unless significant concentrations of monoamines build up (e.g., due to dietary tyramine), in which case MAO-A inhibition is theoretically reversed

How Long Until It Works
- Onset of therapeutic actions usually not immediate, but often delayed 2–4 weeks
- If it is not working within 6–8 weeks, it may require a dosage increase or it may not work at all
- May continue to work for many years to prevent relapse of symptoms

If It Works
- The goal of treatment is complete remission of current symptoms as well as prevention of future relapses
- Treatment most often reduces or even eliminates symptoms, but not a cure since symptoms can recur after medicine stopped
- Continue treatment until all symptoms are gone (remission)
- Once symptoms gone, continue treating for 1 year for the first episode of depression
- For second and subsequent episodes of depression, treatment may need to be indefinite
- Use in anxiety disorders may also need to be indefinite

If It Doesn't Work
- Many patients have only a partial response where some symptoms are improved but others persist (especially insomnia, fatigue, and problems concentrating)
- Other patients may be nonresponders, sometimes called treatment-resistant or treatment-refractory
- Consider increasing dose, switching to another agent or adding an appropriate augmenting agent
- Consider psychotherapy
- Consider evaluation for another diagnosis or for a comorbid condition (e.g., medical illness, substance abuse, etc.)
- Some patients may experience apparent lack of consistent efficacy due to activation of latent or underlying bipolar disorder, and require antidepressant discontinuation and a switch to a mood stabilizer

Best Augmenting Combos for Partial Response or Treatment Resistance
✽ Augmentation of MAOIs has not been systematically studied, and this is something for the expert, to be done with caution and with careful monitoring, but may be somewhat less risky with moclobemide than with other MAO inhibitors

✽ A stimulant such as d-amphetamine or methylphenidate (with caution; may activate bipolar disorder and suicidal ideation)
- Lithium
- Mood-stabilizing anticonvulsants
- Atypical antipsychotics (with special caution for those agents with monoamine reuptake blocking properties, such as ziprasidone and zotepine)

Tests
- Patients should be monitored for changes in blood pressure

SIDE EFFECTS

How Drug Causes Side Effects
- Theoretically due to increases in monoamines in parts of the brain and body and at receptors other than those that cause therapeutic actions (e.g., unwanted actions of serotonin in sleep centers causing insomnia, unwanted actions of norepinephrine on vascular smooth muscle causing changes in blood pressure)
- Side effects are generally immediate, but immediate side effects often disappear in time

Notable Side Effects
- Insomnia, dizziness, agitation, anxiety, restlessness
- Dry mouth, diarrhea, constipation, nausea, vomiting
- Galactorrhea
- Rare hypertension

Life-Threatening or Dangerous Side Effects
- Hypertensive crisis (especially when MAOIs are used with certain tyramine-containing foods – reduced risk compared to irreversible MAOIs)
- Induction of mania
- Rare activation of suicidal ideation and behavior (suicidality) (short-term studies did not show an increase in the risk of suicidality with antidepressants compared to placebo beyond age 24)
- Seizures

Weight Gain
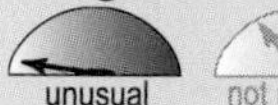

- Reported but not expected

Sedation
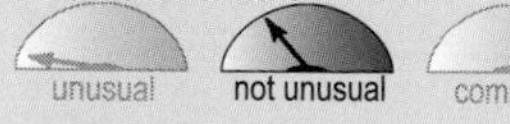

- Occurs in significant minority

What to Do About Side Effects
- Wait
- Wait
- Wait
- Lower the dose
- Switch to an SSRI or newer antidepressant

Best Augmenting Agents for Side Effects
- Trazodone (with caution) for insomnia
- Benzodiazepines for insomnia
- ✻ Single oral or sublingual dose of a calcium channel blocker (e.g., nifedipine) for urgent treatment of hypertension due to drug interaction or dietary tyramine
- Many side effects cannot be improved with an augmenting agent

DOSING AND USE

Usual Dosage Range
- 300–600 mg/day

Dosage Forms
- Tablet 100 mg scored, 150 mg scored

How To Dose
- Initial 300 mg/day in 3 divided doses after a meal; increase dose gradually; maximum dose generally 600 mg/day; minimum dose generally 150 mg/day

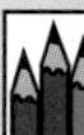

Dosing Tips
- ✻ At higher doses, moclobemide also inhibits MAO-B and thereby loses its selectivity for MAO-A, with uncertain clinical consequences
- ✻ Taking moclobemide after meals as opposed to before may minimize the chances of interactions with tyramine
- May be less toxic in overdose than tricyclic antidepressants and older MAOIs
- Clinical duration of action may be longer than biological half-life and allow twice daily dosing in some patients, or even once daily dosing, especially at lower doses

Overdose
- Agitation, aggression, behavioral disturbances, gastrointestinal irritation

Long-Term Use
- MAOIs may lose efficacy long-term

Habit Forming
- Some patients have developed dependence to MAOIs

How to Stop
- Taper not generally necessary

Pharmacokinetics

- Partially metabolized by CYP450 2C19 and 2D6
- Inactive metabolites
- Elimination half-life approximately 1–4 hours
- Clinical duration of action at least 24 hours

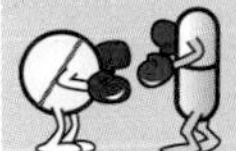

Drug Interactions

- Tramadol may increase the risk of seizures in patients taking an MAO inhibitor
- Can cause a fatal "serotonin syndrome" when combined with drugs that block serotonin reuptake (e.g., SSRIs, SNRIs, sibutramine, tramadol, etc.), so do not use with a serotonin reuptake inhibitor or for up to 5 weeks after stopping the serotonin reuptake inhibitor
- Hypertensive crisis with headache, intracranial bleeding, and death may result from combining MAO inhibitors with sympathomimetic drugs (e.g., amphetamines, methylphenidate, cocaine, dopamine, epinephrine, norepinephrine, and related compounds methyldopa, levodopa, L-tryptophan, L-tyrosine, and phenylalanine)
- Excitation, seizures, delirium, hyperpyrexia, circulatory collapse, coma, and death may result from combining MAO inhibitors with mepiridine or dextromethorphan
- Do not combine with another MAO inhibitor, alcohol, buspirone, bupropion, or guanethidine
- Adverse drug reactions can result from combining MAO inhibitors with tricyclic/tetracyclic antidepressants and related compounds, including carbamazepine, cyclobenzaprine, and mirtazapine, and should be avoided except by experts to treat difficult cases
- MAO inhibitors in combination with spinal anesthesia may cause combined hypotensive effects
- Combination of MAOIs and CNS depressants may enhance sedation and hypotension
- Cimetidine may increase plasma concentrations of moclobemide
- Moclobemide may enhance the effects of nonsteroidal anti-inflammatory drugs such as ibuprofen
- Risk of hypertensive crisis may be increased if moclobemide is used concurrently with levodopa or other dopaminergic agents

Other Warnings/ Precautions

- Use still requires low-tyramine diet, although more tyramine may be tolerated with moclobemide than with other MAO inhibitors before eliciting a hypertensive reaction
- Patients taking MAO inhibitors should avoid high-protein food that has undergone protein breakdown by aging, fermentation, pickling, smoking, or bacterial contamination
- Patients taking MAO inhibitors should avoid cheeses (especially aged varieties), pickled herring, beer, wine, liver, yeast extract, dry sausage, hard salami, pepperoni, Lebanon bologna, pods of broad beans (fava beans), yogurt, and excessive use of caffeine and chocolate
- Patient and prescriber must be vigilant to potential interactions with any drug, including antihypertensives and over-the-counter cough/cold preparations
- Over-the-counter medications to avoid include cough and cold preparations, including those containing dextromethorphan, nasal decongestants (tablets, drops, or spray), hay-fever medications, sinus medications, asthma inhalant medications, anti-appetite medications, weight reducing preparations, "pep" pills
- Use cautiously in hypertensive patients
- Moclobemide is not recommended for use in patients who cannot be monitored closely
- When treating children, carefully weigh the risks and benefits of pharmacological treatment against the risks and benefits of nontreatment with antidepressants and make sure to document this in the patient's chart
- Distribute the brochures provided by the FDA and the drug companies
- Warn patients and their caregivers about the possibility of activating side effects and advise them to report such symptoms immediately
- Monitor patients for activation of suicidal ideation, especially children and adolescents

Do Not Use

- If patient is taking meperidine (pethidine)
- If patient is taking a sympathomimetic agent or taking guanethidine
- If patient is taking another MAOI
- If patient is taking any agent that can inhibit serotonin reuptake (e.g., SSRIs, sibutramine, tramadol, milnacipran, duloxetine, venlafaxine, clomipramine, etc.)
- If patient is in an acute confusional state
- If patient has pheochromocytoma or thyrotoxicosis
- If patient has frequent or severe headaches
- If patient is undergoing elective surgery and requires general anesthesia
- If there is a proven allergy to moclobemide

SPECIAL POPULATIONS

Renal Impairment

- Use with caution

Hepatic Impairment

- Plasma concentrations are increased
- May require one-half to one-third of usual adult dose

Cardiac Impairment

- Cardiac impairment may require lower than usual adult dose
- Patients with angina pectoris or coronary artery disease should limit their exertion

Elderly

- Elderly patients may have greater sensitivity to adverse effects
- Reduction in risk of suicidality with antidepressants compared to placebo in adults age 65 and older

Children and Adolescents

- Not recommended for use in children under age 18
- Carefully weigh the risks and benefits of pharmacological treatment against the risks and benefits of nontreatment with antidepressants and make sure to document this in the patient's chart
- Monitor patients face-to-face regularly, particularly during the first several weeks of treatment
- Use with caution, observing for activation of known or unknown bipolar disorder and/or suicidal ideation, and inform parents or guardians of this risk so they can help observe child or adolescent patients

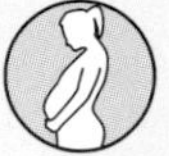

Pregnancy

- Not generally recommended for use during pregnancy, especially during first trimester
- Should evaluate patient for treatment with an antidepressant with a better risk/benefit ratio

Breast Feeding

- Some drug is found in mother's breast milk
- Effects on infant are unknown
- Immediate postpartum period is a high-risk time for depression, especially in women who have had prior depressive episodes, so drug may need to be reinstituted late in the third trimester or shortly after childbirth to prevent a recurrence during the postpartum period
- Should evaluate patient for treatment with an antidepressant with a better risk/benefit ratio

THE ART OF PSYCHOPHARMACOLOGY

Potential Advantages

- Atypical depression
- Severe depression
- Treatment-resistant depression or anxiety disorders

Potential Disadvantages

- Patients noncompliant with dietary restrictions, concomitant drug restrictions, and twice daily dosing after meals

Primary Target Symptoms

- Depressed mood

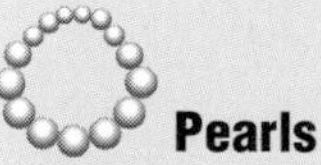

Pearls

- MAOIs are generally reserved for second-line use after SSRIs, SNRIs, and combinations of newer antidepressants have failed
- Patient should be advised not to take any prescription or over-the-counter drugs without consulting his or her doctor because of possible drug interactions with the MAOI

- Headache is often the first symptom of hypertensive crisis
- Moclobemide has a much reduced risk of interactions with tyramine than nonselective MAOIs
- Especially at higher doses of moclobemide, foods with high tyramine need to be avoided: dry sausage, pickled herring, liver, broad bean pods, sauerkraut, cheese, yogurt, alcoholic beverages, nonalcoholic beer and wine, chocolate, caffeine, meat and fish
- The rigid dietary restrictions may reduce compliance

✻ May be a safer alternative to classical irreversible nonselective MAO-A and MAO-B inhibitors with less propensity for tyramine and drug interactions and hepatotoxicity (although not entirely free of interactions)

- May not be as effective at low doses, and may have more side effects at higher doses
- Moclobemide's profile at higher doses may be more similar to classical MAOIs
- MAOIs are a viable second-line treatment option in depression, but are not frequently used

✻ Myths about the danger of dietary tyramine can be exaggerated, but prohibitions against concomitant drugs often not followed closely enough

- Orthostatic hypotension, insomnia, and sexual dysfunction are often the most troublesome common side effects

✻ MAOIs should be for the expert, especially if combining with agents of potential risk (e.g., stimulants, trazodone, TCAs)

✻ MAOIs should not be neglected as therapeutic agents for the treatment-resistant

- Although generally prohibited, a heroic but potentially dangerous treatment for severely treatment-resistant patients is for an expert to give a tricyclic/tetracyclic antidepressant other than clomipramine simultaneously with an MAO inhibitor for patients who fail to respond to numerous other antidepressants
- Use of MAOIs with clomipramine is always prohibited because of the risk of serotonin syndrome and death
- Amoxapine may be the preferred trycyclic/tetracyclic antidepressant to combine with an MAOI in heroic cases due to Its theoretically protective 5HT2A antagonist properties
- If this option is elected, start the MAOI with the tricyclic/tetracyclic antidepressant simultaneously at low doses after appropriate drug washout, then alternately increase doses of these agents every few days to a week as tolerated
- Although very strict dietary and concomitant drug restrictions must be observed to prevent hypertensive crises and serotonin syndrome, the most common side effects of MAOI and tricyclic/tetracyclic combinations may be weight gain and orthostatic hypotension

Suggested Reading

Amrein R, Martin JR, Cameron AM. Moclobemide in patients with dementia and depression. Adv Neurol 1999;80:509–19.

Fulton B, Benfield P. Moclobemide. An update of its pharmacological properties and therapeutic use. Drugs 1996;52:450–74.

Kennedy SH. Continuation and maintenance treatments in major depression: the neglected role of monoamine oxidase inhibitors. J Psychiatry Neurosci 1997;22:127–31.

Lippman SB, Nash K. Monoamine oxidase inhibitor update. Potential adverse food and drug interactions. Drug Saf 1990;5:195–204

Nutt D, Montgomery SA. Moclobemide in the treatment of social phobia. Int Clin Psychopharmacol 1996;11 (Suppl 3):77–82.

MODAFINIL

THERAPEUTICS

Brands
- Provigil
- Alertec
- Modiodal

see index for additional brand names

Generic? No

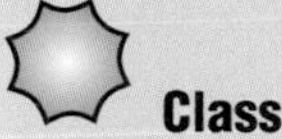

Class
- Wake-promoting

Commonly Prescribed for
(bold for FDA approved)
- **Reducing excessive sleepiness in patients with narcolepsy and shift work sleep disorder**
- **Reducing excessive sleepiness in patients with obstructive sleep apnea/hypopnea syndrome (OSAHS) (adjunct to standard treatment for underlying airway obstruction)**
- Attention deficit hyperactivity disorder (ADHD)
- Fatigue and sleepiness in depression
- Fatigue in multiple sclerosis

How the Drug Works
- Unknown, but clearly different from classical stimulants such as methylphenidate and amphetamine
- Binds to and requires the presence of the dopamine transporter; also requires the presence of alpha adrenergic receptors
- Hypothetically acts as an inhibitor of the dopamine transporter
- Increases neuronal activity selectively in the hypothalamus

✽ Presumably enhances activity in hypothalamic wakefulness center (TMN, tuberomammillary nucleus) within the hypothalamic sleep-wake switch by an unknown mechanism

✽ Activates tuberomammillary nucleus neurons that release histamine

✽ Activates other hypothalamic neurons that release orexin/hypocretin

How Long Until It Works
- Can immediately reduce daytime sleepiness and improve cognitive task performance within 2 hours of first dosing
- Can take several days to optimize dosing and clinical improvement

If It Works
✽ Improves daytime sleepiness and may improve attention as well as fatigue

✽ Does not prevent one from falling asleep when needed
- May not completely normalize wakefulness
- Treat until improvement stabilizes and then continue treatment indefinitely as long as improvement persists

If It Doesn't Work
✽ Change dose; some patients do better with an increased dose but some actually do better with a decreased dose
- Augment or consider an alternative treatment for daytime sleepiness, fatigue, or ADHD

Best Augmenting Combos for Partial Response or Treatment Resistance
✽ Modafinil is itself an adjunct to standard treatments for obstructive sleep apnea/hypopnea syndrome (OSAHS); if continuous positive airway pressure (CPAP) is the treatment of choice, a maximal effort to treat first with CPAP should be made prior to initiating modafinil and CPAP should be continued after initiation of modafinil

✽ Modafinil is itself an augmenting therapy to antidepressants for residual sleepiness and fatigue in major depressive disorder
- Best to attempt another monotherapy prior to augmenting with other drugs in the treatment of sleepiness associated with sleep disorders or problems concentrating in ADHD
- Combination of modafinil with stimulants such as methylphenidate or amphetamine or with atomoxetine for ADHD has not been systematically studied
- However, such combinations may be useful options for experts, with close monitoring, when numerous monotherapies for sleepiness or ADHD have failed

Tests
- None for healthy individuals

SIDE EFFECTS

How Drug Causes Side Effects
- Unknown

- CNS side effects presumably due to excessive CNS actions on various neurotransmitter systems

Notable Side Effects

✻ Headache
- Anxiety, nervousness, insomnia
- Dry mouth, diarrhea, nausea, anorexia
- Pharyngitis, rhinitis, infection
- Hypertension
- Palpitations

Life-Threatening or Dangerous Side Effects

- Transient EKG ischemic changes in patients with mitral valve prolapse or left ventricular hypertrophy have been reported (rare)
- Rare activation of (hypo)mania, anxiety, hallucinations, or suicidal ideation
- Rare severe dermatologic reactions (Stevens-Johnson syndrome and others)

Weight Gain

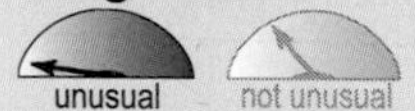

- Reported but not expected

Sedation

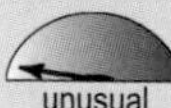
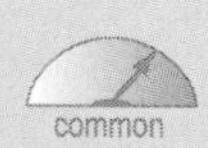

- Reported but not expected
- Patients are usually awakened and some may be activated

What to Do About Side Effects

- Wait
- Lower the dose
- Give only once daily
- Give smaller split doses 2 or more times daily
- For activation or insomnia, do not give in the evening
- If unacceptable side effects persist, discontinue use

Best Augmenting Agents for Side Effects

- Many side effects cannot be improved with an augmenting agent

DOSING AND USE

Usual Dosage Range

- 200 mg/day in the morning

Dosage Forms

- Tablet 100 mg, 200 mg (scored)

How To Dose

- Titration up or down only necessary if not optimally efficacious at the standard starting dose of 200 mg once a day in the morning

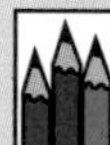

Dosing Tips

✻ For sleepiness, more may be more: higher doses (200–800 mg/day) may be better than lower doses (50–200 mg/day) in patients with daytime sleepiness in sleep disorders

✻ For problems concentrating and fatigue, less may be more: lower doses (50–200 mg/day) may be paradoxically better than higher doses (200–800 mg/day) in some patients
- At high doses, may slightly induce its own metabolism, possibly by actions of inducing CYP450 3A4
- Dose may creep upward in some patients with long-term treatment due to autoinduction; drug holiday may restore efficacy at original dose

Overdose

- No fatalities; agitation, insomnia, increase in hemodynamic parameters

Long-Term Use

- Efficacy in reducing excessive sleepiness in sleep disorders has been demonstrated in 9- to 12-week trials
- Unpublished data show safety for up to 136 weeks
- The need for continued treatment should be reevaluated periodically

Habit Forming

- Schedule IV; may have some potential for abuse but unusual in clinical practice

How to Stop

- Taper not necessary; patients may have sleepiness on discontinuation

Pharmacokinetics

- Metabolized by the liver
- Excreted renally
- Elimination half-life 10–2 hours
- Inhibits CYP450 2C19 (and perhaps 2C9)

- Induces CYP450 3A4 (and slightly 1A2 and 2B6)

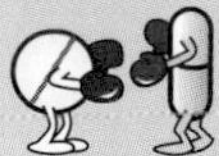

Drug Interactions

- May increase plasma levels of drugs metabolized by CYP450 2C19 (e.g., diazepam, phenytoin, propranolol)
- Modafinil may increase plasma levels of CYP450 2D6 substrates such as tricyclic antidepressants and SSRIs, perhaps requiring downward dose adjustments of these agents
- Modafinil may decrease plasma levels of CYP450 3A4 substrates such as ethinyl estradiol and triazolam
- Due to induction of CYP450 3A4, effectiveness of steroidal contraceptives may be reduced by modafinil, including 1 month after discontinuation
- Inducers or inhibitors of CYP450 3A4 may affect levels of modafinil (e.g., carbamazepine may lower modafinil plasma levels; fluvoxamine and fluoxetine may raise modafinil plasma levels)
- Modafinil may slightly reduce its own levels by autoinduction of CYP450 3A4
- Modafinil may increase clearance of drugs dependent on CYP450 1A2 and reduce their plasma levels
- Patients on modafinil and warfarin should have prothrombin times monitored
- Methylphenidate may delay absorption of modafinil by an hour

❋ However, coadministration with methylphenidate does not significantly change the pharmacokinetics of either modafinil or methylphenidate

❋ Coadministration with dextroamphetamine also does not significantly change the pharmacokinetics of either modafinil or dextroamphetamine

- Interaction studies with MAO inhibitors have not been performed, but MAOIs can be given with modafinil by experts with cautious monitoring

Other Warnings/ Precautions

- Patients with history of drug abuse should be monitored closely
- Modafinil may cause CNS effects similar to those caused by other CNS agents (e.g., changes in mood and, theoretically, activation of psychosis, mania, or suicidal ideation)
- Modafinil should be used in patients with sleep disorders that have been completely evaluated for narcolepsy, obstructive sleep apnea/hypopnea syndrome (OSAHS), and shift work sleep disorder
- In OSAHS patients for whom continuous positive airway pressure (CPAP) is the treatment of choice, a maximal effort to treat first with CPAP should be made prior to initiating modafinil, and then CPAP should be continued after initiating modafinil
- The effectiveness of steroidal contraceptives may be reduced when used with modafinil and for 1 month after discontinuation of modafinil
- Modafinil is not a replacement for sleep

Do Not Use

- If patient has severe hypertension
- If patient has cardiac arrhythmias
- If there is a proven allergy to modafinil

SPECIAL POPULATIONS

Renal Impairment

- Use with caution; dose reduction is recommended

Hepatic Impairment

- Reduce dose by half in severely impaired patients

Cardiac Impairment

- Use with caution
- Not recommended for use in patients with a history of left ventricular hypertrophy, ischemic EKG changes, chest pain, arrhythmias, or recent myocardial infarction

Elderly

- Limited experience in patients over 65
- Clearance of modafinil may be reduced in elderly patients

Children and Adolescents

- Safety and efficacy not established under age 16
- Can be used cautiously by experts for children and adolescents

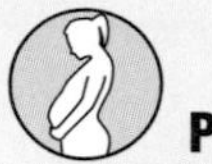

Pregnancy

- Risk Category C [some animal studies show adverse effects; no controlled studies in humans]
- Animal studies were conducted at doses lower than necessary to elucidate the effects of modafinil on the developing fetus
- Use in women of childbearing potential requires weighing potential benefits to the mother against potential risks to the fetus

✻ Generally, modafinil should be discontinued prior to anticipated pregnancies

Breast Feeding

- Unknown if modafinil is secreted in human breast milk, but all psychotropics assumed to be secreted in breast milk

✻ Recommended either to discontinue drug or bottle feed

THE ART OF PSYCHOPHARMACOLOGY

Potential Advantages

- Selective for areas of brain involved in sleep/wake promotion
- Less activating and less abuse potential than stimulants

Potential Disadvantages

- May not work as well as stimulants in some patients

Primary Target Symptoms

- Sleepiness
- Concentration
- Physical and mental fatigue

Pearls

✻ Only agent approved for treating sleepiness associated with obstructive sleep apnea/hypopnea syndrome (OSAHS)

✻ Only agent approved for treating sleepiness associated with shift work sleep disorder

✻ Anecdotal usefulness for jet lag short-term (off-label)

✻ Modafinil is not a replacement for sleep

✻ The treatment for sleep deprivation is sleep, not modafinil

- Controlled studies suggest modafinil improves attention in OSAHS, shift work sleep disorder, and ADHD (both children and adults), but controlled studies of attention have not been performed in major depressive disorder

✻ May be useful to treat fatigue in patients with depression as well as other disorders, such as multiple sclerosis, myotonic dystrophy, HIV/AIDS

- In depression, modafinil's actions on fatigue appear to be independent of actions (if any) on mood
- In depression, modafinil's actions on sleepiness also appear to be independent of actions (if any) on mood but may be linked to actions on fatigue or on global functioning
- Several controlled studies in depression show improvement in sleepiness or global functioning, especially for depressed patients with sleepiness and fatigue
- May be useful adjunct to mood stabilizers for bipolar depression
- May be useful in treating sleepiness associated with opioid analgesia, particularly in end-of-life management
- Subjective sensation associated with modafinil is usually one of normal wakefulness, not of stimulation, although jitteriness can rarely occur
- Anecdotally, some patients may experience wearing off of efficacy over time, especially for off-label uses, with restoration of efficacy after a drug holiday; such wearing off is less likely with intermittent dosing

✻ Compared to stimulants, modafinil has a novel mechanism of action, novel therapeutic uses, and less abuse potential, but is often inaccurately classified as a stimulant

- Alpha 1 antagonists such as prazosin may block the therapeutic actions of modafinil
- The active R-enantiomer of modafinil, also called armodafinil, is in late-stage clinical development

Suggested Reading

Batejat DM, Lagarde DP. Naps and modafinil as countermeasures for the effects of sleep deprivation on cognitive performance. Aviat Space Environ Med 1999;70:493–8.

Bourdon L, Jacobs I, Bateman WA, Vallerand AL. Effect of modafinil on heat production and regulation of body temperatures in cold-exposed humans. Aviat Space Environ Med 1994;65:999–1004.

Cox JM, Pappagallo M. Modafinil: a gift to portmanteau. Am J Hosp Palliat Care 2001;18:408–10.

Jasinski DR, Koyacevic-Ristanovic. Evaluation of the abuse liability of modafinil and other drugs for excessive daytime sleepiness associated with narcolepsy. Clin Neuropharmacol 2000;23:149–56.

Wesensten NJ, Belenky G, Kautz MA, Thorne DR, Reichardt RM, Balkin TJ. Maintaining alertness and performance during sleep deprivation: modafinil versus caffeine. Psychopharmacology (Berl) 2002;159:238–47.

MOLINDONE

THERAPEUTICS

Brands • Moban

see index for additional brand names

Generic? Yes

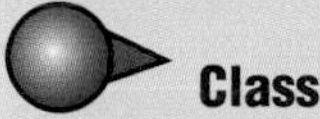

Class

- Conventional antipsychotic (neuroleptic, dopamine 2 antagonist)

Commonly Prescribed for

(bold for FDA approved)

- **Schizophrenia**
- Other psychotic disorders
- Bipolar disorder

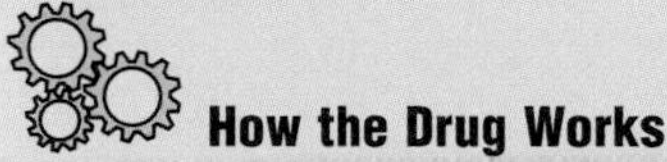

How the Drug Works

- Blocks dopamine 2 receptors, reducing positive symptoms of psychosis

How Long Until It Works

- Psychotic symptoms can improve within 1 week, but it may take several weeks for full effect on behavior

If It Works

- Most often reduces positive symptoms in schizophrenia but does not eliminate them
- Most schizophrenic patients do not have a total remission of symptoms but rather a reduction of symptoms by about a third
- Continue treatment in schizophrenia until reaching a plateau of improvement
- After reaching a satisfactory plateau, continue treatment for at least a year after first episode of psychosis in schizophrenia
- For second and subsequent episodes of psychosis in schizophrenia, treatment may need to be indefinite
- Reduces symptoms of acute psychotic mania but not proven as a mood stabilizer or as an effective maintenance treatment in bipolar disorder
- After reducing acute psychotic symptoms in mania, switch to a mood stabilizer and/or an atypical antipsychotic for mood stabilization and maintenance

If It Doesn't Work

- Consider trying one of the first-line atypical antipsychotics (risperidone, olanzapine, quetiapine, ziprasidone, aripiprazole, paliperidone, amisulpride)
- Consider trying another conventional antipsychotic
- If 2 or more antipsychotic monotherapies do not work, consider clozapine

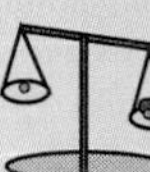

Best Augmenting Combos for Partial Response or Treatment Resistance

- Augmentation of conventional antipsychotics has not been systematically studied
- Addition of a mood stabilizing anticonvulsant such as valproate, carbamazepine, or lamotrigine may be helpful in both schizophrenia and bipolar mania
- Augmentation with lithium in bipolar mania may be helpful
- Addition of a benzodiazepine, especially short-term for agitation

Tests

✻ Since conventional antipsychotics are frequently associated with weight gain, before starting treatment, weigh all patients and determine if the patient is already overweight (BMI 25.0–29.9) or obese (BMI ≥30)

- Before giving a drug that can cause weight gain to an overweight or obese patient, consider determining whether the patient already has pre-diabetes (fasting plasma glucose 100–25 mg/dL), diabetes (fasting plasma glucose >126 mg/dL), or dyslipidemia (increased total cholesterol, LDL cholesterol and triglycerides; decreased HDL cholesterol), and treat or refer such patients for treatment, including nutrition and weight management, physical activity counseling, smoking cessation, and medical management

✻ Monitor weight and BMI during treatment

✻ Consider monitoring fasting triglycerides monthly for several months in patients at high risk for metabolic complications and when initiating or switching antipsychotics

✻ While giving a drug to a patient who has gained >5% of initial weight, consider evaluating for the presence of pre-diabetes, diabetes, or dyslipidemia, or consider switching to a different antipsychotic

- Should check blood pressure in the elderly before starting and for the first few weeks of treatment
- Monitoring elevated prolactin levels of dubious clinical benefit

SIDE EFFECTS

How Drug Causes Side Effects

- By blocking dopamine 2 receptors in the striatum, it can cause motor side effects
- By blocking dopamine 2 receptors in the pituitary, it can cause elevations in prolactin
- By blocking dopamine 2 receptors excessively in the mesocortical and mesolimbic dopamine pathways, especially at high doses, it can cause worsening of negative and cognitive symptoms (neuroleptic-induced deficit syndrome)
- Anticholinergic actions may cause sedation, blurred vision, constipation, dry mouth
- Antihistaminic actions may cause sedation, weight gain
- By blocking alpha 1 adrenergic receptors, it can cause dizziness, sedation, and hypotension
- Mechanism of weight gain and any possible increased incidence of diabetes or dyslipidemia with conventional antipsychotics is unknown

Notable Side Effects

❋ Neuroleptic-induced deficit syndrome
❋ Akathisia
❋ Extrapyramidal symptoms, Parkinsonism, tardive dyskinesia
❋ Galactorrhea, amenorrhea
- Sedation
- Dry mouth, constipation, vision disturbance, urninary retention
- Hypotension, tachycardia

Life-Threatening or Dangerous Side Effects

- Rare neuroleptic malignant syndrome
- Rare leukopenia
- Rare seizures
- Increased risk of death and cerebrovascular events in elderly patients with dementia-related psychosis

Weight Gain

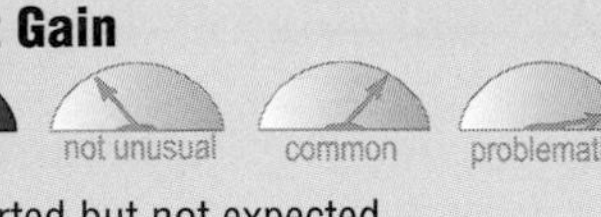

❋ Reported but not expected

Sedation

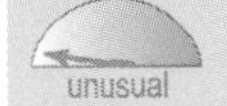

- Many experience and/or can be significant in amount
- Sedation is usually transient

What to Do About Side Effects

- Wait
- Wait
- Wait
- For motor symptoms, add an anticholinergic agent
- Reduce the dose
- For sedation, give at night
- Switch to an atypical antipsychotic
- Weight loss, exercise programs, and medical management for high BMIs, diabetes, dyslipidemia

Best Augmenting Agents for Side Effects

- Benztropine or trihexyphenidyl for motor side effects
- Sometimes amantadine can be helpful for motor side effects
- Benzodiazepines may be helpful for akathisia
- Many side effects cannot be improved with an augmenting agent

DOSING AND USE

Usual Dosage Range

- 40–100 mg/day in divided doses

Dosage Forms

- Tablet 5 mg, 10 mg, 25 mg scored, 50 mg scored, 100 mg scored
- Liquid 20 mg/mL

How To Dose

- Initial 50–75 mg/day; increase to 100 mg/day after 3–4 days; maximum 225 mg/day

Dosing Tips
- Very short half-life, but some patients may only require once daily dosing
- Other patients may do better with 3 or 4 divided doses daily
- Patients receiving atypical antipsychotics may occasionally require a "top up" of a conventional antipsychotic to control aggression or violent behavior

Overdose
- Deaths have occurred; extrapyramidal symptoms, sedation, hypotension, respiratory depression, coma

Long-Term Use
- Some side effects may be irreversible (e.g., tardive dyskinesia)

Habit Forming
- No

How to Stop
- Slow down-titration (over 6–8 weeks), especially when simultaneously beginning a new antipsychotic while switching (i.e., cross-titration)
- Rapid discontinuation may lead to rebound psychosis and worsening of symptoms
- If antiparkinson agents are being used, they should be continued for a few weeks after molindone is discontinued

Pharmacokinetics
- Half-life approximately 1.5 hours

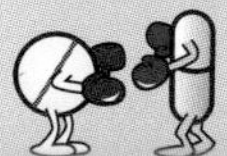

Drug Interactions
- Additive effects may occur if used with CNS depressants
- Some patients taking a neuroleptic and lithium have developed an encephalopathic syndrome similar to neuroleptic malignant syndrome
- Molindone tablets contain calcium sulfate, which may interfere with absorption of phenytoin sodium or tetracyclines
- Combined use with epinephrine may lower blood pressure
- May increase the effects of antihypertensive drugs

Other Warnings/ Precautions
- If signs of neuroleptic malignant syndrome develop, treatment should be immediately discontinued
- Liquid molindone contains sodium metabisulfite, which may cause allergic reactions in some people, especially in asthmatic people
- Use cautiously in patients with alcohol withdrawal or convulsive disorders because of possible lowering of seizure threshold
- Antiemetic effect can mask signs of other disorders or overdose
- Do not use epinephrine in event of overdose as interaction with some pressor agents may lower blood pressure
- Use cautiously in patients with glaucoma, urinary retention
- Observe for signs of ocular toxicity (pigmentary retinopathy, lenticular pigmentation)
- Use only with caution if at all in Parkinson's disease or Lewy body dementia

Do Not Use
- If patient is in a comatose state or has CNS depression
- If there is a proven allergy to molindone

SPECIAL POPULATIONS

Renal Impairment
- Should receive initial lower dose

Hepatic Impairment
- Should receive initial lower dose

Cardiac Impairment
- Use with caution

Elderly
- Should receive initial lower dose
- Although conventional antipsychotics are commonly used for behavioral disturbances in dementia, no agent has been approved for treatment of elderly patients with dementia-related psychosis
- Elderly patients with dementia-related psychosis treated with antipsychotics are at an increased risk of death compared to

placebo, and also have an increased risk of cerebrovascular events

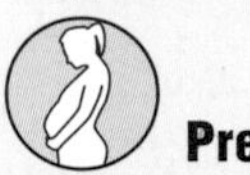

Children and Adolescents

- Safety and efficacy not well established
- Generally consider second-line after atypical antipsychotics

Pregnancy

- Animal studies have not shown adverse effects
- No studies in pregnant women
- Psychotic symptoms may worsen during pregnancy and some form of treatment may be necessary
- Atypical antipsychotics may be preferable to conventional antipsychotics or anticonvulsant mood stabilizers if treatment is required during pregnancy

Breast Feeding

- Unknown if molindone is secreted in human breast milk, but all psychotropics assumed to be secreted in breast milk
- ✻ Recommended either to discontinue drug or bottle feed

THE ART OF PSYCHOPHARMACOLOGY

Potential Advantages

- Some patients benefit from molindone's sedative properties

Potential Disadvantages

- Patients with tardive dyskinesia

Primary Target Symptoms

- Positive symptoms of psychosis
- Motor and autonomic hyperactivity
- Violent or aggressive behavior

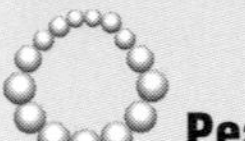

Pearls

- ✻ May cause less weight gain than some other antipsychotics
- Conventional antipsychotics are much less expensive than atypical antipsychotics
- Not shown to be effective for behavioral problems in mental retardation
- Patients have very similar antipsychotic responses to any conventional antipsychotic, which is different from atypical antipsychotics where antipsychotic responses of individual patients can occasionally vary greatly from one atypical antipsychotic to another
- Patients with inadequate responses to atypical antipsychotics may benefit from a trial of augmentation with a conventional antipsychotic such as molindone or from switching to a conventional antipsychotic such as molindone
- However, long-term polypharmacy with a combination of a conventional antipsychotic such as molindone with an atypical antipsychotic may combine their side effects without clearly augmenting the efficacy of either
- Although a frequent practice by some prescribers, adding two conventional antipsychotics together has little rationale and may reduce tolerability without clearly enhancing efficacy

Suggested Reading

Bagnall A, Fenton M, Lewis R, Leitner ML, Kleijnen J. Molindone for schizophrenia and severe mental illness. Cochrane Database Syst Rev 2000;(2):CD002083.

Owen RR Jr, Cole JO. Molindone hydrochloride: a review of laboratory and clinical findings. J Clin Psychopharmacol 1989;9(4):268–76.

THERAPEUTICS

Brands
- Revia (oral)
- Vivitrol (injection)

see index for additional brand names

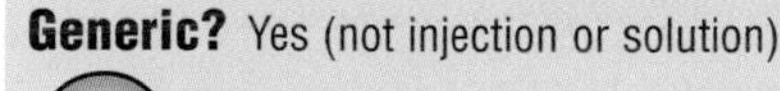

Generic? Yes (not injection or solution)

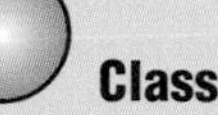

Class
- Alcohol dependence treatment; muopioid receptor antagonist

Commonly Prescribed for
(bold for FDA approved)
- **Alcohol dependence**
- **Blockade of effects of exogenously administered opioids (oral)**

How the Drug Works
- Blocks mu opioid receptors, preventing alcohol or exogenous opioids from binding there and thus preventing the pleasurable effects of alcohol or opioid consumption

How Long Until It Works
- Can begin working within a few days but maximum effects may not be seen for a few weeks

If It Works
- Diminishes rewarding effects of alcohol or opioid consumption
- Reduces cravings, decreases alcohol or opioid consumption

If It Doesn't Work
- Evaluate for and address contributing factors
- Consider switching to another agent
- Consider augmenting with acamprosate

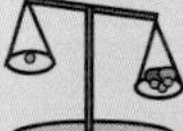

Best Augmenting Combos for Partial Response or Treatment Resistance
- Acamprosate
- Augmentation therapy may be more effective than monotherapy
- Augmentation with behavioral, education, and/or supportive therapy in groups or as an individual is probably key to successful treatment

Tests
- Urine screen for opioids and/or naloxone challenge test prior to initiating treatment for opioid use
- None for use in treating alcohol dependence, although baseline liver function testing, usually obtained anyway for managing alcohol dependence, may be useful

SIDE EFFECTS

How Drug Causes Side Effects
- Blockade of mu opioid receptors

Notable Side Effects
- Nausea, vomiting, decreased appetite
- Dizziness
- Injection site reactions (pain, tenderness, pruritis, induration)

Life-Threatening or Dangerous Side Effects
- Eosinophilic pneumonia
- Hepatocellular injury (at excessive doses)
- Severe injection site reactions requiring surgery

Weight Gain

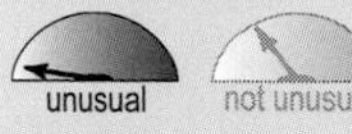

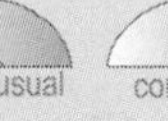

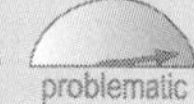

- Reported but not expected

Sedation

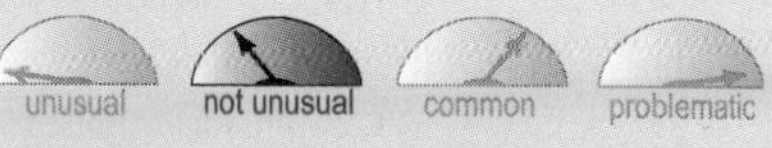

- Occurs in significant minority

What to Do About Side Effects
- Wait
- Adjust dose
- If side effects persist, discontinue use

Best Augmenting Agents for Side Effects
- Dose reduction or switching to another agent may be more effective since most side effects cannot be improved with an augmenting agent

DOSING AND USE

Usual Dosage Range
- Oral: 50 mg/day
- Injection: 380 mg every 4 weeks

Dosage Forms
- Tablet 25 mg, 50 mg, 100 mg
- Oral solution 12 mg/0.6 mL
- Intramuscular formulation 380 mg/vial

How To Dose
- For treating alcohol dependence (oral): recommended dose is 50 mg/day; titration is not required
- For treating alcohol dependence (injection): 380 mg delivered intramuscularly in the gluteal region every 4 weeks; alternate buttocks; must be administered by healthcare professional
- Patient should be opioid free for 7–10 days prior to initiating treatment, as confirmed by negative urine screen and/or naloxone challenge test
- Opioid dependence (oral): initial 25 mg/day; day 2 can increase to 50 mg/day

Dosing Tips
- Providing educational materials and counseling in combination with naltrexone treatment can increase the chances of success
- Individuals who abstain from alcohol for several days prior to initiating treatment with naltrexone may have greater reductions in the number of drinking days as well as number of heavy drinking days, and may also be more likely to abstain completely throughout treatment
- Long-acting naltrexone (injection) must be kept refrigerated
- For long-acting naltrexone (injection), the suspension should be administered immediately after mixing
- Adherence greatly enhanced and assured for 30 days at a time when administering by once monthly depot injection; oral treatment requires 30 decisions to comply in 30 days whereas long-acting injection requires only one decision every 30 days to comply

Overdose
- Nausea, abdominal pain, sedation, dizziness, injection site reactions

Long Term Use
- Has been studied in trials up to one year

Habit Forming
- No

How to Stop
- Taper not necessary

Pharmacokinetics
- Elimination half-life of oral naltrexone is approximately 13 hours
- Elimination half-life of naltrexone via injection is 5–10 days

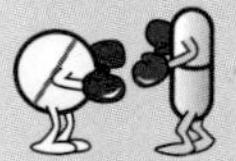

Drug Interactions
- Is hepatically metabolized by dihydrodiol dehydrogenase and not by the CYP450 enzyme system, and thus is unlikely to be affected by drugs that induce or inhibit CYP450 enzymes
- Can block the effects of opioid-containing medications (e.g., some cough and cold remedies, antidiarrheal preparations, opioid analgesics)
- Concomitant administration with acamprosate may increase plasma levels of acamprosate, but this does not appear to be clinically significant and dose adjustment is not recommended

Other Warnings/Precautions
- Can cause hepatocellular injury when given in excessive doses
- To prevent withdrawal in patients dependent on opioids, patients must be opioid free for at least 7–10 days prior to initiating treatment
- Attempts by patients to overcome blockade of opioid receptors by taking large amounts of exogenous opioids could lead to opioid intoxication or even fatal overdose
- Individuals who have been previously treated with naltrexone should be warned that they may respond to lower doses of opioids than previously used, and thus

previous doses may also lead to opioid intoxication
- Individuals receiving naltrexone who require pain management with opioid analgesia may need a higher dose than usual and may experience deeper and more prolonged respiratory depression; pain management with non-opioid or rapid acting opioid analgesics is recommended if possible
- Monitor patients for emergence of depressed mood or suicidality
- Use cautiously in individuals with known psychiatric illness
- Injection should be used cautiously in individuals with thrombocytopenia or any coagulation disorder

Do Not Use
- If patient is taking opioid analgesics
- If patient is currently dependent on opioids or is in acute opiate withdrawal
- If patient has failed the naloxone challenge test or has a positive urine screen for opioids
- If there is a proven allergy to naltrexone
- If there is a proven allergy to polylactide-co-glycolide (PLG), arboxymethylcellulose, or any other components of the diluent (injection)

SPECIAL POPULATIONS

Renal Impairment
- Dose adjustment not generally necessary for mild impairment
- Not studied in moderate to severe renal impairment

Hepatic Impairment
- Has the potential to cause hepatocellular injury when given in excessive doses
- Dose adjustment not generally necessary for mild impairment
- Not studied in severe hepatic impairment
- Contraindicated in acute hepatitis or liver failure

Cardiac Impairment
- Limited available data

Elderly
- Safety and efficacy have not been established
- Some patients may tolerate lower doses better

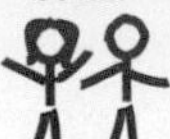

Children and Adolescents
- Safety and efficacy have not been established

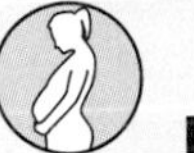

Pregnancy
- Risk Category C [some animal studies show adverse effects; no controlled studies in humans]
- Pregnant women needing to stop drinking may consider behavioral therapy before pharmacotherapy
- Not generally recommended for use during pregnancy, especially during first trimester

Breast Feeding
- Some drug is found in mother's breast milk
- Recommended either to discontinue drug or bottle feed

THE ART OF PSYCHOPHARMACOLOGY

Potential Advantages
- Individuals who are not ready to abstain completely from alcohol
- For binge drinkers

Potential Disadvantages
- Patients who "drink over" their treatment, including their long-acting injection
- Less effective in patients who are not abstinent at the time of treatment initation

Primary Target Symptoms
- Alcohol dependence

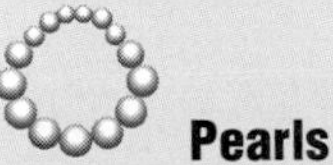

Pearls
- Not only increases total abstinence, but also can reduce days of heavy drinking
- May be a preferred treatment if the goal is reduced-risk drinking (i.e., 3–4 drinks per day in men, maximum 16 drinks per week; 2–3 drinks per day in women, maximum 12 drinks per week)
- Some patients complain of apathy or loss of pleasure with chronic treatment

Suggested Reading

Anton RF, O'Malley SS, Ciraulo DA, et al. Combined pharmacotherapies and behavioral interventions for alcohol dependence: the COMBINE study: a randomized controlled trial. JAMA 2006;295(17):2003–17.

Johansson BA, Berglund M, Lindregn A. Efficacy of maintenance treatment with naltrexone for opioid dependence: a meta-analytical review. Addiction 2006;101(4):491–503.

Mannelli P, Peindl K, Masand PS, Patkar SS. Long-acting injectable naltrexone for the treatment of alcohol dependence. Expert Rev Neurother 2007;7(10):1265–77.

Rosner S, Leucht S, Lehert P, Soyka M. Acamprosate supports abstinence, naltrexone prevents excessive drinking: evidence from a met-analysis with unreported outcomes. J Psychopharmacol 2008;22:11-23.

THERAPEUTICS

Brands • Dutonin

see index for additional brand names

Generic? Yes

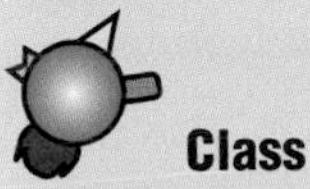

Class

- SARI (serotonin 2 antagonist/reuptake inhibitor); antidepressant

Commonly Prescribed for

(bold for FDA approved)

- **Depression**
- **Relapse prevention in MDD**
- Panic disorder
- Posttraumatic stress disorder (PTSD)

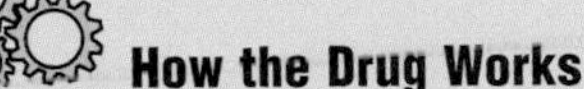

How the Drug Works

- Blocks serotonin 2A receptors potently
- Blocks serotonin reuptake pump (serotonin transporter) and norepinephrine reuptake pump (norepinephrine transporter) less potently

How Long Until It Works

- Can improve insomnia and anxiety early after initiating dosing
- Onset of therapeutic actions usually not immediate, but often delayed 2–4 weeks
- If it is not working within 6–8 weeks for depression, it may require a dosage increase or it may not work at all
- May continue to work for many years to prevent relapse of symptoms

If It Works

- The goal of treatment is complete remission of current symptoms as well as prevention of future relapses
- Treatment most often reduces or even eliminates symptoms, but not a cure since symptoms can recur after medicine stopped
- Continue treatment until all symptoms are gone (remission)
- Once symptoms gone, continue treating for 1 year for the first episode of depression
- For second and subsequent episodes of depression, treatment may need to be indefinite
- Use in anxiety disorders may also need to be indefinite

If It Doesn't Work

- Many patients have only a partial response where some symptoms are improved but others persist (especially insomnia, fatigue, and problems concentrating)
- Other patients may be nonresponders, sometimes called treatment-resistant or treatment-refractory
- Some patients who have an initial response may relapse even though they continue treatment, sometimes called "poop-out"
- Consider increasing dose, switching to another agent or adding an appropriate augmenting agent
- Consider psychotherapy, especially cognitive-behavioral psychotherapies, which have been specifically shown to enhance nefazodone's antidepressant actions
- Consider evaluation for another diagnosis or for a comorbid condition (e.g., medical illness, substance abuse, etc.)
- Some patients may experience apparent lack of consistent efficacy due to activation of latent or underlying bipolar disorder, and require antidepressant discontinuation and a switch to a mood stabilizer

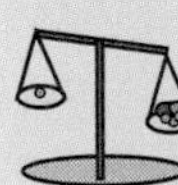

Best Augmenting Combos for Partial Response or Treatment Resistance

- ✱ Venlafaxine and escitalopram may be the best tolerated when switching or augmenting with a serotonin reuptake inhibitor, as neither is a potent CYP450 2D6 inhibitor (use combinations of antidepressants with caution as this may activate bipolar disorder and suicidal ideation)
- Modafinil, especially for fatigue, sleepiness, and lack of concentration
- Mood stabilizers or atypical antipsychotics for bipolar depression, psychotic depression or treatment-resistant depression
- Benzodiazepines for anxiety, but give alprazolam cautiously with nefazodone as alprazolam levels can be much higher in the presence of nefazodone
- Classically, lithium, buspirone, or thyroid hormone

Tests

✻ Liver function testing is not required but is often prudent given the small but finite risk of serious hepatoxicity

✻ However, to date no clinical strategy, including routine liver function tests, has been identified to reduce the risk of irreversible liver failure

SIDE EFFECTS

How Drug Causes Side Effects

- Blockade of alpha adrenergic 1 receptors may explain dizziness, sedation, and hypotension
- A metabolite of nefazodone, mCPP (*meta*-chloro-phenyl-piperazine), can cause side effects if its levels rise significantly

✻ If CYP450 2D6 is absent (7% of Caucasians lack CYP450 2D6) or inhibited (concomitant treatment with CYP450 2D6 inhibitors such as fluoxetine or paroxetine), increased levels of mCPP can form, leading to stimulation of 5HT2C receptors and causing dizziness, insomnia, and agitation

- Most side effects are immediate but often go away with time

Notable Side Effects

- Nausea, dry mouth, constipation, dyspepsia, increased appetite
- Headache, dizziness, vision changes, sedation, insomnia, agitation, confusion, memory impairment
- Ataxia, paresthesia, asthenia
- Cough increased
- Rare postural hypotension

Life-Threatening or Dangerous Side Effects

- Rare seizures
- Rare induction of mania
- Rare activation of suicidal ideation and behavior (suicidality) (short-term studies did not show an increase in the risk of suicidality with antidepressants compared to placebo beyond age 24)
- Rare priapism (no causal relationship established)
- Hepatic failure requiring liver transplant and/or fatal

Weight Gain

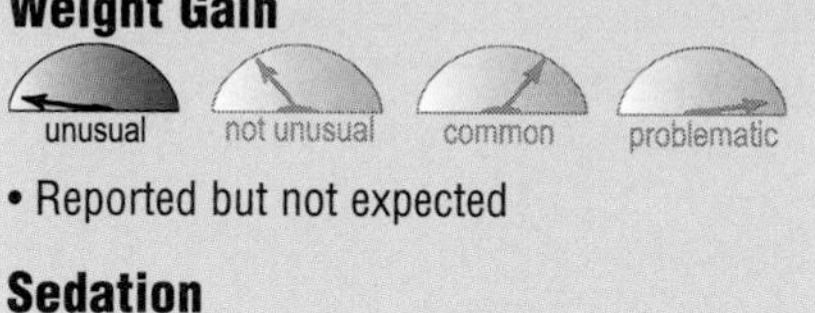

- Reported but not expected

Sedation

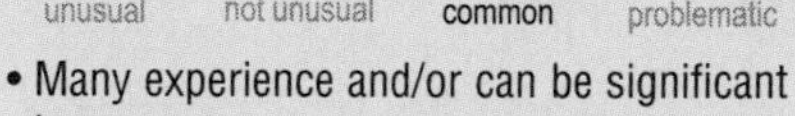

- Many experience and/or can be significant in amount

What to Do About Side Effects

- Wait
- Wait
- Wait
- Take once-daily at night to reduce daytime sedation
- Lower the dose and try titrating again more slowly as tolerated
- Switch to another agent

Best Augmenting Agents for Side Effects

- Often best to try another antidepressant monotherapy prior to resorting to augmentation strategies to treat side effects
- Many side effects cannot be improved with an augmenting agent
- Many side effects are dose-dependent (i.e., they increase as dose increases, or they reemerge until tolerance re-develops)
- Many side effects are time-dependent (i.e., they start immediately upon dosing and upon each dose increase, but go away with time)
- Activation and agitation may represent the induction of a bipolar state, especially a mixed dysphoric bipolar II condition sometimes associated with suicidal ideation, and require the addition of lithium, a mood stabilizer or an atypical antipsychotic, and/or discontinuation of nefazodone

DOSING AND USE

Usual Dosage Range

- 300–600 mg/day

Dosage Forms

- Tablet 50 mg, 100 mg scored, 150 mg scored, 200 mg, 250 mg

How To Dose

- Initial dose 100 mg twice a day; increase by 100–200 mg/day each week until desired efficacy is reached; maximum dose 600 mg twice a day

Dosing Tips

- Take care switching from or adding to SSRIs (especially fluoxetine or paroxetine) because of side effects due to the drug interaction
- Do not underdose the elderly
- Normally twice daily dosing, especially when initiating treatment
- Patients may tolerate all dosing once daily at night once titrated
- Often much more effective at 400–600 mg/day than at lower doses if tolerated
- Slow titration can enhance tolerability when initiating dosing

Overdose

- Rarely lethal; sedation, nausea, vomiting, low blood pressure

Long-Term Use

- Safe

Habit Forming

- No

How to Stop

- Taper is prudent to avoid withdrawal effects, but problems in withdrawal not common

Pharmacokinetics

- Half-life of parent compound is 2–4 hours
- Half-life of active mebatolites up to 12 hours
- Inhibits CYP450 3A4

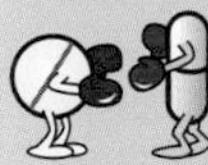

Drug Interactions

- Tramadol increases the risk of seizures in patients taking an antidepressant
- May interact with SSRIs such as paroxetine, fluoxetine, and others that inhibit CYP450 2D6

✻ Since a metabolite of nefazodone, mCPP, is a substrate of CYP450 2D6, combination of 2D6 inhibitors with nefazodone will raise mCPP levels, leading to stimulation of 5HT2C receptors and causing dizziness and agitation

- Can cause a fatal "serotonin syndrome" when combined with MAO inhibitors, so do not use with MAO inhibitors or for at least 14 days after MAOIs are stopped
- Do not start an MAO inhibitor for at least 2 weeks after discontinuing nefazodone
- Via CYP450 3A4 inhibition, nefazodone may increase the half-life of alprazolam and triazolam, so their dosing may need to be reduced by half or more
- Via CYP450 3A4, nefazodone may increase plasma concentrations of buspirone, so buspirone dose may need to be reduced
- Via CYP450 3A4 inhibition, nefazodone could theoretically increase concentrations of certain cholesterol lowering HMG CoA reductase inhibitors, especially simvastatin, atorvastatin, and lovastatin, but not pravastatin or fluvastatin, which would increase the risk of rhabdomyolysis; thus, coadministration of nefazodone with certain HMG CoA reductase inhibitors should proceed with caution
- Via CYP450 3A4 inhibition, nefazodone could theoretically increase the concentrations of pimozide, and cause QTc prolongation and dangerous cardiac arrhythmias
- Nefazodone may reduce clearance of haloperidol, so haloperidol dose may need to be reduced
- It is recommended to discontinue nefazodone prior to elective surgery because of the potential for interaction with general anesthetics

Other Warnings/ Precautions

✻ Hepatotoxicity, sometimes requiring liver transplant and/or fatal, has occurred with nefazodone use. Risk may be one in every 250,000 to 300,000 patient years. Patients should be advised to report symptoms such as jaundice, dark urine, loss of appetite, nausea, and abdominal pain to prescriber immediately. If patient develops signs of hepatocellular injury, such as increased serum AST or serum ALPT levels >3 times the upper limit of normal, nefazodone treatment should be discontinued.

* No risk factor yet predicts who will develop irreversible liver failure with nefazodone and no clinical strategy, including routine monitoring of liver function tests, is known to reduce the risk of liver failure
- Use with caution in patients with history of seizures
- Use with caution in patients with bipolar disorder unless treated with concomitant mood-stabilizing agent
- When treating children, carefully weigh the risks and benefits of pharmacological treatment against the risks and benefits of nontreatment with antidepressants and make sure to document this in the patient's chart
- Distribute the brochures provided by the FDA and the drug companies
- Warn patients and their caregivers about the possibility of activating side effects and advise them to report such symptoms immediately
- Monitor patients for activation of suicidal ideation, especially children and adolescents

Do Not Use
- If patient is taking an MAO inhibitor
- If patient has acute hepatic impairment or elevated baseline serum transaminases
- If patient was previously withdrawn from nefazodone treatment due to hepatic injury
- If patient is taking pimozide, as nefazodone could raise pimozide levels and increase QTc interval, perhaps causing dangerous arrhythmia
- If patient is taking carbamazepine, as this agent can dramatically reduce nefazodone levels and thus interfere with its antidepressant actions
- If there is a proven allergy to nefazodone

SPECIAL POPULATIONS

Renal Impairment
- No dose adjustment necessary

Hepatic Impairment
- Contraindicated in patients with known hepatic impairment

Cardiac Impairment
- Use in patients with cardiac impairment has not been studied, so use with caution because of risk of orthostatic hypotension

Elderly
- Recommended to initiate treatment at half the usual adult dose, but to follow the same titration schedule as with younger patients, including same ultimate dose
- Reduction in risk of suicidality with antidepressants compared to placebo in adults age 65 and older

Children and Adolescents
- Carefully weigh the risks and benefits of pharmacological treatment against the risks and benefits of nontreatment with antidepressants and make sure to document this in the patient's chart
- Monitor patients face-to-face regularly, particularly during the first several weeks of treatment
- Use with caution, observing for activation of known or unknown bipolar disorder and/or suicidal ideation, and inform parents or guardian of this risk so they can help observe child or adolescent patients
- Safety and efficacy have not been established
- Preliminary research indicates efficacy and tolerability of nefazodone in children and adolescents with depression

Pregnancy
- Risk Category C [some animal studies show adverse effects; no controlled studies in humans]
- Not generally recommended for use during pregnancy, especially during first trimester
- Must weigh the risk of treatment (first trimester fetal development, third trimester newborn delivery) to the child against the risk of no treatment (recurrence of depression, maternal health, infant bonding) to the mother and child
- For many patients this may mean continuing treatment during pregnancy

Breast Feeding
- Unknown if nefazodone is secreted in human breast milk, but all psychotropics

assumed to be secreted in breast milk
- Trace amounts may be present in nursing children whose mothers are on nefazodone
- If child becomes irritable or sedated, breast feeding or drug may need to be discontinued
- Immediate postpartum period is a high-risk time for depression, especially in women who have had prior depressive episodes, so drug may need to be reinstituted late in the third trimester or shortly after childbirth to prevent a recurrence during the postpartum period
- Must weigh benefits of breast feeding with risks and benefits of antidepressant treatment versus nontreatment to both the infant and the mother
- For many patients, this may mean continuing treatment during breast feeding

THE ART OF PSYCHOPHARMACOLOGY

Potential Advantages
- Depressed patients with anxiety or insomnia who do not respond to other antidepressants
- Patients with SSRI-induced sexual dysfunction

Potential Disadvantages
- Patients who have difficulty with a long titration period or twice-daily dosing
- Patients with hepatic impairment

Primary Target Symptoms
- Depressed mood
- Sleep disturbance
- Anxiety

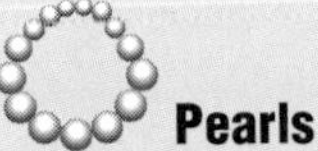

Pearls
- Preliminary data for efficacy in panic disorder and PTSD
- Fluoxetine and paroxetine may not be tolerated when switching or augmenting
- For elderly patients with early dementia and agitated depression, consider nefazodone in the morning and additional trazodone at night
- Anecdotal reports suggest that nefazodone may be effective in treating PMDD
- ✻ Studies suggest that cognitive-behavioral psychotherapy enhances the efficacy of nefazodone in chronic depression
- ✻ Risk of hepatotoxicity makes this agent a second-line choice and has led to its withdrawal from some markets, including the withdrawal of Serzone from the U.S. market
- Rarely, patients may complain of visual "trails" or after-images on nefazodone

Suggested Reading

DeVane CL, Grothe DR, Smith SL. Pharmacology of antidepressants: focus on nefazodone. J Clin Psychiatry 2002; 63(1):10–7.

Dunner DL, Laird LK, Zajecka J, Bailey L, Sussman N, Seabolt JL. Six-year perspectives on the safety and tolerability of nefazodone. J Clin Psychiatry 2002;63(1):32–41.

Khouzam HR. The antidepressant nefazodone. A review of its pharmacology, clinical efficacy, adverse effects, dosage, and administration. J Psychosocial Nursing Ment Health Serv 2000;38:20–25.

Masand PS, Gupta S. Long-term side effects of newer-generation antidepressants: SSRIS, venlafaxine, nefazodone, bupropion, and mirtazapine. Ann Clin Psychiatry 2002; 14:175–82.

Schatzberg AF, Prather MR, Keller MB, Rush AJ, Laird LK, Wright CW. Clinical use of nefazodone in major depression: a 6-year perspective. J Clin Psychiatry 2002; 63(1):18–31.

THERAPEUTICS

Brands • Pamelor

see index for additional brand names

Generic? Yes

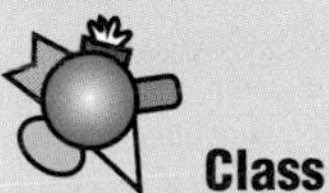

Class

- Tricyclic antidepressant (TCA)
- Predominantly a norepinephrine/ noradrenaline reuptake inhibitor

Commonly Prescribed for

(bold for FDA approved)

- **Major depressive disorder**
- Anxiety
- Insomnia
- Neuropathic pain/chronic pain
- Treatment-resistant depression

How the Drug Works

- Boosts neurotransmitter norepinephrine/ noradrenaline
- Blocks norepinephrine reuptake pump (norepinephrine transporter), presumably increasing noradrenergic neurotransmission
- Since dopamine is inactivated by norepinephrine reuptake in frontal cortex, which largely lacks dopamine transporters, nortriptyline can increase dopamine neurotransmission in this part of the brain
- A more potent inhibitor of norepinephrine reuptake pump than serotonin reuptake pump (serotonin transporter)
- At high doses may also boost neurotransmitter serotonin and presumably increase serotonergic neurotransmission

How Long Until It Works

- May have immediate effects in treating insomnia or anxiety
- Onset of therapeutic actions usually not immediate, but often delayed 2 to 4 weeks
- If it is not working within 6 to 8 weeks for depression, it may require a dosage increase or it may not work at all
- May continue to work for many years to prevent relapse of symptoms

If It Works

- The goal of treatment of depression is complete remission of current symptoms as well as prevention of future relapses
- The goal of treatment of chronic neuropathic pain is to reduce symptoms as much as possible, especially in combination with other treatments
- Treatment of depression most often reduces or even eliminates symptoms, but not a cure since symptoms can recur after medicine stopped
- Treatment of chronic neuropathic pain may reduce symptoms, but rarely eliminates them completely, and is not a cure since symptoms can recur after medicine is stopped
- Continue treatment of depression until all symptoms are gone (remission)
- Once symptoms of depression are gone, continue treating for 1 year for the first episode of depression
- For second and subsequent episodes of depression, treatment may need to be indefinite
- Use in anxiety disorders and chronic pain may also need to be indefinite, but long-term treatment is not well studied in these conditions

If It Doesn't Work

- Many depressed patients have only a partial response where some symptoms are improved but others persist (especially insomnia, fatigue, and problems concentrating)
- Other depressed patients may be nonresponders, sometimes called treatment-resistant or treatment-refractory
- Consider increasing dose, switching to another agent, or adding an appropriate augmenting agent
- Consider psychotherapy
- Consider evaluation for another diagnosis or for a comorbid condition (e.g., medical illness, substance abuse, etc.)
- Some patients may experience apparent lack of consistent efficacy due to activation of latent or underlying bipolar disorder, and require antidepressant discontinuation and a switch to a mood stabilizer

Best Augmenting Combos for Partial Response or Treatment Resistance

- Lithium, buspirone, thyroid hormone (for depression)
- Gabapentin, tiagabine, other anticonvulsants, even opiates if done by

experts while monitoring carefully in difficult cases (for chronic pain)

Tests

* None for healthy individuals, although monitoring of plasma drug levels is available
* Since tricyclic and tetracyclic antidepressants are frequently associated with weight gain, before starting treatment, weigh all patients and determine if the patient is already overweight (BMI 25.0–29.9) or obese (BMI ≥30)
- Before giving a drug that can cause weight gain to an overweight or obese patient, consider determining whether the patient already has pre-diabetes (fasting plasma glucose 100–125 mg/dL), diabetes (fasting plasma glucose >126 mg/dL), or dyslipidemia (increased total cholesterol, LDL cholesterol and triglycerides; decreased HDL cholesterol), and treat or refer such patients for treatment, including nutrition and weight management, physical activity counseling, smoking cessation, and medical management
* Monitor weight and BMI during treatment
* While giving a drug to a patient who has gained >5% of initial weight, consider evaluating for the presence of pre-diabetes, diabetes, or dyslipidemia, or consider switching to a different antidepressant
- EKGs may be useful for selected patients (e.g., those with personal or family history of QTc prolongation; cardiac arrhythmia; recent myocardial infarction; uncompensated heart failure; or taking agents that prolong QTc interval such as pimozide, thioridazine, selected antiarrhythmics, moxifloxacin, sparfloxacin, etc.)
- Patients at risk for electrolyte disturbances (e.g., patients on diuretic therapy) should have baseline and periodic serum potassium and magnesium measurements

SIDE EFFECTS

How Drug Causes Side Effects

- Anticholinergic activity may explain sedative effects, dry mouth, constipation, and blurred vision
- Sedative effects and weight gain may be due to antihistamine properties
- Blockade of alpha adrenergic 1 receptors may explain dizziness, sedation, and hypotension
- Cardiac arrhythmias and seizures, especially in overdose, may be caused by blockade of ion channels

Notable Side Effects

- Blurred vision, constipation, urinary retention, increased appetite, dry mouth, nausea, diarrhea, heartburn, unusual taste in mouth, weight gain
- Fatigue, weakness, dizziness, sedation, headache, anxiety, nervousness, restlessness
- Sexual dysfunction (impotence, change in libido)
- Sweating, rash, itching

Life-Threatening or Dangerous Side Effects

- Paralytic ileus, hyperthermia (TCAs + anticholinergic agents)
- Lowered seizure threshold and rare seizures
- Orthostatic hypotension, sudden death, arrhythmias, tachycardia
- QTc prolongation
- Hepatic failure, extrapyramidal symptoms
- Increased intraocular pressure
- Rare induction of mania
- Rare activation of suicidal ideation and behavior (suicidality) (short-term studies did not show an increase in the risk of suicidality with antidepressants compared to placebo beyond age 24)

Weight Gain

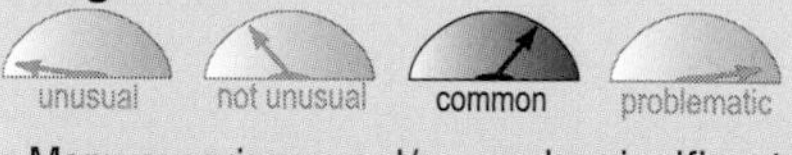

- Many experience and/or can be significant in amount
- Can increase appetite and carbohydrate craving

Sedation

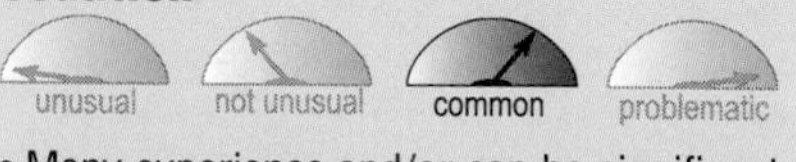

- Many experience and/or can be significant in amount
- Tolerance to sedative effect may develop with long-term use

What to Do About Side Effects

- Wait
- Wait
- Wait
- Lower the dose
- Switch to an SSRI or newer antidepressant

Best Augmenting Agents for Side Effects

- Many side effects cannot be improved with an augmenting agent
- If intolerable anxiety, insomnia, agitation, akathisia, or activation occur either upon dosing initiation or discontinuation, consider the possibility of activated bipolar disorder, and switch to a mood stabilizer or an atypical antipsychotic

DOSING AND USE

Usual Dosage Range

- 75–150 mg/day once daily or in up to 4 divided doses (for depression)
- 50–150 mg/day (for chronic pain)

Dosage Forms

- Capsule 10 mg, 25 mg, 50 mg, 75 mg
- Liquid 10 mg/5 mL

How To Dose

- Initial 10–25 mg/day at bedtime; increase by 25 mg every 3–7 days; can be dosed once daily or in divided doses; maximum dose 300 mg/day
- When treating nicotine dependence, nortriptyline should be initiated 10–28 days before cessation of smoking to achieve steady drug states

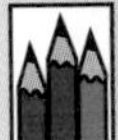

Dosing Tips

- If given in a single dose, should generally be administered at bedtime because of its sedative properties
- If given in split doses, largest dose should generally be given at bedtime because of its sedative properties
- If patients experience nightmares, split dose and do not give large dose at bedtime
- Patients treated for chronic pain may require only lower doses
- Risk of seizure increases with dose

✻ Monitoring plasma levels of nortriptyline is recommended in patients who do not respond to the usual dose or whose treatment is regarded as urgent

- Some formulations of nortriptyline contain sodium bisulphate, which may cause allergic reactions in some patients, perhaps more frequently in asthmatics

Overdose

- Death may occur; CNS depression, convulsions, cardiac dysrhythmias, severe hypotension, EKG changes, coma

Long-Term Use

- Safe

Habit Forming

- No

How to Stop

- Taper to avoid withdrawal effects
- Even with gradual dose reduction some withdrawal symptoms may appear within the first 2 weeks
- Many patients tolerate 50% dose reduction for 3 days, then another 50% reduction for 3 days, then discontinuation
- If withdrawal symptoms emerge during discontinuation, raise dose to stop symptoms and then restart withdrawal much more slowly

Pharmacokinetics

- Substrate for CYP450 2D6
- Nortriptyline is the active metabolite of amitriptyline, formed by demethylation via CYP450 1A2
- Half-life approximately 36 hours

Drug Interactions

- Tramadol increases the risk of seizures in patients taking TCAs
- Use of TCAs with anticholinergic drugs may result in paralytic ileus or hyperthermia
- Fluoxetine, paroxetine, bupropion, duloxetine, and other CYP450 2D6 inhibitors may increase TCA concentrations and cause side effects including dangerous arrhythmias
- Cimetidine may increase plasma concentrations of TCAs and cause anticholinergic symptoms
- Phenothiazines or haloperidol may raise TCA blood concentrations

- May alter effects of antihypertensive drugs; may inhibit hypotensive effects of clonidine
- Use of TCAs with sympathomimetic agents may increase sympathetic activity
- Methylphenidate may inhibit metabolism of TCAs
- Nortriptyline may raise plasma levels of dicumarol
- Activation and agitation, especially following switching or adding antidepressants, may represent the induction of a bipolar state, especially a mixed dysphoric bipolar II condition sometimes associated with suicidal ideation, and require the addition of lithium, a mood stabilizer or an atypical antipsychotic, and/or discontinuation of nortriptyline

Other Warnings/ Precautions

- Add or initiate other antidepressants with caution for up to 2 weeks after discontinuing nortriptyline
- Generally, do not use with MAO inhibitors, including 14 days after MAOIs are stopped; do not start an MAOI until 2 weeks after discontinuing nortriptyline, but see Pearls
- Use with caution in patients with history of seizures, urinary retention, narrow angle-closure glaucoma, hyperthyroidism
- TCAs can increase QTc interval, especially at toxic doses, which can be attained not only by overdose but also by combining with drugs that inhibit TCA metabolism via CYP450 2D6, potentially causing torsade de pointes-type arrhythmia or sudden death
- Because TCAs can prolong QTc interval, use with caution in patients who have bradycardia or who are taking drugs that can induce bradycardia (e.g., beta blockers, calcium channel blockers, clonidine, digitalis)
- Because TCAs can prolong QTc interval, use with caution in patients who have hypokalemia and/or hypomagnesemia or who are taking drugs that can induce hypokalemia and/or magnesemia (e.g., diuretics, stimulant laxatives, intravenous amphotericin B, glucocorticoids, tetracosactide)
- When treating children, carefully weigh the risks and benefits of pharmacological treatment against the risks and benefits of nontreatment with antidepressants and make sure to document this in the patient's chart
- Distribute the brochures provided by the FDA and the drug companies
- Warn patients and their caregivers about the possibility of activating side effects and advise them to report such symptoms immediately
- Monitor patients for activation of suicidal ideation, especially children and adolescents

Do Not Use

- If patient is recovering from myocardial infarction
- If patient is taking agents capable of significantly prolonging QTc interval (e.g., pimozide, thioridazine, selected antiarrhythmics, moxifloxacin, sparfloxacin)
- If there is a history of QTc prolongation or cardiac arrhythmia, recent acute myocardial infarction, uncompensated heart failure
- If patient is taking drugs that inhibit TCA metabolism, including CYP450 2D6 inhibitors, except by an expert
- If there is reduced CYP450 2D6 function, such as patients who are poor 2D6 metabolizers, except by an expert and at low doses
- If there is a proven allergy to nortriptyline or amitriptyline

SPECIAL POPULATIONS

Renal Impairment

- Use with caution; may need to lower dose
- May need to monitor plasma levels

Hepatic Impairment

- Use with caution
- May need to monitor plasma levels
- May require a lower dose with slower titration

Cardiac Impairment

- TCAs have been reported to cause arrhythmias, prolongation of conduction time, orthostatic hypotension, sinus

tachycardia, and heart failure, especially in the diseased heart
- Myocardial infarction and stroke have been reported with TCAs
- TCAs produce QTc prolongation, which may be enhanced by the existence of bradycardia, hypokalemia, congenital or acquired long QTc interval, which should be evaluated prior to administering nortriptyline
- Use with caution if treating concomitantly with a medication likely to produce prolonged bradycardia, hypokalemia, slowing of intracardiac conduction, or prolongation of the QTc interval
- Avoid TCAs in patients with a known history of QTc prolongation, recent acute myocardial infarction, and uncompensated heart failure
- TCAs may cause a sustained increase in heart rate in patients with ischemic heart disease and may worsen (decrease) heart rate variability, an independent risk of mortality in cardiac populations
- Since SSRIs may improve (increase) heart rate variability in patients following a myocardial infarct and may improve survival as well as mood in patients with acute angina or following a myocardial infarction, these are more appropriate agents for cardiac population than tricyclic/tetracyclic antidepressants

✻ Risk/benefit ratio may not justify use of TCAs in cardiac impairment

Elderly

- May be more sensitive to anticholinergic, cardiovascular, hypotensive, and sedative effects
- May require lower dose; it may be useful to monitor plasma levels in elderly patients
- Reduction in risk of suicidality with antidepressants compared to placebo in adults age 65 and older

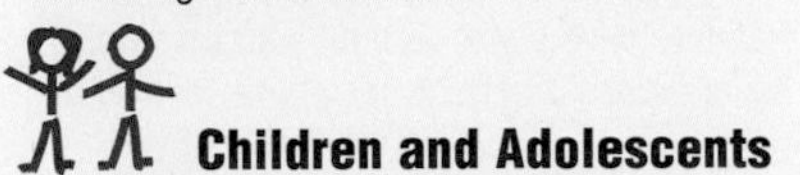

Children and Adolescents

- Carefully weigh the risks and benefits of pharmacological treatment against the risks and benefits of nontreatment with antidepressants and make sure to document this in the patient's chart
- Monitor patients face-to-face regularly, particularly during the first several weeks of treatment
- Use with caution, observing for activation of known or unknown bipolar disorder and/or suicidal ideation, and inform parents or guardian of this risk so they can help observe child or adolescent patients
- Not recommended for use in children under age 12
- Not intended for use under age 6
- Several studies show lack of efficacy of TCAs for depression
- May be used to treat enuresis or hyperactive/impulsive behaviors
- Some cases of sudden death have occurred in children taking TCAs
- Plasma levels may need to be monitored
- Dose in children generally less than 50 mg/day
- May be useful to monitor plasma levels in children and adolescents

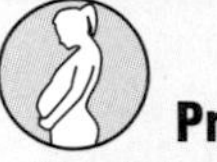

Pregnancy

- Risk Category D [positive evidence of risk to human fetus; potential benefits may still justify its use during pregnancy]
- Crosses the placenta
- Should be used only if potential benefits outweigh potential risks
- Adverse effects have been reported in infants whose mothers took a TCA (lethargy, withdrawal symptoms, fetal malformations)
- Evaluate for treatment with an antidepressant with a better risk/benefit ratio

Breast Feeding

- Some drug is found in mother's breast milk

✻ Recommended either to discontinue drug or bottle feed

- Immediate postpartum period is a high-risk time for depression, especially in women who have had prior depressive episodes, so drug may need to be reinstituted late in the third trimester or shortly after childbirth to prevent a recurrence during the postpartum period
- Must weigh benefits of breast feeding with risks and benefits of antidepressant treatment versus nontreatment to both the infant and the mother
- For many patients this may mean continuing treatment during breast feeding

THE ART OF PSYCHOPHARMACOLOGY

Potential Advantages
- Patients with insomnia
- Severe or treatment-resistant depression
- Patients for whom therapeutic drug monitoring is desirable

Potential Disadvantages
- Pediatric and geriatric patients
- Patients concerned with weight gain
- Cardiac patients

Primary Target Symptoms
- Depressed mood
- Chronic pain

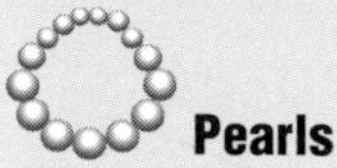

Pearls
- Tricyclic antidepressants are often a first-line treatment option for chronic pain
- Tricyclic antidepressants are no longer generally considered a first-line option for depression because of their side effect profile
- Tricyclic antidepressants continue to be useful for severe or treatment-resistant depression
- Noradrenergic reuptake inhibitors such as nortriptyline can be used as a second-line treatment for smoking cessation, cocaine dependence, and attention deficit disorder
- TCAs may aggravate psychotic symptoms
- Alcohol should be avoided because of additive CNS effects
- Underweight patients may be more susceptible to adverse cardiovascular effects
- Children, patients with inadequate hydration, and patients with cardiac disease may be more susceptible to TCA-induced cardiotoxicity than healthy adults
- For the expert only: although generally prohibited, a heroic but potentially dangerous treatment for severely treatment-resistant patients is for an expert to give a tricyclic/tetracyclic antidepressant other than clomipramine simultaneously with an MAO inhibitor for patients who fail to respond to numerous other antidepressants
- If this option is elected, start the MAOI with the tricyclic/tetracyclic antidepressant simultaneously at low doses after appropriate drug washout, then alternately increase doses of these agents every few days to a week as tolerated
- Although very strict dietary and concomitant drug restrictions must be observed to prevent hypertensive crises and serotonin syndrome, the most common side effects of MAOI and tricyclic/tetracyclic antidepressant combinations may be weight gain and orthostatic hypotension
- Patients on TCAs should be aware that they may experience symptoms such as photosensitivity or blue-green urine
- SSRIs may be more effective than TCAs in women, and TCAs may be more effective than SSRIs in men
- Not recommended for first-line use in children with ADHD because of the availability of safer treatments with better documented efficacy and because of nortriptyline's potential for sudden death in children

❋ Nortriptyline is one of the few TCAs where monitoring of plasma drug levels has been well studied

- Since tricyclic/tetracyclic antidepressants are substrates for CYP450 2D6, and 7% of the population (especially Caucasians) may have a genetic variant leading to reduced activity of 2D6, such patients may not safely tolerate normal doses of tricyclic/tetracyclic antidepressants and may require dose reduction
- Phenotypic testing may be necessary to detect this genetic variant prior to dosing with a tricyclic/tetracyclic antidepressant, especially in vulnerable populations such as children, elderly, cardiac populations, and those on concomitant medications
- Patients who seem to have extraordinarily severe side effects at normal or low doses may have this phenotypic CYP450 2D6 variant and require low doses or switching to another antidepressant not metabolized by 2D6

Suggested Reading

Anderson IM. Meta-analytical studies on new antidepressants. Br Med Bull 2001; 57:161–78.

Anderson IM. Selective serotonin reuptake inhibitors versus tricyclic antidepressants: a meta-analysis of efficacy and tolerability. J Aff Disorders 2000;58:19–36.

Hughes JR, Stead LF, Lancaster T. Antidepressants for smoking cessation. Cochrane Database Syst Rev 2000;4:CD000031.

Wilens TE, Biederman J, Baldessarini RJ, Geller B, Schleifer D, Spencer TJ, Birmajer B, Goldblatt A. Cardiovascular effects of therapeutic doses of tricyclic antidepressants in children and adolescents. J Am Acad Child Adolesc Psychiatry 1996;35(11):1491–501.

OLANZAPINE

THERAPEUTICS

Brands
- Zyprexa
- Olasek
- Ziprexa
- Symbyax (olanzapine-fluoxetine combination)

see index for additional brand names

Generic? Not in U.S., Europe, or Japan

Class

- Atypical antipsychotic (serotonin-dopamine antagonist; second-generation antipsychotic; also a mood stabilizer)

Commonly Prescribed for

(bold for FDA approved)

- **Schizophrenia**
- **Maintaining response in schizophrenia**
- **Acute agitation associated with schizophrenia (intramuscular)**
- **Acute mania/mixed mania (monotherapy and adjunct to lithium or valproate)**
- **Bipolar maintenance**
- **Acute agitation associated with bipolar I mania (intramuscular)**
- **Bipolar depression [in combination with fluoxetine (Symbyax)]**
- Other psychotic disorders
- Unipolar depression unresponsive to antidepressants
- Behavioral disturbances in dementias
- Behavioral disturbances in children and adolescents
- Disorders associated with problems with impulse control
- Borderline personality disorder

How the Drug Works

- Blocks dopamine 2 receptors, reducing positive symptoms of psychosis and stabilizing affective symptoms
- Blocks serotonin 2A receptors, causing enhancement of dopamine release in certain brain regions and thus reducing motor side effects and possibly improving cognitive and affective symptoms
- Interactions at a myriad of other neurotransmitter receptors may contribute to olanzapine's efficacy

✱ Specifically, antagonist actions at 5HT2C receptors may contribute to efficacy for cognitive and affective symptoms in some patients

✱ 5HT2C antagonist actions plus serotonin reuptake blockade of fluoxetine add to the actions of olanzapine when given as Symbyax (olanzapine-fluoxetine combination)

How Long Until It Works

- Psychotic and manic symptoms can improve within 1 week, but it may take several weeks for full effect on behavior as well as on cognition and affective stabilization
- Classically recommended to wait at least 4–6 weeks to determine efficacy of drug, but in practice some patients require up to 16–20 weeks to show a good response, especially on cognitive symptoms
- IM formulation can reduce agitation in 15–30 minutes

If It Works

- Most often reduces positive symptoms in schizophrenia but does not eliminate them
- Can improve negative symptoms, as well as aggressive, cognitive, and affective symptoms in schizophrenia
- Most schizophrenic patients do not have a total remission of symptoms but rather a reduction of symptoms by about a third
- Perhaps 5–15% of schizophrenic patients can experience an overall improvement of greater than 50–60%, especially when receiving stable treatment for more than a year
- Such patients are considered super-responders or "awakeners" since they may be well enough to be employed, live independently, and sustain long-term relationships
- Many bipolar patients may experience a reduction of symptoms by half or more
- Continue treatment until reaching a plateau of improvement
- After reaching a satisfactory plateau, continue treatment for at least a year after first episode of psychosis
- For second and subsequent episodes of psychosis, treatment may need to be indefinite
- Even for first episodes of psychosis, it may be preferable to continue treatment indefinitely to avoid subsequent episodes

- Treatment may not only reduce mania but also prevent recurrences of mania in bipolar disorder

If It Doesn't Work

- Try one of the other atypical antipsychotics (risperidone, quetiapine, ziprasidone, aripiprazole, paliperidone, amisulpride)
- If 2 or more antipsychotic monotherapies do not work, consider clozapine
- If no first-line atypical antipsychotic is effective, consider higher doses or augmentation with valproate or lamotrigine
- Some patients may require treatment with a conventional antipsychotic
- Consider noncompliance and switch to another antipsychotic with fewer side effects or to an antipsychotic that can be given by depot injection
- Consider initiating rehabilitation and psychotherapy
- Consider presence of concomitant drug abuse

Best Augmenting Combos for Partial Response or Treatment Resistance

- Valproic acid (valproate, divalproex, divalproex ER)
- Other mood-stabilizing anticonvulsants (carbamazepine, oxcarbazepine, lamotrigine)
- Lithium
- Benzodiazepines
- Fluoxetine and other antidepressants may be effective augmenting agents to olanzapine for bipolar depression, psychotic depression, and for unipolar depression not responsive to antidepressants alone (e.g., olanzapine-fluoxetine combination)

Tests

Before starting an atypical antipsychotic

* Weigh all patients and track BMI during treatment
- Get baseline personal and family history of diabetes, obesity, dyslipidemia, hypertension, and cardiovascular disease
* Get waist circumference (at umbilicus), blood pressure, fasting plasma glucose, and fasting lipid profile
- Determine if the patient is
  - overweight (BMI 25.0–29.9)
  - obese (BMI ≥30)
  - has pre-diabetes (fasting plasma glucose 100–25 mg/dL)
  - has diabetes (fasting plasma glucose >126 mg/dL)
  - has hypertension (BP >140/90 mm Hg)
  - has dyslipidemia (increased total cholesterol, LDL cholesterol, and triglycerides; decreased HDL cholesterol)
- Treat or refer such patients for treatment, including nutrition and weight management, physical activity counseling, smoking cessation, and medical management

Monitoring after starting an atypical antipsychotic

* BMI monthly for 3 months, then quarterly
* Consider monitoring fasting triglycerides monthly for several months in patients at high risk for metabolic complications and when initiating or switching antipsychotics
* Blood pressure, fasting plasma glucose, fasting lipids within 3 months and then annually, but earlier and more frequently for patients with diabetes or who have gained >5% of initial weight
- Treat or refer for treatment and consider switching to another atypical antipsychotic for patients who become overweight, obese, pre-diabetic, diabetic, hypertensive, or dyslipidemic while receiving an atypical antipsychotic
* Even in patients without known diabetes, be vigilant for the rare but life threatening onset of diabetic ketoacidosis, which always requires immediate treatment, by monitoring for the rapid onset of polyuria, polydipsia, weight loss, nausea, vomiting, dehydration, rapid respiration, weakness and clouding of sensorium, even coma
- Patients with liver disease should have blood tests a few times a year

SIDE EFFECTS

How Drug Causes Side Effects

- By blocking histamine 1 receptors in the brain, it can cause sedation and possibly weight gain
- By blocking alpha 1 adrenergic receptors, it can cause dizziness, sedation, and hypotension

- By blocking muscarinic 1 receptors, it can cause dry mouth, constipation, and sedation
- By blocking dopamine 2 receptors in the striatum, it can cause motor side effects (unusual)
- Mechanism of weight gain and increased incidence of diabetes and dyslipidemia with atypical antipsychotics is unknown but insulin regulation may be impaired by blocking pancreatic M3 muscarinic receptors

Notable Side Effects

✱ Probably increases risk for diabetes mellitus and dyslipidemia
- Dizziness, sedation
- Dry mouth, constipation, dyspepsia, weight gain
- Peripheral edema
- Joint pain, back pain, chest pain, extremity pain, abnormal gait, ecchymosis
- Tachycardia
- Orthostatic hypotension, usually during initial dose titration
- Rare tardive dyskinesia (much reduced risk compared to conventional antipsychotics)
- Rare rash on exposure to sunlight

Life-Threatening or Dangerous Side Effects

- Hyperglycemia, in some cases extreme and associated with ketoacidosis or hyperosmolar coma or death, has been reported in patients taking atypical antipsychotics
- Rare neuroleptic malignant syndrome (much reduced risk compared to conventional antipsychotics)
- Rare seizures
- Increased risk of death and cerebrovascular events in elderly patients with dementia-related psychosis

Weight Gain

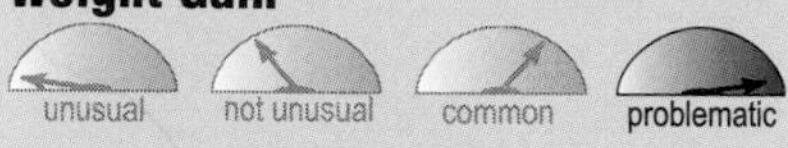

- Frequent and can be significant in amount
- Can become a health problem in some
- More than for some other antipsychotics, but never say always as not a problem in everyone

Sedation

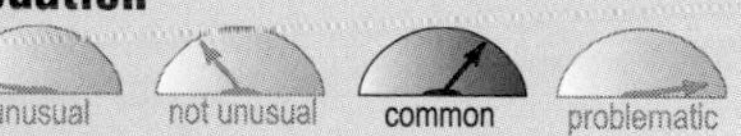

- Many patients experience and/or can be significant in amount
- Usually transient
- May be less than for some antipsychotics, more than for others

What to Do About Side Effects

- Wait
- Wait
- Wait
- Take at bedtime to help reduce daytime sedation
- Anticholinergics may reduce motor side effects such as akathisia when present, but rarely necessary
- Weight loss, exercise programs, and medical management for high BMIs, diabetes, dyslipidemia
- Switch to another atypical antipsychotic

Best Augmenting Agents for Side Effects

- Benztropine or trihexyphenidyl for motor side effects
- Many side effects cannot be improved with an augmenting agent

DOSING AND USE

Usual Dosage Range

- 10–20 mg/day (oral or intramuscular)
- 6–12 mg olanzapine / 25–50 mg fluoxetine (olanzapine-fluoxetine combination)

Dosage Forms

- Tablets 2.5 mg, 5 mg, 7.5 mg, 10 mg, 15 mg, 20 mg
- Orally disintegrating tablets 5 mg, 10 mg, 15 mg, 20 mg
- Intramuscular formulation 5 mg/mL, each vial contains 10 mg (available in some countries)
- Olanzapine-fluoxetine combination capsule (mg equivalent olanzapine/mg equivalent fluoxetine) 6 mg/25 mg, 6 mg/50 mg, 12 mg/25 mg, 12 mg/50 mg

How To Dose

- Initial 5–10 mg once daily orally; increase by 5 mg/day once a week until desired

efficacy is reached; maximum approved dose is 20 mg/day
- For intramuscular formulation, recommended initial dose 10 mg; second injection of 5–10 mg may be administered 2 hours after first injection; maximum daily dose of olanzapine is 20 mg, with no more than 3 injections per 24 hours
- For olanzapine-fluoxetine combination, recommended initial dose 6 mg/25 mg once daily in evening; increase dose based on efficacy and tolerability; maximum generally 18 mg/75 mg

Dosing Tips

✻ **More may be more:** raising usual dose above 15 mg/day can be useful for acutely ill and agitated patients and some treatment-resistant patients, gaining efficacy without many more side effects

✻ Some heroic uses for patients who do not respond to other antipsychotics can occasionally justify dosing over 30 mg/day

- Usual doses (>15 mg/day range) can be among the most costly among atypical antipsychotics, and dosing >30 mg/day can be very expensive
- Rather than raise the dose above these levels in acutely agitated patients requiring acute antipsychotic actions, consider augmentation with a benzodiazepine or conventional antipsychotic, either orally or intramuscularly
- Rather than raise the dose above these levels in partial responders, consider augmentation with a mood-stabilizing anticonvulsant, such as valproate or lamotrigine
- Clearance of olanzapine is slightly reduced in women compared to men, so women may need lower doses than men
- Children and elderly should generally be dosed at the lower end of the dosage spectrum

✻ Olanzapine intramuscularly can be given short-term, both to initiate dosing with oral olanzapine or another oral antipsychotic and to treat breakthrough agitation in patients maintained on oral antipsychotics

Overdose

- Rarely lethal in monotherapy overdose; sedation, slurred speech

Long-Term Use

- Approved to maintain response in long-term treatment of schizophrenia
- Approved for long-term maintenance in bipolar disorder
- Often used for long-term maintenance in various behavioral disorders

Habit Forming

- No

How to Stop

- Slow down-titration of oral formulation (over 6–8 weeks), especially when simultaneously beginning a new antipsychotic while switching (i.e., cross-titration)
- Rapid oral discontinuation may lead to rebound psychosis and worsening of symptoms

Pharmacokinetics

- Metabolites are inactive
- Parent drug has 21–54 hour half-life

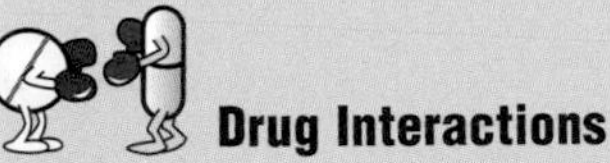

Drug Interactions

- May increase effect of antihypertensive agents
- May antagonize levodopa, dopamine agonists
- Dose may need to be lowered if given with CYP450 1A2 inhibitors (e.g., fluvoxamine); raised if given in conjunction with CYP450 1A2 inducers (e.g., cigarette smoke, carbamazepine)

Other Warnings/ Precautions

- Use with caution in patients with conditions that predispose to hypotension (dehydration, overheating)
- Use with caution in patients with prostatic hypertrophy, narrow angle-closure glaucoma, paralytic ileus
- Patients receiving the intramuscular formulation of olanzapine should be observed closely for hypotension
- Intramuscular formulation is not generally recommended to be administered with parenteral benzodiazepines; if patient requires a parenteral benzodiazepine it should be given at least 1 hour after intramuscular olanzapine

- Olanzapine should be used cautiously in patients at risk for aspiration pneumonia, as dysphagia has been reported

Do Not Use

- If there is a known risk of narrow angle-closure glaucoma (intramuscular formulation)
- If patient has unstable medical condition (e.g., acute myocardial infarction, unstable angina pectoris, severe hypotension and/or bradycardia, sick sinus syndrome, recent heart surgery) (intramuscular formulation)
- If there is a proven allergy to olanzapine

SPECIAL POPULATIONS

Renal Impairment

- No dose adjustment required for oral formulation
- Not removed by hemodialysis
- For intramuscular formulation, consider lower starting dose (5 mg)

Hepatic Impairment

- May need to lower dose
- Patients with liver disease should have liver function tests a few times a year
- For moderate to severe hepatic impairment, starting oral dose 5 mg; increase with caution
- For intramuscuar formulation, consider lower starting dose (5 mg)

Cardiac Impairment

- Drug should be used with caution because of risk of orthostatic hypotension

Elderly

- Some patients may tolerate lower doses better
- Increased incidence of stroke
- For intramuscular formulation, recommended starting dose is 2.5–5 mg; a second injection of 2.5–5 mg may be administered 2 hours after first injection; no more than 3 injections should be administered within 24 hours
- Although atypical antipsychotics are commonly used for behavioral disturbances in dementia, no agent has been approved for treatment of elderly patients with dementia-related psychosis
- Elderly patients with dementia-related psychosis treated with atypical antipsychotics are at an increased risk of death compared to placebo, and also have an increased risk of cerebrovascular events

Children and Adolescents

- Not officially recommended under age 18; however, olanzapine is often used for patients under 18
- Clinical experience and early data suggest olanzapine is probably safe and effective for behavioral disturbances in children and adolescents
- Children and adolescents using olanzapine may need to be monitored more often than adults
- Intramuscular formulation has not been studied in patients under 18 and is not recommended for use in this population

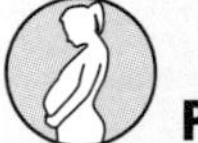

Pregnancy

- Risk Category C [some animal studies show adverse effects; no controlled studies in humans]
- Psychotic symptoms may worsen during pregnancy, and some form of treatment may be necessary
- Early findings of infants exposed to olanzapine in utero currently do not show adverse consequences
- Olanzapine may be preferable to anticonvulsant mood stabilizers if treatment is required during pregnancy

Breast Feeding

- Unknown if olanzapine is secreted in human breast milk, but all psychotropics assumed to be secreted in breast milk

✻ Recommended either to discontinue drug or bottle feed

- Infants of women who choose to breast feed while on olanzapine should be monitored for possible adverse effects

THE ART OF PSYCHOPHARMACOLOGY

Potential Advantages

* Some cases of psychosis and bipolar disorder refractory to treatment with other antipsychotics
* Often a preferred augmenting agent in bipolar depression or treatment-resistant unipolar depression
* Patients needing rapid onset of antipsychotic action without drug titration
• Patients switching from intramuscular olanzapine to an oral preparation

Potential Disadvantages

• Patients concerned about gaining weight
* Patients with diabetes mellitus, obesity, and/or dyslipidemia

Primary Target Symptoms

• Positive symptoms of psychosis
• Negative symptoms of psychosis
• Cognitive symptoms
• Unstable mood (both depressed mood and mania)
• Aggressive symptoms

Pearls

• Recent landmark head to head study in schizophrenia suggests greater effectiveness (i.e., lower dropouts of all causes) at moderately high doses compared to some other atypical and conventional antipsychotics at moderate doses
• Same recent head to head study in schizophrenia suggests greater efficacy but greater metabolic side effects compared to some other atypical and conventional antipsychotics
• Well accepted for use in schizophrenia and bipolar disorder, including difficult cases
* Documented utility in treatment-refractory cases, especially at higher doses
* Documented efficacy as augmenting agent to SSRIs (fluoxetine) in nonpsychotic treatment-resistant major depressive disorder
* Documented efficacy in bipolar depression, especially in combination with fluoxetine
• More weight gain than many other antipsychotics —does not mean every patient gains weight
• Motor side effects unusual at low- to mid-doses
• Less sedation than for some other antipsychotics, more than for others
* Controversial as to whether olanzapine has more risk of diabetes and dyslipidemia than other antipsychotics
• One of the most expensive atypical antipsychotics within the usual therapeutic dosing range
• Cigarette smoke can decrease olanzapine levels and patients may require a dose increase if they begin or increase smoking
* One of only two atypical antipsychotics with a short-acting intramuscular dosage formulation
• Long-acting intramuscular dosage formulation is in late-stage clinical development

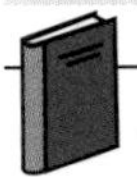

Suggested Reading

Duggan L, Fenton M, Dardennes RM, El-Dosoky A, Indran S. Olanzapine for schizophrenia. Cochrane Database Syst Rev 2003;(1):CD001359.

Lieberman JA, Stroup TS, McEvoy JP, Swartz MS, Rosenheck RA, Perkins DO, et al. Effectiveness of antipsychotic drugs in patients with chronic schizophrenia. N Engl J Med 2005;353(12):1209–23.

Nasrallah HA. Atypical antipsychotic-induced metabolic side effects: insights from receptor-binding profiles. Mol Psychiatry 2008;13(1):27–35.

Smith LA, Cornelius V, Warnock A, Tacchi MJ, Taylor D. Pharmacological interventions for acute bipolar mania: a systematic review of randomized placebo-controlled trials. Bipolar Disord 2007;9(6):551–60.

THERAPEUTICS

Brands • Serax

see index for additional brand names

Generic? Yes

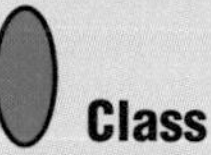

Class

• Benzodiazepine (anxiolytic)

Commonly Prescribed for

(bold for FDA approved)

- **Anxiety**
- **Anxiety associated with depression**
- **Alcohol withdrawal**

How the Drug Works

- Binds to benzodiazepine receptors at the GABA-A ligand-gated chloride channel complex
- Enhances the inhibitory effects of GABA
- Boosts chloride conductance through GABA-regulated channels
- Inhibits neuronal activity presumably in amygdala-centered fear circuits to provide therapeutic benefits in anxiety disorders

How Long Until It Works

- Some immediate relief with first dosing is common; can take several weeks with daily dosing for maximal therapeutic benefit

If It Works

- For short-term symptoms of anxiety – after a few weeks, discontinue use or use on an "as-needed" basis
- For chronic anxiety disorders, the goal of treatment is complete remission of symptoms as well as prevention of future relapses
- For chronic anxiety disorders, treatment most often reduces or even eliminates symptoms, but not a cure since symptoms can recur after medicine stopped
- For long-term symptoms of anxiety, consider switching to an SSRI or SNRI for long-term maintenance
- If long-term maintenance with a benzodiazepine is necessary, continue treatment for 6 months after symptoms resolve, and then taper dose slowly
- If symptoms reemerge, consider treatment with an SSRI or SNRI, or consider restarting the benzodiazepine; sometimes benzodiazepines have to be used in combination with SSRIs or SNRIs for best results

If It Doesn't Work

- Consider switching to another agent or adding an appropriate augmenting agent
- Consider psychotherapy, especially cognitive behavioral psychotherapy
- Consider presence of concomitant substance abuse
- Consider presence of oxazepam abuse
- Consider another diagnosis, such as a comorbid medical condition

Best Augmenting Combos for Partial Response or Treatment Resistance

- Benzodiazepines are frequently used as augmenting agents for antipsychotics and mood stabilizers in the treatment of psychotic and bipolar disorders
- Benzodiazepines are frequently used as augmenting agents for SSRIs and SNRIs in the treatment of anxiety disorders
- Not generally rational to combine with other benzodiazepines
- Caution if using as an anxiolytic concomitantly with other sedative hypnotics for sleep

Tests

- In patients with seizure disorders, concomitant medical illness, and/or those with multiple concomitant long-term medications, periodic liver tests and blood counts may be prudent

SIDE EFFECTS

How Drug Causes Side Effects

- Same mechanism for side effects as for therapeutic effects – namely due to excessive actions at benzodiazepine receptors
- Long-term adaptations in benzodiazepine receptors may explain the development of dependence, tolerance, and withdrawal
- Side effects are generally immediate, but immediate side effects often disappear in time

Notable Side Effects

- ✽ Sedation, fatigue, depression
- ✽ Dizziness, ataxia, slurred speech, weakness
- ✽ Forgetfulness, confusion
- ✽ Hyperexcitability, nervousness
- Rare hallucinations, mania
- Rare hypotension
- Hypersalivation, dry mouth

Life-Threatening or Dangerous Side Effects

- Respiratory depression, especially when taken with CNS depressants in overdose
- Rare hepatic dysfunction, renal dysfunction, blood dyscrasias

Weight Gain

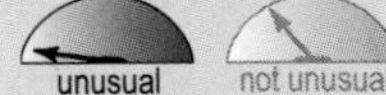

- Reported but not expected

Sedation

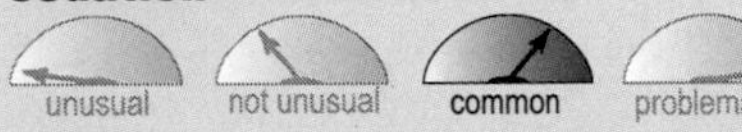

- Many experience and/or can be significant in amount
- Especially at initiation of treatment or when dose increases
- Tolerance often develops over time

What to Do About Side Effects

- Wait
- Wait
- Wait
- Lower the dose
- Take largest dose at bedtime to avoid sedative effects during the day
- Switch to another agent
- Administer flumazenil if side effects are severe or life-threatening

Best Augmenting Agents for Side Effects

- Many side effects cannot be improved with an augmenting agent

DOSING AND USE

Usual Dosage Range

- Mild to moderate anxiety: 30–60 mg/day in 3–4 divided doses
- Severe anxiety, anxiety associated with alcohol withdrawal: 45–120 mg/day in 3–4 divided doses

Dosage Forms

- Capsule 10 mg, 15 mg, 30 mg
- Tablet 15 mg

How To Dose

- Titration generally not necessary

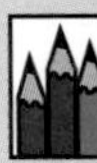

Dosing Tips

- Use lowest possible effective dose for the shortest possible period of time (a benzodiazepine-sparing strategy)
- 15-mg tablet contains tartrazine, which may cause allergic reactions in certain patients, particularly those who are sensitive to aspirin
- For interdose symptoms of anxiety, can either increase dose or maintain same total daily dose but divide into more frequent doses
- Can also use an as-needed occasional "top up" dose for interdose anxiety
- Because anxiety disorders can require higher doses, the risk of dependence may be greater in these patients
- Some severely ill patients may require doses higher than the generally recommended maximum dose
- Frequency of dosing in practice is often greater than predicted from half-life, as duration of biological activity is often shorter than pharmacokinetic terminal half-life

Overdose

- Fatalities can occur; hypotension, tiredness, ataxia, confusion, coma

Long-Term Use

- Risk of dependence, particularly for treatment periods longer than 12 weeks and especially in patients with past or current polysubstance abuse

Habit Forming

- Oxazepam is a Schedule IV drug
- Patients may develop dependence and/or tolerance with long-term use

How to Stop

- Patients with history of seizure may seize upon withdrawal, especially if withdrawal is abrupt
- Taper by 15 mg every 3 days to reduce chances of withdrawal effects
- For difficult to taper cases, consider reducing dose much more slowly once reaching 45 mg/day, perhaps by as little as 10 mg per week or less
- For other patients with severe problems discontinuing a benzodiazepine, dosing may need to be tapered over many months (i.e., reduce dose by 1% every 3 days by crushing tablet and suspending or dissolving in 100 mL of fruit juice and then disposing of 1 mL while drinking the rest; 3–7 days later, dispose of 2 mL, and so on). This is both a form of very slow biological tapering and a form of behavioral desensitization
- Be sure to differentiate reemergence of symptoms requiring reinstitution of treatment from withdrawal symptoms
- Benzodiazepine-dependent anxiety patients and insulin-dependent diabetics are not addicted to their medications. When benzodiazepine-dependent patients stop their medication, disease symptoms can reemerge, disease symptoms can worsen (rebound), and/or withdrawal symptoms can emerge

Pharmacokinetics

- Elimination half-life 3–21 hours
- No active metabolites

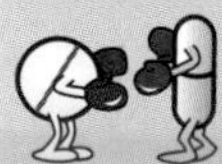

Drug Interactions

- Increased depressive effects when taken with other CNS depressants

Other Warnings/ Precautions

- Dosage changes should be made in collaboration with prescriber
- Use with caution in patients with pulmonary disease; rare reports of death after initiation of benzodiazepines in patients with severe pulmonary impairment
- History of drug or alcohol abuse often creates greater risk for dependency
- Some depressed patients may experience a worsening of suicidal ideation
- Some patients may exhibit abnormal thinking or behavioral changes similar to those caused by other CNS depressants (i.e., either depressant actions or disinhibiting actions)

Do Not Use

- If patient has narrow angle-closure glaucoma
- If there is a proven allergy to oxazepam or any benzodiazepine

SPECIAL POPULATIONS

Renal Impairment

- Use with caution; oxazepam levels may be increased

Hepatic Impairment

- Use with caution; oxazepam levels may be increased
- Because of its short half-life and inactive metabolites, oxazepam may be a preferred benzodiazepine in some patients with liver disease

Cardiac Impairment

- Benzodiazepines have been used to treat anxiety associated with acute myocardial infarction

Elderly

- Initial 30 mg in 3 divided doses; can be increased to 30–60 mg/day in 3–4 divided doses

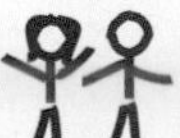

Children and Adolescents

- Safety and efficacy not established under age 6
- No clear dosing guidelines for children ages 6–12
- Long-term effects of oxazepam in children/adolescents are unknown
- Should generally receive lower doses and be more closely monitored

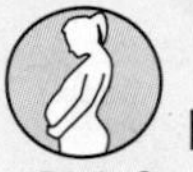

Pregnancy

- Risk Category D [positive evidence of risk to human fetus; potential benefits may still justify its use during pregnancy]
- Possible increased risk of birth defects when benzodiazepines taken during pregnancy
- Because of the potential risks, oxazepam is not generally recommended as treatment for anxiety during pregnancy, especially during the first trimester
- Drug should be tapered if discontinued
- Infants whose mothers received a benzodiazepine late in pregnancy may experience withdrawal effects
- Neonatal flaccidity has been reported in infants whose mothers took a benzodiazepine during pregnancy
- Seizures, even mild seizures, may cause harm to the embryo/fetus

Breast Feeding

- Some drug is found in mother's breast milk
- ✻ Recommended either to discontinue drug or bottle feed
- Effects on infant have been observed and include feeding difficulties, sedation, and weight loss

THE ART OF PSYCHOPHARMACOLOGY

Potential Advantages

- Rapid onset of action

Potential Disadvantages

- Euphoria may lead to abuse
- Abuse especially risky in past or present substance abusers

Primary Target Symptoms

- Panic attacks
- Anxiety
- Agitation

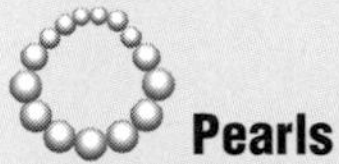

Pearls

- Can be a very useful adjunct to SSRIs and SNRIs in the treatment of numerous anxiety disorders
- Not effective for treating psychosis as a monotherapy, but can be used as an adjunct to antipsychotics
- Not effective for treating bipolar disorder as a monotherapy, but can be used as an adjunct to mood stabilizers and antipsychotics
- ✻ Because of its short half-life and inactive metabolites, oxazepam may be preferred over some benzodiazepines for patients with liver disease
- Oxazepam may be preferred over some other benzodiazepines for the treatment of delirium
- Can both cause and treat depression in different patients
- When using to treat insomnia, remember that insomnia may be a symptom of some other primary disorder itself, and thus warrant evaluation for comorbid psychiatric and/or medical conditions

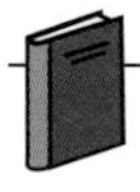

Suggested Reading

Ayd FJ Jr. Oxazepam: update 1989. Int Clin Psychopharmacol 1990;5:1–15.

Garattini S. Biochemical and pharmacological properties of oxazepam. Acta Psychiatr Scand Suppl 1978;274:9–18.

Greenblatt DJ. Clinical pharmacokinetics of oxazepam and lorazepam. Clin Pharmacokinet 1981;6:89–105.

THERAPEUTICS

Brands • Trileptal

see index for additional brand names

Generic? Yes

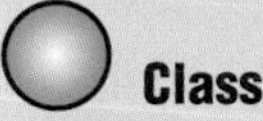

Class

- Anticonvulsant, voltage-sensitive sodium channel antagonist

Commonly Prescribed for

(bold for FDA approved)

- **Partial seizures in adults with epilepsy (monotherapy or adjunctive)**
- **Partial seizures in children ages 4–16 with epilepsy (monotherapy or adjunctive)**
- Bipolar disorder

How the Drug Works

✻ Acts as a use-dependent blocker of voltage-sensitive sodium channels

✻ Interacts with the open channel conformation of voltage-sensitive sodium channels

✻ Interacts at a specific site of the alpha pore-forming subunit of voltage-sensitive sodium channels

- Inhibits release of glutamate

How Long Until It Works

- For acute mania, effects should occur within a few weeks
- May take several weeks to months to optimize an effect on mood stabilization
- Should reduce seizures by 2 weeks

If It Works

- The goal of treatment is complete remission of symptoms (e.g., seizures, mania)
- Continue treatment until all symptoms are gone or until improvement is stable and then continue treating indefinitely as long as improvement persists
- Continue treatment indefinitely to avoid recurrence of mania and seizures

If It Doesn't Work (for bipolar disorder)

✻ Many patients only have a partial response where some symptoms are improved but others persist or continue to wax and wane without stabilization of mood

- Other patients may be nonresponders, sometimes called treatment-resistant or treatment-refractory
- Consider increasing dose, switching to another agent or adding an appropriate augmenting agent
- Consider adding psychotherapy
- For bipolar disorder, consider the presence of noncompliance and counsel patient
- Switch to another mood stabilizer with fewer side effects
- Consider evaluation for another diagnosis or for a comorbid condition (e.g., medical illness, substance abuse, etc.)

Best Augmenting Combos for Partial Response or Treatment Resistance

- Oxcarbazepine is itself a second-line augmenting agent for numerous other anticonvulsants, lithium, and atypical antipsychotics in treating bipolar disorder, although its use in bipolar disorder is not yet well-studied
- Oxcarbazepine may be a second- or third-line augmenting agent for antipsychotics in treating schizophrenia, although its use in schizophrenia is also not yet well-studied

Tests

- Consider monitoring sodium levels because of possibility of hyponatremia, especially during the first 3 months

SIDE EFFECTS

How Drug Causes Side Effects

- CNS side effects theoretically due to excessive actions at voltage-sensitive sodium channels

Notable Side Effects

✻ Sedation, dizziness, headache, ataxia, nystagmus, abnormal gait, confusion, nervousness, fatigue

✻ Nausea, vomiting, abdominal pain, dyspepsia

- Diplopia, vertigo, abnormal vision

✻ Rash

Life-Threatening or Dangerous Side Effects

- Hyponatremia
- Rare activation of suicidal ideation and behavior (suicidality)

Weight Gain

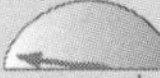
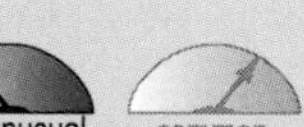

- Occurs in significant minority
- Some patients experience increased appetite

Sedation

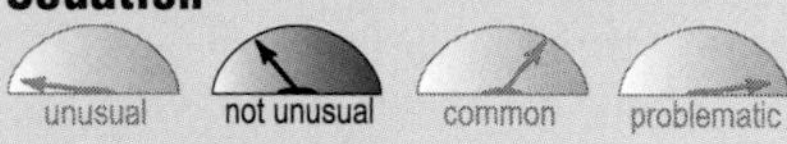

- Occurs in significant minority
- Dose-related
- Less than carbamazepine
- More when combined with other anticonvulsants
- Can wear off with time, but may not wear off at high doses

What to Do About Side Effects

- Wait
- Wait
- Wait
- Switch to another agent

Best Augmenting Agents for Side Effects

- Many side effects cannot be improved with an augmenting agent

DOSING AND USE

Usual Dosage Range

- 1,200–2,400 mg/day

Dosage Forms

- Tablet 150 mg, 300 mg, 600 mg
- Liquid 300 mg/5 mL

How To Dose

- Monotherapy for seizures or bipolar disorder: initial 600 mg/day in 2 doses; increase every 3 days by 300 mg/day; maximum dose generally 2,400 mg/day
- Adjunctive: initial 600 mg/day in 2 doses; each week can increase by 600 mg/day; recommended dose 1,200 mg/day; maximum dose generally 2,400 mg/day
- When converting from adjunctive to monotherapy in the treatment of epilepsy, titrate concomitant drug down over 3–6 weeks while titrating oxcarbazepine up over 2–4 weeks, with an initial daily oxcarbazepine dose of 600 mg divided in 2 doses

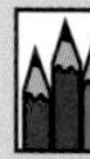

Dosing Tips

✻ Doses of oxcarbazepine need to be about one-third higher than those of carbamazepine for similar results
- Usually administered as adjunctive medication to other anticonvulsants, lithium, or atypical antipsychotics for bipolar disorder
- Side effects may increase with dose
- Although increased efficacy for seizures is seen at 2,400 mg/day compared to 1,200 mg/day, CNS side effects may be intolerable at the higher dose
- Liquid formulation can be administered mixed in a glass of water or directly from the oral dosing syringe supplied
- Slow dose titration may delay onset of therapeutic action but enhance tolerability to sedating side effects
- Should titrate slowly in the presence of other sedating agents, such as other anticonvulsants, in order to best tolerate additive sedative side effects

Overdose

- No fatalities reported

Long-Term Use

- Safe
- Monitoring of sodium may be required, especially during the first 3 months

Habit Forming

- No

How to Stop

- Taper
- Epilepsy patients may seize upon withdrawal, especially if withdrawal is abrupt

✻ Rapid discontinuation may increase the risk of relapse in bipolar disorder
- Discontinuation symptoms uncommon

Pharmacokinetics

- Metabolized in the liver
- Renally excreted
- Inhibits CYP450 2C19
- ✻ Oxcarbazepine is a prodrug for 10-hydroxy carbazepine
- ✻ This main active metabolite is sometimes called the monohydroxy derivative or MHD, and is also known as licarbazepine
- ✻ Half-life of parent drug is approximately 2 hours; half-life of MHD is approximately 9 hours; thus oxcarbazepine is essentially a prodrug rapidly converted to its MHD, licarbazepine
- A mild inducer of CYP450 3A4

Drug Interactions

- Depressive effects may be increased by other CNS depressants (alcohol, MAOIs, other anticonvulsants, etc.)
- Strong inducers of CYP450 cytochromes (e.g., carbamazepine, phenobarbital, phenytoin, and primidone) can decrease plasma levels of the active metabolite MHD
- Verapamil may decrease plasma levels of the active metabolite MHD
- Oxcarbazepine can decrease plasma levels of hormonal contraceptives and dihydropyridine calcium antagonists
- Oxcarbazepine at doses greater than 1,200 mg/day may increase plasma levels of phenytoin, possibly requiring dose reduction of phenytoin

Other Warnings/ Precautions

- Because oxcarbazepine has a tricyclic chemical structure, it is not recommended to be taken with MAOIs, including 14 days after MAOIs are stopped; do not start an MAOI until 2 weeks after discontinuing oxcarbazepine
- Because oxcarbazepine can lower plasma levels of hormonal contraceptives, it may also reduce their effectiveness
- May exacerbate narrow angle-closure glaucoma
- May need to restrict fluids and/or monitor sodium because of risk of hyponatremia
- Use cautiously in patients who have demonstrated hypersensitivity to carbamazepine
- Warn patients and their caregivers about the possibility of activation of suicidal ideation and advise them to report such side effects immediately

Do Not Use

- If patient is taking an MAOI
- If there is a proven allergy to any tricyclic compound
- If there is a proven allergy to oxcarbazepine

SPECIAL POPULATIONS

Renal Impairment

- Oxcarbazepine is renally excreted
- Elimination half-life of active metabolite MHD is increased
- Reduce initial dose by half; may need to use slower titration

Hepatic Impairment

- No dose adjustment recommended for mild to moderate hepatic impairment

Cardiac Impairment

- No dose adjustment recommended

Elderly

- Older patients may have reduced creatinine clearance and require reduced dosing
- Elderly patients may be more susceptible to adverse effects
- Some patients may tolerate lower doses better

Children and Adolescents

- Approved as adjunctive therapy or monotherapy for partial seizures in children 4 and older
- Ages 4–16 (adjunctive): initial 8–10 mg/kg per day or less than 600 mg/day in 2 doses; increase over 2 weeks to 900 mg/day (20–29 kg), 1,200 mg/day (29.1–39 kg), or 1,800 mg per day (>39 kg)
- When converting from adjunctive to monotherapy, titrate concomitant drug down over 3–6 weeks while titrating oxcarbazepine up by no more than 10 mg/kg per day each week, with an initial daily oxcarbazepine dose of 8–10 mg/kg per day divided in 2 doses

- Monotherapy: Initial 8–10 mg/kg per day in 2 doses; increase every 3 days by 5 mg/kg per day; recommended maintenance dose dependent on weight
- 0–20 kg (600–900 mg per day); 21–30 kg (900–1,200 mg per day); 31–40 kg (900–1,500 mg per day); 41–45 kg (1,200–1,500 mg per day); 46–55 kg (1,200–1,800 mg per day); 56–65 kg (1,200–2,100 mg per day); over 65 kg (1,500–2,100 mg)
- Children below age 8 may have increased clearance compared to adults

Pregnancy

- Risk Category C [some animal studies show adverse effects; no controlled studies in humans]

✻ Oxcarbazepine is structurally similar to carbamazepine, which is thought to be teratogenic in humans

✻ Use during first trimester may raise risk of neural tube defects (e.g., spina bifida) or other congenital anomalies

- Use in women of childbearing potential requires weighing potential benefits to the mother against the risks to the fetus

✻ If drug is continued, perform tests to detect birth defects

✻ If drug is continued, start on folate 1 mg/day to reduce risk of neural tube defects

- Antiepileptic Drug Pregnancy Registry: (888) 233-2334
- Taper drug if discontinuing

✻ For bipolar patients, oxcarbazepine should generally be discontinued before anticipated pregnancies

- Seizures, even mild seizures, may cause harm to the embryo/fetus
- Recurrent bipolar illness during pregnancy can be quite disruptive

✻ For bipolar patients, given the risk of relapse in the postpartum period, some form of mood stabilizer treatment may need to be restarted immediately after delivery if patient is unmedicated during pregnancy

✻ Atypical antipsychotics may be preferable to lithium or anticonvulsants such as oxcarbazepine if treatment of bipolar disorder is required during pregnancy

- Bipolar symptoms may recur or worsen during pregnancy and some form of treatment may be necessary

Breast Feeding

- Some drug is found in mother's breast milk

✻ Recommended either to discontinue drug or bottle feed

- If drug is continued while breast feeding, infant should be monitored for possible adverse effects
- If infant shows signs of irritability or sedation, drug may need to be discontinued
- Bipolar disorder may recur during the postpartum period, particularly if there is a history of prior postpartum episodes of either depression or psychosis

✻ Relapse rates may be lower in women who receive prophylactic treatment for postpartum episodes of bipolar disorder

- Atypical antipsychotics and anticonvulsants such as valproate may be safer than oxcarbazepine during the postpartum period when breast feeding

THE ART OF PSYCHOPHARMACOLOGY

Potential Advantages

- Treatment-resistant bipolar and psychotic disorders
- Those unable to tolerate carbamazepine but who respond to carbamazepine

Potential Disadvantages

- Patients at risk for hyponatremia

Primary Target Symptoms

- Incidence of seizures
- Severity of seizures
- Unstable mood, especially mania

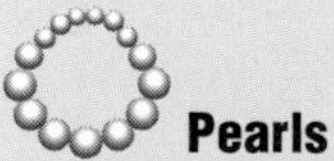

Pearls

✻ Some evidence of effectiveness in treating acute mania; included in American Psychiatric Association's bipolar treatment guidelines as an option for acute treatment and maintenance treatment of bipolar disorder

- Some evidence of effectiveness as adjunctive treatment in schizophrenia and schizoaffective disorders

- Oxcarbazepine is the 10-keto analog of carbamazepine, but not a metabolite of carbamazepine
- Less well investigated in bipolar disorder than carbamazepine

✽ Oxcarbazepine seems to have the same mechanism of therapeutic action as carbamazepine but with fewer side effects

✽ Specifically, risk of leukopenia, aplastic anemia, agranulocytosis, elevated liver enzymes, or Stevens-Johnson syndrome and serious rash associated with carbamazepine does not seem to be associated with oxcarbazepine

- Skin rash reactions to carbamazepine may resolve in 75% of patients with epilepsy when switched to oxcarbazepine; thus, 25% of patients who experience rash with carbamazepine may also experience it with oxcarbazepine
- Oxcarbazepine has much less prominent actions on CYP 450 enzyme systems than carbamazepine, and thus fewer drug-drug interactions
- Specifically, oxcarbazepine and its active metabolite, the monohydroxy derivative (MHD), cause less enzyme induction of CYP450 3A4 than the structurally-related carbamazepine
- The active metabolite MHD, also called licarbazepine, is a racemic mixture of 80% S-MHD (active) and 20% R-MHD (inactive)
- R, S-licarbazepine is also in clinical development as a novel mood stabilizer
- The active S enantiomer of licarbazepine is another related compound in development as yet another novel mood stabilizer

✽ Most significant risk of oxcarbazepine may be clinically significant hyponatremia (sodium level <125 m mol/L), most likely occurring within the first 3 months of treatment, and occurring in 2–3% of patients

- Unknown if this risk is higher than for carbamazepine

✽ Since SSRIs can sometimes also reduce sodium due to SIADH (syndrome of inappropriate antidiuretic hormone production), patients treated with combinations of oxcarbazepine and SSRIs should be carefully monitored, especially in the early stages of treatment

- By analogy with carbamazepine, could theoretically be useful in chronic neuropathic pain

Suggested Reading

Beydoun A. Safety and efficacy of oxcarbazepine: results of randomized, double-blind trials. Pharmacotherapy 2000; 20(8 Pt 2):152S–158S.

Centorrino F, Albert MJ, Berry JM, Kelleher JP, Fellman V, Line G, Koukopoulos AE, Kidwell JE, Fogarty KV, Baldessarini RJ. Oxcarbazepine: clinical experience with hospitalized psychiatric patients. Bipolar Disord 2003;5:370–4.

Dietrich DE, Kropp S, Emrich HM. Oxcarbazepine in affective and schizoaffective disorders. Pharmacopsychiatry 2001;34:242–50.

Glauser TA. Oxcarbazepine in the treatment of epilepsy. Pharmacotherapy 2001;21:904–19.

Hellewell JS. Oxcarbazepine (Trileptal) in the treatment of bipolar disorders: a review of efficacy and tolerability. J Affect Disord 2002;72(Suppl 1):S23–34.

THERAPEUTICS

Brands • INVEGA

see index for additional brand names

Generic? No

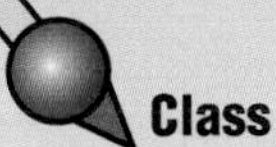

Class

- Atypical antipsychotic (serotonin-dopamine antagonist; second-generation antipsychotics; also a mood stabilizer)

Commonly Prescribed for

(bold for FDA approved)

- **Schizophrenia**
- **Maintaining response in schizophrenia**
- Other psychotic disorders
- Bipolar disorder
- Behavioral disturbances in dementia
- Behavioral disturbances in children and adolescents
- Disorders associated with problems with impulse control

How the Drug Works

- Blocks dopamine 2 receptors, reducing positive symptoms of psychosis and stabilizing affective symptoms
- Blocks serotonin 2A receptors, causing enhancement of dopamine release in certain brain regions and thus reducing motor side effects and possibly improving cognitive and affective symptoms

* Alpha 2 antagonist properties may contribute to antidepressant actions

How Long Until It Works

- Psychotic symptoms can improve within 1 week, but it may take several weeks for full effect on behavior as well as on cognition
- Classically recommended to wait at least 4–6 weeks to determine efficacy of drug, but in practice some patients may require up to 16–20 weeks to show a good response, especially on cognitive symptoms

If It Works

- Most often reduces positive symptoms but does not eliminate them
- Can improve negative symptoms, as well as aggressive, cognitive, and affective symptoms in schizophrenia
- Most schizophrenia patients do not have a total remission of symptoms but rather a reduction of symptoms by about a third
- Perhaps 5–15% of schizophrenia patients can experience an overall improvement of greater than 50–60%, especially when receiving stable treatment for more than a year
- Such patients are considered super-responders or "awakeners" since they may be well enough to be employed, live independently, and sustain long-term relationships
- Continue treatment until reaching a plateau of improvement
- After reaching a satisfactory plateau, continue treatment for at least a year after first episode of psychosis
- For second and subsequent episodes of psychosis, treatment may need to be indefinite
- Even for first episodes of psychosis, it may be preferable to continue treatment

If It Doesn't Work

- Try one of the other atypical antipsychotics (risperidone, olanzapine, quetiapine, ziprasidone, aripiprazole, amisulpride)
- If 2 or more antipsychotic monotherapies do not work, consider clozapine
- If no first-line atypical antipsychotic is effective, consider higher doses or augmentation with valproate or lamotrigine
- Some patients may require treatment with a conventional antipsychotic
- Consider noncompliance and switch to another antipsychotic with fewer side effects or to an antipsychotic that can be given by depot injection (a depot formulation of paliperidone is in development)
- Consider initiating rehabilitation and psychotherapy
- Consider presence of concomitant drug abuse

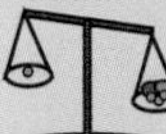

Best Augmenting Combos for Partial Response or Treatment Resistance

- Valproic acid (valproate, divalproex, divalproex ER)

- Other mood-stabilizing anticonvulsants (carbamazepine, oxcarbazepine, lamotrigine)
- Lithium
- Benzodiazepines

Tests

Before starting an atypical antipsychotic:

✽ Weigh all patients and track BMI during treatment
- Get baseline personal and family history of diabetes, obesity, dyslipidemia, hypertension, and cardiovascular disease

✽ Get waist circumference (at umbilicus), blood pressure, fasting plasma glucose, and fasting lipid profile
- Determine if the patient is
  - overweight (BMI 25.0–29.9)
  - obese (BMI >30)
  - has pre-diabetes (fasting plasma glucose 100–25 mg/dL)
  - has diabetes (fasting plasma glucose >126 mg/dL)
  - has hypertension (BP >140/90 mm Hg)
  - has dyslipidemia (increased total cholesterol, LDL cholesterol, and triglycerides; decreased HDL cholesterol)
- Treat or refer such patients for treatment, including nutrition and weight management, physical activity counseling, smoking cessation, and medical management

Monitoring after starting an atypical antipsychotic:

✽ BMI monthly for 3 months, than quarterly

✽ Consider monitoring fasting triglycerides monthly for several months in patients at high risk for metabolic complications and when initiating or switching antipsychotics

✽ Blood pressure, fasting plasma glucose, fasting lipids within 3 months and then annually, but earlier and more frequently for patients with diabetes or who have gained >5% of initial weight
- Treat or refer for treatment and consider switching to another atypical antipsychotic for patients who become overweight, obese, pre-diabetic, diabetic, hypertensive, or dyslipidemic while receiving an atypical antipsychotic

✽ Even in patients without known diabetes, be vigilant for the rare but life-threatening onset of diabetic ketoacidosis, which always requires immediate treatment, by monitoring for the rapid onset of polyuria, polydipsia, weight loss, nausea, vomiting, dehydration, rapid respiration, weakness and clouding of sensorium, even coma
- Should check blood pressure in the elderly before starting and for the first few weeks of treatment
- Monitoring elevated prolactin levels of dubious clinical benefit

SIDE EFFECTS

How Drug Causes Side Effects

- By blocking alpha 1 adrenergic receptors, it can cause dizziness, sedation, and hypotension
- By blocking dopamine 2 receptors in the striatum, it can cause motor side effects, especially at high doses
- By blocking dopamine 2 receptors in the pituitary, it can cause elevations in prolactin
- Mechanism of weight gain and increased incidence of diabetes and dyslipidemia with atypical antipsychotics is unknown

Notable Side Effects

✽ Dose-dependent extrapyramidal symptoms

✽ Hyperprolactinemia

✽ May increase risk for diabetes and dyslipidemia
- Rare tardive dyskinesia (much reduced risk compared to conventional antipsychotics)
- Sedation, hypersalivation
- Orthostatic hypotension
- Tachycardia

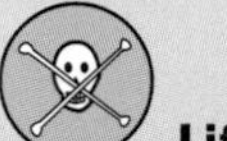

Life-Threatening or Dangerous Side Effects

- Hyperglycemia, in some cases extreme and associated with ketoacidosis or hyperosmolar coma or death, has been reported in patients taking atypical antipsychotics
- Increased risk of death and cerebrovascular events in elderly patients with dementia-related psychosis
- Rare neuroleptic malignant syndrome (much reduced risk compared to conventional antipsychotics)
- Rare seizures

Weight Gain

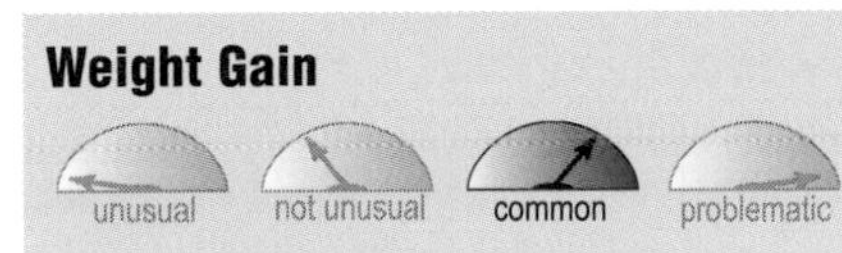

- Many patients experience and/or can be significant in amount
- May be dose-dependent
- May be less than for some antipsychotics, more than for others

Sedation

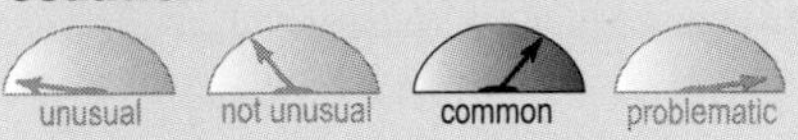

- Many experience and/or can be significant in amount
- May be dose-dependent
- May be less than for some antipsychotics, more than for others

What to Do About Side Effects

- Wait
- Wait
- Wait
- Anticholinergics may reduce motor side effects when present
- Weight loss, exercise programs, and medical management for high BMIs, diabetes, dyslipidemia
- Switch to another atypical antipsychotic

Best Augmenting Agents for Side Effects

- Benztropine or trihexyphenidyl for motor side effects
- Many side effects cannot be improved with an augmenting agent

DOSING AND USE

Usual Dosage Range

- 6 mg/day

Dosage Forms

- Tablet (extended-release) 3 mg, 6 mg, 9 mg

How To Dose

- Initial dose 6 mg/day taken in the morning
- Can increase by 3 mg/day every 5 days; maximum dose generally 12 mg/day

Dosing Tips

- Tablet should not be divided or chewed, but rather should only be swallowed whole
- Tablet does not change shape in the GI tract and generally should not be used in patients with gastrointestinal narrowing because of the risk of intestinal obstruction
- Some patients may benefit from doses above 6 mg/day; alternatively, for some patients 3 mg/day may be sufficient
- There is a dose-dependent increase in some side effects, including extrapyramidal symptoms and weight gain, above 6 mg/day
- Rather than raise the dose above these levels in acutely agitated patients requiring acute antipsychotic actions, consider augmentation with a benzodiazepine or conventional antipsychotic, either orally or intramuscularly
- Rather than raise the dose above these levels in partial responders, consider augmentation with a mood-stabilizing anticonvulsant, such as valproate or lamotrigine
- Children and elderly should generally be dosed at the lower end of the dosage spectrum

Overdose

- Extrapyramidal symptoms, gait unsteadiness, sedation, tachycardia, hypotension, QT prolongation

Long Term Use

- Approved for maintenance in schizophrenia

Habit Forming

- No

How to Stop

- Down-titration of oral formulation, especially when simultaneously beginning a new antipsychotic while switching (i.e., cross-titration)
- Rapid oral discontinuation may lead to rebound psychosis and worsening of symptoms

Pharmacokinetics

- Active metabolite of risperidone
- Half-life approximately 23 hours

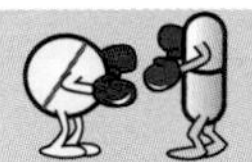

Drug Interactions

- May increase effects of antihypertensive agents
- May antagonize levodopa, dopamine agonists
- May enhance QTc prolongation of other drugs capable of prolonging QTc interval

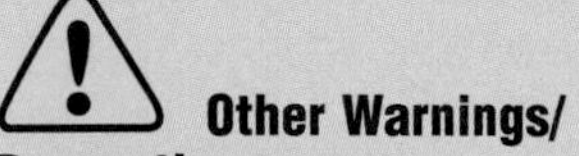

Other Warnings/ Precautions

- Use with caution in patients with conditions that predispose to hypotension (dehydration, overheating)
- Dysphagia has been associated with antipsychotic use, and paliperidone should be used cautiously in patients at risk for aspiration pneumonia
- Paliperidone prolongs QTc interval more than some other antipsychotics
- Priapism has been reported with other antipsychotics, including risperidone

Do Not Use

- If patient is taking agents capable of significantly prolonging QTc interval (e.g., pimozide, thioridazine, selected antiarrhythmics, moxifloxacin, sparfloxacin)
- If there is a history of QTc prolongation or cardiac arrhythmia, recent acute myocardial infarction, uncompensated heart failure
- If patient has a preexisting severe gastrointestinal narrowing
- If there is a proven allergy to paliperidone or risperidone

SPECIAL POPULATIONS

Renal Impairment

- For mild impairment, maximum recommended dose 6 mg/day
- For moderate to severe impairment, maximum recommended dose 3 mg/day

Hepatic Impairment

- No dose adjustment necessary for mild to moderate impairment
- Use in individuals with severe hepatic impairment has not been studied

Cardiac Impairment

- Drug should be used with caution because of risk of orthostatic hypotension

Elderly

- Some patients may tolerate lower doses better
- Although atypical antipsychotics are commonly used for behavioral disturbances in dementia, no agent has been approved for treatment of elderly patients with dementia-related psychosis
- Elderly patients with dementia-related psychosis treated with atypical antipsychotics are at an increased risk of death compared to placebo, and also have an increased risk of cerebrovascular events

Children and Adolescents

- Safety and efficacy have not been established
- Children and adolescents using paliperidone may need to be monitored more often than adults

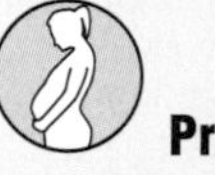

Pregnancy

- Risk Category C [some animal studies show adverse effects; no controlled studies in humans]
- Psychotic symptoms may worsen during pregnancy and some form of treatment may be necessary
- Paliperidone may be preferable to anticonvulsant mood stabilizers if treatment is required during pregnancy
- Effects of hyperprolactinemia on the fetus are unknown

Breast Feeding

- Some drug is found in mother's breast milk
- Recommended either to discontinue drug or bottle feed
- Infants of women who choose to breast feed while on paliperidone should be monitored for possible adverse effects

THE ART OF PSYCHOPHARMACOLOGY

Potential Advantages

- Some cases of psychosis and bipolar disorder refractory to treatment with other antipsychotics
- Patients requiring rapid onset of antipsychotic action without dosage titration

Potential Disadvantages

- Patients for whom elevated prolactin may not be desired (e.g., possibly pregnant patients; pubescent girls with amenorrhea; postmenopausal women with low estrogen who do not take estrogen replacement therapy)

Primary Target Symptoms

- Positive symptoms of psychosis
- Negative symptoms of psychosis
- Cognitive symptoms
- Unstable mood (both depression and mania)
- Aggressive symptoms

Pearls

- Some patients respond to paliperidone or tolerate paliperidone better than the parent drug risperidone
- Hyperprolactinemia in women with low estrogen may accelerate osteoporosis
- Less weight gain than some antipsychotics, more than others
- May cause more motor side effects than some other atypical antipsychotics, especially when administered to patients with Parkinson's disease or Lewy body dementia
- Trilayer tablet consists of 3 compartments (2 containing drug, 1 a "push" compartment) and an orifice at the head of the first drug compartment; water fills the push compartment and gradually pushes drug up and out of the tablet through the orifice

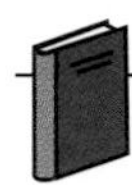

Suggested Reading

Meltzer HY, Bobo WV, Nuamah IF, et al. Efficacy and tolerability of oral paliperidone extended-release tablets in the treatment of acute schizophrenia: pooled data from three 6-week, placebo-controlled studies. J Clin Psychiatry 2008 May 6:e1–e13 [Epub ahead of print].

Nasrallah HA. Atypical antipsychotic-induced metabolic side effects: insights from receptor-binding profiles. Mol Psychiatry 2008;13(1):27–35.

Nussbaum A, Stroup TS. Paliperidone for schizophrenia. Cochrane Database Syst Rev 2008;16(2):CD006369.

THERAPEUTICS

Brands
- Paxil
- Paxil CR

see index for additional brand names

Generic? Yes

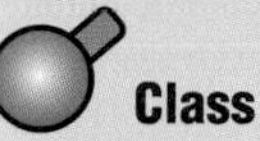

Class

- SSRI (selective serotonin reuptake inhibitor); often classified as an antidepressant, but it is not just an antidepressant

Commonly Prescribed for

(bold for FDA approved)

- **Major depressive disorder (paroxetine and paroxetine CR)**
- **Obsessive-compulsive disorder (OCD)**
- **Panic disorder (paroxetine and paroxetine CR)**
- **Social anxiety disorder (social phobia) (paroxetine and paroxetine CR)**
- **Posttraumatic stress disorder (PTSD)**
- **Generalized anxiety disorder (GAD)**
- **Premenstrual dysphoric disorder (PMDD) (paroxetine CR)**

How the Drug Works

- Boosts neurotransmitter serotonin
- Blocks serotonin reuptake pump (serotonin transporter)
- Desensitizes serotonin receptors, especially serotonin 1A autoreceptors
- Presumably increases serotonergic neurotransmission
- Paroxetine also has mild anticholinergic actions
- Paroxetine may have mild norepinephrine reuptake blocking actions

How Long Until It Works

- ✻ Some patients may experience relief of insomnia or anxiety early after initiation of treatment
- Onset of therapeutic actions usually not immediate, but often delayed 2–4 weeks
- If it is not working within 6–8 weeks for depression, it may require a dosage increase or it may not work at all
- By contrast, for generalized anxiety, onset of response and increases in remission rates may still occur after 8 weeks of treatment and for up to 6 months after initiating dosing
- May continue to work for many years to prevent relapse of symptoms

If It Works

- The goal of treatment is complete remission of current symptoms as well as prevention of future relapses
- Treatment most often reduces or even eliminates symptoms, but not a cure since symptoms can recur after medicine stopped
- Continue treatment until all symptoms are gone (remission) or significantly reduced (e.g., OCD, PTSD)
- Once symptoms are gone, continue treating for 1 year for the first episode of depression
- For second and subsequent episodes of depression, treatment may need to be indefinite
- Use in anxiety disorders may also need to be indefinite

If It Doesn't Work

- Many patients only have a partial response where some symptoms are improved but others persist (especially insomnia, fatigue, and problems concentrating in depression)
- Other patients may be nonresponders, sometimes called treatment-resistant or treatment-refractory
- Some patients who have an initial response may relapse even though they continue treatment, sometimes called "poop-out"
- Consider increasing dose, switching to another agent or adding an appropriate augmenting agent
- Consider psychotherapy
- Consider evaluation for another diagnosis or for a comorbid condition (e.g., medical illness, substance abuse, etc.)
- Some patients may experience apparent lack of consistent efficacy due to activation of latent or underlying bipolar disorder, and require antidepressant discontinuation and a switch to a mood stabilizer

Best Augmenting Combos for Partial Response or Treatment Resistance

- Trazodone, especially for insomnia
- Bupropion, mirtazapine, reboxetine, or atomoxetine (add with caution and at lower

doses since paroxetine could theoretically raise atomoxetine levels); use combinations of antidepressants with caution as this may activate bipolar disorder and suicidal ideation
- Modafinil, especially for fatigue, sleepiness, and lack of concentration
- Mood stabilizers or atypical antipsychotics for bipolar depression, psychotic depression, treatment-resistant depression, or treatment-resistant anxiety disorders
- Benzodiazepines
- If all else fails for anxiety disorders, consider gabapentin or tiagabine
- Hypnotics for insomnia
- Classically, lithium, buspirone, or thyroid hormone

Tests
- None for healthy individuals

SIDE EFFECTS

How Drug Causes Side Effects
- Theoretically due to increases in serotonin concentrations at serotonin receptors in parts of the brain and body other than those that cause therapeutic actions (e.g., unwanted actions of serotonin in sleep centers causing insomnia, unwanted actions of serotonin in the gut causing diarrhea, etc.)
- Increasing serotonin can cause diminished dopamine release and might contribute to emotional flattening, cognitive slowing, and apathy in some patients
- Most side effects are immediate but often go away with time, in contrast to most therapeutic effects which are delayed and are enhanced over time

✻ Paroxetine's weak antimuscarinic properties can cause constipation, dry mouth, sedation

Notable Side Effects
- Sexual dysfunction (men: delayed ejaculation, erectile dysfunction; men and women: decreased sexual desire, anorgasmia)
- Gastrointestinal (decreased appetite, nausea, diarrhea, constipation, dry mouth)
- Mostly central nervous system (insomnia but also sedation, agitation, tremors, headache, dizziness)
- Note: patients with diagnosed or undiagnosed bipolar or psychotic disorders may be more vulnerable to CNS-activating actions of SSRIs
- Autonomic (sweating)
- Bruising and rare bleeding
- Rare hyponatremia (mostly in elderly patients and generally reversible on discontinuation of paroxetine)

Life-Threatening or Dangerous Side Effects
- Rare seizures
- Rare induction of mania
- Rare activation of suicidal ideation and behavior (suicidality) (short-term studies did not show an increase in the risk of suicidality with antidepressants compared to placebo beyond age 24)

Weight Gain

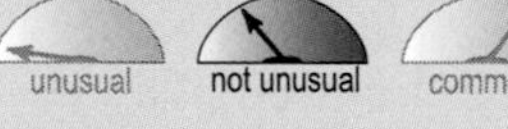

- Occurs in significant minority

Sedation

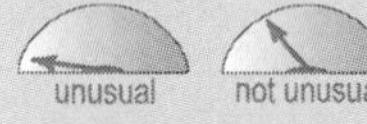

- Many experience and/or can be significant in amount
- Generally transient

What to Do About Side Effects
- Wait
- Wait
- Wait
- If paroxetine is sedating, take at night to reduce daytime drowsiness
- Reduce dose to 5–10 mg (12.5 mg for CR) until side effects abate, then increase as tolerated, usually to at least 20 mg (25 mg CR)
- In a few weeks, switch or add other drugs

Best Augmenting Agents for Side Effects
- Often best to try another SSRI or another antidepressant monotherapy prior to resorting to augmentation strategies to treat side effects
- Trazodone or a hypnotic for insomnia
- Bupropion, sildenafil, vardenafil, or tadalafil for sexual dysfunction

- Bupropion for emotional flattening, cognitive slowing, or apathy
- Mirtazapine for insomnia, agitation, and gastrointestinal side effects
- Benzodiazepines for jitteriness and anxiety, especially at initiation of treatment and especially for anxious patients
- Many side effects are dose-dependent (i.e., they increase as dose increases, or they reemerge until tolerance redevelops)
- Many side effects are time-dependent (i.e., they start immediately upon dosing and upon each dose increase, but go away with time)
- Activation and agitation may represent the induction of a bipolar state, especially a mixed dysphoric bipolar II condition sometimes associated with suicidal ideation, and require the addition of lithium, a mood stabilizer or an atypical antipsychotic, and/or discontinuation of paroxetine

DOSING AND USE

Usual Dosage Range

- Depression: 20–50 mg (25–62.5 mg CR)

Dosage Forms

- Tablets 10 mg scored, 20 mg scored, 30 mg, 40 mg
- Controlled-release tablets 12.5 mg, 25 mg
- Liquid 10 mg/5 mL – 250 mL bottle

How To Dose

- Depression: initial 20 mg (25 mg CR); usually wait a few weeks to assess drug effects before increasing dose, but can increase by 10 mg/day (12.5 mg/day CR) once a week; maximum generally 50 mg/day (62.5 mg/day CR); single dose
- Panic disorder: initial 10 mg/day (12.5 mg/day CR); usually wait a few weeks to assess drug effects before increasing dose, but can increase by 10 mg/day (12.5 mg/day CR) once a week; maximum generally 60 mg/day (75 mg/day CR); single dose
- Social anxiety disorder: initial 20 mg/day (25 mg/day CR); usually wait a few weeks to assess drug effects before increasing dose, but can increase by 10 mg/day (12.5 mg/day CR) once a week; maximum 60 mg/day (75 mg/day CR); single dose
- Other anxiety disorders: initial 20 mg/day (25 mg/day CR); usually wait a few weeks to assess drug effects before increasing dose, but can increase by 10 mg/day (12.5 mg/day CR) once a week; maximum 60 mg/day (75 mg/day CR); single dose

Dosing Tips

- 20-mg tablet is scored, so to save costs, give 10 mg as half of 20-mg tablet, since 10-mg and 20-mg tablets cost about the same in many markets
- Given once daily, often at bedtime, but any time of day tolerated
- 20 mg/day (25 mg/day CR) is often sufficient for patients with social anxiety disorder and depression
- Other anxiety disorders, as well as difficult cases in general, may require higher dosing
- Occasional patients are dosed above 60 mg/day (75 mg/day CR), but this is for experts and requires caution
- If intolerable anxiety, insomnia, agitation, akathisia, or activation occur either upon dosing initiation or discontinuation, consider the possibility of activated bipolar disorder and switch to a mood stabilizer or an atypical antipsychotic
- Liquid formulation easiest for doses below 10 mg when used for cases that are very intolerant to paroxetine or especially for very slow down-titration during discontinuation for patients with withdrawal symptoms
- Paroxetine CR tablets not scored, so chewing or cutting in half can destroy controlled-release properties
- Unlike other SSRIs and antidepressants where dosage increments can be double and triple the starting dose, paroxetine's dosing increments are in 50% increments (i.e., 20, 30, 40; or 25, 37.5, 50 CR)
- Paroxetine inhibits its own metabolism and thus plasma concentrations can double when oral doses increase by 50%; plasma concentrations can increase 2–7-fold when oral doses are doubled

✻ Main advantage of CR is reduced side effects, especially nausea and perhaps sedation, sexual dysfunction, and withdrawal

* For patients with severe problems discontinuing paroxetine, dosing may need to be tapered over many months (i.e., reduce dose by 1% every 3 days by crushing tablet and suspending or dissolving in 100 mL of fruit juice and then disposing of 1 mL while drinking the rest; 3–7 days later, dispose of 2 mL, and so on). This is both a form of very slow biological tapering and a form of behavioral desensitization
- For some patients with severe problems discontinuing paroxetine, it may be useful to add an SSRI with a long half-life, especially fluoxetine, prior to taper of paroxetine; while maintaining fluoxetine dosing, first slowly taper paroxetine and then taper fluoxetine
- Be sure to differentiate between re-emergence of symptoms requiring re-institution of treatment and withdrawal symptoms

Overdose
- Rarely lethal in monotherapy overdose; vomiting, sedation, heart rhythm disturbances, dilated pupils, dry mouth

Long-Term Use
- Safe

Habit Forming
- No

How to Stop
- Taper to avoid withdrawal effects (dizziness, nausea, stomach cramps, sweating, tingling, dysesthesias)
- Many patients tolerate 50% dose reduction for 3 days, then another 50% reduction for 3 days, then discontinuation
- If withdrawal symptoms emerge during discontinuation, raise dose to stop symptoms and then restart withdrawal much more slowly

* Withdrawal effects can be more common or more severe with paroxetine than with some other SSRIs
- Paroxetine's withdrawal effects may be related in part to the fact that it inhibits its own metabolism
- Thus, when paroxetine is withdrawn, the rate of its decline can be faster as it stops inhibiting its metabolism
- Controlled-release paroxetine may slow the rate of decline and thus reduce withdrawal reactions in some patients
- Readaptation of cholinergic receptors after prolonged blockade may contribute to withdrawal effects of paroxetine

Pharmacokinetics
- Inactive metabolites
- Half-life approximately 24 hours
- Inhibits CYP450 2D6

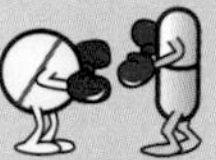

Drug Interactions
- Tramadol increases the risk of seizures in patients taking an antidepressant
- Can increase tricyclic antidepressant levels; use with caution with tricyclic antidepressants or when switching from a TCA to paroxetine
- Can cause a fatal "serotonin syndrome" when combined with MAO inhibitors, so do not use with MAO inhibitors or for at least 14 days after MAOIs are stopped
- Do not start an MAO inhibitor for at least 2 weeks after discontinuing paroxetine
- May displace highly protein bound drugs (e.g., warfarin)
- There are reports of elevated theophylline levels associated with paroxetine treatment, so it is recommended that theophylline levels be monitored when these drugs are administered together
- May increase anticholinergic effects of procyclidine and other drugs with anticholinergic properties
- Can rarely cause weakness, hyperreflexia, and incoordination when combined with sumatriptan or possibly with other triptans, requiring careful monitoring of patient
- Possible increased risk of bleeding, especially when combined with anticoagulants (e.g., warfarin, NSAIDs)
- Via CYP450 2D6 inhibition, paroxetine could theoretically interfere with the analgesic actions of codeine, and increase the plasma levels of some beta blockers and of atomoxetine
- Via CYP450 2D6 inhibition, paroxetine could theoretically increase concentrations of thioridazine and cause dangerous cardiac arrhythmias

- Paroxetine increases pimozide levels, and pimozide prolongs QT interval, so concomitant use of pimozide and paroxetine is contraindicated

Other Warnings/ Precautions

- Add or initiate other antidepressants with caution for up to 2 weeks after discontinuing paroxetine
- Use with caution in patients with history of seizures
- Use with caution in patients with bipolar disorder unless treated with concomitant mood stabilizing agent
- When treating children, carefully weigh the risks and benefits of pharmacological treatment against the risks and benefits of nontreatment with antidepressants and make sure to document this in the patient's chart
- Distribute the brochures provided by the FDA and the drug companies
- Warn patients and their caregivers about the possibility of activating side effects and advise them to report such symptoms immediately
- Monitor patients for activation of suicidal ideation, especially children and adolescents

Do Not Use

- If patient is taking an MAO inhibitor
- If patient is taking thioridazine
- If patient is taking pimozide
- If there is a proven allergy to paroxetine

SPECIAL POPULATIONS

Renal Impairment

- Lower dose [initial 10 mg/day (12.5 mg CR), maximum 40 mg/day (50 mg/day CR)]

Hepatic Impairment

- Lower dose [initial 10 mg/day (12.5 mg CR), maximum 40 mg/day (50 mg/day CR)]

Cardiac Impairment

- Preliminary research suggests that paroxetine is safe in these patients
- Treating depression with SSRIs in patients with acute angina or following myocardial infarction may reduce cardiac events and improve survival as well as mood

Elderly

- Lower dose [initial 10 mg/day (12.5 mg CR), maximum 40 mg/day (50 mg/day CR)]
- Reduction in risk of suicidality with antidepressants compared to placebo in adults age 65 and older

Children and Adolescents

- Carefully weigh the risks and benefits of pharmacological treatment against the risks and benefits of nontreatment with antidepressants and make sure to document this in the patient's chart
- Monitor patients face-to-face regularly, particularly during the first several weeks of treatment
- Use with caution, observing for activation of known or unknown bipolar disorder and/or suicidal ideation, and inform parents or guardian of this risk so they can help observe child or adolescent patients
- Not specifically approved, but preliminary evidence suggests efficacy in children and adolescents with OCD, social phobia, or depression

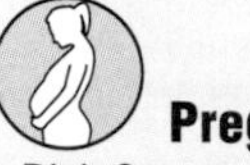

Pregnancy

- Risk Category D [positive evidence of risk to human fetus; potential benefits may still justify its use during pregnancy]
- Not generally recommended for use during pregnancy, especially during first trimester
- Epidemiological data have shown an increased risk of cardiovascular malformations (primarily ventricular and atrial septal defects) in infants born to women who took paroxetine during the first trimester
- Unless the benefits of paroxetine to the mother justify continuing treatment, consider discontinuing paroxetine or switching to another antidepressant
- Paroxetine use late in pregnancy may be associated with higher risk of neonatal complications, including respiratory distress

- At delivery there may be more bleeding in the mother and transient irritability or sedation in the newborn
- Must weigh the risk of treatment (first trimester fetal development, third trimester newborn delivery) to the child against the risk of no treatment (recurrence of depression, maternal health, infant bonding) to the mother and child
- For many patients this may mean continuing treatment during pregnancy
- SSRI use beyond the 20th week of pregnancy may be associated with increased risk of pulmonary hypertension in newborns
- Neonates exposed to SSRIs or SNRIs late in the third trimester have developed complications requiring prolonged hospitalization, respiratory support, and tube feeding; reported symptoms are consistent with either a direct toxic effect of SSRIs and SNRIs or, possibly, a drug discontinuation syndrome, and include respiratory distress, cyanosis, apnea, seizures, temperature instability, feeding difficulty, vomiting, hypoglycemia, hypotonia, hypertonia, hyperreflexia, tremor, jitteriness, irritability, and constant crying

Breast Feeding

- Some drug is found in mother's breast milk
- Trace amounts may be present in nursing children whose mothers are on paroxetine
- If child becomes irritable or sedated, breast feeding or drug may need to be discontinued
- Immediate postpartum period is a high-risk time for depression, especially in women who have had prior depressive episodes, so drug may need to be reinstituted late in the third trimester or shortly after childbirth to prevent a recurrence during the postpartum period
- Must weigh benefits of breast feeding with risks and benefits of antidepressant treatment versus nontreatment to both the infant and the mother
- For many patients, this may mean continuing treatment during breast feeding

THE ART OF PSYCHOPHARMACOLOGY

Potential Advantages

- Patients with anxiety disorders and insomnia
- Patients with mixed anxiety/depression

Potential Disadvantages

- Patients with hypersomnia
- Alzheimer/cognitive disorders
- Patients with psychomotor retardation, fatigue, and low energy

Primary Target Symptoms

- Depressed mood
- Anxiety
- Sleep disturbance, especially insomnia
- Panic attacks, avoidant behavior, re-experiencing, hyperarousal

Pearls

* Often a preferred treatment of anxious depression as well as major depressive disorder comorbid with anxiety disorders
* Withdrawal effects may be more likely than for some other SSRIs when discontinued (especially akathisia, restlessness, gastrointestinal symptoms, dizziness, tingling, dysesthesias, nausea, stomach cramps, restlessness)
- Inhibits own metabolism, so dosing is not linear
* Paroxetine has mild anticholinergic actions that can enhance the rapid onset of anxiolytic and hypnotic efficacy but also cause mild anticholinergic side effects
- Can cause cognitive and affective "flattening"
- May be less activating than other SSRIs
- Paroxetine is a potent CYP450 2D6 inhibitor
- SSRIs may be less effective in women over 50, especially if they are not taking estrogen
- SSRIs may be useful for hot flushes in perimenopausal women
- Some anecdotal reports suggest greater weight gain and sexual dysfunction than some other SSRIs, but the clinical significance of this is unknown
- For sexual dysfunction, can augment with bupropion, sildenafil, tadalafil, or switch to a non-SSRI such as bupropion or mirtazapine

- Some postmenopausal women's depression will respond better to paroxetine plus estrogen augmentation than to paroxetine alone
- Nonresponse to paroxetine in elderly may require consideration of mild cognitive impairment or Alzheimer disease
- CR formulation may enhance tolerability, especially for nausea
- Can be better tolerated than some SSRIs for patients with anxiety and insomnia and can reduce these symptoms early in dosing

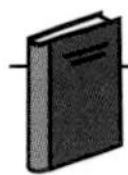

Suggested Reading

Bourin M, Chue P, Guillon Y. Paroxetine: a review. CNS Drug Rev 2001;7:25–47.

Edwards JG, Anderson I. Systematic review and guide to selection of selective serotonin reuptake inhibitors. Drugs 1999;57:507–533.

Green B. Focus on paroxetine. Curr Med Res Opin 2003;19:13–21.

Wagstaff AJ, Cheer SM, Matheson AJ, Ormrod D, Goa KL. Paroxetine: an update of its use in psychiatric disorders in adults. Drugs 2002;62:655–703.

THERAPEUTICS

Brands • Lullan

see index for additional brand names

Generic? No

Class

- Atypical antipsychotic (serotonin-dopamine antagonist, second-generation antipsychotic)

Commonly Prescribed for

(bold for FDA approved)

- Schizophrenia (Japan)

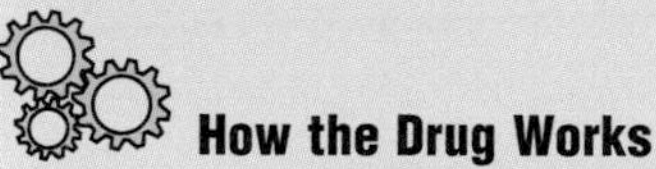

How the Drug Works

- Blocks dopamine 2 receptors, reducing positive symptoms of psychosis
- Blocks serotonin 2A receptors, causing enhancement of dopamine release in certain brain regions and thus reducing motor side effects and possibly improving cognitive and affective symptoms

✻ Interactions at 5HT1A receptors may contribute to efficacy for cognitive and affective symptoms in some patients

How Long Until It Works

- Psychotic symptoms can improve within 1 week, but it may take several weeks for full effect on behavior as well as on cognition and affective stabilization
- Classically recommended to wait at least 4–6 weeks to determine efficacy of drug, but in practice some patients require up to 16–20 weeks to show a good response, especially on cognitive symptoms

If It Works

- Most often reduces positive symptoms in schizophrenia but does not eliminate them
- Can improve negative symptoms, as well as aggressive, cognitive, and affective symptoms in schizophrenia
- Most schizophrenic patients do not have a total remission of symptoms but rather a reduction of symptoms by about a third
- Perhaps 5–15% of schizophrenic patients can experience an overall improvement of greater than 50–60%, especially when receiving stable treatment for more than a year
- Such patients are considered super-responders or "awakeners" since they may be well enough to be employed, live independently, and sustain long-term relationships
- Continue treatment until reaching a plateau of improvement
- After reaching a satisfactory plateau, continue treatment for at least a year after first episode of psychosis
- For second and subsequent episodes of psychosis, treatment may need to be indefinite
- Even for first episodes of psychosis, it may be preferable to continue treatment

If It Doesn't Work

- Consider trying one of the first-line atypical antipsychotics (e.g. risperidone, olanzapine, quetiapine, aripiprazole, paliperidone)
- If 2 or more antipsychotic monotherapies do not work, consider clozapine
- If no first-line atypical antipsychotic is effective, consider higher doses or augmentation with valproate or lamotrigine
- Some patients may require treatment with a conventional antipsychotic
- Consider noncompliance and switch to another antipsychotic with fewer side effects or to an antipsychotic that can be given by depot injection
- Consider initiating rehabilitation and psychotherapy
- Consider presence of concomitant drug abuse

Best Augmenting Combos for Partial Response or Treatment Resistance

- Augmentation of perospirone has not been systematically studied
- Addition of a benzodiazepine, especially short-term for agitation
- Addition of a mood-stabilizing anticonvulsant such as valproate, carbamazepine, or lamotrigine may theoretically be helpful in both schizophrenia and bipolar mania
- Augmentation with lithium in bipolar mania may be helpful

Tests

✻ Potential of weight gain, diabetes, and dyslipidemia associated with perospirone has not been systematically studied, but patients should be monitored the same as for other atypical antipsychotics

Before starting an atypical antipsychotic

- ✻ Weigh all patients and track BMI during treatment
- Get baseline personal and family history of diabetes, obesity, dyslipidemia, hypertension, and cardiovascular disease
- ✻ Get waist circumference (at umbilicus), blood pressure, fasting plasma glucose, and fasting lipid profile
- Determine if patient is
  - overweight (BMI 25.0–29.9)
  - obese (BMI ≥30)
  - has pre-diabetes (fasting plasma glucose 100–25 mg/dL)
  - has diabetes (fasting plasma glucose >126 mg/dL)
  - has hypertension (BP >140/90 mm Hg)
  - has dyslipidemia (increased total cholesterol, LDL cholesterol, and triglycerides; decreased HDL cholesterol)
- Treat or refer such patients for treatment, including nutrition and weight management, physical activity counseling, smoking cessation, and medical management

Monitoring after starting an atypical antipsychotic

- ✻ BMI monthly for 3 months, then quarterly
- ✻ Consider monitoring fasting triglycerides monthly for several months in patients at high risk for metabolic complications and when initiating or switching antipsychotics
- ✻ Blood pressure, fasting plasma glucose, fasting lipids within 3 months and then annually, but earlier and more frequently for patients with diabetes or who have gained >5% of initial weight
- Treat or refer for treatment and consider switching to another atypical antipsychotic for patients who become overweight, obese, pre-diabetic, diabetic, hypertensive, or dyslipidemic while receiving an atypical antipsychotic
- ✻ Even in patients without known diabetes, be vigilant for the rare but life threatening onset of diabetic ketoacidosis, which always requires immediate treatment, by monitoring for the rapid onset of polyuria, polydipsia, weight loss, nausea, vomiting, dehydration, rapid respiration, weakness and clouding of sensorium, even coma
- Should check blood pressure in the elderly before starting and for the first few weeks of treatment

SIDE EFFECTS

How Drug Causes Side Effects

- By blocking dopamine 2 receptors in the striatum, it can cause motor side effects
- By blocking dopamine 2 receptors in the pituitary, it can cause increased prolactin (unusual)
- Mechanism of weight gain and increased incidence of diabetes and dyslipidemia with some atypical antipsychotics is unknown
- Receptor binding portfolio of perospirone is not well-characterized

Notable Side Effects

- ✻ Extrapyramidal symptoms, akathisia
- ✻ Insomnia
- Sedation, anxiety, weakness, headache, anorexia, constipation
- Theoretically, tardive dyskinesia (should be reduced risk compared to conventional antipsychotics)
- Elevated creatine phosphokinase levels

Life-Threatening or Dangerous Side Effects

- Rare neuroleptic malignant syndrome
- Theoretically, seizures are rarely associated with atypical antipsychotics
- Increased risk of death and cerebrovascular events in elderly patients with dementia-related psychosis

Weight Gain

- ✻ Not well characterized

Sedation

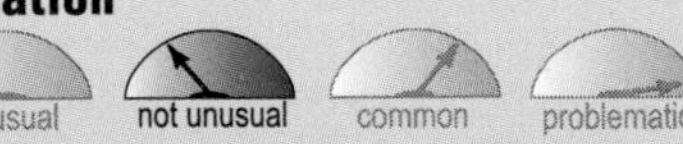

- Occurs in significant minority

What to Do About Side Effects

- Wait
- Wait
- Wait
- For motor symptoms, add an anticholinergic agent
- Reduce the dose
- Switch to another atypical antipsychotic

Best Augmenting Agents for Side Effects

- Benztropine or trihexyphenidyl for motor side effects
- Sometimes amantadine can be helpful for motor side effects
- Benzodiazepines may be helpful for akathisia
- Many side effects cannot be improved with an augmenting agent

DOSING AND USE

Usual Dosage Range

- 8–48 mg/day in 3 divided doses

Dosage Forms

- Tablet 4 mg, 8 mg

How To Dose

- Begin at 4 mg 3 times a day, increasing as tolerated up to 16 mg 3 times a day

Dosing Tips

- Some patients have been treated with up to 96 mg/day in 3 divided doses
- Unknown whether dosing frequency can be reduced to once or twice daily, but by analogy with other agents in this class with half-lives shorter than 24 hours, this may be possible

Overdose

- Not reported

Long-Term Use

- Long-term studies not reported, but as for other atypical antipsychotics, long-term use for treatment of schizophrenia is common

Habit Forming

- No

How to Stop

- Slow down-titration (over 6–8 weeks), especially when simultaneously beginning a new antipsychotic while switching (i.e., cross-titration)
- Rapid discontinuation may lead to rebound psychosis and worsening of symptoms
- If antiparkinson agents are being used, they should be continued for a few weeks after perospirone is discontinued

Pharmacokinetics

- Metabolized primarily by CYP450 3A4
- No active metabolites

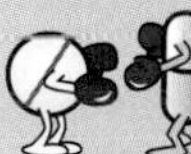

Drug Interactions

- Ketaconazole and possibly other CYP450 3A4 inhibitors such as nefazodone, fluvoxamine, and fluoxetine may increase plasma levels of perospirone
- Carbamazepine and possibly other inducers of CYP450 3A4 may decrease plasma levels of perospirone

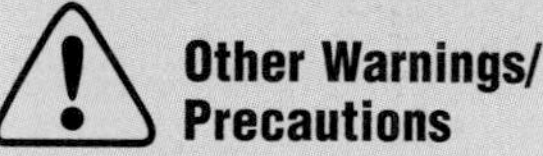

Other Warnings/ Precautions

- Not reported

Do Not Use

- If there is a proven allergy to perospirone

SPECIAL POPULATIONS

Renal Impairment

- Use with caution

Hepatic Impairment

- Use with caution

Cardiac Impairment

- Use with caution

Elderly

- Some patients may tolerate lower doses better
- Although atypical antipsychotics are commonly used for behavioral disturbances in dementia, no agent has been approved for treatment of elderly patients with dementia-related psychosis
- Elderly patients with dementia-related psychosis treated with atypical antipsychotics are at an increased risk of death compared to placebo, and also have an increased risk of cerebrovascular events

Children and Adolescents

- Use with caution

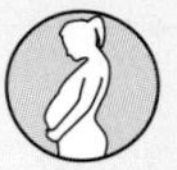

Pregnancy

- Psychotic symptoms may worsen during pregnancy and some form of treatment may be necessary

Breast Feeding

- Unknown if perospirone is secreted in human breast milk, but all psychotropics assumed to be secreted in breast milk
- ✻ Recommended either to discontinue drug or bottle feed
- Infants of women who choose to breast feed should be monitored for possible adverse effects

THE ART OF PSYCHOPHARMACOLOGY

Potential Advantages

- In Japan, studies suggest efficacy for negative symptoms of schizophrenia

Potential Disadvantages

- Patients who have difficulty complying with three times daily administration

Primary Target Symptoms

- Positive symptoms of psychosis
- Negative symptoms of psychosis
- Affective symptoms (depression, anxiety)
- Cognitive symptoms

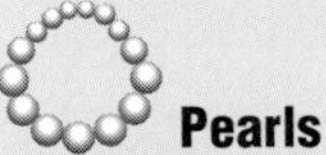

Pearls

- Extrapyramidal symptoms may be more frequent than with some other atypical antipsychotics
- Potent 5HT1A binding properties may be helpful for improving cognitive symptoms of schizophrenia in long-term treatment
- Theoretically, should be effective in acute bipolar mania

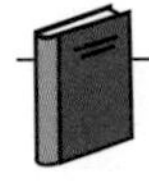

Suggested Reading

Ohno Y. Pharmacological characteristics of perospirone hydrochloride, a novel antipsychotic agent. Nippon Yakurigaku Zasshi 2000;116(4):225–31.

PERPHENAZINE

THERAPEUTICS

Brands • Trilafon
see index for additional brand names

Generic? Yes

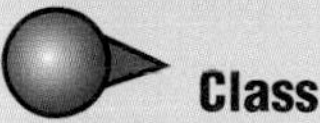

Class
- Conventional antipsychotic (neuroleptic, phenothiazine, dopamine 2 antagonist, antiemetic)

Commonly Prescribed for
(bold for FDA approved)
- **Schizophrenia**
- **Nausea, vomiting**
- Other psychotic disorders
- Bipolar disorder

How the Drug Works
- Blocks dopamine 2 receptors, reducing positive symptoms of psychosis
- Combination of dopamine D2, histamine H1, and cholinergic M1 blockade in the vomiting center may reduce nausea and vomiting

How Long Until It Works
- Psychotic symptoms can improve within 1 week, but may take several weeks for full effect on behavior
- Injection: initial effect after 10 minutes, peak after 1–2 hours
- Actions on nausea and vomiting are immediate

If It Works
- Most often reduces positive symptoms in schizophrenia but does not eliminate them
- Most schizophrenic patients do not have a total remission of symptoms but rather a reduction of symptoms by about a third
- Continue treatment in schizophrenia until reaching a plateau of improvement
- After reaching a satisfactory plateau, continue treatment for at least a year after first episode of psychosis in schizophrenia
- For second and subsequent episodes of psychosis in schizophrenia, treatment may need to be indefinite
- Reduces symptoms of acute psychotic mania but not proven as a mood stabilizer or as an effective maintenance treatment in bipolar disorder
- After reducing acute psychotic symptoms in mania, switch to a mood stabilizer and/or an atypical antipsychotic for mood stabilization and maintenance

If It Doesn't Work
- Consider trying one of the first-line atypical antipsychotics (risperidone, olanzapine, quetiapine, ziprasidone, aripiprazole, paliperidone, amisulpride)
- Consider trying another conventional antipsychotic
- If 2 or more antipsychotic monotherapies do not work, consider clozapine

Best Augmenting Combos for Partial Response or Treatment Resistance
- Augmentation of conventional antipsychotics has not been systematically studied
- Addition of a mood-stabilizing anticonvulsant such as valproate, carbamazepine, or lamotrigine may be helpful in both schizophrenia and bipolar mania
- Augmentation with lithium in bipolar mania may be helpful
- Addition of a benzodiazepine, especially short-term for agitation

Tests
✻ Since conventional antipsychotics are frequently associated with weight gain, before starting treatment, weigh all patients and determine if the patient is already overweight (BMI 25.0–29.9) or obese (BMI ≥30)
- Before giving a drug that can cause weight gain to an overweight or obese patient, consider determining whether the patient already has pre-diabetes (fasting plasma glucose 100–25 mg/dL), diabetes (fasting plasma glucose >126 mg/dL), or dyslipidemia (increased total cholesterol, LDL cholesterol and triglycerides; decreased HDL cholesterol), and treat or refer such patients for treatment, including nutrition and weight management, physical activity counseling, smoking cessation, and medical management

✻ Monitor weight and BMI during treatment

✻ Consider monitoring fasting triglycerides monthly for several months in patients at high risk for metabolic complications and when initiating or switching antipsychotics
✻ While giving a drug to a patient who has gained >5% of initial weight, consider evaluating for the presence of pre-diabetes, diabetes, or dyslipidemia, or consider switching to a different antipsychotic
- Should check blood pressure in the elderly before starting and for the first few weeks of treatment
- Monitoring elevated prolactin levels of dubious clinical benefit
- Phenothiazines may cause false-positive phenylketonuria results

SIDE EFFECTS

How Drug Causes Side Effects

- By blocking dopamine 2 receptors in the striatum, it can cause motor side effects
- By blocking dopamine 2 receptors in the pituitary, it can cause elevations in prolactin
- By blocking dopamine 2 receptors excessively in the mesocortical and mesolimbic dopamine pathways, especially at high doses, it can cause worsening of negative and cognitive symptoms (neuroleptic-induced deficit syndrome)
- Anticholinergic actions may cause sedation, blurred vision, constipation, dry mouth
- Antihistaminic actions may cause sedation, weight gain
- By blocking alpha 1 adrenergic receptors, it can cause dizziness, sedation, and hypotension
- Mechanism of weight gain and any possible increased incidence of diabetes or dyslipidemia with conventional antipsychotics is unknown

Notable Side Effects

✻ Neuroleptic-induced deficit syndrome
✻ Akathisia
✻ Extrapyramidal symptoms, Parkinsonism, tardive dyskinesia
✻ Galactorrhea, amenorrhea
- Dizziness, sedation
- Dry mouth, constipation, urinary retention, blurred vision
- Decreased sweating
- Sexual dysfunction
- Hypotension, tachycardia, syncope
- Weight gain

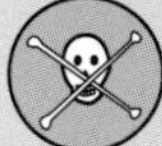

Life-Threatening or Dangerous Side Effects

- Rare neuroleptic malignant syndrome
- Rare jaundice, agranulocytosis
- Rare seizures
- Increased risk of death and cerebrovascular events in elderly patients with dementia-related psychosis

Weight Gain

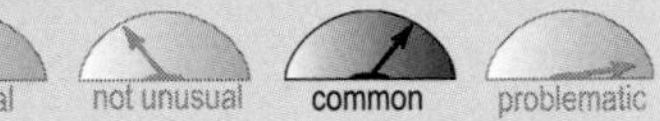

- Many experience and/or can be significant in amount

Sedation

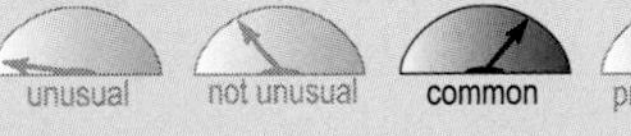

- Many experience and/or can be significant in amount
- Sedation is usually transient

What to Do About Side Effects

- Wait
- Wait
- Wait
- For motor symptoms, add an anticholinergic agent
- Reduce the dose
- For sedation, give at night
- Switch to an atypical antipsychotic
- Weight loss, exercise programs, and medical management for high BMIs, diabetes, dyslipidemia

Best Augmenting Agents for Side Effects

- Benztropine or trihexyphenidyl for motor side effects
- Sometimes amantadine can be helpful for motor side effects
- Benzodiazepines may be helpful for akathisia
- Many side effects cannot be improved with an augmenting agent

DOSING AND USE

Usual Dosage Range
- Psychosis: oral: 12–24 mg/day; 16–64 mg/day in hospitalized patients
- Nausea/vomiting: 8–16 mg/day oral, 5 mg intramuscularly

Dosage Forms
- Tablet 2 mg, 4 mg, 8 mg, 16 mg
- Injection 5 mg/mL

How To Dose
- Oral: Psychosis: 4–8 mg 3 times a day; 8–16 mg 2 times a day to 4 times a day in hospitalized patients; maximum 64 mg/day
- Oral: Nausea/vomiting: 8–16 mg/day in divided doses; maximum 24 mg/day
- Intramuscular: Psychosis: initial 5 mg; can repeat every 6 hours, maximum 15 mg/day (30 mg/day in hospitalized patients)

Dosing Tips
- Injection contains sulfites that may cause allergic reactions, particularly in patients with asthma
- Oral perphenazine is less potent than the injection, so patients should receive equal or higher dosage when switched from injection to tablet

Overdose
- Extrapyramidal symptoms, coma, hypotension, sedation, seizures, respiratory depression

Long-Term Use
- Some side effects may be irreversible (e.g., tardive dyskinesia)

Habit Forming
- No

How to Stop
- Slow down-titration of oral formulation (over 6–8 weeks), especially when simultaneously beginning a new antipsychotic while switching (i.e., cross-titration)
- Rapid oral discontinuation may lead to rebound psychosis and worsening of symptoms
- If antiparkinson agents are being used, they should be continued for a few weeks after perphenazine is discontinued

Pharmacokinetics
- Half-life approximately 9.5 hours

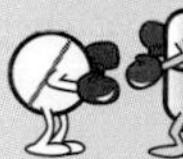

Drug Interactions
- May decrease the effects of levodopa, dopamine agonists
- May increase the effects of antihypertensive drugs except for guanethidine, whose antihypertensive actions perphenazine may antagonize
- Additive effects may occur if used with CNS depressants
- Anticholinergic effects may occur if used with atropine or related compounds
- Some patients taking a neuroleptic and lithium have developed an encephalopathic syndrome similar to neuroleptic malignant syndrome
- Epinephrine may lower blood pressure; diuretics and alcohol may increase risk of hypotension

Other Warnings/ Precautions
- If signs of neruoleptic malignant syndrome develop, treatment should be immediately discontinued
- Use cautiously in patients with respiratory disorders
- Use cautiously in patients with alcohol withdrawal or convulsive disorders because of possible lowering of seizure threshold
- Do not use epinephrine in event of overdose as interaction with some pressor agents may lower blood pressure
- Avoid undue exposure to sunlight
- Avoid extreme heat exposure
- Use with caution in patients with respiratory disorders, glaucoma or urinary retention
- Antiemetic effect of perphenazine may mask signs of other disorders or overdose; suppression of cough reflex may cause asphyxia
- Observe for signs of ocular toxicity (corneal and lenticular deposits)

- Use only with caution if at all in Parkinson's disease or Lewy body dementia

Do Not Use
- If patient is in a comatose state or has CNS depression
- If there is the presence of blood dyscrasias, subcortical brain damage, bone marrow depression, or liver disease
- If there is a proven allergy to perphenazine
- If there is a known sensitivity to any phenothiazine

SPECIAL POPULATIONS

Renal Impairment
- Use with caution

Hepatic Impairment
- Use with caution; may not be recommended as long-term treatment because perphenazine may increase risk of further liver damage

Cardiac Impairment
- Cardiovascular toxicity can occur, especially orthostatic hypotension

Elderly
- Lower doses should be used and patient should be monitored closely
- Although conventional antipsychotics are commonly used for behavioral disturbances in dementia, no agent has been approved for treatment of elderly patients with dementia-related psychosis
- Elderly patients with dementia-related psychosis treated with antipsychotics are at an increased risk of death compared to placebo, and also have an increased risk of cerebrovascular events

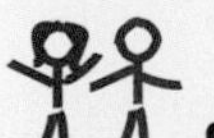

Children and Adolescents
- Not recommended for use in children under age 12
- Over age 12: if given intramuscularly, should receive lowest adult dose
- Generally consider second-line after atypical antipsychotics

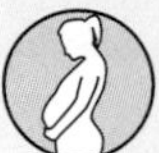

Pregnancy
- Risk Category C [some animal studies show adverse effects; no controlled studies in humans]
- Reports of extrapyramidal symptoms, jaundice, hyperreflexia, hyporeflexia in infants whose mothers took a phenothiazine during pregnancy
- Perphenazine should only be used during pregnancy if clearly needed
- Psychotic symptoms may worsen during pregnancy and some form of treatment may be necessary
- Atypical antipsychotics may be preferable to conventional antipsychotics or anticonvulsant mood stabilizers if treatment is required during pregnancy

Breast Feeding
- Unknown if perphenazine is secreted in human breast milk, but all psychotropics assumed to be secreted in breast milk
- ✻ Recommended either to discontinue drug or bottle feed

THE ART OF PSYCHOPHARMACOLOGY

Potential Advantages
- Intramuscular formulation for emergency use

Potential Disadvantages
- Patients with tardive dyskinesia
- Children
- Elderly

Primary Target Symptoms
- Positive symptoms of psychosis
- Motor and autonomic hyperactivity
- Violent or aggressive behavior

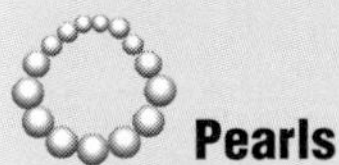

Pearls
- Recent landmark head to head study in schizophrenia suggests comparable effectiveness with some atypical antipsychotics
- Perphenazine is a higher potency phenothiazine
- Less risk of sedation and orthostatic hypotension but greater risk of

extrapyramidal symptoms than with low potency phenothiazines
- Conventional antipsychotics are much less expensive than atypical antipsychotics
- Patients have very similar antipsychotic responses to any conventional antipsychotic, which is different from atypical antipsychotics where antipsychotic responses of individual patients can occasionally vary greatly from one atypical antipsychotic to another
- Patients with inadequate responses to atypical antipsychotics may benefit from a trial of augmentation with a conventional antipsychotic such as perphenazine or from switching to a conventional antipsychotic such as perphenazine
- However, long-term polypharmacy with a combination of a conventional antipsychotic such as perphenazine with an atypical antipsychotic may combine their side effects without clearly augmenting the efficacy of either
- Although a frequent practice by some prescribers, adding 2 conventional antipsychotics together has little rationale and may reduce tolerability without clearly enhancing efficacy
- Availability of alternative treatments and risk of tardive dyskinesia make utilization of perphenazine for nausea and vomiting a short-term and second-line treatment option

Suggested Reading

Dencker SJ, Gios I, Martensson E, Norden T, Nyberg G, Persson R, Roman G, Stockman O, Syard KO. A long-term cross-over pharmacokinetic study comparing perphenazine decanoate and haloperidol decanoate in schizophrenic patients. Psychopharmacology (Berl) 1994;114:24–30.

Frankenburg FR. Choices in antipsychotic therapy in schizophrenia. Harv Rev Psychiatry 1999;6:241–9.

Lieberman JA, Stroup TS, McEvoy JP, Swartz MS, Rosenheck RA, Perkins DO, et al. Effectiveness of antipsychotic drugs in patients with chronic schizophrenia. N Engl J Med 2005;353(12):1209–23.

Quraishi S, David A. Depot perphenazine decanoate and enanthate for schizophrenia. Cochrane Database Syst Rev 2000;(2):CD001717.

THERAPEUTICS

Brands
- Nardil
- Nardelzine

see index for additional brand names

Generic? Yes

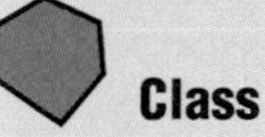

Class
- Monoamine oxidase inhibitor (MAOI)

Commonly Prescribed for
(bold for FDA approved)
- **Depressed patients characterized as "atypical," "nonendogenous," or "neurotic"**
- Treatment-resistant depression
- Treatment-resistant panic disorder
- Treatment-resistant social anxiety disorder

How the Drug Works
- Irreversibly blocks monoamine oxidase (MAO) from breaking down norepinephrine, serotonin, and dopamine
- This presumably boosts noradrenergic, serotonergic, and dopaminergic neurotransmission

How Long Until It Works
- Onset of therapeutic actions usually not immediate, but often delayed 2–4 weeks
- If it is not working within 6–8 weeks, it may require a dosage increase or it may not work at all
- May continue to work for many years to prevent relapse of symptoms

If It Works
- The goal of treatment is complete remission of current symptoms as well as prevention of future relapses
- Treatment most often reduces or even eliminates symptoms, but not a cure since symptoms can recur after medicine stopped
- Continue treatment until all symptoms are gone (remission)
- Once symptoms gone, continue treating for 1 year for the first episode of depression
- For second and subsequent episodes of depression, treatment may need to be indefinite
- Use in anxiety disorders may also need to be indefinite

If It Doesn't Work
- Many patients only have a partial response where some symptoms are improved but others persist (especially insomnia, fatigue, and problems concentrating)
- Other patients may be nonresponders, sometimes called treatment-resistant or treatment-refractory
- Some patients who have an initial response may relapse even though they continue treatment, sometimes called "poop-out"
- Consider increasing dose, switching to another agent, or adding an appropriate augmenting agent
- Consider psychotherapy
- Consider evaluation for another diagnosis or for a comorbid condition (e.g., medical illness, substance abuse, etc.)
- Some patients may experience apparent lack of consistent efficacy due to activation of latent or underlying bipolar disorder, and require antidepressant discontinuation and a switch to a mood stabilizer

Best Augmenting Combos for Partial Response or Treatment Resistance
❋ Augmentation of MAOIs has not been systematically studied, and this is something for the expert, to be done with caution and with careful monitoring

❋ A stimulant such as d-amphetamine or methylphenidate (with caution; may activate bipolar disorder and suicidal ideation; may elevate blood pressure)
- Lithium
- Mood-stabilizing anticonvulsants
- Atypical antipsychotics (with special caution for those agents with monoamine reuptake blocking properties, such as ziprasidone and zotepine)

Tests
- Patients should be monitored for changes in blood pressure
- Patients receiving high doses or long-term treatment should have hepatic function evaluated periodically

❋ Since MAO inhibitors are frequently associated with weight gain, before starting treatment, weigh all patients and determine

if the patient is already overweight (BMI 25.0–29.9) or obese (BMI ≥30)
- Before giving a drug that can cause weight gain to an overweight or obese patient, consider determining whether the patient already has pre-diabetes (fasting plasma glucose 100–25 mg/dL), diabetes (fasting plasma glucose >126 mg/dL), or dyslipidemia (increased total cholesterol, LDL cholesterol and triglycerides; decreased HDL cholesterol), and treat or refer such patients for treatment, including nutrition and weight management, physical activity counseling, smoking cessation, and medical management

✻ Monitor weight and BMI during treatment

✻ While giving a drug to a patient who has gained >5% of initial weight, consider evaluating for the presence of pre-diabetes, diabetes, or dyslipidemia, or consider switching to a different antidepressant

SIDE EFFECTS

How Drug Causes Side Effects
- Theoretically due to increases in monoamines in parts of the brain and body and at receptors other than those that cause therapeutic actions (e.g., unwanted actions of serotonin in sleep centers causing insomnia, unwanted actions of norepinephrine on vascular smooth muscle causing changes in blood pressure, etc.)
- Side effects are generally immediate, but immediate side effects often disappear in time

Notable Side Effects
- Dizziness, sedation, headache, sleep disturbances, fatigue, weakness, tremor, movement problems, blurred vision, increased sweating
- Constipation, dry mouth, nausea, change in appetite, weight gain
- Sexual dysfunction
- Orthostatic hypotension (dose-related); syncope may develop at high doses

Life-Threatening or Dangerous Side Effects
- Hypertensive crisis (especially when MAOIs are used with certain tyramine-containing foods or prohibited drugs)
- Induction of mania
- Rare activation of suicidal ideation and behavior (suicidality) (short-term studies did not show an increase in the risk of suicidality with antidepressants compared to placebo beyond age 24)
- Seizures
- Hepatotoxicity

Weight Gain

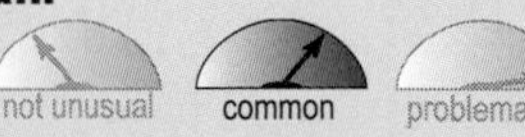

- Many experience and/or can be significant in amount

Sedation

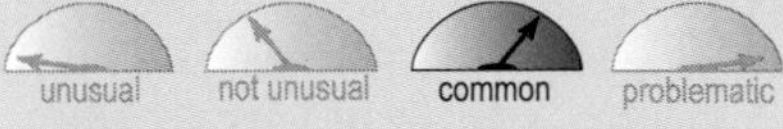

- Many experience and/or can be significant in amount
- Can also cause activation

What to Do About Side Effects
- Wait
- Wait
- Wait
- Lower the dose
- Take at night if daytime sedation
- Switch after appropriate washout to an SSRI or newer antidepressant

Best Augmenting Agents for Side Effects
- Trazodone (with caution) for insomnia
- Benzodiazepines for insomnia

✻ Single oral or sublingual dose of a calcium channel blocker (e.g., nifedipine) for urgent treatment of hypertension due to drug interaction or dietary tyramine

- Many side effects cannot be improved with an augmenting agent

DOSING AND USE

Usual Dosage Range
- 45–75 mg/day

Dosage Forms
- Tablet 15 mg

How To Dose
- Initial 45 mg/day in 3 divided doses; increase to 60–90 mg/day; after desired

therapeutic effect is achieved lower dose as far as possible

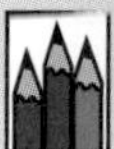

Dosing Tips

- Once dosing is stabilized, some patients may tolerate once or twice daily dosing rather than 3-times-a-day dosing
- Orthostatic hypotension, especially at high doses, may require splitting into 4 daily doses
- Patients receiving high doses may need to be evaluated periodically for effects on the liver
- Little evidence to support efficacy of phenelzine below doses of 45 mg/day

Overdose

- Death may occur; dizziness, ataxia, sedation, headache, insomnia, restlessness, anxiety, irritability, cardiovascular effects, confusion, respiratory depression, coma

Long-Term Use

- May require periodic evaluation of hepatic function
- MAOIs may lose efficacy long-term

Habit Forming

- Some patients have developed dependence to MAOIs

How to Stop

- Generally no need to taper, as the drug wears off slowly over 2–3 weeks

Pharmacokinetics

- Clinical duration of action may be up to 21 days due to irreversible enzyme inhibition

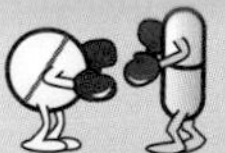

Drug Interactions

- Tramadol may increase the risk of seizures in patients taking an MAO inhibitor
- Can cause a fatal "serotonin syndrome" when combined with drugs that block serotonin reuptake (e.g., SSRIs, SNRIs, sibutramine, tramadol, etc.), so do not use with a serotonin reuptake inhibitor or for up to 5 weeks after stopping the serotonin reuptake inhibitor
- Hypertensive crisis with headache, intracranial bleeding, and death may result from combining MAO inhibitors with sympathomimetic drugs (e.g., amphetamines, methylphenidate, cocaine, dopamine, epinephrine, norepinephrine, and related compounds methyldopa, levodopa, L-tryptophan, L-tyrosine, and phenylalanine)
- Excitation, seizures, delirium, hyperpyrexia, circulatory collapse, coma, and death may result from combining MAO inhibitors with mepiridine or dextromethorphan
- Do not combine with another MAO inhibitor, alcohol, buspirone, bupropion, or guanethidine
- Adverse drug reactions can result from combining MAO inhibitors with tricyclic/tetracyclic antidepressants and related compounds, including carbamazepine, cyclobenzaprine, and mirtazapine, and should be avoided except by experts to treat difficult cases
- MAO inhibitors in combination with spinal anesthesia may cause combined hypotensive effects
- Combination of MAOIs and CNS depressants may enhance sedation and hypotension

Other Warnings/ Precautions

- Use requires low tyramine diet
- Patients taking MAO inhibitors should avoid high protein food that has undergone protein breakdown by aging, fermentation, pickling, smoking, or bacterial contamination
- Patients taking MAO inhibitors should avoid cheeses (especially aged varieties), pickled herring, beer, wine, liver, yeast extract, dry sausage, hard salami, pepperoni, Lebanon bologna, pods of broad beans (fava beans), yogurt, and excessive use of caffeine and chocolate
- Patient and prescriber must be vigilant to potential interactions with any drug, including antihypertensives and over-the-counter cough/cold preparations
- Over-the-counter medications to avoid include cough and cold preparations, including those containing dextromethorphan, nasal decongestants (tablets, drops, or spray), hay-fever medications, sinus medications, asthma inhalant medications, anti-appetite

medications, weight reducing preparations, "pep" pills
- Hypoglycemia may occur in diabetic patients receiving insulin or oral antidiabetic agents
- Use cautiously in patients receiving reserpine, anesthetics, disulfiram, metrizamide, anticholinergic agents
- Phenelzine is not recommended for use in patients who cannot be monitored closely
- When treating children, carefully weigh the risks and benefits of pharmacological treatment against the risks and benefits of nontreatment with antidepressants and make sure to document this in the patient's chart
- Distribute the brochures provided by the FDA and the drug companies
- Warn patients and their caregivers about the possibility of activating side effects and advise them to report such symptoms immediately
- Monitor patients for activation of suicidal ideation, especially children and adolescents

Do Not Use
- If patient is taking meperidine (pethidine)
- If patient is taking a sympathomimetic agent or taking guanethidine
- If patient is taking another MAOI
- If patient is taking any agent that can inhibit serotonin reuptake (e.g., SSRIs, sibutramine, tramadol, milnacipran, duloxetine, venlafaxine, clomipramine, etc.)
- If patient is taking diuretics, dextromethorphan, buspirone, bupropion
- If patient has pheochromocytoma
- If patient has cardiovascular or cerebrovascular disease
- If patient has frequent or severe headaches
- If patient is undergoing elective surgery and requires general anesthesia
- If patient has a history of liver disease or abnormal liver function tests
- If patient is taking a prohibited drug
- If patient is not compliant with a low-tyramine diet
- If there is a proven allergy to phenelzine

SPECIAL POPULATIONS

Renal Impairment
- Use with caution – drug may accumulate in plasma
- May require lower than usual adult dose

Hepatic Impairment
- Phenelzine should not be used

Cardiac Impairment
- Contraindicated in patients with congestive heart failure or hypertension
- Any other cardiac impairment may require lower than usual adult dose
- Patients with angina pectoris or coronary artery disease should limit their exertion

Elderly
- Initial dose 7.5 mg/day; increase every few days by 7.5–15 mg/day
- Elderly patients may have greater sensitivity to adverse effects
- Reduction in risk of suicidality with antidepressants compared to placebo in adults age 65 and older

Children and Adolescents
- Not recommended for use under age 16
- Carefully weigh the risks and benefits of pharmacological treatment against the risks and benefits of nontreatment with antidepressants and make sure to document this in the patient's chart
- Monitor patients face-to-face regularly, particularly during the first several weeks of treatment
- Use with caution, observing for activation of known or unknown bipolar disorder and/or suicidal ideation, and inform parents or guardian of this risk so they can help observe child or adolescent patients

Pregnancy
- Risk Category C [some animal studies show adverse effects; no controlled studies in humans]
- Not generally recommended for use during pregnancy, especially during first trimester
- Possible increased incidence of fetal malformations if phenelzine is taken during the first trimester

- Should evaluate patient for treatment with an antidepressant with a better risk/benefit ratio

Breast Feeding

- Some drug is found in mother's breast milk
- If child becomes irritable or sedated, breast feeding or drug may need to be discontinued
- Immediate postpartum period is a high-risk time for depression, especially in women who have had prior depressive episodes, so drug may need to be reinstituted late in the third trimester or shortly after childbirth to prevent a recurrence during the postpartum period
- Should evaluate patient for treatment with an antidepressant with a better risk/benefit ratio

THE ART OF PSYCHOPHARMACOLOGY

Potential Advantages

- Atypical depression
- Severe depression
- Treatment-resistant depression or anxiety disorders

Potential Disadvantages

- Requires compliance to dietary restrictions, concomitant drug restrictions
- Patients with cardiac problems or hypertension
- Multiple daily doses

Primary Target Symptoms

- Depressed mood
- Somatic symptoms
- Sleep and eating disturbances
- Psychomotor retardation
- Morbid preoccupation

Pearls

- MAOIs are generally reserved for second-line use after SSRIs, SNRIs, and combinations of newer antidepressants have failed
- Patient should be advised not to take any prescription or over-the-counter drugs without consulting their doctor because of possible drug interactions with the MAOI
- Headache is often the first symptom of hypertensive crisis
- Foods generally to avoid as they are usually high in tyramine content: dry sausage, pickled herring, liver, broad bean pods, sauerkraut, cheese, yogurt, alcoholic beverages, nonalcoholic beer and wine, chocolate, caffeine, meat and fish
- The rigid dietary restrictions may reduce compliance
- Mood disorders can be associated with eating disorders (especially in adolescent females), and phenelzine can be used to treat both depression and bulimia
- MAOIs are a viable second-line treatment option in depression, but are not frequently used
- ✱ Myths about the danger of dietary tyramine can be exaggerated, but prohibitions against concomitant drugs often not followed closely enough
- Orthostatic hypotension, insomnia, and sexual dysfunction are often the most troublesome common side effects
- ✱ MAOIs should be for the expert, especially if combining with agents of potential risk (e.g., stimulants, trazodone, TCAs)
- ✱ MAOIs should not be neglected as therapeutic agents for the treatment-resistant
- Although generally prohibited, a heroic but potentially dangerous treatment for severely treatment-resistant patients is for an expert to give a tricyclic/tetracyclic antidepressant other than clomipramine simultaneously with an MAO inhibitor for patients who fail to respond to numerous other antidepressants
- Use of MAOIs with clomipramine is always prohibited because of the risk of serotonin syndrome and death
- Amoxapine may be the preferred trycyclic/tetracyclic antidepressant to combine with an MAOI in heroic cases due to its theoretically protective 5HT2A antagonist properties
- If this option is elected, start the MAOI with the tricyclic/tetracyclic antidepressant simultaneously at low doses after appropriate drug washout, then alternately increase doses of these agents every few days to a week as tolerated

- Although very strict dietary and concomitant drug restrictions must be observed to prevent hypertensive crises and serotonin syndrome, the most common side effects of MAOI and tricyclic/tetracyclic combinations may be weight gain and orthostatic hypotension

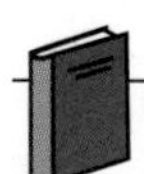

Suggested Reading

Kennedy SH. Continuation and maintenance treatments in major depression: the neglected role of monoamine oxidase inhibitors. J Psychiatry Neurosci 1997;22:127–31.

Lippman SB, Nash K. Monoamine oxidase inhibitor update. Potential adverse food and drug interactions. Drug Saf 1990;5:195–204.

Parsons B, Quitkin FM, McGrath PJ, Stewart JW, Tricamo E, Ocepek-Welikson K, Harrison W, Rabkin JG, Wager SG, Nunes E. Phenelzine, imipramine, and placebo in borderline patients meeting criteria for atypical depression. Psychopharmacol Bull 1989; 25:524–34.

THERAPEUTICS

Brands • Orap

see index for additional brand names

Generic? Not in U.S.

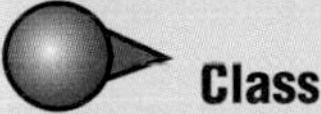

Class

- Tourette's syndrome/tic suppressant; conventional antipsychotic (neuroleptic, dopamine 2 antagonist)

Commonly Prescribed for

(bold for FDA approved)

- **Suppression of motor and phonic tics in patients with Tourette syndrome who have failed to respond satisfactorily to standard treatment**
- Psychotic disorders in patients who have failed to respond satisfactorily to standard treatment

How the Drug Works

- Blocks dopamine 2 receptors in the nigrostriatal dopamine pathway, reducing tics in Tourette's syndrome
- When used for psychosis, can block dopamine 2 receptors in the mesolimbic dopamine pathway, reducing positive symptoms of psychosis

How Long Until It Works

- Relief from tics may occur more rapidly than antipsychotic actions
- Psychotic symptoms can improve within 1 week, but it may take several weeks for full effect on behavior

If It Works

✽ Is a second-line treatment option for Tourette's syndrome

✽ Is a secondary or tertiary treatment option for psychosis or other behavioral disorders

- Should evaluate for switching to an antipsychotic with a better/risk benefit ratio

If It Doesn't Work

- Consider trying one of the first-line atypical antipsychotics (risperidone, olanzapine, quetiapine, ziprasidone, aripiprazole, paliperidone, amisulpride)
- Consider trying another conventional antipsychotic
- If 2 or more antipsychotic monotherapies do not work, consider clozapine

Best Augmenting Combos for Partial Response or Treatment Resistance

✽ Augmentation of pimozide has not been systematically studied and can be dangerous, especially with drugs that can either prolong QTc interval or raise pimozide plasma levels

Tests

✽ Baseline EKG and serum potassium levels should be determined

✽ Periodic evaluation of EKG and serum potassium levels, especially during dose titration

- Serum magnesium levels may also need to be monitored

✽ Since conventional antipsychotics are frequently associated with weight gain, before starting treatment, weigh all patients and determine if the patient is already overweight (BMI 25.0–29.9) or obese (BMI ≥30)

- Before giving a drug that can cause weight gain to an overweight or obese patient, consider determining whether the patient already has pre-diabetes (fasting plasma glucose 100–25 mg/dL), diabetes (fasting plasma glucose >126 mg/dL), or dyslipidemia (increased total cholesterol, LDL cholesterol and triglycerides; decreased HDL cholesterol), and treat or refer such patients for treatment, including nutrition and weight management, physical activity counseling, smoking cessation, and medical management

✽ Monitor weight and BMI during treatment

✽ Consider monitoring fasting triglycerides monthly for several months in patients at high risk for metabolic complications and when initiating or switching antipsychotics

✽ While giving a drug to a patient who has gained >5% of initial weight, consider evaluating for the presence of pre-diabetes, diabetes, or dyslipidemia, or consider switching to a different antipsychotic

- Should check blood pressure in the elderly before starting and for the first few weeks of treatment
- Monitoring elevated prolactin levels of dubious clinical benefit

SIDE EFFECTS

How Drug Causes Side Effects

- By blocking dopamine 2 receptors in the striatum, it can cause motor side effects
- By blocking dopamine 2 receptors in the pituitary, it can cause elevations in prolactin
- By blocking dopamine 2 receptors excessively in the mesocortical and mesolimbic dopamine pathways, especially at high doses, it can cause worsening of negative and cognitive symptoms (neuroleptic-induced deficit syndrome)
- Anticholinergic actions may cause sedation, blurred vision, constipation, dry mouth
- Antihistaminic actions may cause sedation, weight gain
- By blocking alpha 1 adrenergic receptors, it can cause dizziness, sedation, and hypotension
- Mechanism of weight gain and any possible increased incidence of diabetes or dyslipidemia with conventional antipsychotics is unknown

❋ Mechanism of potentially dangerous QTc prolongation may be related to actions at ion channels

Notable Side Effects

❋ Neuroleptic-induced deficit syndrome
❋ Akathisia
❋ Extrapyramidal symptoms, Parkinsonism, tardive dyskinesia
❋ Hypotension

- Sedation, akinesia
- Galactorrhea, amenorrhea
- Dry mouth, constipation, blurred vision
- Sexual dysfunction

❋ Weight gain

Life-Threatening or Dangerous Side Effects

- Rare neuroleptic malignant syndrome
- Rare seizures

❋ Dose-dependent QTc prolongation

- Ventricular arrhythmias and sudden death
- Increased risk of death and cerebrovascular events in elderly patients with dementia-related psychosis

Weight Gain

unusual not unusual common problematic

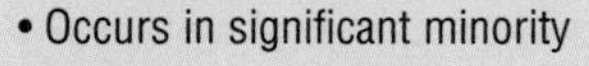

- Occurs in significant minority

Sedation

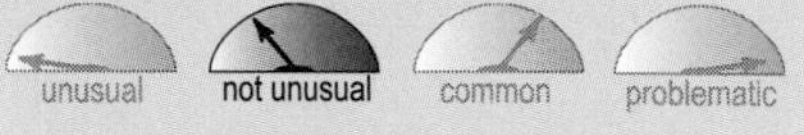

- Occurs in significant minority

What to Do About Side Effects

- Wait
- Wait
- Wait
- For motor symptoms, add an anticholinergic agent
- Reduce the dose
- For sedation, give at night
- Switch to an atypical antipsychotic
- Weight loss, exercise programs, and medical management for high BMIs, diabetes, dyslipidemia

Best Augmenting Agents for Side Effects

❋ Augmentation of pimozide has not been systematically studied and can be dangerous, especially with drugs that can either prolong QTc interval or raise pimozide plasma levels

DOSING AND USE

Usual Dosage Range

- Less than 10 mg/day

Dosage Forms

- Tablet 1 mg scored, 2 mg scored

How To Dose

- Initial 1–2 mg/day in divided doses; can increase dose every other day; maximum 10 mg/day or 0.2 mg/kg per day
- Children: initial 0.05 mg/kg per day at night; can increase every 3 days; maximum 10 mg/day or 0.2 mg/kg per day

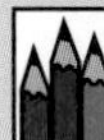

Dosing Tips

❋ The effects of pimozide on the QTc interval are dose-dependent, so start low and go slow while carefully monitoring QTc interval

Overdose
- Deaths have occurred; extrapyramidal symptoms, EKG changes, hypotension, respiratory depression, coma

Long-Term Use
- Some side effects may be irreversible (e.g., tardive dyskinesia)

Habit Forming
- No

How to Stop
- Slow down-titration (over 6 to 8 weeks), especially when simultaneously beginning a new antipsychotic while switching (i.e., cross-titration)
- Rapid discontinuation may lead to rebound psychosis and worsening of symptoms
- If antiparkinson agents are being used, they should be continued for a few weeks after pimozide is discontinued

Pharmacokinetics
- Metabolized by CYP450 3A and to a lesser extent by CYP450 1A2
- Mean elimination half-life approximately 55 hours

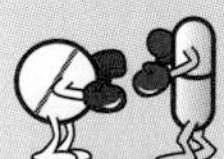

Drug Interactions
- May decrease the effects of levodopa, dopamine agonists
- May enhance QTc prolongation of other drugs capable of prolonging QTc interval
- May increase the effects of antihypertensive drugs

✻ Use with CYP450 3A4 inhibitors (e.g., drugs such as fluoxetine, sertraline, fluvoxamine, and nefazodone; foods such as grapefruit juice) can raise pimozide levels and increase the risks of dangerous arrhythmias

- Use of pimozide and fluoxetine may lead to bradycardia
- Additive effects may occur if used with CNS depressants
- Some patients taking a neuroleptic and lithium have developed an encephalopathic syndrome similar to neuroleptic malignant syndrome
- Combined use with epinephrine may lower blood pressure

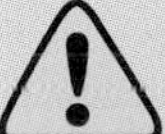

Other Warnings/ Precautions
- If signs of neuroleptic malignant syndrome develop, treatment should be immediately discontinued
- Use cautiously in patients with alcohol withdrawal or convulsive disorders because of possible lowering of seizure threshold
- Antiemetic effect can mask signs of other disorders or overdose
- Do not use epinephrine in event of overdose as interaction with some pressor agents may lower blood pressure
- Use only with caution if at all in Parkinson's disease or Lewy body dementia
- Because pimozide may dose-dependently prolong QTc interval, use with caution in patients who have bradycardia or who are taking drugs that can induce bradycardia (e.g., beta blockers, calcium channel blockers, clonidine, digitalis)
- Because pimozide may dose-dependently prolong QTc interval, use with caution in patients who have hypokalemia and/or hypomagnesemia or who are taking drugs that can induce hypokalemia and/or magnesemia (e.g., diuretics, stimulant laxatives, intravenous amphotericin B, glucocorticoids, tetracosactide)
- Pimozide can increase tumors in mice (dose-related effect)

✻ Pimozide can increase the QTc interval and potentially cause arrhythmia or sudden death, especially in combination with drugs that raise its levels

Do Not Use
- If patient is in a comatose state or has CNS depression

✻ If patient is taking an agent capable of significanty prolonging QTc interval (e.g., thioridazine, selected antiarrhythmics, moxifoxacin, and sparfloxacin)

✻ If there is a history of QTc prolongation or cardiac arrhythmia, recent acute myocardial infarction, uncompensated heart failure

- If patient is taking drugs that can cause tics

✻ If patient is taking drugs that inhibit pimozide metabolism, such as macrolide antibiotics, azole antifungal agents (ketoconazole, itraconazole), protease

inhibitors, nefazodone, fluvoxamine, fluoxetine, sertaline, etc.
- If there is a proven allergy to pimozide
- If there is a known sensitivity to other antipsychotics

SPECIAL POPULATIONS

Renal Impairment
- Use with caution

Hepatic Impairment
- Use with caution

Cardiac Impairment
- Pimozide produces a dose-dependent prolongation of QTc interval, which may be enhanced by the existence of bradycardia, hypokalemia, congenital or acquired long QTc interval, which should be evaluated prior to administering pimozide
- Use with caution if treating concomitantly with a medication likely to produce prolonged bradycardia, hypokalemia, slowing of intracardiac conduction, or prolongation of the QTc interval
- Avoid pimozide in patients with a known history of QTc prolongation, recent acute myocardial infarction, and uncompensated heart failure

Elderly
- Some patients may tolerate lower doses better
- Although conventional antipsychotics are commonly used for behavioral disturbances in dementia, no agent has been approved for treatment of elderly patients with dementia-related psychosis
- Elderly patients with dementia-related psychosis treated with antipsychotics are at an increased risk of death compared to placebo, and also have an increased risk of cerebrovascular events

Children and Adolescents
- Safety and efficacy established for patients over age 12
- Preliminary data show similar safety for patients age 2–12 as for patients over 12
- Generally use second-line after atypical antipsychotics and other conventional antipsychotics

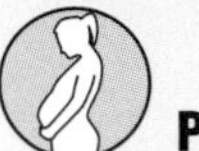

Pregnancy
- Risk Category C [some animal studies show adverse effects; no controlled studies in humans]
- Renal papillary abnormalities have been seen in rats during pregnancy
- No studies in pregnant women
- Psychotic symptoms may worsen during pregnancy and some form of treatment may be necessary
- Atypical antipsychotics may be preferable to conventional antipsychotics or anticonvulsant mood stabilizers if treatment is required during pregnancy
- Should evaluate for an antipsychotic with a better risk/benefit ratio if treatment required during pregnancy

Breast Feeding
- Unknown if pimozide is secreted in human breast milk, but all psychotropics assumed to be secreted in breast milk
- Not recommended for use because of potential for tumorigenicity or cardiovascular effects on infant

✱ Recommended either to discontinue drug or bottle feed

THE ART OF PSYCHOPHARMACOLOGY

Potential Advantages
- Only for patients who respond to this agent and not to other antipsychotics

Potential Disadvantages
- Vulnerable populations such as children and elderly
- Patients on other drugs

Primary Target Symptoms
- Vocal and motor tics in patients who fail to respond to treatment with other antipsychotics
- Psychotic symptoms in patients who fail to respond to treatment with other antipsychotics

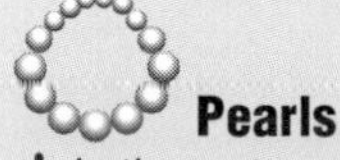

Pearls

- * In the past, was a first-line choice for Tourette's syndrome and for certain behavioral disorders, including monosymptomatic hypochondriasis; however, it is now recognized that the benefits of pimozide generally do not outweigh its risks in most patients
- * Because of its effects on the QTc interval, pimozide is not intended for use unless other options for tic disorders (or psychotic disorders) have failed

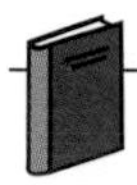

Suggested Reading

Shapiro AK, Shapiro E, Fulop G. Pimozide treatment of tic and Tourette disorders. Pediatrics 1987;79(6):1032–9.

Sultana A, McMonagle T. Pimozide for schizophrenia or related psychoses. Cochrane Database Syst Rev 2000;(3):CD001949.

Tueth MJ, Cheong JA. Clinical uses of pimozide. South Med J 1993;86(3):344–9.

THERAPEUTICS

Brands • Piportil

see index for additional brand names

Generic? No

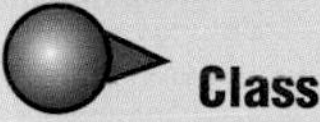

Class

- Conventional antipsychotic (neuroleptic, phenothiazine, dopamine 2 antagonist)

Commonly Prescribed for

(bold for FDA approved)

- Maintenance treatment of schizophrenia
- Other psychotic disorders
- Bipolar disorder

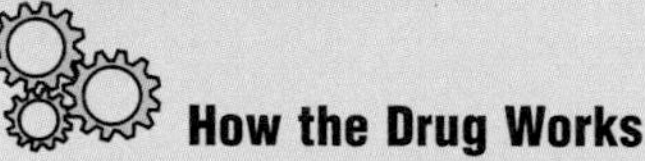

How the Drug Works

- Blocks dopamine 2 receptors, reducing positive symptoms of psychosis

How Long Until It Works

- Psychotic symptoms can improve within 1 week, but it may take several weeks for full effect on behavior

If It Works

- Most often reduces positive symptoms in schizophrenia but does not eliminate them
- Most schizophrenic patients do not have a total remission of symptoms but rather a reduction of symptoms by about a third
- Continue treatment in schizophrenia until reaching a plateau of improvement
- After reaching a satisfactory plateau, continue treatment for at least a year after first episode of psychosis in schizophrenia
- For second and subsequent episodes of psychosis in schizophrenia, treatment may need to be indefinite
- Reduces symptoms of acute psychotic mania but not proven as a mood stabilizer or as an effective maintenance treatment in bipolar disorder
- After reducing acute psychotic symptoms in mania, switch to a mood stabilizer and/or an atypical antipsychotic for mood stabilization and maintenance

If It Doesn't Work

- Consider trying one of the first-line atypical antipsychotics (risperidone, olanzapine, quetiapine, ziprasidone, aripiprazole, paliperidone, amisulpride)
- Consider trying another conventional antipsychotic
- If 2 or more antipsychotic monotherapies do not work, consider clozapine

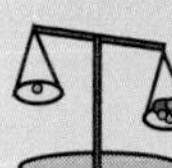

Best Augmenting Combos for Partial Response or Treatment Resistance

- Augmentation of conventional antipsychotics has not been systematically studied
- Addition of a mood stabilizing anticonvulsant such as valproate, carbamazepine, or lamotrigine may be helpful in both schizophrenia and bipolar mania
- Augmentation with lithium in bipolar mania may be helpful
- Addition of a benzodiazepine, especially short-term for agitation

Tests

❋ Since conventional antipsychotics are frequently associated with weight gain, before starting treatment, weigh all patients and determine if the patient is already overweight (BMI 25.0–29.9) or obese (BMI ≥30)

- Before giving a drug that can cause weight gain to an overweight or obese patient, consider determining whether the patient already has pre-diabetes (fasting plasma glucose 100–25 mg/dL), diabetes (fasting plasma glucose >126 mg/dL), or dyslipidemia (increased total cholesterol, LDL cholesterol and triglycerides; decreased HDL cholesterol), and treat or refer such patients for treatment, including nutrition and weight management, physical activity counseling, smoking cessation, and medical management

❋ Monitor weight and BMI during treatment

❋ Consider monitoring fasting triglycerides monthly for several months in patients at high risk for metabolic complications and when initiating or switching antipsychotics

❋ While giving a drug to a patient who has gained >5% of initial weight, consider evaluating for the presence of pre-diabetes, diabetes, or dyslipidemia, or consider switching to a different antipsychotic

- Should check blood pressure in the elderly before starting and for the first few weeks

- Monitoring elevated prolactin levels of dubious clinical benefit
- Phenothiazines may cause false-positive phenylketonuria results

SIDE EFFECTS

How Drug Causes Side Effects

- By blocking dopamine 2 receptors in the striatum, it can cause motor side effects
- By blocking dopamine 2 receptors in the pituitary, it can cause elevations in prolactin
- By blocking dopamine 2 receptors excessively in the mesocortical and mesolimbic dopamine pathways, especially at high doses, it can cause worsening of negative and cognitive symptoms (neuroleptic-induced deficit syndrome)
- Anticholinergic actions may cause sedation, blurred vision, constipation, dry mouth
- Antihistaminic actions may cause sedation, weight gain
- By blocking alpha 1 adrenergic receptors, it can cause dizziness, sedation, and hypotension
- Mechanism of weight gain and any possible increased incidence of diabetes or dyslipidemia with conventional antipsychotics is unknown

Notable Side Effects

✱ Excitement, insomnia, restlessness
✱ Rare tardive dyskinesia (risk increases with duration of treatment and with dose)
✱ Galactorrhea, amenorrhea
- Dry mouth, nausea, blurred vision, sweating, appetite change
- Sexual dysfunction (impotence)
- Hypotension, arrhythmia, tachycardia
- Weight gain
- Rare rash

Life-Threatening or Dangerous Side Effects

- Rare neuroleptic malignant syndrome
- Jaundice, leucopenia
- Rare seizures
- Increased risk of death and cerebrovascular events in elderly patients with dementia-related psychosis

Weight Gain

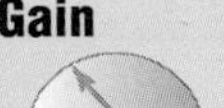
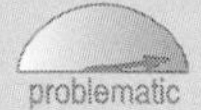

- Many experience and/or can be significant in amount

Sedation

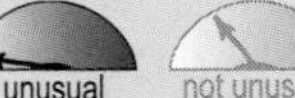
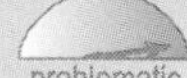

- Reported but not expected

What to Do About Side Effects

- Wait
- Wait
- Wait
- For motor symptoms, add an anticholinergic agent
- Reduce the dose
- For sedation, take at night
- Switch to an atypical antipsychotic
- Weight loss, exercise programs, and medical management for high BMIs, diabetes, dyslipidemia

Best Augmenting Agents for Side Effects

- Benztropine or trihexyphenidyl for motor side effects
- Sometimes amantadine can be helpful for motor side effects
- Benzodiazepines may be helpful for akathisia
- Many side effects cannot be improved with an augmenting agent

DOSING AND USE

Usual Dosage Range

- 50–100 mg once a month

Dosage Forms

- Injection 50 mg/mL

How To Dose

- Initial 25 mg; can be increased by 25–50 mg; maximum 200 mg once a month
- Drug should be administerd intramuscularly in the gluteal region

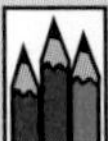

Dosing Tips

✱ Only available as long acting intramuscular formulation and not as oral formulation

- The peak of action generally occurs after 9–10 days
- May need to treat with an oral antipsychotic for 1–2 weeks when initiating treatment
- One of the few conventional antipsychotics available in a depot formulation lasting for up to a month

Overdose

- Sedation, tachycardia, extrapyramidal symptoms, arrhythmia, hypothermia, EKG changes, hypotension

Long-Term Use

- Some side effects may be irreversible (e.g., tardive dyskinesia)

Habit Forming

- No

How to Stop

- If antiparkinson agents are being used, they should be continued for a few weeks after pipothiazine is discontinued

Pharmacokinetics

- Onset of action of palmitic ester formulation within 2–3 days
- Duration of action of palmitic ester formulation 3–6 weeks

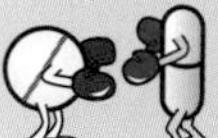

Drug Interactions

- Use with tricyclic antidepressants may increase risk of cardiac symptoms
- CNS effects may be increased if used with other CNS depressants
- May increase the effects of antihypertensive agents
- May decrease the effects of amphetamines, levodopa, dopamine agonists, clonidine, guanethidine, adrenaline
- Effects may be reduced by anticholinergic agents
- Antacids, antiparkinson drugs, and lithium may reduce pipothiazine absorption
- Combined use with epinephrine may lower blood pressure
- Some patients taking a neuroleptic and lithium have developed an encephalopathic syndrome similar to neuroleptic malignant syndrome

Other Warnings/ Precautions

- Patients may be more sensitive to extreme temperatures
- Use with caution in patients with Parkinson's disease, Lewy body dementia, or extrapyramidal symptoms with previous treatments
- Avoid undue exposure to sunlight
- Use with caution in patients with respiratory disease, Lewy body dementia, narrow angle-closure glaucoma (including family history), alcohol withdrawal syndrome, brain damage, epilepsy, hypothyroidism, myaesthenia gravis, prostatic hypertrophy, thyrotoxicosis
- Contact with skin can cause rash
- Antiemetic effect can mask signs of other disorders or overdose
- Do not use epinephrine in event of overdose as interaction with some pressor agents may lower blood pressure

Do Not Use

- If patient is comatose
- If there is cerebral atherosclerosis
- If patient has phaeochromocytoma
- If patient has renal or liver failure, blood dyscrasias
- If patient has severe cardiac impairment
- If patient has subcortical brain damage
- If there is a proven allergy to pipothiazine
- If there is a known sensitivity to any phenothiazine

SPECIAL POPULATIONS

Renal Impairment

- Use with caution

Hepatic Impairment

- Use with caution

Cardiac Impairment

- Use with caution

Elderly

- Elderly patients do not metabolize the drug as quickly
- Dose should be reduced
- Recommended starting dose 5–10 mg
- Although conventional antipsychotics are commonly used for behavioral

disturbances in dementia, no agent has been approved for treatment of elderly patients with dementia-related psychosis
- Elderly patients with dementia-related psychosis treated with antipsychotics are at an increased risk of death compared to placebo, and also have an increased risk of cerebrovascular events

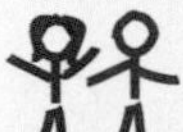

Children and Adolescents
- Not recommended for use in children

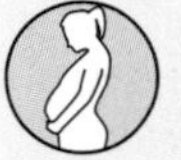

Pregnancy
- Risk Category C [some animal studies show adverse effects; no controlled studies in humans]
- Reports of extrapyramidal symptoms, jaundice, hyperreflexia, hyporeflexia in infants whose mothers took a phenothiazine during pregnancy
- Not recommended unless absolutely necessary
- Psychotic symptoms may worsen during pregnancy and some form of treatment may be necessary
- Atypical antipsychotics may be preferable to conventional antipsychotics or anticonvulsant mood stabilizers if treatment is required during pregnancy

Breast Feeding
- Unknown if pipothiazine is secreted in human breast milk, but all psychotropics assumed to be secreted in breast milk

✻ Recommended either to discontinue drug or bottle feed

THE ART OF PSYCHOPHARMACOLOGY

Potential Advantages
- Noncompliant patients

Potential Disadvantages
- Patients who need immediate onset of antipsychotic actions

Primary Target Symptoms
- Positive symptoms of psychosis
- Negative symptoms of psychosis
- Aggressive symptoms

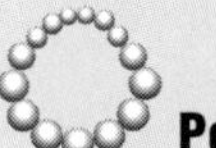

Pearls
- Pipothiazine is a higher potency phenothiazine
- Less risk of sedation and orthostatic hypotension but greater risk of extrapyramidal symptoms than with low potency phenothiazines

✻ Only available in long-acting parenteral formulation

- Generally, patients must be stabilized on an oral antipsychotic prior to switching to parenteral long-acting pipothiazine
- Patients have very similar antipsychotic responses to any conventional antipsychotic, which is different from atypical antipsychotics where antipsychotic responses of individual patients can occasionally vary greatly from one atypical antipsychotic to another
- Patients with inadequate responses to atypical antipsychotics may benefit from a trial of augmentation with a conventional antipsychotic such as pipothiazine or from switching to a conventional antipsychotic such as pipothiazine
- However, long-term polypharmacy with a combination of a conventional antipsychotic with an atypical antipsychotic such as pipothiazine may combine their side effects without clearly augmenting the efficacy of either
- Although a frequent practice by some prescribers, adding 2 conventional antipsychotics together has little rationale and may reduce tolerability without clearly enhancing efficacy

Suggested Reading

Leong OK, Wong KE, Tay WK, Gill RC. A comparative study of pipothiazine palmitate and fluphenazine decanoate in the maintenance of remission of schizophrenia. Singapore Med J 1989;30(5):436–40.

Quraishi S, David A. Depot pipothiazine palmitate and undecylenate for schizophrenia. Cochrane Database Syst Rev 2001;(3):CD001720.

Schmidt K. Pipothiazine palmitate: a versatile, sustained-action neuroleptic in psychiatric practice. Curr Med Res Opin 1986;10(5):326–9.

THERAPEUTICS

Brands • Lyrica
see index for additional brand names

Generic? No

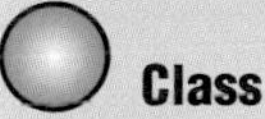

Class

- Anticonvulsant, antineuralgic for chronic pain, alpha 2 delta ligand at voltage-sensitive calcium channels

Commonly Prescribed for

(bold for FDA approved)

- **Diabetic peripheral neuropathy**
- **Postherpetic neuralgia**
- **Fibromyalgia**
- **Partial seizures in adults (adjunctive)**
- Peripheral neuropathic pain
- Generalized anxiety disorder
- Panic disorder
- Social anxiety disorder

How the Drug Works

- Is a leucine analogue and is transported both into the blood from the gut and also across the blood-brain barrier into the brain from the blood by the system L transport system (a sodium independent transporter) as well as by additional sodium-dependent amino acid transporter systems

✻ Binds to the alpha 2 delta subunit of voltage-sensitive calcium channels

- This closes N and P/Q presynaptic calcium channels, diminishing excessive neuronal activity and neurotransmitter release
- Although structurally related to gamma-aminobutyric acid (GABA), no known direct actions on GABA or its receptors

How Long Until It Works

- Can reduce neuropathic pain and anxiety within a week
- Should reduce seizures by 2 weeks
- If it is not producing clinical benefits within 6–8 weeks, it may require a dosage increase or it may not work at all

If It Works

- The goal of treatment of neuropathic pain, seizures, and anxiety disorders is to reduce symptoms as much as possible, and if necessary in combination with other treatments
- Treatment of neuropathic pain most often reduces but does not eliminate all symptoms and is not a cure since symptoms usually recur after medicine stopped
- Continue treatment until all symptoms are gone or until improvement is stable and then continue treating indefinitely as long as improvement persists

If It Doesn't Work (for neuropathic pain)

- Many patients only have a partial response where some symptoms are improved but others persist
- Other patients may be nonresponders, sometimes called treatment-resistant or treatment-refractory
- Consider increasing dose, switching to another agent or adding an appropriate augmenting agent
- Consider biofeedback or hypnosis for pain
- Consider psychotherapy for anxiety
- Consider the presence of noncompliance and counsel patient
- Consider evaluation for another diagnosis or for a comorbid condition (e.g., medical illness, substance abuse, etc.)

Best Augmenting Combos for Partial Response or Treatment Resistance

✻ In addition to being a first-line treatment for neuropathic pain and anxiety disorders, pregabalin is itself an augmenting agent to numerous other anticonvulsants in treating epilepsy

- For postherpetic neuralgia, pregabalin can decrease concomitant opiate use

✻ For neuropathic pain, tricyclic antidepressants and SNRIs as well as tiagabine, other anticonvulsants, and even opiates can augment pregabalin if done by experts while carefully monitoring in difficult cases

- For anxiety, SSRIs, SNRIs, or benzodiazepines can augment pregabalin

Tests

- None for healthy individuals

SIDE EFFECTS

How Drug Causes Side Effects
- CNS side effects may be due to excessive blockade of voltage-sensitive calcium channels

Notable Side Effects
✻ Sedation, dizziness
- Ataxia, fatigue, tremor, dysarthria, paraesthesia, memory impairment, coordination abnormal, impaired attention, confusion, euphoric mood, irritability
- Vomiting, dry mouth, constipation, weight gain, increased appetite, flatulence
- Blurred vision, diplopia
- Peripheral edema
- Libido decreased, erectile dysfunction

Life-Threatening or Dangerous Side Effects
- Rare activation of suicidal ideation and behavior (suicidality)

Weight Gain
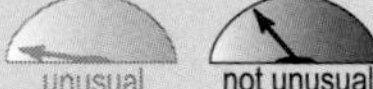

- Occurs in significant minority

Sedation
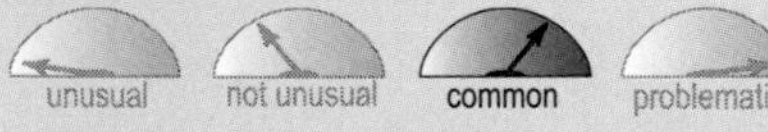

- Many experience and/or can be significant in amount
- Dose-related
- Can wear off with time

What to Do About Side Effects
- Wait
- Wait
- Wait
- Take more of the dose at night to reduce daytime sedation
- Lower the dose
- Switch to another agent

Best Augmenting Agents for Side Effects
- Many side effects cannot be improved with an augmenting agent

DOSING AND USE

Usual Dosage Range
- 150–600 mg/day in 2–3 doses

Dosage Forms
- Capsule 25 mg, 50 mg, 75 mg, 100 mg, 150 mg, 200 mg, 225 mg, 300 mg

How To Dose
- Neuropathic pain: initial 150 mg/day in 2–3 doses; can increase to 300 mg/day in 2–3 doses after 3–7 days; can increase to 600 mg/day in 2–3 doses after 7 more days; maximum dose generally 600 mg/day
- Seizures: initial 150 mg/day in 2–3 doses; can increase to 300 mg/day in 2–3 doses after 7 days; can increase to 600 mg/day in 2–3 doses after 7 more days; maximum dose generally 600 mg/day

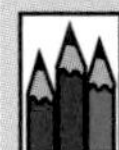

Dosing Tips
✻ Generally given in one-third to one-sixth the dose of gabapentin
- If pregabalin is added to a second sedating agent, such as another anticonvulsant, a benzodiazepine, or an opiate, the titration period should be at least a week to improve tolerance to sedation
- Most patients need to take pregabalin only twice daily
- At the high end of the dosing range, tolerability may be enhanced by splitting dose into 3 or more divided doses
- For intolerable sedation, can give most of the dose at night and less during the day
- To improve slow-wave sleep, may only need to take pregabalin at bedtime
- May be taken with or without food

Overdose
- No fatalities

Long-Term Use
- Safe

Habit Forming
- No

How to Stop
- Taper over a minimum of 1 week
- Epilepsy patients may seize upon withdrawal, especially if withdrawal is abrupt
- Discontinuation symptoms uncommon

Pharmacokinetics

- Pregabalin is not metabolized but excreted intact renally
- Elimination half-life approximately 5–7 hours

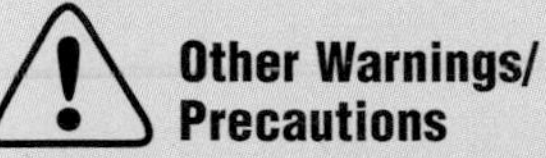

Drug Interactions

- Pregabalin has not been shown to have significant pharmacokinetic drug interactions
- Because pregabalin is excreted unchanged, it is unlikely to have significant pharmacokinetic drug interactions
- May add to or potentiate the sedative effects of oxycodone, lorazepam, and alcohol

Other Warnings/ Precautions

- Dizziness and sedation could increase the chances of accidental injury (falls) in the elderly
- Increased incidence of hemangiosarcoma at high doses in mice involves platelet changes and associated endothelial cell proliferation not present in rats or humans; no evidence to suggest an associated risk for humans
- Warn patients and their caregivers about the possibility of activation of suicidal ideation and advise them to report such side effects immediately

Do Not Use

- If there is a proven allergy to pregabalin or gabapentin
- If patient has a problem of galactose intolerance, the Lapp lactase deficiency, or glucose-galactose malabsorption

SPECIAL POPULATIONS

Renal Impairment

- Pregabalin is renally excreted, so the dose may need to be lowered
- Dosing can be adjusted according to creatinine clearance, such that patients with clearance below 15 mL/min should receive 25–75 mg/day in 1 dose, patients with clearance between 15–29 mL/min should receive 25–150 mg/day in 1–2 doses, and patients with clearance between 30–59 mL/min should receive 75–300 mg/day in 2–3 doses
- Starting dose should be at the bottom of the range; titrate as usual up to maximum dose
- Can be removed by hemodialysis; patients receiving hemodialysis may require a supplemental dose of pregabalin following hemodialysis (25–100 mg)

Hepatic Impairment

- Dose adjustment not necessary

Cardiac Impairment

- No specific recommendations

Elderly

- Some patients may tolerate lower doses better
- Elderly patients may be more susceptible to adverse effects

Children and Adolescents

- Safety and efficacy have not been established
- Use should be reserved for the expert

Pregnancy

- Risk Category C [some animal studies show adverse effects; no controlled studies in humans]
- Use in women of childbearing potential requires weighing potential benefits to the mother against the risks to the fetus
- Antiepileptic Drug Pregnancy Registry: (888) 233-2334
- Taper drug if discontinuing
- Seizures, even mild seizures, may cause harm to the embryo/fetus

Breast Feeding

- Unknown if pregabalin is secreted in human breast milk, but all psychotropics assumed to be secreted in breast milk

✻ Recommended either to discontinue drug or bottle feed

- If drug is continued while breast feeding, infant should be monitored for possible adverse effects

- If infant becomes irritable or sedated, breast feeding or drug may need to be discontinued

THE ART OF PSYCHOPHARMACOLOGY

Potential Advantages

- First-line for diabetic peripheral neuropathy
- Fibromyalgia
- Anxiety disorders
- Sleep
- Has relatively mild side effect profile
- Has few pharmacokinetic drug interactions
- More potent and probably better tolerated than gabapentin

Potential Disadvantages

- Requires 2–3 times a day dosing
- Not yet approved for anxiety disorders
- Not yet available in the United States

Primary Target Symptoms

- Seizures
- Pain
- Anxiety

Pearls

✻ First treatment approved for fibromyalgia
✻ One of the first treatments approved for neuropathic pain associated with diabetic peripheral neuropathy
- Also approved in postherpetic neuralgia
- Improves sleep disruption as well as pain in patients with painful diabetic peripheral neuropathy or postherpetic neuralgia
- Improves sleep disruption as well as pain associated with fibromyalgia
- Well-studied in epilepsy, peripheral neuropathic pain, and generalized anxiety disorder (GAD), and actually approved for GAD in Europe

✻ Off-label use for generalized anxiety disorder, panic disorder, and social anxiety disorder may be justified
- May have uniquely robust therapeutic actions for both the somatic and the psychic symptoms of generalized anxiety disorder

✻ Off-label use as an adjunct for bipolar disorder may not be justified
✻ One of the few agents that enhances slow-wave delta sleep, which may be helpful in chronic neuropathic pain syndromes
- Pregabalin is generally well-tolerated, with only mild adverse effects

✻ Although no head-to-head studies, appears to be better tolerated and more consistently efficacious at high doses than gabapentin
✻ Drug absorption and clinical efficacy may be more consistent at high doses for pregabalin compared to gabapentin because of the higher potency of pregabalin and the fact that, unlike gabapentin, it is transported by more than one transport system

Suggested Reading

Hovinga CA. Novel anticonvulsant medications in development. Expert Opin Investig Drugs 2002;11:1387–406.

Lauria-Horner BA, Pohl RB. Pregabalin: a new anxiolytic. Expert Opin Investig Drugs 2003; 12:663–72.

Stahl SM. Anticonvulsants and the relief of chronic pain: pregabalin and gabapentin as alpha(2)delta ligands at voltage-gated calcium channels. J Clin Psychiatry 2004;65:596–7.

Stahl SM. Anticonvulsants as anxiolytics, part 2: Pregabalin and gabapentin as alpha(2)delta ligands at voltage-gated calcium channels. J Clin Psychiatry 2004;65:460–1.

THERAPEUTICS

Brands
- Triptil
- Vivactil

see index for additional brand names

Generic? Yes

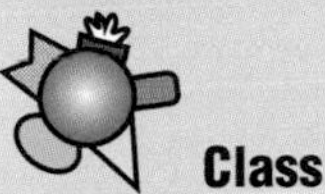

Class
- Tricyclic antidepressant (TCA)
- Predominantly a norepinephrine/noradrenaline reuptake inhibitor

Commonly Prescribed for
(bold for FDA approved)
- **Mental depression**
- Treatment-resistant depression

How the Drug Works
- Boosts neurotransmitter norepinephrine/noradrenaline
- Blocks norepinephrine reuptake pump (norepinephrine transporter), presumably increasing noradrenergic neurotransmission
- Since dopamine is inactivated by norepinephrine reuptake in frontal cortex, which largely lacks dopamine transporters, protriptyline can increase dopamine neurotransmission in this part of the brain
- A more potent inhibitor of norepinephrine reuptake pump than serotonin reuptake pump (serotonin transporter)
- At high doses may also boost neurotransmitter serotonin and presumably increase serotonergic neurotransmission

How Long Until It Works
✻ Some evidence it may have an early onset of action with improvement in activity and energy as early as 1 week
- Onset of therapeutic actions usually not immediate, but often delayed 2 to 4 weeks
- If it is not working within 6 to 8 weeks for depression, it may require a dosage increase or it may not work at all
- May continue to work for many years to prevent relapse of symptoms

If It Works
- The goal of treatment is complete remission of current symptoms as well as prevention of future relapses
- Treatment most often reduces or even eliminates symptoms, but not a cure since symptoms can recur after medicine stopped
- Continue treatment until all symptoms are gone (remission)
- Once symptoms gone, continue treating for 1 year for the first episode of depression
- For second and subsequent episodes of depression, treatment may need to be indefinite
- Use in anxiety disorders may also need to be indefinite

If It Doesn't Work
- Many patients only have a partial response where some symptoms are improved but others persist (especially insomnia, fatigue, and problems concentrating)
- Other patients may be nonresponders, sometimes called treatment-resistant or treatment-refractory
- Consider increasing dose, switching to another agent or adding an appropriate augmenting agent
- Consider psychotherapy
- Consider evaluation for another diagnosis or for a comorbid condition (e.g., medical illness, substance abuse, etc.)
- Some patients may experience apparent lack of consistent efficacy due to activation of latent or underlying bipolar disorder, and require antidepressant discontinuation and a switch to a mood stabilizer

Best Augmenting Combos for Partial Response or Treatment Resistance
- Lithium, buspirone, thyroid hormone

Tests
- None for healthy individuals

✻ Since tricyclic and tetracyclic antidepressants are frequently associated with weight gain, before starting treatment, weigh all patients and determine if the patient is already overweight (BMI 25.0–29.9) or obese (BMI ≥30)
- Before giving a drug that can cause weight gain to an overweight or obese patient, consider determining whether the patient

already has pre-diabetes (fasting plasma glucose 100–25 mg/dL), diabetes (fasting plasma glucose >126 mg/dL), or dyslipidemia (increased total cholesterol, LDL cholesterol and triglycerides; decreased HDL cholesterol), and treat or refer such patients for treatment, including nutrition and weight management, physical activity counseling, smoking cessation, and medical management

❋ Monitor weight and BMI during treatment

❋ While giving a drug to a patient who has gained >5% of initial weight, consider evaluating for the presence of pre-diabetes, diabetes, or dyslipidemia, or consider switching to a different antidepressant

- EKGs may be useful for selected patients (e.g., those with personal or family history of QTc prolongation; cardiac arrhythmia; recent myocardial infarction; uncompensated heart failure; or taking agents that prolong QTc interval such as pimozide, thioridazine, selected antiarrhythmics, moxifloxacin, sparfloxacin, etc.)
- Patients at risk for electrolyte disturbances (e.g., patients on diuretic therapy) should have baseline and periodic serum potassium and magnesium measurements

SIDE EFFECTS

How Drug Causes Side Effects

❋ Anticholinergic activity for protriptyline may be more potent than for some other TCAs and may explain sedative effects, dry mouth, constipation, blurred vision, tachycardia, and hypotension

- Sedative effects and weight gain may be due to antihistamine properties
- Blockade of alpha adrenergic 1 receptors may explain dizziness, sedation, and hypotension
- Cardiac arrhythmias, especially in overdose, may be caused by blockade of ion channels

Notable Side Effects

- Blurred vision, constipation, urinary retention, increased appetite, dry mouth, nausea, diarrhea, heartburn, unusual taste in mouth, weight gain
- Fatigue, weakness, dizziness, sedation, headache, anxiety, nervousness, restlessness
- Sexual dysfunction (impotence, change in libido)
- Sweating, rash, itching

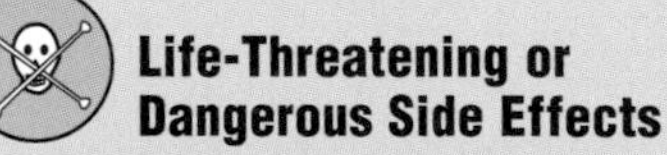

Life-Threatening or Dangerous Side Effects

- Paralytic ileus, hyperthermia (TCAs + anticholinergic agents)
- Lowered seizure threshold and rare seizures
- Orthostatic hypotension, sudden death, arrhythmias, tachycardia
- QTc prolongation
- Hepatic failure, extrapyramidal symptoms
- Increased intraocular pressure
- Rare induction of mania
- Rare activation of suicidal ideation and behavior (suidicality) (short-term studies did not show an increase in the risk of suicidality with antidepressants compared to placebo beyond age 24)

Weight Gain

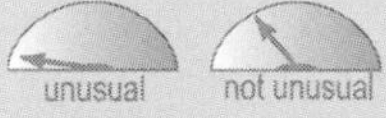

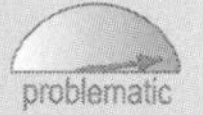

- Many experience and/or can be significant in amount
- Can increase appetite and carbohydrate craving

Sedation

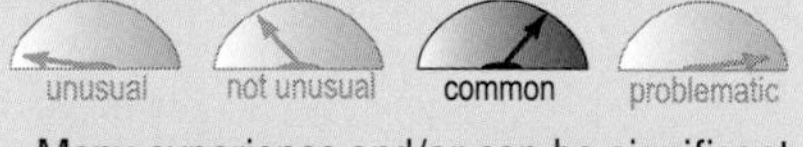

- Many experience and/or can be significant in amount

❋ Not as sedating as other TCAs; more likely to be activating than other TCAs

What to Do About Side Effects

- Wait
- Wait
- Wait
- Lower the dose
- Switch to an SSRI or newer antidepressant

Best Augmenting Agents for Side Effects

- Trazodone or a hypnotic for insomnia
- Benzodiazepines for agitation and anxiety
- Many side effects cannot be improved with an augmenting agent

DOSING AND USE

Usual Dosage Range
- 15–40 mg/day in 3–4 divided doses

Dosage Forms
- Tablets 5 mg, 10 mg

How To Dose
- Initial 15 mg/day in divided doses; increase morning dose as needed; maximum dose 60 mg/day

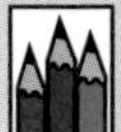

Dosing Tips
- ✻ Be aware that among this class of agents (tricyclic/tetracyclic antidepressants), protriptyline has uniquely low dosing (15–40 mg/day for protriptyline compared to 75–300 mg/day for most other tricyclic/tetracyclic antidepressants)
- ✻ Be aware that among this class of agents (tricyclic/tetracyclic antidepressants), protriptyline has uniquely frequent dosing (3–4 times a day compared to once daily for most other tricyclic/tetracyclic antidepressants)
- If intolerable anxiety, insomnia, agitation, akathisia, or activation occur either upon dosing initiation or discontinuation, consider the possibility of activated bipolar disorder, and switch to a mood stabilizer or an atypical antipsychotic

Overdose
- Death may occur; CNS depression, convulsions, cardiac dysrhythmias, severe hypotension, EKG changes, coma

Long-Term Use
- Safe

Habit Forming
- No

How to Stop
- Taper to avoid withdrawal effects
- Even with gradual dose reduction some withdrawal symptoms may appear within the first 2 weeks
- Many patients tolerate 50% dose reduction for 3 days, then another 50% reduction for 3 days, then discontinuation
- If withdrawal symptoms emerge during discontinuation, raise dose to stop symptoms and then restart withdrawal much more slowly

Pharmacokinetics
- Substrate for CYP450 2D6
- Half-life approximately 74 hours

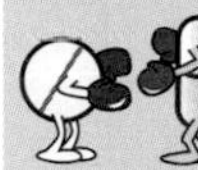

Drug Interactions
- Tramadol increases the risk of seizures in patients taking TCAs
- Use of TCAs with anticholinergic drugs may result in paralytic ileus or hyperthermia
- Fluoxetine, paroxetine, bupropion, duloxetine, and other 2D6 inhibitors may increase TCA concentrations
- Cimetidine may increase plasma concentrations of TCAs and cause anti-cholinergic symptoms
- Phenothiazines or haloperidol may raise TCA blood concentrations
- May alter effects of antihypertensive drugs; may inhibit hypotensive effects of clonidine
- Use with sympathomimetic agents may increase sympathetic activity
- Methylphenidate may inhibit metabolism of TCAs
- Activation and agitation, especially following switching or adding antidepressants, may represent the induction of a bipolar state, especially a mixed dysphoric bipolar II condition sometimes associated with suicidal ideation, and require the addition of lithium, a mood stabilizer or an atypical antipsychotic, and/or discontinuation of protriptyline

Other Warnings/ Precautions
- Add or initiate other antidepressants with caution for up to 2 weeks after discontinuing protriptyline
- Generally, do not use with MAO inhibitors, including 14 days after MAOIs are stopped; do not start an MAOI until 2 weeks after discontinuing protriptyline
- Use with caution in patients with history of seizures, urinary retention, narrow angle-closure glaucoma, hyperthyroidism
- TCAs can increase QTc interval, especially at toxic doses, which can be attained not only by overdose but also by combining

with drugs that inhibit TCA metabolism via CYP450 2D6, potentially causing torsade de pointes-type arrhythmia or sudden death
- Because TCAs can prolong QTc interval, use with caution in patients who have bradycardia or who are taking drugs that can induce bradycardia (e.g., beta blockers, calcium channel blockers, clonidine, digitalis)
- Because TCAs can prolong QTc interval, use with caution in patients who have hypokalemia and/or hypomagnesemia or who are taking drugs that can induce hypokalemia and/or magnesemia (e.g., diuretics, stimulant laxatives, intravenous amphotericin B, glucocorticoids, tetracosactide)
- When treating children, carefully weigh the risks and benefits of pharmacological treatment against the risks and benefits of nontreatment with antidepressants and make sure to document this in the patient's chart
- Distribute the brochures provided by the FDA and the drug companies
- Warn patients and their caregivers about the possibility of activating side effects and advise them to report such symptoms immediately
- Monitor patients for activation of suicidal ideation, especially children and adolescents

Do Not Use

- If patient is recovering from myocardial infarction
- If patient is taking agents capable of significantly prolonging QTc interval (e.g., pimozide, thioridazine, selected antiarrhythmics, moxifloxacin, sparfloxacin)
- If there is a history of QTc prolongation or cardiac arrhythmia, recent acute myocardial infarction, uncompensated heart failure
- If patient is taking drugs that inhibit TCA metabolism, including CYP450 2D6 inhibitors, except by an expert
- If there is reduced CYP450 2D6 function, such as patients who are poor 2D6 metabolizers, except by an expert and at low doses
- If there is a proven allergy to protriptyline

SPECIAL POPULATIONS

Renal Impairment

- Use with caution; may need to lower dose
- Patient may need to be monitored closely

Hepatic Impairment

- Use with caution; may need to lower dose
- Patient may need to be monitored closely

Cardiac Impairment

- TCAs have been reported to cause arrhythmias, prolongation of conduction time, orthostatic hypotension, sinus tachycardia, and heart failure, especially in the diseased heart
- Myocardial infarction and stroke have been reported with TCAs
- TCAs produce QTc prolongation, which may be enhanced by the existence of bradycardia, hypokalemia, congenital or acquired long QTc interval, which should be evaluated prior to administering protriptyline
- Use with caution if treating concomitantly with a medication likely to produce prolonged bradycardia, hypokalemia, slowing of intracardiac conduction, or prolongation of the QTc interval
- Avoid TCAs in patients with a known history of QTc prolongation, recent acute myocardial infarction, and uncompensated heart failure
- TCAs may cause a sustained increase in heart rate in patients with ischemic heart disease and may worsen (decrease) heart rate variability, an independent risk of mortality in cardiac populations
- Since SSRIs may improve (increase) heart rate variability in patients following a myocardial infarct and may improve survival as well as mood in patients with acute angina or following a myocardial infarction, these are more appropriate agents for cardiac population than tricyclic/tetracyclic antidepressants

❋ Risk/benefit ratio may not justify use of TCAs in cardiac impairment

Elderly

- May be more sensitive to anticholinergic, cardiovascular, hypotensive, and sedative effects

- Recommended dose is between 15–20 mg/day; doses >20 mg/day require close monitoring of patient
- Reduction in risk of suicidality with antidepressants compared to placebo in adults age 65 and older

Children and Adolescents

- Carefully weigh the risks and benefits of pharmacological treatment against the risks and benefits of nontreatment with antidepressants and make sure to document this in the patient's chart
- Monitor patients face-to-face regularly, particularly during the first several weeks of treatment
- Use with caution, observing for activation of known or unknown bipolar disorder and/or suicidal ideation, and inform parents or guardian of this risk so they can help observe child or adolescent patients
- Not recommended for use under age 12
- Not intended for use under age 6
- Several studies show lack of efficacy of TCAs for depression
- Some cases of sudden death have occurred in children taking TCAs
- Recommended dose: 15–20 mg/day

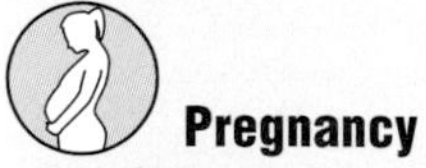

Pregnancy

- Risk Category C [some animal studies show adverse effects; no controlled studies in humans]
- Crosses the placenta
- Adverse effects have been reported in infants whose mothers took a TCA (lethargy, withdrawal symptoms, fetal malformations)
- Must weigh the risk of treatment (first trimester fetal development, third trimester newborn delivery) to the child against the risk of no treatment (recurrence of depression, maternal health, infant bonding) to the mother and child
- For many patients this may mean continuing treatment during pregnancy

Breast Feeding

- Some drug is found in mother's breast milk
- ✻ Recommended either to discontinue drug or bottle feed
- Immediate postpartum period is a high-risk time for depression, especially in women who have had prior depressive episodes, so drug may need to be reinstituted late in the third trimester or shortly after childbirth to prevent a recurrence during the postpartum period
- Must weigh benefits of breast feeding with risks and benefits of antidepressant treatment versus nontreatment to both the infant and the mother
- For many patients this may mean continuing treatment during breast feeding

THE ART OF PSYCHOPHARMACOLOGY

Potential Advantages

- Severe or treatment-resistant depression
- Withdrawn, anergic patients

Potential Disadvantages

- Pediatric, geriatric, and cardiac patients
- Patients concerned with weight gain
- Patients noncompliant with 3–4 times daily dosing

Primary Target Symptoms

- Depressed mood

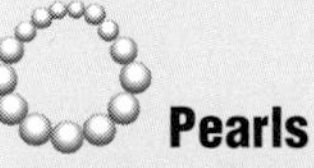

Pearls

- Tricyclic antidepressants are no longer generally considered a first-line treatment option for depression because of their side effect profile
- Tricyclic antidepressants continue to be useful for severe or treatment-resistant depression
- ✻ Has some potential advantages for withdrawn, anergic patients
- ✻ May have a more rapid onset of action than some other TCAs
- ✻ May aggravate agitation and anxiety more than some other TCAs
- ✻ May have more anticholinergic side effects, hypotension, and tachycardia than some other TCAs
- Noradrenergic reuptake inhibitors such as protriptyline can be used as a second-line treatment for smoking cessation, cocaine dependence, and attention deficit disorder
- TCAs may aggravate psychotic symptoms
- Alcohol should be avoided because of additive CNS effects

- Underweight patients may be more susceptible to adverse cardiovascular effects
- Children, patients with inadequate hydration, and patients with cardiac disease may be more susceptible to TCA-induced cardiotoxicity than healthy adults
- For the expert only: a heroic treatment (but potentially dangerous) for severely treatment-resistant patients is to give simultaneously with monoamine oxidase inhibitors for patients who fail to respond to numerous other antidepressants, but generally recommend a different TCA than protriptyline for this use
- If this option is elected, start the MAOI with the tricyclic/tetracyclic antidepressant simultaneously at low doses after appropriate drug washout, then alternately increase doses of these agents every few days to a week as tolerated
- Although very strict dietary and concomitant drug restrictions must be observed to prevent hypertensive crises and serotonin syndrome, the most common side effects of MAOI and tricyclic/tetracyclic antidepressant combinations may be weight gain and orthostatic hypotension
- Patients on TCAs should be aware that they may experience symptoms such as photosensitivity or blue-green urine
- SSRIs may be more effective than TCAs in women, and TCAs may be more effective than SSRIs in men
- Since tricyclic/tetracyclic antidepressants are substrates for CYP450 2D6, and 7% of the population (especially Caucasians) may have a genetic variant leading to reduced activity of 2D6, such patients may not safely tolerate normal doses of tricyclic/tetracyclic antidepressants and may require dose reduction
- Phenotypic testing may be necessary to detect this genetic variant prior to dosing with a tricyclic/tetracyclic antidepressant, especially in vulnerable populations such as children, elderly, cardiac populations, and those on concomitant medications
- Patients who seem to have extraordinarily severe side effects at normal or low doses may have this phenotypic CYP450 2D6 variant and require low doses or switching to another antidepressant not metabolized by 2D6

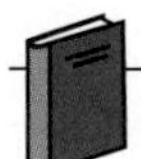

Suggested Reading

Anderson IM. Meta-analytical studies on new antidepressants. Br Med Bull 2001;57:161–78.

Anderson IM. Selective serotonin reuptake inhibitors versus tricyclic antidepressants: a meta-analysis of efficacy and tolerability. J Aff Disorders 2000;58:19–36.

Rudorfer MV, Potter WZ. Metabolism of tricyclic antidepressants. Cell Mol Neurobiol 1999;19(3):373–409.

QUAZEPAM

THERAPEUTICS

Brands • Doral

see index for additional brand names

Generic? No

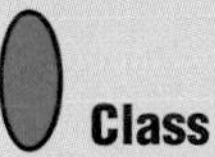

Class

• Benzodiazepine (hypnotic)

Commonly Prescribed for

(bold for FDA approved)

• **Short-term treatment of insomnia**

How the Drug Works

• Binds to benzodiazepine receptors at the GABA-A ligand-gated chloride channel complex
• Enhances the inhibitory effects of GABA
• Boosts chloride conductance through GABA-regulated channels
• Inhibitory actions in sleep centers may provide sedative hypnotic effects

How Long Until It Works

• Generally takes effect in less than an hour

If It Works

• Improves quality of sleep
• Effects on total wake-time and number of nighttime awakenings may be decreased over time

If It Doesn't Work

• If insomnia does not improve after 7–10 days, it may be a manifestation of a primary psychiatric or physical illness such as obstructive sleep apnea or restless leg syndrome, which requires independent evaluation
• Increase the dose
• Improve sleep hygiene
• Switch to another agent

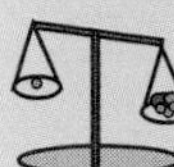

Best Augmenting Combos for Partial Response or Treatment Resistance

• Generally, best to switch to another agent
• Trazodone
• Agents with antihistamine actions (e.g., diphenhydramine, tricyclic antidepressants)

Tests

• In patients with seizure disorders, concomitant medical illness, and/or those with multiple concomitant long-term medications, periodic liver tests and blood counts may be prudent

SIDE EFFECTS

How Drug Causes Side Effects

• Same mechanism for side effects as for therapeutic effects – namely due to excessive actions at benzodiazepine receptors
• Actions at benzodiazepine receptors that carry over to the next day can cause daytime sedation, amnesia, and ataxia
• Long-term adaptations in benzodiazepine receptors may explain the development of dependence, tolerance, and withdrawal

Notable Side Effects

✻ Sedation, fatigue, depression
✻ Dizziness, ataxia, slurred speech, weakness
✻ Forgetfulness, confusion
✻ Hyperexcitability, nervousness
• Rare hallucinations, mania
• Rare hypotension
• Hypersalivation, dry mouth
• Rebound insomnia when withdrawing from long-term treatment

Life-Threatening or Dangerous Side Effects

• Respiratory depression, especially when taken with CNS depressants in overdose
• Rare hepatic dysfunction, renal dysfunction, blood dyscrasias

Weight Gain

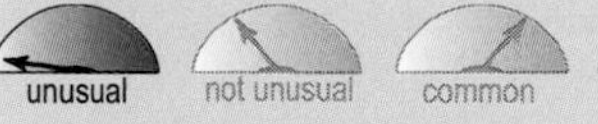

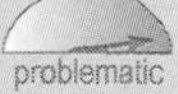

• Reported but not expected

Sedation

unusual not unusual

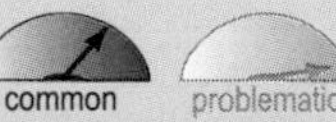

• Many experience and/or can be significant in amount

What to Do About Side Effects

- Wait
- To avoid problems with memory, only take quazepam if planning to have a full night's sleep
- Lower the dose
- Switch to a shorter-acting sedative hypnotic
- Switch to a non-benzodiazepine hypnotic
- Administer flumazenil if side effects are severe or life-threatening

Best Augmenting Agents for Side Effects

- Many side effects cannot be improved with an augmenting agent

DOSING AND USE

Usual Dosage Range

- 15 mg/day at bedtime

Dosage Forms

- Tablet 7.5 mg, 15 mg

How To Dose

- 15 mg/day at bedtime; increase to 30 mg/day if ineffective; maximum dose 30 mg/day

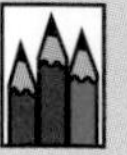

Dosing Tips

- Use lowest possible effective dose and assess need for continued treatment regularly
- Quazepam should generally not be prescribed in quantities greater than a 1-month supply
- Patients with lower body weights may require lower doses
- Risk of dependence may increase with dose and duration of treatment

Overdose

- No death reported in monotherapy; sedation, respiratory depression, poor coordination, confusion, coma

Long-Term Use

- Not generally intended for use beyond 4 weeks

* Because of its relatively longer half-life, quazepam may cause some daytime sedation and/or impaired motor/cognitive function, and may do so progressively over time

Habit Forming

- Quazepam is a Schedule IV drug
- Some patients may develop dependence and/or tolerance; risk may be greater with higher doses
- History of drug addiction may increase risk of dependence

How to Stop

- If taken for more than a few weeks, taper to reduce chances of withdrawal effects
- Patients with seizure history may seize upon sudden withdrawal
- Rebound insomnia may occur the first 1–2 nights after stopping
- For patients with severe problems discontinuing a benzodiazepine, dosing may need to be tapered over many months (i.e., reduce dose by 1% every 3 days by crushing tablet and suspending or dissolving in 100 mL of fruit juice and then disposing of 1 mL while drinking the rest; 3–7 days later, dispose of 2 mL, and so on). This is both a form of very slow biological tapering and a form of behavioral desensitization

Pharmacokinetics

- Half life 25–41 hours
- Active metabolite
- Metabolized in part by CYP450 3A4

Drug Interactions

- Increased depressive effects when taken with other CNS depressants
- Effects of quazepam may be increased by CYP450 3A4 inhibitors such as nefazodone or fluvoxamine

Other Warnings/ Precautions

- Insomnia may be a symptom of a primary disorder, rather than a primary disorder itself
- Some patients may exhibit abnormal thinking or behavioral changes similar to those caused by other CNS depressants (i.e., either depressant actions or disinhibiting actions)

- Some depressed patients may experience a worsening of suicidal ideation
- Use only with extreme caution in patients with impaired respiratory function or obstructive sleep apnea
- Quazepam should be administered only at bedtime

Do Not Use

- If patient is pregnant
- If patient has narrow angle-closure glaucoma
- If there is a proven allergy to quazepam or any benzodiazepine

SPECIAL POPULATIONS

Renal Impairment

- Recommended dose: 7.5 mg/day

Hepatic Impairment

- Recommended dose: 7.5 mg/day

Cardiac Impairment

- Benzodiazepines have been used to treat insomnia associated with acute myocardial infarction

Elderly

- Recommended dose: 7.5 mg/day
- If 15 mg/day is given initially, try to reduce the dose to 7.5 mg/day after the first 1–2 nights

Children and Adolescents

- Safety and efficacy have not been established
- Long-term effects of quazepam in children/adolescents are unknown
- Should generally receive lower doses and be more closely monitored

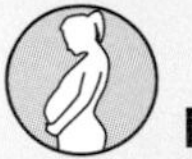

Pregnancy

- Risk Category X [positive evidence of risk to human fetus; contraindicated for use in pregnancy]
- Infants whose mothers received a benzodiazepine late in pregnancy may experience withdrawal effects
- Neonatal flaccidity has been reported in infants whose mothers took a benzodiazepine during pregnancy

Breast Feeding

- Some drug is found in mother's breast milk
- ✻ Recommended either to discontinue drug or bottle feed
- Effects on infant have been observed and include feeding difficulties, sedation, and weight loss

THE ART OF PSYCHOPHARMACOLOGY

Potential Advantages

- Transient insomnia

Potential Disadvantages

- Chronic nightly insomnia

Primary Target Symptoms

- Time to sleep onset
- Total night sleep
- Nighttime awakening

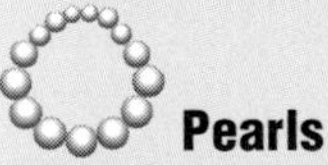

Pearls

- ✻ Because quazepam tends to accumulate over time, perhaps not the best hypnotic for chronic nightly use
- If tolerance develops, it may result in increased anxiety during the day and/or increased wakefulness during the latter part of the night
- Quazepam has a longer half-life than some other sedative hypnotics, so it may be less likely to cause rebound insomnia on discontinuation
- ✻ Long-term accumulation of quazepam and its active metabolites may cause insidious onset of confusion or falls, especially in the elderly

Suggested Reading

Ankier SI, Goa KL. Quazepam. A preliminary review of its pharmacodynamic and pharmacokinetic properties, and therapeutic efficacy in insomnia. Drugs 1988;35:42–62.

Hilbert JM, Battista D. Quazepam and flurazepam: differential pharmacokinetic and pharmacodynamic characteristics. J Clin Psychiatry 1991;52(Suppl):21–6.

Kales A. Quazepam: hypnotic efficacy and side effects. Pharmacotherapy 1990;10:1–10.

Kirkwood CK. Management of insomnia. J Am Pharm Assoc (Wash) 1999;39:688–96.

Roth T, Roehrs TA. A review of the safety profiles of benzodiazepine hypnotics. J Clin Psychiatry 1991;52 (Suppl):38–41.

QUETIAPINE

THERAPEUTICS

Brands • Seroquel
• Seroquel XR

see index for additional brand names

Generic? Not in U.S., Europe, or Japan

Class

- Atypical antipsychotic (serotonin-dopamine antagonist; second-generation antipsychotic; also a mood stabilizer)

Commonly Prescribed for

(bold for FDA approved)

- **Acute schizophrenia (quetiapine, quetiapine XR)**
- **Schizophrenia maintenance (quetiapine XR)**
- **Acute mania (quetiapine and quetiapine XR, monotherapy and adjunct to lithium or valproate)**
- **Bipolar maintenance (quetiapine, quetiapine XR)**
- **Bipolar depression (quetiapine, quetiapine XR)**
- Major depressive disorder
- Other psychotic disorders
- Mixed mania
- Behavioral disturbances in dementias
- Behavioral disturbances in Parkinson's disease and Lewy body dementia
- Psychosis associated with levodopa treatment in Parkinson's disease
- Behavioral disturbances in children and adolescents
- Disorders associated with problems with impulse control
- Severe treatment-resistant anxiety

How the Drug Works

- Blocks dopamine 2 receptors, reducing positive symptoms of psychosis and stabilizing affective symptoms
- Blocks serotonin 2A receptors, causing enhancement of dopamine release in certain brain regions and thus reducing motor side effects and possibly improving cognitive and affective symptoms
- Interactions at a myriad of other neurotransmitter receptors may contribute to quetiapine's efficacy

✻ Specifically, actions at 5HT1A receptors may contribute to efficacy for cognitive and affective symptoms in some patients, especially at moderate to high doses

How Long Until It Works

- Psychotic and manic symptoms can improve within 1 week, but it may take several weeks for full effect on behavior as well as on cognition and affective stabilization
- Classically recommended to wait at least 4–6 weeks to determine efficacy of drug, but in practice some patients require up to 16–20 weeks to show a good response, especially on cognitive symptoms

If It Works

- Most often reduces positive symptoms in schizophrenia but does not eliminate them
- Can improve negative symptoms, as well as aggressive, cognitive, and affective symptoms in schizophrenia
- Most schizophrenic patients do not have a total remission of symptoms but rather a reduction of symptoms by about a third
- Perhaps 5–15% of schizophrenic patients can experience an overall improvement of greater than 50–60%, especially when receiving stable treatment for more than a year
- Such patients are considered super-responders or "awakeners" since they may be well enough to be employed, live independently, and sustain long-term relationships
- Many bipolar patients may experience a reduction of symptoms by half or more
- Continue treatment until reaching a plateau of improvement
- After reaching a satisfactory plateau, continue treatment for at least a year after first episode of psychosis
- For second and subsequent episodes of psychosis, treatment may need to be indefinite
- Even for first episodes of psychosis, it may be preferable to continue treatment indefinitely to avoid subsequent episodes
- Treatment may not only reduce mania but also prevent recurrences of mania in bipolar disorder

If It Doesn't Work

- Try one of the other atypical antipsychotics (risperidone, olanzapine, ziprasidone, aripiprazole, paliperidone, amisulpride)
- If 2 or more antipsychotic monotherapies do not work, consider clozapine
- If no first-line atypical antipsychotic is effective, consider higher doses or augmentation with valproate or lamotrigine
- Some patients may require treatment with a conventional antipsychotic
- Consider noncompliance and switch to another antipsychotic with fewer side effects or to an antipsychotic that can be given by depot injection
- Consider initiating rehabilitation and psychotherapy
- Consider presence of concomitant drug abuse

Best Augmenting Combos for Partial Response or Treatment Resistance

- Valproic acid (valproate, divalproex, divalproex ER)
- Other mood stabilizing anticonvulsants (carbamazepine, oxcarbazepine, lamotrigine)
- Lithium
- Benzodiazepines

Tests

Before starting an atypical antipsychotic

✻ Weigh all patients and track BMI during treatment
- Get baseline personal and family history of diabetes, obesity, dyslipidemia, hypertension, and cardiovascular disease

✻ Get waist circumference (at umbilicus), blood pressure, fasting plasma glucose, and fasting lipid profile
- Determine if the patient is
  - overweight (BMI 25.0–29.9)
  - obese (BMI ≥30)
  - has pre-diabetes (fasting plasma glucose 100–25 mg/dL)
  - has diabetes (fasting plasma glucose >126 mg/dL)
  - has hypertension (BP >140/90 mm Hg)
  - has dyslipidemia (increased total cholesterol, LDL cholesterol, and triglycerides; decreased HDL cholesterol)
- Treat or refer such patients for treatment, including nutrition and weight management, physical activity counseling, smoking cessation, and medical management

Monitoring after starting an atypical antipsychotic

✻ BMI monthly for 3 months, then quarterly

✻ Consider monitoring fasting triglycerides monthly for several months in patients at high risk for metabolic complications and when initiating or switching antipsychotics

✻ Blood pressure, fasting plasma glucose, fasting lipids within 3 months and then annually, but earlier and more frequently for patients with diabetes or who have gained >5% of initial weight
- Treat or refer for treatment and consider switching to another atypical antipsychotic for patients who become overweight, obese, pre-diabetic, diabetic, hypertensive, or dyslipidemic while receiving an atypical antipsychotic

✻ Even in patients without known diabetes, be vigilant for the rare but life threatening onset of diabetic ketoacidosis, which always requires immediate treatment, by monitoring for the rapid onset of polyuria, polydipsia, weight loss, nausea, vomiting, dehydration, rapid respiration, weakness and clouding of sensorium, even coma
- Although U.S. manufacturer recommends 6-month eye checks for cataracts, clinical experience suggests this may be unnecessary

SIDE EFFECTS

How Drug Causes Side Effects

- By blocking histamine 1 receptors in the brain, it can cause sedation and possibly weight gain
- By blocking alpha 1 adrenergic receptors, it can cause dizziness, sedation, and hypotension
- By blocking muscarinic 1 receptors, it can cause dry mouth, constipation, and sedation
- By blocking dopamine 2 receptors in the striatum, it can cause motor side effects (rare)
- Mechanism of weight gain and increased incidence of diabetes and dyslipidemia with atypical antipsychotics is unknown

Notable Side Effects

✱ May increase risk for diabetes and dyslipidemia
✱ Dizziness, sedation
- Dry mouth, constipation, dyspepsia, abdominal pain, weight gain
- Tachycardia
- Orthostatic hypotension, usually during initial dose titration
- Theoretical risk of tardive dyskinesia

Life-Threatening or Dangerous Side Effects

- Hyperglycemia, in some cases extreme and associated with ketoacidosis or hyperosmolar coma or death, has been reported in patients taking atypical antipsychotics
- Rare neuroleptic malignant syndrome (much reduced risk compared to conventional antipsychotics)
- Rare seizures
- Increased risk of death and cerebrovascular events in elderly patients with dementia-related psychosis

Weight Gain

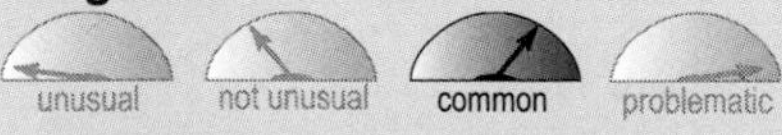

- Many patients experience and/or can be significant in amount at effective antipsychotic doses
- Can become a health problem in some
- May be less than for some antipsychotics, more than for others

Sedation

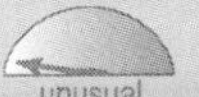

- Frequent and can be significant in amount
- Some patients may not tolerate it
- More than for some other antipsychotics, but never say always as not a problem in everyone
- Can wear off over time
- Can reemerge as dose increases and then wear off again over time
- Not necessarily increased as dose is raised

What to Do About Side Effects

- Wait
- Wait
- Wait
- Usually dosed twice daily, so take more of the total daily dose at bedtime to help reduce daytime sedation
- Start dosing low and increase slowly as side effects wear off at each dosing increment
- Weight loss, exercise programs, and medical management for high BMIs, diabetes, dyslipidemia
- Switch to another atypical antipsychotic

Best Augmenting Agents for Side Effects

- Many side effects cannot be improved with an augmenting agent

DOSING AND USE

Usual Dosage Range

- 400–800 mg/day in 1 (quetiapine XR) or 2 (quetiapine) doses for schizophrenia
- 400–800 mg/day in 1 (quetiapine XR) or 2 (quetiapine) doses for bipolar mania
- 300 mg once daily for bipolar depression

Dosage Forms

- Tablets 25 mg, 50 mg, 100 mg, 200 mg, 300 mg, 400 mg
- Extended-release tablets 200 mg, 300 mg, 400 mg

How To Dose

- (according to manufacturer for quetiapine in schizophrenia): initial 25 mg/day twice a day; increase by 25–50 mg twice a day each day until desired efficacy is reached; maximum approved dose 800 mg/day
- In practice, can start adults with schizophrenia under age 65 with same doses as recommended for acute bipolar mania
- (according to manufacturer for quetiapine in acute bipolar mania): initiate in twice daily doses, totaling 100 mg/day on day 1, increasing to 400 mg/day on day 4 in increments of up to 100 mg/day; further dosage adjustments up to 800 mg/day by day 6 should be in increments of no greater than 200 mg/day
- Bipolar depression for quetiapine and quetiapine XR: once daily at bedtime; titrate as needed to reach 300 mg/day by day 4
- Quetiapine XR in schizophrenia and acute mania: initial 300 mg once daily, preferably

in the evening; can increase by 300 mg/day each day until desired efficacy is reached; maximum approved dose 800 mg/day

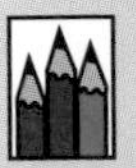

Dosing Tips

* ✻ **More may be much more:** Clinical practice suggests quetiapine often underdosed, then switched prior to adequate trials
* Clinical practice suggests that at low doses it may be a sedative hypnotic, possibly due to potent H1 antihistamine actions, but this is an expensive use for which there are many other options
* ✻ Initial target dose of 400–800 mg/day should be reached in most cases to optimize the chances of success in treating acute psychosis and acute mania, but many patients are not adequately dosed in clinical practice
* Many patients do well with immediate-release as a single daily oral dose, usually at bedtime
* May be lower cost than some other atypical antipsychotics at 200 mg twice daily, but higher doses can be among the most costly for atypical antipsychotics
* Recommended titration to 400 mg/day by the fourth day can often be achieved when necessary to control acute symptoms
* Rapid dose escalation in manic or psychotic patients may lesson sedative side effects
* ✻ Higher doses generally achieve greater response for manic or psychotic symptoms
* In contrast, some patients with bipolar depression may respond well to doses less than 300 mg/day and as little as 25 mg/day
* Dosing in major depression may be even lower than in bipolar depression, and dosing may be even lower still in generalized anxiety disorder
* Rapid dose escalation in manic or psychotic patients may lesson sedative side effects
* ✻ Occasional patients may require more than 800–1,000 mg/day
* Rather than raise the dose above these levels in acutely agitated patients requiring acute antipsychotic actions, consider augmentation with a benzodiazepine or conventional antipsychotic, either orally or intramuscularly
* Rather than raise the dose above these levels in partial responders, consider augmentation with a mood-stabilizing anticonvulsant such as valproate or lamotrigine
* Children and elderly should generally be dosed at the lower end of the dosage spectrum
* Quetiapine XR is controlled-release and therefore should not be chewed or crushed but rather should be swallowed whole
* Quetiapine XL is in late-stage clinical development and may generate increased concentrations of active metabolite norquetiapine, with theoretically improved profile for affective and anxiety disorders

Overdose

* Rarely lethal in monotherapy overdose; sedation, slurred speech, hypotension

Long-Term Use

* Approved for long-term maintenance in schizophrenia and bipolar disorder, and often used for long-term maintenance in various behavioral disorders

Habit Forming

* No

How to Stop

* Slow down-titration (over 6–8 weeks), especially when simultaneously beginning a new antipsychotic while switching (i.e., cross-titration)
* Rapid discontinuation may lead to rebound psychosis and worsening of symptoms

Pharmacokinetics

* Metabolites are inactive
* Parent drug has 6–7 hour half-life

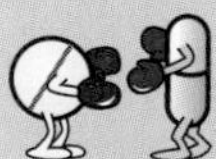

Drug Interactions

* CYP450 3A inhibitors and CYP450 2D6 inhibitors may reduce clearance of quetiapine and thus raise quetiapine plasma levels, but dosage reduction of quetiapine usually not necessary
* May increase effect of antihypertensive agents

Other Warnings/ Precautions

- In the U.S., manufacturer recommends examination for cataracts before and every 6 months after initiating quetiapine, but this does not seem to be necessary in clinical practice
- Quetiapine should be used cautiously in patients at risk for aspiration pneumonia, as dysphagia has been reported

SPECIAL POPULATIONS

Renal Impairment

- No dose adjustment required

Hepatic Impairment

- Downward dose adjustment may be necessary

Cardiac Impairment

- Drug should be used with caution because of risk of orthostatic hypotension

Elderly

- Lower dose is generally used (e.g., 25–100 mg twice a day), although higher doses may be used if tolerated
- Although atypical antipsychotics are commonly used for behavioral disturbances in dementia, no agent has been approved for treatment of elderly patients with dementia-related psychosis
- Elderly patients with dementia-related psychosis treated with atypical antipsychotics are at an increased risk of death compared to placebo, and also have an increased risk of cerebrovascular events

Children and Adolescents

- Not officially recommended for patients under age 18
- Clinical experience and early data suggest quetiapine may be safe and effective for behavioral disturbances in children and adolescents
- Children and adolescents using quetiapine may need to be monitored more often than adults
- Use with caution, observing for activation of suicidal ideation, and inform parents or guardian of this risk so they can help observe child or adolescent patients
- May tolerate lower doses better

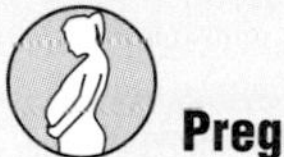

Pregnancy

- Risk Category C [some animal studies show adverse effects; no controlled studies in humans]
- Psychotic symptoms may worsen during pregnancy and some form of treatment may be necessary
- Quetiapine may be preferable to anticonvulsant mood stabilizers if treatment is required during pregnancy

Breast Feeding

- Unknown if quetiapine is secreted in human breast milk, but all psychotropics assumed to be secreted in breast milk
- Recommended either to discontinue drug or bottle feed
- Infants of women who choose to breast feed while on quetiapine should be monitored for possible adverse effects

THE ART OF PSYCHOPHARMACOLOGY

Potential Advantages

- Bipolar depression
- Some cases of psychosis and bipolar disorder refractory to treatment with other antipsychotics

✻ Patients with Parkinson's disease who need an antipsychotic or mood stabilizer

✻ Patients with Lewy body dementia who need an antipsychotic or mood stabilizer

Potential Disadvantages

- Patients requiring rapid onset of action
- Patients who have difficulty tolerating sedation

Primary Target Symptoms

- Positive symptoms of psychosis
- Negative symptoms of psychosis
- Cognitive symptoms
- Unstable mood (both depression and mania)
- Aggressive symptoms
- Insomnia and anxiety

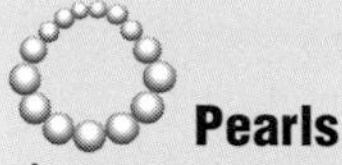

Pearls

* ✻ May be the preferred antipsychotic for psychosis in Parkinson's disease and Lewy body dementia
* Anecdotal reports of efficacy in treatment-refractory cases and positive symptoms of psychoses other than schizophrenia
* ✻ Efficacy may be underestimated for psychosis and mania since quetiapine is often under-dosed in clinical practice
* ✻ Approved in bipolar depression
* The active metabolite of quetiapine, norquetiapine, has the additional properties of norepinephrine reuptake inhibition and antagonism of 5HT2C receptors, which may contribute to therapeutic effects for mood and cognition
* Dosing differs depending on the indication, with high-dose mechanisms including robust blockade of D2 receptors above 60% occupancy and equal or greater 5HT2A blockade; medium dose mechanisms including moderate amounts of NET inhibition combined with 5HT2C antagonism and 5HT1A partial agonism; and low dose mechanisms including H1 antagonism and 5HT1A partial agonism and, to a lesser extent, NET inhibition and 5HT2C antagonism
* More sedation than some other antipsychotics, which may be of benefit in acutely manic or psychotic patients but not for stabilized patients in long-term maintenance
* ✻ Essentially no motor side effects or prolactin elevation
* May have less weight gain than some antipsychotics, more than others
* ✻ Controversial as to whether quetiapine has more or less risk of diabetes and dyslipidemia than some other antipsychotics
* Can be a more expensive atypical antipsychotic than some others when dosed appropriately in schizophrenia or acute mania; some patients respond to moderate doses, which are less expensive
* Commonly used at low doses to augment other atypical antipsychotics, but such antipsychotic polypharmacy has not been systematically studied and can be quite expensive
* Anecdotal reports of efficacy in posttraumatic stress disorder, including symptoms of sleep disturbance and anxiety
* Quetiapine XL is in late-stage clinical development for major depression and generalized anxiety disorder

Suggested Reading

Keating GM, Robinson DM. Quetiapine: A review of its use in the treatment of bipolar depression. Drugs 2007;67(7):1077–95.

Lieberman JA, Stroup TS, McEvoy JP. Effectiveness of antipsychotic drugs in patients with chronic schizophrenia. N Engl J Med 2005;353(12):1209–23.

Nasrallah HA. Atypical antipsychotic-induced metabolic side effects: insights from receptor-binding profiles. Mol Psychiatry 2008;13(1):27–35.

Smith LA, Cornelius V, Warnock A, Tacchi MJ, Taylor D. Pharmacological interventions for acute bipolar mania: a systematic review of randomized placebo-controlled trials. Bipolar Disord 2007;9(6):551–60.

Srisurapanont M, Disayavanish C, Taimkaew K. Quetiapine for schizophrenia. Cochrane Database Syst Rev 2000;3:CD000967.

RAMELTEON

THERAPEUTICS

Brands • Rozerem

see index for additional brand names

Generic? No

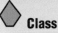

Class

- Melatonin 1 and 2 receptor agonist

Commonly Prescribed for

(bold for FDA approved)

- **Insomnia (difficulty with sleep onset)**
- Primary insomnia
- Chronic insomnia
- Transient insomnia
- Insomnia associated with shift work, jet lag, or circadian rhythm disturbances

How the Drug Works

- Binds selectively to melatonin 1 and melatonin 2 receptors as a full agonist

How Long Until It Works

- Generally takes effect in less than an hour

If It Works

- Reduces time to sleep onset
- Increases total sleep time
- May improve quality of sleep

If It Doesn't Work

- If insomnia does not improve after 7–10 days, it may be a manifestation of a primary psychiatric or physical illness such as obstructive sleep apnea or restless leg syndrome, which requires independent evaluation
- Increase the dose
- Improve sleep hygiene
- Switch to another agent

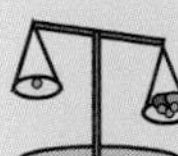

Best Augmenting Combos for Partial Response or Treatment Resistance

- Generally, best to switch to another agent
- Eszopiclone, zolpidem
- Trazodone
- Agents with antihistamine actions (e.g., diphenhydramine, tricyclic antidepressants)

Tests

- None for healthy individuals
- For patients presenting with unexplained amenorrhea, galactorrhea, decreased libido, or problems with fertility, could consider measuring prolactin and testosterone levels

SIDE EFFECTS

How Drug Causes Side Effects

- Actions at melatonin receptors that carry over to the next day could theoretically cause daytime sedation, fatigue, and sluggishness, but this is not common

Notable Side Effects

* Sedation
* Dizziness
* Fatigue
* Headache

Life-Threatening or Dangerous Side Effects

- Respiratory depression, especially when taken with other CNS depressants in overdose

Weight Gain

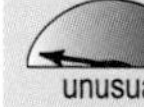

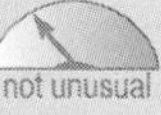

common

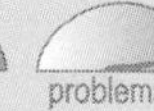

- Reported but not expected

Sedation

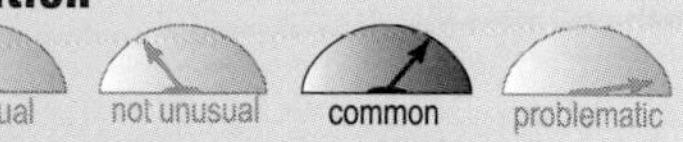

- Many experience and/or can be significant in amount
- May experience sedation or sleepiness immediately after dosing, but not commonly after awakening from a night's sleep

What to Do About Side Effects

- Wait
- To avoid problems with memory, only take ramelteon if planning to have a full night's sleep
- Lower the dose
- Switch to a non-benzodiazepine sedative hypnotic

Best Augmenting Agents for Side Effects
- Many side effects cannot be improved with an augmenting agent

DOSING AND USE

Usual Dosage Range
- 8 mg at bedtime

Dosage Forms
- Tablet 8 mg

How To Dose
- No titration, take dose at bedtime

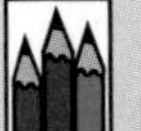

Dosing Tips
- Unusual lack of apparent dose response curve
- Doses between 4 mg and 64 mg may have similar effects on sleep and similar side effects
- Doses up to 160 mg were studied without apparent abuse liability
- Suggests therapeutic effects may be mediated by an "on-off" type of therapeutic effect on a sleep switch that works at any dose over a certain threshold
- Since ramelteon has very low oral bioavailability and thus highly variable absorption, a substantial dose range may be required to generate sufficient absorption in various patients
- Thus, "one size does not fit all" despite approval at only one dose without titration (i.e., 8 mg)
- Suggest increasing dose before concluding lack of efficacy
- Do not administer with or immediately after a high fat meal as this may delay its onset of action or diminish its efficacy

Overdose
- No reports of ramelteon overdose
- No safety or tolerability concerns in studies up to 160 mg

Long-Term Use
- No reports of dependence, tolerance, or abuse liability
- Not restricted to short-term use but few long-term studies

Habit Forming
- No

How to Stop
- No evidence of rebound insomnia the first night after stopping
- No need to taper dose

Pharmacokinetics
- Metabolized predominantly by CYP450 1A2
- CYP450 3A4 and 2C are also involved in metabolism of ramelteon
- Mean elimination half-life of parent drug 1–2.6 hours
- Mean elimination half-life of major metabolite, M-II, is 2–5 hours

Drug Interactions
- Inhibitors of CYP450 1A2, such as fluvoxamine, could increase plasma levels of ramelteon
- Inducers of CYP450, such as rifampin, could decrease plasma levels of ramelteon
- Inhibitors of CYP450 3A4, such as ketoconazole, could increase plasma levels of ramelteon
- Inhibitors of CYP450 2C9, such as fluconazole, could increase plasma levels of ramelteon
- Exercise caution if combining with alcohol
- No interaction with fluoxetine (CYP450 2D6 inhibitor)

Other Warnings/ Precautions
- Insomnia may be a symptom of a primary disorder, rather than a primary disorder itself
- Use only with extreme caution in patients with impaired respiratory function or obstructive sleep apnea
- Ramelteon should only be administered at bedtime
- May decrease testosterone levels or increase prolactin levels, but the clinical significance of this is unknown

Do Not Use
- With fluvoxamine
- In patients with severe hepatic impairment
- If there is a proven allergy to ramelteon

SPECIAL POPULATIONS

Renal Impairment
- Dose adjustment not generally necessary

Hepatic Impairment
- Use with caution in patients with moderate hepatic impairment
- Not recommended for use in patients with severe impairment

Cardiac Impairment
- Dosage adjustment may not be necessary

Elderly
- No adjustment necessary
- Greater absorption and higher plasma drug concentrations but no increase in side effects

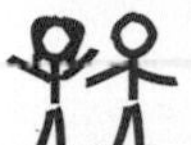

Children and Adolescents
- Safety and efficacy have not been established

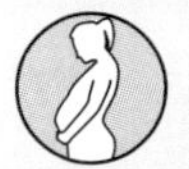

Pregnancy
- Risk Category C [some animal studies show adverse effects; no controlled studies in humans]

Breast Feeding
- Unknown if ramelteon is secreted in human breast milk, but all psychotropics assumed to be secreted in breast milk

✽ Recommended either to discontinue drug or bottle feed

THE ART OF PSYCHOPHARMACOLOGY

Potential Advantages
- Those who require long-term treatment
- Those who need a hypnotic but have a past history of substance abuse
- Possibly for circadian rhythm disturbances

Potential Disadvantages
- More expensive than some other hypnotics
- For patients who require sedation

Primary Target Symptoms
- Time to sleep onset

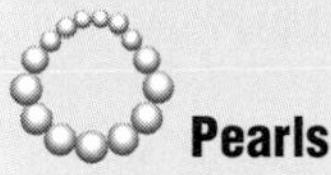

Pearls
- First in a new class of agents, chronohypnotics, that act upon circadian rhythms by stimulating melatonin receptors in the brain's "pacemaker," namely the suprachiasmatic nucleus
- Theoretically, stimulation of melatonin 1 receptors mediates the suppressive effects of melatonin on the suprachiasmatic nucleus
- Theoretically, stimulation of melatonin 2 receptors mediates the phase-shifting effect of melatonin
- Ramelteon may act by promoting the proper maintenance of circadian rhythms underlying a normal sleep-wake cycle
- Thus, ramelteon may also prove effective for treatment of circadian rhythm disturbances such as shift work sleep disorder and jet lag
- Lack of actions on GABA systems, which may be related to lack of apparent abuse liability
- Only approved hypnotic agent that is not scheduled and is considered to have no abuse liability
- No evidence that ramelteon worsens apnea/hypopnea index in chronic obstructive pulmonary disease or in obstructive sleep apnea, but not recommended in severe cases

✽ May be preferred over benzodiazepines because of its rapid onset of action, short duration of effect, and safety profile
- Rebound insomnia does not appear to be common
- May have fewer carryover side effects than some other sedative hypnotics

Suggested Reading

Erman M, Seiden D, Zammit G, Sainati S, Zhang J. An efficacy, safety, and dose-response study of Ramelteon in patients with chronic primary insomnia. Sleep Med 2006;7(1):17–24.

Kato K, Hirai K, Nishiyama K, Uchikawa O, Fukatsu K, Okhawa S, et al. Neurochemical properties of ramelteon (TAK-375), a selective MT1/MT2 receptor agonist. Neuropharmacology 2005;48(2):301–10.

McGechan A, Wellington K. Ramelteon. CNS Drugs 2005;19(12):1057–65.

Pandi-Perumal SR, Zisapel N, Srinivasan V, Cardinali DP. Melatonin and sleep in aging population. Exp Gerontol 2005;40(12):911–25.

THERAPEUTICS

Brands • Norebox
• Edronax

see index for additional brand names

Generic? No

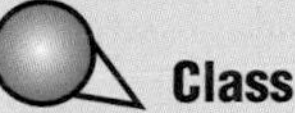

Class

- Selective norepinephrine reuptake inhibitor (NRI); antidepressant

Commonly Prescribed for

(bold for FDA approved)

- Major depressive disorder
- Dysthymia
- Panic disorder
- Attention deficit hyperactivity disorder (ADHD)

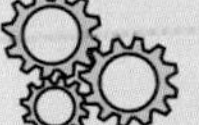

How the Drug Works

- Boosts neurotransmitter norepinephrine/ noradrenaline and may also increase dopamine in prefrontal cortex
- Blocks norepinephrine reuptake pump (norepinephrine transporter)
- Presumably, this increases noradrenergic neurotransmission
- Since dopamine is inactivated by norepinephrine reuptake in frontal cortex which largely lacks dopamine transporters, reboxetine can increase dopamine neurotransmission in this part of the brain

How Long Until It Works

- Onset of therapeutic actions usually not immediate, but often delayed 2–4 weeks
- If it is not working within 6–8 weeks for depression, it may require a dosage increase or it may not work at all
- May continue to work for many years to prevent relapse of symptoms

If It Works

- The goal of treatment is complete remission of current symptoms as well as prevention of future relapses
- Treatment most often reduces or even eliminates symptoms, but not a cure since symptoms can recur after medicine stopped
- Continue treatment until all symptoms are gone (remission)
- Once symptoms gone, continue treating for 1 year for the first episode of depression
- For second and subsequent episodes of depression, treatment may need to be indefinite

If It Doesn't Work

- Many patients only have a partial response where some symptoms are improved but others persist (especially insomnia, fatigue, and problems concentrating)
- Other patients may be nonresponders, sometimes called treatment-resistant or treatment-refractory
- Consider increasing dose, switching to another agent or adding an appropriate augmenting agent
- Consider psychotherapy
- Consider evaluation for another diagnosis or for a comorbid condition (e.g., medical illness, substance abuse, etc.)
- Some patients may experience apparent lack of consistent efficacy due to activation of latent or underlying bipolar disorder, and require antidepressant discontinuation and a switch to a mood stabilizer

Best Augmenting Combos for Partial Response or Treatment Resistance

- Trazodone, especially for insomnia
- SSRIs, SNRIs, mirtazapine (use combinations of antidepressants with caution as this may activate bipolar disorder and suicidal ideation)
- Modafinil, especially for fatigue, sleepiness, and lack of concentration
- Mood stabilizers or atypical antipsychotics for bipolar depression, psychotic depression or treatment-resistant depression
- Benzodiazepines for anxiety
- Hypnotics for insomnia
- Classically, lithium, buspirone, or thyroid hormone

Tests

- None for healthy individuals

SIDE EFFECTS

How Drug Causes Side Effects

- Norepinephrine increases in parts of the brain and body and at receptors other than

those that cause therapeutic actions (e.g., unwanted actions of norepinephrine on acetylcholine release causing constipation and dry mouth, etc.)
- Most side effects are immediate but often go away with time

Notable Side Effects
- Insomnia, dizziness, anxiety, agitation
- Dry mouth, constipation
- Urinary hesitancy, urinary retention
- Sexual dysfunction (impotence)
- Dose-dependent hypotension

Life-Threatening or Dangerous Side Effects
- Rare seizures
- Rare induction of mania
- Rare activation of suicidal ideation and behavior (suicidality) (short-term studies did not show an increase in the risk of suicidality with antidepressants compared to placebo beyond age 24)

Weight Gain
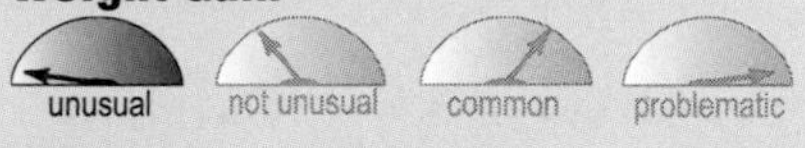

- Reported but not expected

Sedation
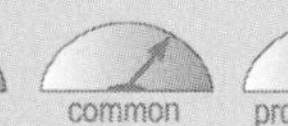

- Reported but not expected

What to Do About Side Effects
- Wait
- Wait
- Wait
- Lower the dose
- In a few weeks, switch or add other drugs

Best Augmenting Agents for Side Effects
- For urinary hesitancy, give an alpha 1 blocker such as tamsulosin
- Often best to try another antidepressant monotherapy prior to resorting to augmentation strategies to treat side effects
- Trazodone or a hypnotic for drug-induced insomnia
- Benzodiazepines for drug-induced anxiety and activation
- Mirtazapine for drug-induced insomnia or anxiety
- Many side effects are dose-dependent (i.e., they increase as dose increases, or they reemerge until tolerance redevelops)
- Many side effects are time-dependent (i.e., they start immediately upon dosing and upon each dose increase, but go away with time)
- Activation and agitation may represent the induction of a bipolar state, especially a mixed dysphoric bipolar II condition sometimes associated with suicidal ideation, and require the addition of lithium, a mood stabilizer or an atypical antipsychotic, and/or discontinuation of reboxetine

DOSING AND USE

Usual Dosage Range
- 8 mg/day in 2 doses (10 mg usual maximum daily dose)

Dosage Forms
- Tablet 2 mg, 4 mg scored

How To Dose
- Initial 2 mg/day twice a day for 1 week, 4 mg/day twice a day for second week

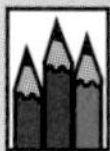

Dosing Tips
- When switching from another antidepressant or adding to another antidepressant, dosing may need to be lower and titration slower to prevent activating side effects (e.g., 2 mg in the daytime for 2–3 days, then 2 mg bid for 1–2 weeks)
- Give second daily dose in late afternoon rather than at bedtime to avoid undesired activation or insomnia in the evening
- May not need full dose of 8 mg/day when given in conjunction with another antidepressant
- Some patients may need 10 mg/day or more if well-tolerated without orthostatic hypotension and if additional efficacy is seen at high doses in difficult cases
- Early dosing in patients with panic and anxiety may need to be lower and titration slower, perhaps with the use of

concomitant short-term benzodiazepines to increase tolerability

Overdose
- Postural hypotension, anxiety, hypertension

Long-Term Use
- Safe

Habit Forming
- No

How to Stop
- Taper not necessary

Pharmacokinetics
- Metabolized by CYP450 3A4
- Inhibits CYP450 2D6 and 3A4 at high doses
- Elimination half-life approximately 13 hours

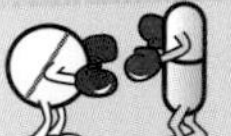

Drug Interactions
- Tramadol increases the risk of seizures in patients taking an antidepressant
- May need to reduce reboxetine dose or avoid concomitant use with inhibitors of CYP450 3A4, such as azole and antifungals, macrolide antibiotics, fluvoxamine, nefazodone, fluoxetine, sertraline, etc.
- Via CYP450 2D6 inhibition, reboxetine could theoretically interfere with the analgesic actions of codeine, and increase the plasma levels of some beta blockers and of atomoxetine and TCAs
- Via CYP450 2D6 inhibition, reboxetine could theoretically increase concentrations of thioridazine and cause dangerous cardiac arrhythmias
- Via CYP450 3A4 inhibition, reboxetine may increase the levels of alprazolam, buspirone, and triazolam
- Via CYP450 3A4 inhibition, reboxetine could theoretically increase concentrations of certain cholesterol lowering HMG CoA reductase inhibitors, especially simvastatin, atorvastatin, and lovastatin, but not pravastatin or fluvastatin, which would increase the risk of rhabdomyolysis; thus, coadministration of reboxetine with certain HMG CoA reductase inhibitors should proceed with caution
- Via CYP450 3A4 inhibition, reboxetine could theoretically increase the concentrations of pimozide, and cause QTc prolongation and dangerous cardiac arrhythmias
- Use with ergotamine may increase blood pressure
- Hypokalemia may occur if reboxetine is used with diuretics
- Do not use with MAO inhibitors, including 14 days after MAOIs are stopped

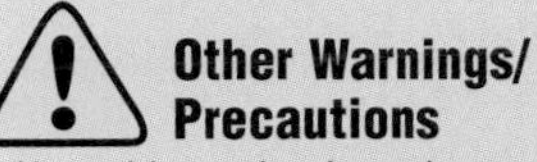

Other Warnings/ Precautions
- Use with caution in patients with bipolar disorder unless treated with concomitant mood-stabilizing agent
- Use with caution in patients with urinary retention, benign prostatic hyperplasia, glaucoma, epilepsy
- Use with caution with drugs that lower blood pressure
- When treating children, carefully weigh the risks and benefits of pharmacological treatment against the risks and benefits of nontreatment with antidepressants and make sure to document this in the patient's chart
- Distribute the brochures provided by the FDA and the drug companies
- Warn patients and their caregivers about the possibility of activating side effects and advise them to report such symptoms immediately
- Monitor patients for activation of suicidal ideation, especially children and adolescents

Do Not Use
- If patient has narrow angle-closure glaucoma
- If patient is taking an MAO inhibitor
- If patient is taking pimozide or thioridazine
- If there is a proven allergy to reboxetine

SPECIAL POPULATIONS

Renal Impairment
- Plasma concentrations are increased
- May need to lower dose

Hepatic Impairment
- Plasma concentrations are increased
- May need to lower dose

Cardiac Impairment
- Use with caution

Elderly
- Lower dose is recommended (4–6 mg/day)
- Reduction in risk of suicidality with antidepressants compared to placebo in adults age 65 and older

Children and Adolescents
- Carefully weigh the risks and benefits of pharmacological treatment against the risks and benefits of nontreatment with antidepressants and make sure to document this in the patient's chart
- Monitor patients face-to-face regularly, particularly during the first several weeks of treatment
- Use with caution, observing for activation of known or unknown bipolar disorder and/or suicidal ideation, and inform parents or guardians of this risk so they can help observe child or adolescent patients
- No guidelines for children; safety and efficacy have not been established

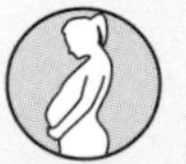

Pregnancy
- No controlled studies in humans
- Not generally recommended for use during pregnancy, especially during first trimester
- Must weigh the risk of treatment (first trimester fetal development, third trimester newborn delivery) to the child against the risk of no treatment (recurrence of depression, maternal health, infant bonding) to the mother and child
- For many patients this may mean continuing treatment during pregnancy

Breast Feeding
- Some drug is found in mother's breast milk
- Immediate postpartum period is a high-risk time for depression, especially in women who have had prior depressive episodes, so drug may need to be reinstituted late in the third trimester or shortly after childbirth to prevent a recurrence during the postpartum period
- Must weigh benefits of breast feeding with risks and benefits of antidepressant treatment versus nontreatment to both the infant and the mother
- For many patients, this may mean continuing treatment during breast feeding

THE ART OF PSYCHOPHARMACOLOGY

Potential Advantages
- Tired, unmotivated patients
- Patients with cognitive disturbances
- Patients with psychomotor retardation

Potential Disadvantages
- Patients unable to comply with twice-daily dosing
- Patients unable to tolerate activation

Primary Target Symptoms
- Depressed mood
- Energy, motivation, and interest
- Suicidal ideation
- Cognitive disturbance
- Psychomotor retardation

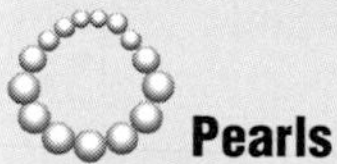

Pearls
- May be effective if SSRIs have failed or for SSRI "poop-out"

✽ May be more likely than SSRIs to improve social and work functioning
- Reboxetine is a mixture of an active and an inactive enantiomer, and the active enantiomer may be developed in future clinical testing

✽ Side effects may appear "anticholinergic," but reboxetine does not directly block muscarinic receptors
- Constipation, dry mouth, and urinary retention are noradrenergic, due in part to peripheral alpha 1 receptor stimulation causing decreased acetylcholine release

✽ Thus, antidotes for these side effects can be alpha 1 antagonists such as tamsulosin, especially for urinary retention in men over 50 with borderline urine flow
- Novel use of reboxetine may be for attention deficit disorder, analogous to the actions of another norepinephrine selective reuptake inhibitor, atomoxetine, but few controlled studies
- Another novel use may be for neuropathic pain, alone or in combination with other antidepressants, but few controlled studies
- Some studies suggest efficacy in panic disorder

Suggested Reading

Fleishaker JC. Clinical pharmacokinetics of reboxetine, a selective norepinephrine reuptake inhibitor for the treatment of patients with depression. Clin Pharmacokinet 2000;39(6):413–27.

Kasper S, el Giamal N, Hilger E. Reboxetine: the first selective noradrenaline re-uptake inhibitor. Expert Opin Pharmacother 2000;1(4):771–82.

Keller M. Role of serotonin and noradrenaline in social dysfunction: a review of data on reboxetine and the Social Adaptation Self-evaluation Scale (SASS). Gen Hosp Psychiatry 2001;23(1):15–9.

Tanum L. Reboxetine: tolerability and safety profile in patients with major depression. Acta Psychiatr Scand Suppl 2000;402:37–40.

THERAPEUTICS

Brands • Risperdal • CONSTA

see index for additional brand names

Generic? Yes

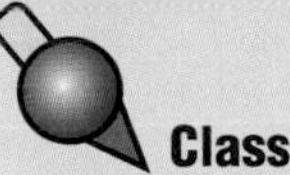

Class

- Atypical antipsychotic (serotonin-dopamine antagonist; second-generation antipsychotic; also a mood stabilizer)

Commonly Prescribed for

(bold for FDA approved)

- **Schizophrenia, ages 13 and older (oral, long-acting microspheres intramuscularly)**
- **Delaying relapse in schizophrenia (oral)**
- **Other psychotic disorders (oral)**
- **Acute mania/mixed mania, ages 10 and older (oral, monotherapy and adjunct to lithium or valproate)**
- **Autism-related irritability in children ages 5–16**
- Bipolar maintenance
- Bipolar depression
- Behavioral disturbances in dementias
- Behavioral disturbances in children and adolescents
- Disorders associated with problems with impulse control

How the Drug Works

- Blocks dopamine 2 receptors, reducing positive symptoms of psychosis and stabilizing affective symptoms
- Blocks serotonin 2A receptors, causing enhancement of dopamine release in certain brain regions and thus reducing motor side effects and possibly improving cognitive and affective symptoms
- Interactions at a myriad of other neurotransmitter receptors may contribute to risperidone's efficacy

✻ Specifically, alpha 2 antagonist properties may contribute to antidepressant actions

How Long Until It Works

- Psychotic and manic symptoms can improve within 1 week, but it may take several weeks for full effect on behavior as well as on cognition and affective stabilization
- Classically recommended to wait at least 4–6 weeks to determine efficacy of drug, but in practice some patients require up to 16–20 weeks to show a good response, especially on cognitive symptoms

If It Works

- Most often reduces positive symptoms in schizophrenia but does not eliminate them
- Can improve negative symptoms, as well as aggressive, cognitive, and affective symptoms in schizophrenia
- Most schizophrenic patients do not have a total remission of symptoms but rather a reduction of symptoms by about a third
- Perhaps 5–15% of schizophrenic patients can experience an overall improvement of greater than 50–60%, especially when receiving stable treatment for more than a year
- Such patients are considered super-responders or "awakeners" since they may be well enough to be employed, live independently, and sustain long-term relationships
- Many bipolar patients may experience a reduction of symptoms by half or more
- Continue treatment until reaching a plateau of improvement
- After reaching a satisfactory plateau, continue treatment for at least a year after first episode of psychosis
- For second and subsequent episodes of psychosis, treatment may need to be indefinite
- Even for first episodes of psychosis, it may be preferable to continue treatment indefinitely to avoid subsequent episodes
- Treatment may not only reduce mania but also prevent recurrences of mania in bipolar disorder

If It Doesn't Work

- Try one of the other atypical antipsychotics (olanzapine, quetiapine, ziprasidone, aripiprazole, paliperidone, amisulpride)
- If 2 or more antipsychotic monotherapies do not work, consider clozapine
- If no first-line atypical antipsychotic is effective, consider higher doses or augmentation with valproate or lamotrigine
- Some patients may require treatment with a conventional antipsychotic
- Consider noncompliance and switch to another antipsychotic with fewer side

effects or to an antipsychotic that can be given by depot injection
- Consider initiating rehabilitation and psychotherapy
- Consider presence of concomitant drug abuse

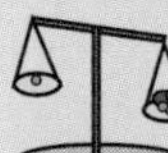

Best Augmenting Combos for Partial Response or Treatment Resistance

- Valproic acid (valproate, divalproex, divalproex ER)
- Other mood stabilizing anticonvulsants (carbamazepine, oxcarbazepine, lamotrigine)
- Lithium
- Benzodiazepines

Tests

Before starting an atypical antipsychotic

✻ Weigh all patients and track BMI during treatment
- Get baseline personal and family history of diabetes, obesity, dyslipidemia, hypertension, and cardiovascular disease

✻ Get waist circumference (at umbilicus), blood pressure, fasting plasma glucose, and fasting lipid profile
- Determine if the patient is
  - overweight (BMI 25.0–29.9)
  - obese (BMI ≥30)
  - has pre-diabetes (fasting plasma glucose 100–25 mg/dL)
  - has diabetes (fasting plasma glucose >126 mg/dL)
  - has hypertension (BP >140/90 mm Hg)
  - has dyslipidemia (increased total cholesterol, LDL cholesterol, and triglycerides; decreased HDL cholesterol)
- Treat or refer such patients for treatment, including nutrition and weight management, physical activity counseling, smoking cessation, and medical management

Monitoring after starting an atypical antipsychotic

✻ BMI monthly for 3 months, then quarterly

✻ Consider monitoring fasting triglycerides monthly for several months in patients at high risk for metabolic complications and when initiating or switching antipsychotics

✻ Blood pressure, fasting plasma glucose, fasting lipids within 3 months and then annually, but earlier and more frequently for patients with diabetes or who have gained >5% of initial weight
- Treat or refer for treatment and consider switching to another atypical antipsychotic for patients who become overweight, obese, pre-diabetic, diabetic, hypertensive, or dyslipidemic while receiving an atypical antipsychotic

✻ Even in patients without known diabetes, be vigilant for the rare but life-threatening onset of diabetic ketoacidosis, which always requires immediate treatment, by monitoring for the rapid onset of polyuria, polydipsia, weight loss, nausea, vomiting, dehydration, rapid respiration, weakness and clouding of sensorium, even coma
- Should check blood pressure in the elderly before starting and for the first few weeks of treatment
- Monitoring elevated prolactin levels of dubious clinical benefit

SIDE EFFECTS

How Drug Causes Side Effects

- By blocking alpha 1 adrenergic receptors, it can cause dizziness, sedation, and hypotension
- By blocking dopamine 2 receptors in the striatum, it can cause motor side effects, especially at high doses
- By blocking dopamine 2 receptors in the pituitary, it can cause elevations in prolactin
- Mechanism of weight gain and increased incidence of diabetes and dyslipidemia with atypical antipsychotics is unknown

Notable Side Effects

✻ May increase risk for diabetes and dyslipidemia

✻ Dose-dependent extrapyramidal symptoms

✻ Dose-related hyperprolactinemia
- Rare tardive dyskinesia (much reduced risk compared to conventional antipsychotics)
- Dizziness, insomnia, headache, anxiety, sedation
- Nausea, constipation, abdominal pain, weight gain
- Rare orthostatic hypotension, usually during initial dose titration
- Tachycardia, sexual dysfunction

Life-Threatening or Dangerous Side Effects

- Hyperglycemia, in some cases extreme and associated with ketoacidosis or hyperosmolar coma or death, has been reported in patients taking atypical antipsychotics
- Increased risk of death and cerebrovascular events in elderly patients with dementia-related psychosis
- Rare neuroleptic malignant syndrome (much reduced risk compared to conventional antipsychotics)
- Rare seizures

Weight Gain

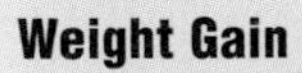

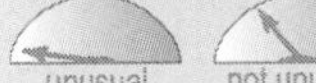

unusual | not unusual | **common** | problematic

- Many patients experience and/or can be significant in amount
- Can become a health problem in some
- May be less than for some antipsychotics, more than for others

Sedation

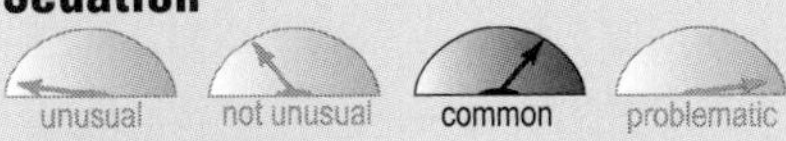

unusual | not unusual | **common** | problematic

- Many patients experience and/or can be significant in amount
- Usually transient
- May be less than for some antipsychotics, more than for others

What to Do About Side Effects

- Wait
- Wait
- Wait
- Take at bedtime to help reduce daytime sedation
- Anticholinergics may reduce motor side effects when present
- Weight loss, exercise programs, and medical management for high BMIs, diabetes, dyslipidemia
- Switch to another atypical antipsychotic

Best Augmenting Agents for Side Effects

- Benztropine or trihexyphenidyl for motor side effects
- Many side effects cannot be improved with an augmenting agent

DOSING AND USE

Usual Dosage Range

- 2–8 mg/day orally for acute psychosis and bipolar disorder
- 0.5–2.0 mg/day orally for children and elderly
- 25–50 mg depot intramuscularly every 2 weeks

Dosage Forms

- Tablets 0.25 mg, 0.5 mg, 1 mg, 2 mg, 3 mg, 4 mg, 6 mg
- Orally disintegrating tablets 0.5 mg, 1 mg, 2 mg
- Liquid 1 mg/mL–30 mL bottle
- Risperidone long-acting depot microspheres formulation for deep intramuscular administration 25 mg vial/kit, 37.5 mg vial/kit, 50 mg vial/kit

How To Dose

- In adults with psychosis in nonemergent settings, initial dosage recommendation is 1 mg/day orally in 2 divided doses
- Increase each day by 1 mg/day orally until desired efficacy is reached
- Maximum generally 16 mg/day orally
- Typically maximum effect is seen at 4–8 mg/day orally
- Can be administered on a once daily schedule as well as twice daily orally
- Long-acting risperidone is not recommended for patients who have not first demonstrated tolerability to oral risperidone
- Long-acting risperidone should be administered every 2 weeks by deep intramuscular gluteal injection
- Oral antipsychotic medication should be given with the first injection of long-acting risperidone and continued for 3 weeks, then discontinued
- Long-acting risperidone should only be administered by a health care professional
- Typically maximum effect with long-acting risperidone is seen at 25–50 mg every 2 weeks; maximum recommended dose is 50 mg every 2 weeks
- Titration of long-acting risperidone should occur at intervals of no less than 4 weeks
- Two different dosage strengths of long-acting risperidone should not be combined in a single administration

Dosing Tips – Oral Formulation

- ✻ **Less may be more:** lowering the dose in some patients with stable efficacy but side effects may reduce side effects without loss of efficacy, especially for doses over 6 mg/day orally
- ✻ Target doses for best efficacy/best tolerability in many adults with psychosis or bipolar disorder may be 2–6 mg/day (average 4.5 mg/day) orally
- Patients who respond to these doses may have one of the lowest drug costs among the atypical antipsychotics
- Low doses may not be adequate in difficult patients
- Rather than raise the dose above these levels in acutely agitated patients requiring acute antipsychotic actions, consider augmentation with a benzodiazepine or conventional antipsychotic, either orally or intramuscularly
- Rather than raise the dose above these levels in partial responders, consider augmentation with a mood stabilizing anticonvulsant, such as valproate or lamotrigine
- Approved for use up to 16 mg/day orally, but data suggest that risk of extrapyramidal symptoms is increased above 6 mg/day
- Risperidone oral solution is not compatible with cola or tea
- Children and elderly may need to have oral twice daily dosing during initiation and titration of drug dosing and then can switch to oral once daily when maintenance dose is reached
- Children and elderly should generally be dosed at the lower end of the dosage spectrum

Dosing Tips – Long-Acting Microsphere Depot Formulation

- ✻ When initiating long-acting risperidone formulation by intramuscular injection, onset of action can be delayed for 2 weeks while microspheres are being absorbed
- ✻ For antipsychotic coverage during initiation of long-acting risperidone, continue ongoing treatment with an oral antipsychotic or initiate treatment with some oral antipsychotic for 3 weeks
- Steady-state plasma concentrations are reached after 4 injections of long-acting risperidone and maintained for 4–6 weeks after the last injection
- For missed long-acting risperidone injections 2 or more weeks late (i.e., 28 or more days following last injection), may need to provide antipsychotic coverage with oral administration for 3 weeks while reinitiating injections
- For missed long-acting risperidone injections up to 2 weeks late (i.e., within 28 days of last injection), may not need to provide oral coverage
- Long-acting risperidone must be kept refrigerated
- Must deliver each syringe in full since drug is not in a solution (i.e., half a syringe is not necessarily half the drug dose)

Overdose

- Rarely lethal in monotherapy overdose; sedation, rapid heartbeat, convulsions, low blood pressure, difficulty breathing

Long-Term Use

- Approved to delay relapse in long-term treatment of schizophrenia
- Often used for long-term maintenance in bipolar disorder and various behavioral disorders

Habit Forming

- No

How to Stop

- Slow down-titration of oral formulation (over 6–8 weeks), especially when simultaneously beginning a new antipsychotic while switching (i.e., cross-titration)
- Rapid oral discontinuation may lead to rebound psychosis and worsening of symptoms

Pharmacokinetics

- Metabolites are active
- Metabolized by CYP450 2D6
- Parent drug of oral formulation has 20–24 hour half-life
- Long-acting risperidone has 3–6 day half-life
- Long-acting risperidone has elimination phase of approximately 7–8 weeks after last injection

Drug Interactions

- May increase effect of antihypertensive agents
- May antagonize levodopa, dopamine agonists
- Clearance of risperidone may be reduced and thus plasma levels increased by clozapine; dosing adjustment usually not necessary
- Coadministration with carbamazepine may decrease plasma levels of risperidone
- Coadministration with fluoxetine and paroxetine may increase plasma levels of risperidone
- Since risperidone is metabolized by CYP450 2D6, any agent that inhibits this enzyme could theoretically raise risperidone plasma levels; however, dose reduction of risperidone is usually not necessary when such combinations are used

Other Warnings/ Precautions

- Use with caution in patients with conditions that predispose to hypotension (dehydration, overheating)
- Risperidone should be used cautiously in patients at risk for aspiration pneumonia, as dysphagia has been reported
- Priapism has been reported

Do Not Use

- If there is a proven allergy to risperidone or paliperidone

SPECIAL POPULATIONS

Renal Impairment

- Initial 0.5 mg orally twice a day for first week; increase to 1 mg twice a day during second week
- Long-acting risperidone should not be administered unless patient has demonstrated tolerability of at least 2 mg/day orally
- Long-acting risperidone should be dosed at 25 mg every 2 weeks; oral administration should be continued for 3 weeks after the first injection

Hepatic Impairment

- Initial 0.5 mg orally twice a day for first week; increase to 1 mg twice a day during second week
- Long-acting risperidone should not be administered unless patient has demonstrated tolerability of at least 2 mg/day orally
- Long-acting risperidone should be dosed at 25 mg every 2 weeks; oral administration should be continued for 3 weeks after the first injection

Cardiac Impairment

- Drug should be used with caution because of risk of orthostatic hypotension

✻ When administered to elderly patients with atrial fibrillation, may increase the chances of stroke

Elderly

- Initial 0.5 mg orally twice a day; increase by 0.5 mg twice a day; titrate once a week for doses above 1.5 mg twice a day
- Recommended dose of long-acting risperidone is 25 mg every 2 weeks; oral administration should be continued for 3 weeks after the first injection
- Although atypical antipsychotics are commonly used for behavioral disturbances in dementia, no agent has been approved for treatment of elderly patients with dementia-related psychosis
- Elderly patients with dementia-related psychosis treated with atypical antipsychotics are at an increased risk of death compared to placebo, and also have an increased risk of cerebrovascular events

Children and Adolescents

✻ Approved for use in schizophrenia (ages 13 and older), mania/mixed episodes (ages 10 and older), and irritability associated with autism (ages 5–16)

✻ Risperidone is the most frequently used atypical antipsychotic in children and adolescents

- Clinical experience and early data suggest risperidone is safe and effective for behavioral disturbances in children and adolescents

- Children and adolescents using risperidone may need to be monitored more often than adults

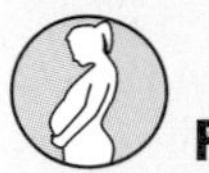

Pregnancy

- Risk Category C [some animal studies show adverse effects; no controlled studies in humans]
- Psychotic symptoms may worsen during pregnancy and some form of treatment may be necessary
- Early findings of infants exposed to risperidone in utero do not show adverse consequences
- Risperidone may be preferable to anticonvulsant mood stabilizers if treatment is required during pregnancy
- Effects of hyperprolactinemia on the fetus are unknown

Breast Feeding

- Some drug is found in mother's breast milk
- ✱ Recommended either to discontinue drug or bottle feed
- Infants of women who choose to breast feed while on risperidone should be monitored for possible adverse effects

THE ART OF PSYCHOPHARMACOLOGY

Potential Advantages

- Some cases of psychosis and bipolar disorder refractory to treatment with other antipsychotics
- ✱ Often a preferred treatment for dementia with aggressive features
- ✱ Often a preferred atypical antipsychotic for children with behavioral disturbances of multiple causations
- ✱ Noncompliant patients (long-acting risperidone)
- ✱ Long-term outcomes may be enhanced when compliance is enhanced (long-acting risperidone)

Potential Disadvantages

- Patients for whom elevated prolactin may not be desired (e.g., possibly pregnant patients; pubescent girls with amenorrhea; postmenopausal women with low estrogen who do not take estrogen replacement therapy)

Primary Target Symptoms

- Positive symptoms of psychosis
- Negative symptoms of psychosis
- Cognitive functioning
- Unstable mood (both depression and mania)
- Aggressive symptoms

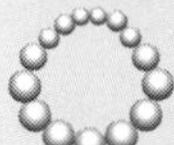

Pearls

- ✱ One of only two atypical antipsychotics with an indication in children
- ✱ Well accepted for treatment of behavioral symptoms in children and adolescents, but may have more sedation and weight gain in pediatric populations than in adult populations
- ✱ Well accepted for treatment of agitation and aggression in elderly demented patients
- Many anecdotal reports of utility in treatment-refractory cases and for positive symptoms of psychosis in disorders other than schizophrenia
- Hyperprolactinemia in women with low estrogen may accelerate osteoporosis
- Less weight gain than some antipsychotics, more than others
- Less sedation than some antipsychotics, more than others
- Risperidone is one of the least expensive atypical antipsychotics within the usual therapeutic dosing range
- Increased risk of stroke may be most relevant in the elderly with atrial fibrillation
- ✱ Controversial as to whether risperidone has more or less risk of diabetes and dyslipidemia than some other antipsychotics
- May cause more motor side effects than some other atypical antipsychotics, especially when administered to patients with Parkinson's disease or Lewy body dementia
- ✱ Only atypical antipsychotic with a long-acting depot formulation

Suggested Reading

Lieberman JA, Stroup TS, McEvoy JP. Effectiveness of antipsychotic drugs in patients with chronic schizophrenia. N Engl J Med 2005;353(12):1209–23.

Moller HJ. Long-acting injectable risperidone for the treatment of schizophrenia: clinical perspectives. Drugs 2007;67(11):1541–66.

Nasrallah HA. Atypical antipsychotic-induced metabolic side effects: insights from receptor-binding profiles. Mol Psychiatry 2008;13(1):27–35.

Scott LJ, Dhillon S. Risperidone: a review of its use in the treatment of irritability associated with autistic disorder in children and adolescents Paediatr Drs 2007;9(5):343–54.

Smith LA, Cornelius V, Warnock A, Tacchi MJ, Taylor D. Pharmacological interventions for acute bipolar mania: a systematic review of randomized placebo-controlled trials. Bipolar Disord 2007;9(6):551–60.

THERAPEUTICS

Brands • Exelon

see index for additional brand names

Generic? No

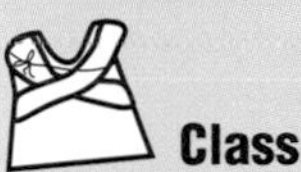

Class

- Cholinesterase inhibitor (acetylcholinesterase inhibitor and butyrylcholinesterase inhibitor); cognitive enhancer

Commonly Prescribed for

(bold for FDA approved)

- **Alzheimer disease (mild to moderate)**
- **Parkinson's disease dementia (mild to moderate)**
- Memory disorders in other conditions
- Mild cognitive impairment

How the Drug Works

✻ Pseudoirreversibly inhibits centrally active acetylcholinesterase (AChE), making more acetylcholine available
- Increased availability of acetylcholine compensates in part for degenerating cholinergic neurons in neocortex that regulate memory

✻ Inhibits butyrylcholinesterase (BuChE)
- May release growth factors or interfere with amyloid deposition

How Long Until It Works

- May take up to 6 weeks before any improvement in baseline memory or behavior is evident
- May take months before any stabilization in degenerative course is evident

If It Works

- May improve symptoms and slow progression of disease, but does not reverse the degenerative process

If It Doesn't Work

- Consider adjusting dose, switching to a different cholinesterase inhibitor or adding an appropriate augmenting agent
- Reconsider diagnosis and rule out other conditions such as depression or a dementia other than Alzheimer disease

Best Augmenting Combos for Partial Response or Treatment Resistance

✻ Atypical antipsychotics to reduce behavioral disturbances

✻ Antidepressants if concomitant depression, apathy, or lack of interest

✻ Memantine for moderate to severe Alzheimer disease
- Divalproex, carbamazepine, or oxcarbazepine for behavioral disturbances

Tests

- None for healthy individuals

SIDE EFFECTS

How Drug Causes Side Effects

- Peripheral inhibition of acetylcholinesterase can cause gastrointestinal side effects
- Peripheral inhibition of butyrylcholinesterase can cause gastrointestinal side effects
- Central inhibition of acetylcholinesterase may contribute to nausea, vomiting, weight loss, and sleep disturbances

Notable Side Effects

✻ Nausea, diarrhea, vomiting, appetite loss, weight loss, dyspepsia, increased gastric acid secretion
- Headache, dizziness
- Fatigue, asthenia, sweating

Life-Threatening or Dangerous Side Effects

- Rare seizures
- Rare syncope

Weight Gain

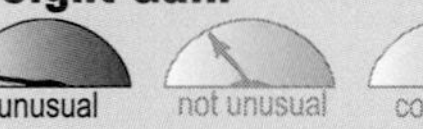

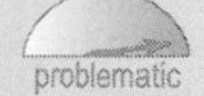

- Reported but not expected
- Some patients may experience weight loss

Sedation

unusual not unusual common problematic

- Reported but not expected

What to Do About Side Effects

- Wait

- Wait
- Wait
- Use slower dose titration
- Consider lowering dose, switching to a different agent or adding an appropriate augmenting agent

Best Augmenting Agents for Side Effects

- Many side effects cannot be improved with an augmenting agent

DOSING AND USE

Usual Dosage Range

- Oral: 6–12 mg in 2 doses
- Transdermal: 9.5 mg/24 hours once daily

Dosage Forms

- Capsule 1.5 mg, 3 mg, 4.5 mg, 6 mg
- Liquid 2 mg/mL – 120 mL bottle
- Transdermal 9 mg/5 cm^2 (4.6 mg/24 hours), 18 mg/10 cm^2 (9.5 mg/24 hours)

How To Dose

- Oral: initial 1.5 mg twice daily; increase by 3 mg every 2 weeks; titrate to tolerability; maximum dose generally 6 mg twice daily
- Transdermal: initial 4.6 mg/24 hours; after 4 weeks increase to 9.5 mg/24 hours, which is the maximum recommended dose

Dosing Tips

- Incidence of nausea is generally higher during the titration phase than during maintenance treatment
- ✻ If restarting treatment after a lapse of several days or more, dose titration should occur as when starting drug for the first time
- Oral doses between 6–12 mg/day have been shown to be more effective than doses between 1–4 mg/day
- Recommended to take oral rivastigmine with food
- Rapid dose titration increases the incidence of gastrointestinal side effects
- For transdermal formulation, dose increases should occur after a minimum of 4 weeks at the previous dose and only if the previous dose was well tolerated
- Transdermal patch should only be applied to dry, intact skin on the upper torso or another area unlikely to rub against tight clothing
- Plasma exposure with transdermal rivastigmine is 20–30% lower when applied to the abdomen or thigh as compared to the upper back, chest, or upper arm
- New application site should be selected for each day; patch should be applied at approximately the same time every day; only one patch should be applied at a time; patches should not be cut; new patch should not be applied to the same spot for at least 14 days
- Avoid touching the exposed (sticky) side of the patch, and after application, wash hands with soap and water; do not touch eyes until after hands have been washed
- Switching from oral formulation to transdermal formulation: patients receiving oral rivastigmine <6 mg/day can switch to 4.6 mg/24 hours transdermal; patients receiving oral rivastigmine 6–12 mg/day can switch to 9.5 mg/24 hours transdermal; apply the first patch on the day following the last oral dose
- Probably best to utilize highest tolerated dose within the usual dosage range
- ✻ When switching to another cholinesterase inhibitor, probably best to cross-titrate from one to the other to prevent precipitous decline in function if the patient washes out of one drug entirely

Overdose

- Can be lethal; nausea, vomiting, excess salivation, sweating, hypotension, bradycardia, collapse, convulsions, muscle weakness (weakness of respiratory muscles can lead to death)

Long-Term Use

- Drug may lose effectiveness in slowing degenerative course of Alzheimer disease after 6 months
- Can be effective in many patients for several years

Habit Forming

- No

How to Stop

- Taper not necessary

- Discontinuation may lead to notable deterioration in memory and behavior which may not be restored when drug is restarted or another cholinesterase inhibitor is initiated

Pharmacokinetics

- Elimination half-life 1–2 hours
- Not hepatically metabolized; no CYP450-mediated pharmacokinetic drug interactions

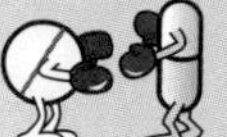

Drug Interactions

- Rivastigmine may increase the effects of anesthetics and should be discontinued prior to surgery
- Rivastigmine may interact with anticholinergic agents and the combination may decrease the efficacy of both
- Clearance of rivastigmine may be increased by nicotine
- May have synergistic effect if administered with cholinomimetics (e.g., bethanechol)
- Bradycardia may occur if combined with beta blockers
- Theoretically, could reduce the efficacy of levodopa in Parkinson's disease
- Not rational to combine with another cholinesterase inhibitor

Other Warnings/ Precautions

- May exacerbate asthma or other pulmonary disease
- Increased gastric acid secretion may increase the risk of ulcers
- Bradycardia or heart block may occur in patients with or without cardiac impairment

✻ Severe vomiting with esophageal rupture may occur if rivastigmine therapy is resumed without retitrating the drug to full dosing

- Individuals with low body weight may be at greater risk for adverse effects

Do Not Use

- If there is a proven allergy to rivastigmine or other carbamates

SPECIAL POPULATIONS

Renal Impairment

- Dose adjustment not necessary; titrate to point of tolerability

Hepatic Impairment

- Dose adjustment not necessary; titrate to point of tolerability

Cardiac Impairment

- Should be used with caution
- Syncopal episodes have been reported with the use of rivastigmine

Elderly

- Some patients may tolerate lower doses better

Children and Adolescents

- Safety and efficacy have not been established

Pregnancy

- Risk Category B [animal studies do not show adverse effects; no controlled studies in humans]

✻ Not recommended for use in pregnant women or women of childbearing potential

Breast Feeding

- Unknown if rivastigmine is secreted in human breast milk, but all psychotropics assumed to be secreted in breast milk

✻ Recommended either to discontinue drug or bottle feed

- Rivastigmine is not recommended for use in nursing women

THE ART OF PSYCHOPHARMACOLOGY

Potential Advantages

- Theoretically, butyrylcholinesterase inhibition centrally could enhance therapeutic efficacy
- May be useful in some patients who do not respond to or do not tolerate other cholinesterase inhibitors
- Later stages or rapidly progressive Alzheimer disease

Potential Disadvantages

- Theoretically, butyrylcholinesterase inhibition peripherally could enhance side effects

Primary Target Symptoms

- Memory loss in Alzheimer disease
- Behavioral symptoms in Alzheimer disease
- Memory loss in other dementias

Pearls

- Dramatic reversal of symptoms of Alzheimer disease is not generally seen with cholinesterase inhibitors
- Can lead to therapeutic nihilism among prescribers and lack of an appropriate trial of a cholinesterase inhibitor

✻ Perhaps only 50% of Alzheimer patients are diagnosed, and only 50% of those diagnosed are treated, and only 50% of those treated are given a cholinesterase inhibitor, and then only for 200 days in a disease that lasts 7–10 years

- Must evaluate lack of efficacy and loss of efficacy over months, not weeks

✻ Treats behavioral and psychological symptoms of Alzheimer dementia as well as cognitive symptoms (i.e., especially apathy, disinhibition, delusions, anxiety, lack of cooperation, pacing)

- Patients who themselves complain of memory problems may have depression, whereas patients whose spouses or children complain of the patient's memory problems may have Alzheimer disease
- Treat the patient but ask the caregiver about efficacy
- What you see may depend upon how early you treat
- The first symptoms of Alzheimer disease are generally mood changes; thus, Alzheimer disease may initially be diagnosed as depression
- Women may experience cognitive symptoms in perimenopause as a result of hormonal changes that are not a sign of dementia or Alzheimer disease
- Aggressively treat concomitant symptoms with augmentation (e.g., atypical antipsychotics for agitation, antidepressants for depression)
- If treatment with antidepressants fails to improve apathy and depressed mood in the elderly, it is possible that this represents early Alzheimer disease and a cholinesterase inhibitor like rivastigmine may be helpful
- What to expect from a cholinesterase inhibitor:
  - Patients do not generally improve dramatically although this can be observed in a significant minority of patients
  - Onset of behavioral problems and nursing home placement can be delayed
  - Functional outcomes, including activities of daily living, can be preserved
  - Caregiver burden and stress can be reduced
- Delay in progression in Alzheimer disease is not evidence of disease-modifying actions of cholinesterase inhibition
- Cholinesterase inhibitors like rivastigmine depend upon the presence of intact targets for acetylcholine for maximum effectiveness and thus may be most effective in the early stages of Alzheimer disease
- The most prominent side effects of rivastigmine are gastrointestinal effects, which are usually mild and transient

✻ May cause more gastrointestinal side effects than some other cholinesterase inhibitors, especially if not slowly titrated

- At recommended doses, transdermal formulation may have lower incidence of gastrointestinal side effects than oral formulation
- Use with caution in underweight or frail patients
- Weight loss can be a problem in Alzheimer patients with debilitation and muscle wasting
- Women over 85, particularly with low body weights, may experience more adverse effects
- For patients with intolerable side effects, generally allow a washout period with resolution of side effects prior to switching to another cholinesterase inhibitor
- Cognitive improvement may be linked to substantial (>65%) inhibition of acetylcholinesterase
- Rivastigmine may be more selective for the form of acetylcholinesterase in hippocampus (G1)

✻ More potent inhibitor of the G1 form of acetylcholinesterase enzyme, found in high concentrations in Alzheimer patient's brains, than the G4 form of the enzyme
- Butyrylcholinesterase action in the brain may not be relevant in individuals without Alzheimer disease or in early Alzheimer disease; in the later stages of the disease, enzyme actively increases as gliosis occurs
- Rivastigmine's effects on butyrylcholinesterase may be more relevant in later stages of Alzheimer disease, when gliosis is occurring

✻ May be more useful for later stages or for more rapidly progressive forms of Alzheimer disease, when gliosis increases butyrlylcholinesterase

✻ Butyrylcholinesterase actively could interfere with amyloid plaque formation, which contains this enzyme
- Some Alzheimer patients who fail to respond to another cholinesterase inhibitor may respond when switched to rivastigmine
- Some Alzheimer patients who fail to respond to rivastigmine may respond to another cholinesterase inhibitor
- To prevent potential clinical deterioration, generally switch from long-term treatment with one cholinesterase inhibitor to another without a washout period

✻ May slow the progression of mild cognitive impairment to Alzheimer disease

✻ May be useful for dementia with Lewy bodies (DLB, constituted by early loss of attentiveness and visual perception with possible hallucinations, Parkinson-like movement problems, fluctuating cognition such as daytime drowsiness and lethargy, staring into space for long periods, episodes of disorganized speech)
- May decrease delusion, apathy, agitation, and hallucinations in dementia with Lewy bodies

✻ May be useful for vascular dementia (e.g., acute onset with slow stepwise progression that has plateaus, often with gait abnormalities, focal signs, imbalance, and urinary incontinence)
- May be helpful for dementia in Down's syndrome
- Suggestions of utility in some cases of treatment-resistant bipolar disorder
- Theoretically, may be useful for ADHD, but not yet proven
- Theoretically, could be useful in any memory condition characterized by cholinergic deficiency (e.g., some cases of brain injury, cancer chemotherapy-induced cognitive changes, etc.)

Suggested Reading

Bentue-Ferrer D, Tribut O, Polard E, Allain H. Clinically significant drug interactions with cholinesterase inhibitors: a guide for neurologists. CNS Drugs 2003;17:947–63.

Bonner LT, Peskind ER. Pharmacologic treatments of dementia. Med Clin North Am 2002;86:657–74.

Jones RW. Have cholinergic therapies reached their clinical boundary in Alzheimer's disease? Int J Geriatr Psychiatry 2003;18(Suppl 1): S7–S13.

Stahl SM. Cholinesterase inhibitors for Alzheimer's disease. Hosp Pract (Off Ed) 1998;33:131–6.

Stahl SM. The new cholinesterase inhibitors for Alzheimer's disease, part 1. J Clin Psychiatry 2000;61:710–11.

Stahl SM. The new cholinesterase inhibitors for Alzheimer's disease, part 2. J Clin Psychiatry 2000;61:813–14.

Williams BR, Nazarians A, Gill MA. A review of rivastigmine: a reversible cholinesterase inhibitor. Clin Ther 2003;25:1634–53.

THERAPEUTICS

Brands
- EMSAM
- Eldepryl

see index for additional brand names

Generic? Yes (oral only)

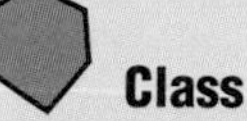

Class
- Transdermal: tissue selective monoamine oxidase (MAO) inhibitor (MAO-A and MAO-B inhibitor in brain and relatively selective MAO-B inhibitor in gut)
- Oral: selective MAO-B inhibitor

Commonly Prescribed for
(bold for FDA approved)
- **Major depressive disorder (transdermal)**
- **Oral: Parkinson's disease or symptomatic Parkinsonism (adjunctive)**
- Treatment-resistant depression
- Panic disorder (transdermal)
- Social anxiety disorder (transdermal)
- Treatment-resistant anxiety disorders (transdermal)
- Alzheimer disease and other dementias (oral)

How the Drug Works
- Transdermal selegiline (recommended doses): in the brain, irreversibly inhibits both MAO-A and MAO-B from breaking down norepinephrine, serotonin, and dopamine, which presumably boosts noradrenergic, serotonergic, and dopaminergic neurotransmission
- Transdermal selegiline (recommended doses): in the gut, is a relatively selective irreversible inhibitor of MAO-B (intestine and liver), reducing the chances of dietary interactions with the MAO-A substrate tyramine
- Oral: at recommended doses, selectively and irreversibly blocks MAO-B, which presumably boosts dopaminergic neurotransmission
- Oral: above recommended doses, irreversibly blocks both MAO-A and MAO-B from breaking down norepinephrine, serotonin, and dopamine while simultaneously blocking metabolism of tyramine in the gut
- Thus, high dose oral administration is not tissue selective and is not MAO-A sparing in the gut, and may interact with tyramine-containing foods to cause hypertension

How Long Until It Works
- Onset of therapeutic actions in depression with transdermal administration is usually not immediate, but often delayed 2–4 weeks or longer
- If it is not working for depression within 6–8 weeks, it may require a dosage increase or it may not work at all
- May continue to work in depression for many years to prevent relapse of symptoms
- Can enhance the actions of levodopa in Parkinson's disease within a few weeks of initiating oral dosing
- Theoretical slowing of functional loss in both Parkinson's disease and Alzheimer disease is a provocative possibility under investigation and would take many months or more than a year to observe

If It Works
- The goal of treatment in depression is complete remission of current symptoms as well as prevention of future relapses
- Treatment of depression most often reduces or even eliminates symptoms, but not a cure since symptoms can recur after medicine stopped
- Continue treatment of depression until all symptoms of depression are gone (remission)
- Once symptoms of depression are gone, continue treating for 1 year for the first episode of depression
- For second and subsequent episodes of depression, treatment may need to be indefinite
- Continue use in Parkinson's disease as long as there is evidence that selegiline is favorably enhancing the actions of levodopa
- Use of selegiline to slow functional loss in Parkinson's disease or Alzheimer disease would be long-term if proven effective for this use

If It Doesn't Work
- Many depressed patients only have a partial response where some symptoms are improved but others persist (especially insomnia, fatigue, and problems concentrating)

- Other depressed patients may be nonresponders, sometimes called treatment-resistant or treatment-refractory
- Some depressed patients who have an initial response may relapse even though they continue treatment, sometimes called "poop out"
- For depression, consider increasing dose, switching to another agent or adding an appropriate augmenting agent, psychotherapy, and evaluation for another diagnosis or for a comorbid condition (e.g., medical illness, substance abuse, etc.)
- Some patients may experience apparent lack of consistent efficacy due to activation of latent or underlying bipolar disorder, and require antidepressant discontinuation and a switch to a mood stabilizer
- Use alternate treatments for Parkinson's disease or Alzheimer's disease

Best Augmenting Combos for Partial Response or Treatment Resistance

✻ Augmentation of selegiline has not been systematically studied in depression, and this is something for the expert, to be done with caution and with careful monitoring

- A stimulant such as d-amphetamine or methylphenidate (with caution and by experts only as use of stimulants with selegiline is listed as a warning; may activate bipolar disorder and suicidal ideation; may elevate blood pressure)
- Lithium
- Mood-stabilizing anticonvulsants
- Atypical antipsychotics (with special caution for those agents with monoamine reuptake blocking properties, such as ziprasidone and zotepine)
- Carbidopa-levodopa (for Parkinson's disease)

Tests

- Patients should be monitored for changes in blood pressure
- Although preliminary evidence from clinical trials suggests little or no weight gain, nonselective MAO inhibitors are frequently associated with weight gain. Thus, before starting treatment for depression with high doses of selegiline, weigh all patients and determine if the patient is already overweight (BMI >25.0–29.9) or obese (BMI ≥30)
- Before giving a drug that can cause weight gain to an overweight or obese patient, consider determining whether the patient already has pre-diabetes (fasting plasma glucose 100–25 mg/dl), diabetes (fasting plasma glucose >126 mg/dl), or dyslipidemia (increased total cholesterol, LDL cholesterol and triglycerides; decreased HDL cholesterol), and treat or refer such patients for treatment including nutrition and weight management, physical activity counseling, smoking cessation, and medical management

✻ Monitor weight and BMI during treatment

✻ While giving a drug to a patient who has gained >5% of initial weight, consider evaluating for the presence of pre-diabetes, diabetes, or dyslipidemia, or consider switching to a different antidepressant

SIDE EFFECTS

How Drug Causes Side Effects

- At recommended transdermal doses, norepinephrine, serotonin and dopamine increase in parts of the brain and at receptors other than those that cause therapeutic actions
- At high transdermal doses, loss of tissue selectivity and loss of MAO-A sparing actions in the gut may enhance the possibility of dietary tyramine interactions if MAO-B inhibition occurs in the gut
- At recommended oral doses, dopamine increases in parts of the brain and body and at receptors other than those that cause therapeutic actions
- Side effects are generally immediate, but immediate side effects often disappear in time

Notable Side Effects

- Transdermal: application site reactions, headache, insomnia, diarrhea, dry mouth
- Oral: exacerbation of levodopa side effects, especially nausea, dizziness, abdominal pain, dry mouth, headache, dyskinesia, confusion, hallucinations, vivid dreams

Life-Threatening or Dangerous Side Effects

- Transdermal: hypertensive crisis was not observed with preliminary experience in clinical trials, even in patients who were not following a low tyramine diet
- Oral: hypertensive crisis (especially when MAOIs are used with certain tryamine-containing foods or prohibited drugs) – reduced risk at low oral doses compared to nonselective MAOIs
- Theoretically, when used at high doses may induce seizures and mania as do nonselective MAOIs
- Rare activation of suicidal ideation and behavior (suicidality) (short-term studies did not show an increase in the risk of suicidality with antidepressants compared to placebo beyond age 24)

Weight Gain

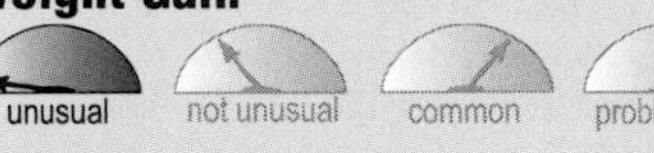

- Transdermal: Reported but not expected; some patients may experience weight loss
- Oral: Occurs in significant minority

Sedation

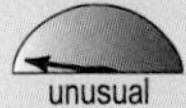

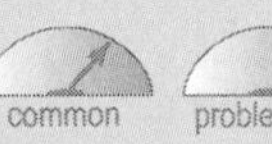

- Reported but not expected
- Can be activating in some patients

What to Do About Side Effects

- Wait
- Wait
- Wait
- Lower the dose
- Switch after appropriate washout to an SSRI or newer antidepressant (depression)
- Switch to other anti-parkinsonian therapies (Parkinson's disease)

Best Augmenting Agents for Side Effects

- Trazodone (with caution) for insomnia in depression
- Benzodiazepines for insomnia in depression
- Single oral or sublingual dose of a calcium channel blocker (e.g., nifedipine) for urgent treatment of hypertension due to drug interaction or dietary tyramine
- Many side effects cannot be improved with an augmenting agent, especially at lower doses

DOSING AND USE

Usual Dosage Range

- Depression (transdermal): 6 mg/24 hours–12 mg/24 hours
- Depression (oral): 30–60 mg/day
- Parkinson's disease/Alzheimer disease: 5–10 mg/day

Dosage Forms

- Transdermal patch 20 mg/20 cm² (6 mg/24 hours), 30 mg/30 cm² (9 mg/24 hours), 40 mg/40cm² (12 mg/24 hours)
- Capsule 5 mg
- Tablet 5 mg scored

How To Dose

- Depression (transdermal): Initial 6 mg/24 hours; can increase by 3 mg/24 hours every 2 weeks; maximum dose generally 12 mg/24 hours
- Parkinson's disease: Initial 2.5 mg/day twice daily; increase to 5 mg twice daily; reduce dose of levodopa after 2–3 days

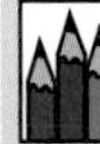

Dosing Tips

- Transdermal patch contains 1 mg of selegiline per 1 cm² and delivers approximately 0.3 mg of selegiline per cm² over 24 hours
- Patch is available in three sizes – 20 mg/20 cm², 30 mg/30 cm², and 40 mg/40 cm² – that deliver doses of approximately 6 mg, 9 mg, and 12 mg, respectively, over 24 hours
- At 6 mg/24 hours (transdermal) dietary adjustments are not generally required
- Dietary modifications to restrict tyramine intake from foods are recommended for doses above 6 mg/24 hours (transdermal)
- Transdermal patch should only be applied to dry, intact skin on the upper torso, upper thigh, or outer surface of the upper arm
- New application site should be selected for each day; patch should be applied at approximately the same time every day;

only one patch should be applied at a time; patches should not be cut
- Avoid touching the exposed (sticky) side of the patch, and after application, wash hands with soap and water; do not touch eyes until after hands have been washed
- Heat could theoretically increase the amount of selegiline absorbed from the transdermal patch, so patients should avoid exposing the application site to external sources of direct heat (e.g., heating pads, prolonged direct sunlight)
- Although there is theoretically a three day reservoir of drug in each patch, multiday administration from a single patch is generally not recommended and has not been tested; because of residual drug in the patch after 24 hours of administration, discard used patches in a manner that prevents accidental application or ingestion by children, pets, or others
- For Parkinson's disease, oral dosage above 10 mg/day generally not recommended
- Dosage of carbidopa-levodopa can at times be reduced by 10–30% after 2–3 days of administering oral selegiline 5–10 mg/day in Parkinson's disease
- At doses above 10 mg/day (oral), selegiline may become nonselective and inhibit both MAO-A and MAO-B
- At doses above 30 mg/day (oral), selegiline may have antidepressant properties
- Patients receiving high oral doses may need to be evaluated periodically for effects on the liver
- Doses above 10 mg/day (oral) may increase the risk of hypertensive crisis, tyramine interactions, and drug interactions similar to those of phenelzine and tranylcypromine

Overdose
- Overdose with the transdermal formulation is likely to produce substantial amounts of MAO-A inhibition as well as MAO-B inhibition, and should be treated the same as overdose with a nonselective oral MAO inhibitor
- Dizziness, anxiety, ataxia, insomnia, sedation, irritability, headache; cardiovascular effects, confusion, respiratory depression, coma

Long-Term Use
- Long-term use has not been systematically studied although generally recommended for chronic use as for other antidepressants

Habit Forming
- Lack of evidence for abuse potential with transdermal selegiline despite its metabolism to l-amphetamine and l-methamphetamine
- Some patients have developed dependence to other MAOIs

How to Stop
- Transdermal: MAO inhibition slowly recovers over 2–3 weeks after patch removed
- Oral: Generally no need to taper, as the drug wears off slowly over 2–3 weeks

Pharmacokinetics
- Clinical duration of action may be up to 21 days due to irreversible enzyme inhibition
- Major metabolite of selegiline is desmethylselegiline; other metabolites are l-methamphetamine and l-amphetamine
- Because first-pass metabolism is not extensive with transdermal dosing, this results in notably higher exposure to selegiline and lower exposure to metabolites as compared to oral dosing
- With transdermal selegiline, 25–30% of selegiline content is delivered systemically over 24 hours from each patch
- Mean half life of transdermal selegiline is approximately 18–25 hours
- Steady-state mean elimination half-life of oral selegiline is approximately 10 hours

Drug Interactions
- Many misunderstandings about what drugs can be combined with MAO inhibitors
- Theoretically and especially at high doses, selegiline could cause a fatal "serotonin syndrome" when combined with drugs that block serotonin reuptake (e.g., SSRIs, SNRIs, sibutramine, tramadol, clomipramine, etc), so do not use with a serotonin reuptake inhibitors for up to 5 half lives after stopping the serotonin reuptake inhibitor (i.e., "wash-in" of selegiline should be about 1 week after

discontinuing most agents [except 5 weeks or more after discontinuing fluoxetine because of its long half-life and that of its active metabolite])
- When discontinuing selegiline ("wash-out" period), wait two weeks before starting another antidepressant in order to allow enough time for the body to regenerate MAO enzyme
- Transdermal: no pharmacokinetic drug interactions present in studies with alprazolam, ibuprofen, levothyroxine, olanzapine, risperidone and warfarin
- Tramadol may increase the risk of seizures in patients taking an MAO inhibitor
- Selegiline may interact with opiate agonists to cause agitation, hallucination, or death
- Hypertensive crisis with headache, intracranial bleeding, and death may result from combining nonselective MAO inhibitors with sympathomimetic drugs (e.g., amphetamines, methylphenidate, cocaine, dopamine, epinephrine, nonepinephrine, and related compounds methyldopa, levodopa, L-tryptophan, L-tyrosine, and phenylalanine
- Excitation, seizures, delirium, hyperpyrexia, circulatory collapse, coma, and death may result from combining nonselective MAO inhibitors with mepiridine or dextromethorphan
- Do not combine with another MAO inhibitor, alcohol, buspirone, bupropion, or guanethidine
- Adverse drug reactions can result from combining MAO inhibitors with tricyclic/tetracyclic antidepressants and related compounds, including carbamazepine, cyclobenzaprine, and mirtazapine, and should be avoided except by experts to treat difficult cases
- Carbamazepine increases plasma levels of selegiline and is contraindicated with MAOIs
- MAO inhibitors in combination with spinal anesthesia may cause combined hypotensive effects
- Combination of MAOIs and CNS depressants may enhance sedation and hypotension

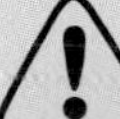

Other Warnings/ Precautions

- Ingestion of a "high tyramine meal" is generally defined as 40 mg or more of tyramine in the fasted state
- Studies show that 200–400 mg of tyramine in the fasted state (and even more ingestion of tyramine in the fed state) may be required for a hypertensive response with administration of the low dose transdermal patch (20 mg); thus, no dietary precautions are required at this dose
- Tyramine sensitivity of the low dose transdermal patch (20 mg) may be comparable to that of low dose oral selegiline (10 mg) with neither causing a hypertensive reaction to high tyramine meals
- Tyramine sensitivity and hypertensive responses to the high dose transdermal patch (40 mg) may occur with administration of 70–100 mg of tyramine in the fasted state, so dietary restrictions may also not be necessary at 30 mg or 40 mg of transdermal administration of selegiline
- However, insufficient studies have been performed to be sure of the safety of transdermal administration at 30 mg or 40 mg, so dietary restrictions of tyramine are still recommended at these higher doses
- Oral administration of nonselective irreversible MAO inhibitors generally requires adherence to a low tyramine diet
- Ingestion of a "high-tyramine meal" defined as 40 mg or more of tyramine in the fasted state or as little as ingestion of 10 mg of tyramine in the fasted state can cause hypertensive reactions in patients taking a nonselective irreversible MAO inhibitor orally
- Foods to avoid for oral administration of nonselective irreversible MAO inhibitors include: dried, aged, smoked, fermented, spoiled, or improperly stored meat, poultry, and fish; broad bean pods; aged cheeses; tap and nonpasteurized beers; marmite; sauerkraut; soy products/tofu
- These restrictions are generally recommended for patients taking the higher doses of transdermal selegiline (30 mg and 40 mg transdermally) but not

for the lower doses of transdermal selegiline (20 mg transdermally) or for the low dose orally (10 mg)
- Transdermal: studies of low-dose transdermal administration of selegiline (20 mg) failed to show changes in systolic or diastolic blood pressure or pulse when administered to normal volunteers taking either pseudoephedrine 60 mg three times a day for 2 days or 25 mg of phenylpropanolamine (no longer commercially available in the US) every 4 hours for 1 day
- However, sufficient safety information is not available to recommend administration of pseudoephedrine without a precaution; blood pressure should be monitored if low dose transdermal selegiline is given at all with pseudoephedrine
- Pseudoephedrine may need to be avoided when administering transdermal selegiline, particularly at higher doses of selegiline or in vulnerable patients with hypertension
- Although risk may be reduced with transdermal administration of selegiline, patient and prescriber must be vigilant to potential interactions with any drug, including antihypertensives and over-the-counter cough/cold preparations
- Over-the-counter medications to avoid or use with caution under the care of an expert include cough and cold preparations, including those containing dextromethorphan, nasal decongestants (tablets, drops, or spray), hay-fever medications, sinus medications, asthma inhalant medications, anti-appetite medications, weight reducing preparations, "pep" pills
- Hypoglycemia may occur in diabetic patients receiving insulin or oral antidiabetic agents
- Use cautiously in patients receiving reserpine, anesthetics, disulfiram, metrizamide, anticholinergic agents
- Selegiline is not recommended for use in patients who cannot be monitored closely
- Only use sympathomimetic agents or guanethidine with oral doses of selegiline below 10 mg/day
- When treating children, carefully weigh the risks and benefits of pharmacological treatment against the risks and benefits of nontreatment with antidepressants and make sure to document this in the patient's chart
- Distribute the brochures provide by the FDA and the drug companies
- Warn patients and their caregivers about the possibility of activating side effects and advise them to report such symptoms immediately
- Monitor patients for activation of suicidal ideation, especially children and adolescents

Do Not Use
- If patient is taking meperidine (pethidine)
- If patient is taking a sympathomimetic agent or taking guanethidine
- If patient is taking another MAOI
- If patient is taking any agent that can inhibit serotonin reuptake (e.g., SSRIs, sibutramine, tramadol, milnacipran, duloxetine, venlafaxine, clomipramine, etc.)
- If patient is taking diuretics, dextromethorphan, buspirone, bupropion
- If patient is taking St. John's wort, cyclobenzaprine, methadone, propoxyphene
- If patient has pheochromocytoma
- If patient is undergoing elective surgery and requires general anesthesia
- If there is a proven allergy to selegiline

SPECIAL POPULATIONS

Renal Impairment
- No dose adjustment necessary for transdermal administration in patients with mild to moderate renal impairment
- Use oral administration with caution – drug may accumulate in plasma in patients with renal impairment
- Oral administration may require lower than usual adult dose

Hepatic Impairment
- No dose adjustment necessary for transdermal administration in patients with mild to moderate hepatic impairment
- Oral administration may require lower than usual adult dose

Cardiac Impairment
- May require lower than usual adult dose
- Observe closely for orthostatic hypotension

Elderly
- Recommended dose for patients over 65 years old is 20 mg
- Dose increases in the elderly should be made with caution and patients should be observed for postural changes in blood pressure throughout treatment
- Reduction in risk of suicidality with antidepressants compared to placebo in adults age 65 and older

Children and Adolescents
- Not recommended for use in children under 18
- Use with caution, observing for activation of known or unknown bipolar disorder and/or suicidal ideation, and inform parents or guardians of this risk so they can help observe child or adolescent patients
- Carefully weigh the risks and benefits of pharmacological treatment against the risks and benefits of nontreatment with antidepressants and make sure to document this in the patient's chart
- Monitor patients face-to-face regularly, particularly during the first several weeks of treatment

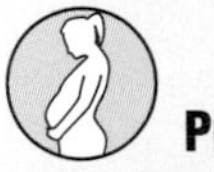

Pregnancy
- Risk Category C [some animal studies show adverse effects; no controlled studies in humans]
- Not generally recommended for use during pregnancy, especially during first trimester
- Should evaluate patient for treatment with an antidepressant with a better risk/benefit ratio

Breast Feeding
- Some drug is found in mother's breast milk
- Immediate postpartum period is a high-risk time for depression, especially in women who have had prior depressive episodes, so drug may need to be reinstituted late in the third trimester or shortly after childbirth to prevent a recurrence during the postpartum period
- Should evaluate patient for treatment with an antidepressant with a better risk/benefit ratio

THE ART OF PSYCHOPHARMACOLOGY

Potential Advantages
- Treatment-resistant depression
- Patients with atypical depression (hypersomnia, hyperphagia)
- Patients who wish to avoid weight gain and sexual dysfunction
- Parkinson's patients inadequately responsive to levodopa

Potential Disadvantages
- Noncompliant patients
- Patients with motor complications and fluctuations on levodopa treatment
- Patients with cardiac problems or hypertension

Primary Target Symptoms
- Depressed mood (depression)
- Somatic symptoms (depression)
- Sleep and eating disturbances (depression)
- Psychomotor disturbances (depression)
- Motor symptoms (Parkinson's disease)

Pearls
- Transdermal administration may allow freedom from dietary restrictions
- Transdermal selegiline theoretically appealing as a triple action agent (serotonin, norepinephrine and dopamine) for treatment-refractory and difficult cases of depression
- Transdermal selegiline may have low risk of weight gain and sexual dysfunction, and may be useful for cognitive dysfunction in attention deficit disorder and other cognitive disorders, as it increases dopamine and is metabolized to l-amphetamine and l-methamphetamine
- Low dose oral administration generally used as an adjunctive treatment for Parkinson's disease after other drugs have lost efficacy
- At oral doses used for Parkinson's disease, virtually no risk of interactions with food
- Neuroprotective effects are possible but unproved

✻ Enhancement of levodopa action can occur for Parkinson's patients at low oral doses, but antidepressant actions probably require high oral doses that do not have the potential tissue selectivity and lack of dietary restrictions of the low dose transdermal formulation

* ✻ High doses may lose safety features
* MAOIs are generally reserved for second-line use after SSRIs, SNRIs, and combinations of newer antidepressants have failed
* Patient should be advised not to take any prescription or over-the-counter drugs without consulting their doctor because of possible drug interactions
* Headache is often the first symptom of hypertensive crisis
* Myths about the danger of dietary tyramine can be exaggerated, but prohibitions against concomitant drugs often not followed closely enough
* ✻ Combining multiple psychotropic agents with MAOIs should be for the expert, especially if combining with agents of potential risk (e.g., stimulants, trazodone, TCAs)
* ✻ MAOIs should not be neglected as therapeutic agents for the treatment-resistant

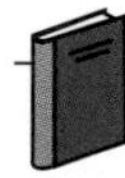

Suggested Reading

Bodkin JA, Amsterdam JD. Transdermal selegiline in major depression: a double-blind, placebo-controlled, parallel-group study in outpatients. Am J Psychiatry 2002;159(11):1869–75.

Kennedy SH. Continuation and maintenance treatments in major depression: the neglected role of monoamine oxidase inhibitors. J Psychiatry Neurosci 1997;22:127–31.

Shulman KI, Walker SE. A reevaluation of dietary restrictions for irreversible monoamine oxidase inhibitors. Psychiatr Ann 2001;31:378–84.

THERAPEUTICS

Brands • Zoloft
see index for additional brand names

Generic? Yes

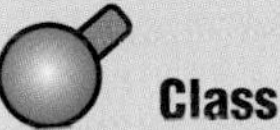

Class

- SSRI (selective serotonin reuptake inhibitor); often classified as an antidepressant, but it is not just an antidepressant

Commonly Prescribed for

(bold for FDA approved)

- **Major depressive disorder**
- **Premenstrual dysphoric disorder (PMDD)**
- **Panic disorder**
- **Posttraumatic stress disorder (PTSD)**
- **Social anxiety disorder (social phobia)**
- **Obsessive-compulsive disorder (OCD)**
- Generalized anxiety disorder (GAD)

How the Drug Works

- Boosts neurotransmitter serotonin
- Blocks serotonin reuptake pump (serotonin transporter)
- Desensitizes serotonin receptors, especially serotonin 1A receptors
- Presumably increases serotonergic neurotransmission

✻ Sertraline also has some ability to block dopamine reuptake pump (dopamine transporter), which could increase dopamine neurotransmission and contribute to its therapeutic actions

- Sertraline also has mild antagonist actions at sigma receptors

How Long Until It Works

✻ Some patients may experience increased energy or activation early after initiation of treatment

- Onset of therapeutic actions usually not immediate, but often delayed 2–4 weeks
- If it is not working within 6–8 weeks, it may require a dosage increase or it may not work at all
- May continue to work for many years to prevent relapse of symptoms

If It Works

- The goal of treatment is complete remission of current symptoms as well as prevention of future relapses
- Treatment most often reduces or even eliminates symptoms, but not a cure since symptoms can recur after medicine stopped
- Continue treatment until all symptoms are gone (remission) or significantly reduced (e.g., OCD, PTSD)
- Once symptoms gone, continue treating for 1 year for the first episode of depression
- For second and subsequent episodes of depression, treatment may need to be indefinite
- Use in anxiety disorders may also need to be indefinite

If It Doesn't Work

- Many patients only have a partial response where some symptoms are improved but others persist (especially insomnia, fatigue, and problems concentrating in depression)
- Other patients may be nonresponders, sometimes called treatment-resistant or treatment-refractory
- Some patients who have an initial response may relapse even though they continue treatment, sometimes called "poop-out"
- Consider increasing dose, switching to another agent or adding an appropriate augmenting agent
- Consider psychotherapy
- Consider evaluation for another diagnosis or for a comorbid condition (e.g., medical illness, substance abuse, etc.)
- Some patients may experience apparent lack of consistent efficacy due to activation of latent or underlying bipolar disorder, and require antidepressant discontinuation and a switch to a mood stabilizer

Best Augmenting Combos for Partial Response or Treatment Resistance

- Trazodone, especially for insomnia
- In the U.S., sertraline (Zoloft) is commonly augmented with bupropion (Wellbutrin) with good results in a combination anecdotally called "Well-loft" (use combinations of antidepressants with caution as this may activate bipolar disorder and suicidal ideation)

- Mirtazapine, reboxetine, or atomoxetine (add with caution and at lower doses since sertraline could theoretically raise atomoxetine levels); use combinations of antidepressants with caution as this may activate bipolar disorder and suicidal ideation
- Modafinil, especially for fatigue, sleepiness, and lack of concentration
- Mood stabilizers or atypical antipsychotics for bipolar depression, psychotic depression, treatment-resistant depression, or treatment-resistant anxiety disorders
- Benzodiazepines
- If all else fails for anxiety disorders, consider gabapentin or tiagabine
- Hypnotics for insomnia
- Classically, lithium, buspirone, or thyroid hormone

Tests

- None for healthy individuals

SIDE EFFECTS

How Drug Causes Side Effects

- Theoretically due to increases in serotonin concentrations at serotonin receptors in parts of the brain and body other than those that cause therapeutic actions (e.g., unwanted actions of serotonin in sleep centers causing insomnia, unwanted actions of serotonin in the gut causing diarrhea, etc.)

* Increasing serotonin can cause diminished dopamine release and might contribute to emotional flattening, cognitive slowing, and apathy in some patients, although this could theoretically be diminished in some patients by sertraline's dopamine reuptake blocking properties

- Most side effects are immediate but often go away with time, in contrast to most therapeutic effects which are delayed and are enhanced over time
- Sertraline's possible dopamine reuptake blocking properties could contribute to agitation, anxiety, and undesirable activation, especially early in dosing

Notable Side Effects

- Sexual dysfunction (men: delayed ejaculation, erectile dysfunction; men and women: decreased sexual desire, anorgasmia)
- Gastrointestinal (decreased appetite, nausea, diarrhea, constipation, dry mouth)
- Mostly central nervous system (insomnia but also sedation, agitation, tremors, headache, dizziness)
- Note: patients with diagnosed or undiagnosed bipolar or psychotic disorders may be more vulnerable to CNS-activating actions of SSRIs
- Autonomic (sweating)
- Bruising and rare bleeding
- Rare hyponatremia (mostly in elderly patients and generally reversible on discontinuation of sertraline)
- Rare hypotension

Life-Threatening or Dangerous Side Effects

- Rare seizures
- Rare induction of mania
- Rare activation of suicidal ideation and behavior (suicidality) (short-term studies did not show an increase in the risk of suicidality with antidepressants compared to placebo beyond age 24)

Weight Gain

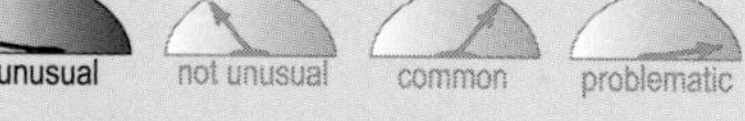

- Reported but not expected
- Some patients may actually experience weight loss

Sedation

unusual not unusual common

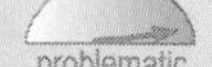

- Reported but not expected
- Possibly activating in some patients

What to Do About Side Effects

- Wait
- Wait
- Wait
- If sertraline is activating, take in the morning to help reduce insomnia
- Reduce dose to 25 mg or even 12.5 mg until side effects abate, then increase dose as tolerated, usually to at least 50 mg/day
- In a few weeks, switch or add other drugs

Best Augmenting Agents for Side Effects

- Often best to try another SSRI or another antidepressant monotherapy prior to resorting to augmentation strategies to treat side effects
- Trazodone or a hypnotic for insomnia
- Bupropion, sildenafil, vardenafil or tadalafil for sexual dysfunction
- Bupropion for emotional flattening, cognitive slowing, or apathy
- Mirtazapine for insomnia, agitation, and gastrointestinal side effects
- Benzodiazepines for jitteriness and anxiety, especially at initiation of treatment and especially for anxious patients
- Many side effects are dose-dependent (i.e., they increase as dose increases, or they reemerge until tolerance redevelops)
- Many side effects are time-dependent (i.e., they start immediately upon dosing and upon each dose increase, but go away with time)
- Activation and agitation may represent the induction of a bipolar state, especially a mixed dysphoric bipolar II condition sometimes associated with suicidal ideation, and require the addition of lithium, a mood stabilizer or an atypical antipsychotic, and/or discontinuation of sertraline

DOSING AND USE

Usual Dosage Range

- 50–200 mg/day

Dosage Forms

- Tablets 25 mg scored, 50 mg scored, 100 mg
- Oral solution 20 mg/mL

How To Dose

- Depression and OCD: initial 50 mg/day; usually wait a few weeks to assess drug effects before increasing dose, but can increase once a week; maximum generally 200 mg/day; single dose
- Panic, PTSD, and social anxiety: initial 25 mg/day; increase to 50 mg/day after 1 week thereafter, usually wait a few weeks to assess drug effects before increasing dose; maximum generally 200 mg/day; single dose
- PMDD: initial 50 mg/day; can dose daily through the menstrual cycle or limit to the luteal phase
- Oral solution: mix with 4 oz of water, ginger ale, lemon/lime soda, lemonade, or orange juice only; drink immediately after mixing

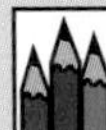

Dosing Tips

- All tablets are scored, so to save costs, give 50 mg as half of 100-mg tablet, since 100-mg and 50-mg tablets cost about the same in many markets
- Give once daily, often in the mornings to reduce chances of insomnia
- Many patients ultimately require more than 50 mg dose per day
- Some patients are dosed above 200 mg
- Evidence that some treatment-resistant OCD patients may respond safely to doses up to 400 mg/day, but this is for experts and use with caution
- The more anxious and agitated the patient, the lower the starting dose, the slower the titration, and the more likely the need for a concomitant agent such as trazodone or a benzodiazepine
- If intolerable anxiety, insomnia, agitation, akathisia, or activation occur either upon dosing initiation or discontinuation, consider the possibility of activated bipolar disorder and switch to a mood stabilizer or atypical antipsychotic
- Utilize half a 25-mg tablet (12.5 mg) when initiating treatment in patients with a history of intolerance to previous antidepressants

Overdose

- Rarely lethal in monotherapy overdose; vomiting, sedation, heart rhythm disturbances, dilated pupils, agitation; fatalities have been reported in sertraline overdose combined with other drugs or alcohol

Long-Term Use

- Safe

Habit Forming

- No

How to Stop

- Taper to avoid withdrawal effects (dizziness, nausea, stomach cramps, sweating, tingling, dysesthesias)
- Many patients tolerate 50% dose reduction for 3 days, then another 50% reduction for 3 days, then discontinuation
- If withdrawal symptoms emerge during discontinuation, raise dose to stop symptoms and then restart withdrawal much more slowly

Pharmacokinetics

- Parent drug has 22–36 hour half-life
- Metabolite half-life 62–104 hours
- Inhibits CYP450 2D6 (weakly at low doses)
- Inhibits CYP450 3A4 (weakly at low doses)

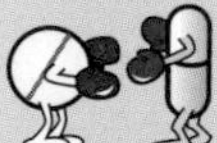

Drug Interactions

- Tramadol increases the risk of seizures in patients taking an antidepressant
- Can increase tricyclic antidepressant levels; use with caution with tricyclic antidepressants or when switching from a TCA to sertraline
- Can cause a fatal "serotonin syndrome" when combined with MAO inhibitors, so do not use with MAO inhibitors or for at least 14 days after MAOIs are stopped
- Do not start an MAO inhibitor for at least 2 weeks after discontinuing sertraline
- May displace highly protein bound drugs (e.g., warfarin)
- Can rarely cause weakness, hyperreflexia, and incoordination when combined with sumatriptan or possibly with other triptans, requiring careful monitoring of patient
- Possible increased risk of bleeding, especially when combined with anticoagulants (e.g., warfarin, NSAIDs)
- Via CYP450 2D6 inhibition, sertraline could theoretically interfere with the analgesic actions of codeine, and increase the plasma levels of some beta blockers and of atomoxetine
- Via CYP450 2D6 inhibition sertraline could theoretically increase concentrations of thioridazine and cause dangerous cardiac arrhythmias
- Via CYP450 3A4 inhibition, sertraline may increase the levels of alprazolam, buspirone, and triazolam
- Via CYP450 3A4 inhibition, sertraline could theoretically increase concentrations of certain cholesterol lowering HMG CoA reductase inhibitors, especially simvastatin, atorvastatin, and lovastatin, but not pravastatin or fluvastatin, which would increase the risk of rhabdomyolysis; thus, coadministration of sertraline with certain HMG CoA reductase inhibitors should proceed with caution
- Via CYP450 3A4 inhibition, sertraline could theoretically increase the concentrations of pimozide, and cause QTc prolongation and dangerous cardiac arrhythmias

Other Warnings/ Precautions

- Add or initiate other antidepressants with caution for up to 2 weeks after discontinuing sertraline
- Use with caution in patients with history of seizures
- Use with caution in patients with bipolar disorder unless treated with concomitant mood stabilizing agent
- When treating children, carefully weigh the risks and benefits of pharmacological treatment against the risks and benefits of nontreatment with antidepressants and make sure to document this in the patient's chart
- Distribute the brochures provided by the FDA and the drug companies
- Warn patients and their caregivers about the possibility of activating side effects and advise them to report such symptoms immediately
- Monitor patients for activation of suicidal ideation, especially children and adolescents

Do Not Use

- If patient is taking an MAO inhibitor
- If patient is taking pimozide
- If patient is taking thioridazine
- Use of sertraline oral concentrate is contraindicated with disulfiram due to the alcohol content of the concentrate
- If there is a proven allergy to sertraline

SPECIAL POPULATIONS

Renal Impairment

- No dose adjustment
- Not removed by hemodialysis

Hepatic Impairment
- Lower dose or give less frequently, perhaps by half

Cardiac Impairment
- Proven cardiovascular safety in depressed patients with recent myocardial infarction or angina
- Treating depression with SSRIs in patients with acute angina or following myocardial infarction may reduce cardiac events and improve survival as well as mood

Elderly
- Some patients may tolerate lower doses and/or slower titration better
- Reduction in risk of suicidality with antidepressants compared to placebo in adults age 65 and older

Children and Adolescents
- Carefully weigh the risks and benefits of pharmacological treatment against the risks and benefits of nontreatment with antidepressants and make sure to document this in the patient's chart
- Monitor patients face-to-face regularly, particularly during the first several weeks of treatment
- Use with caution, observing for activation of known or unknown bipolar disorder and/or suicidal ideation, and inform parents or guardian of this risk so they can help observe child or adolescent patients
- Approved for use in OCD
- Ages 6–12: initial dose 25 mg/day
- Ages 13 and up: adult dosing
- Long-term effects, particularly on growth, have not been studied

Pregnancy
- Risk Category C [some animal studies show adverse effects; no controlled studies in humans]
- Not generally recommended for use during pregnancy, especially during first trimester
- Nonetheless, continuous treatment during pregnancy may be necessary and has not been proven to be harmful to the fetus
- At delivery there may be more bleeding in the mother and transient irritability or sedation in the newborn
- Must weigh the risk of treatment (first trimester fetal development, third trimester newborn delivery) to the child against the risk of no treatment (recurrence of depression, maternal health, infant bonding) to the mother and child
- For many patients this may mean continuing treatment during pregnancy
- SSRI use beyond the 20th week of pregnancy may be associated with increased risk of pulmonary hypertension in newborns
- Neonates exposed to SSRIs or SNRIs late in the third trimester have developed complications requiring prolonged hospitalization, respiratory support, and tube feeding; reported symptoms are consistent with either a direct toxic effect of SSRIs and SNRIs or, possibly, a drug discontinuation syndrome, and include respiratory distress, cyanosis, apnea, seizures, temperature instability, feeding difficulty, vomiting, hypoglycemia, hypotonia, hypertonia, hyperreflexia, tremor, jitteriness, irritability, and constant crying

Breast Feeding
- Some drug is found in mother's breast milk
- Trace amounts may be present in nursing children whose mothers are on sertraline
- Sertraline has shown efficacy in treating postpartum depression
- If child becomes irritable or sedated, breast feeding or drug may need to be discontinued
- Immediate postpartum period is a high-risk time for depression, especially in women who have had prior depressive episodes, so drug may need to be reinstituted late in the third trimester or shortly after childbirth to prevent a recurrence during the postpartum period
- Must weigh benefits of breast feeding with risks and benefits of antidepressant treatment versus nontreatment to both the infant and the mother
- For many patients, this may mean continuing treatment during breast feeding

THE ART OF PSYCHOPHARMACOLOGY

Potential Advantages
- Patients with atypical depression (hypersomnia, increased appetite)

- Patients with fatigue and low energy
- Patients who wish to avoid hyperprolactinemia (e.g., pubescent children, girls and women with galactorrhea, girls and women with unexplained amenorrhea, postmenopausal women who are not taking estrogen replacement therapy)
- Patients who are sensitive to the prolactin-elevating properties of other SSRIs (sertraline is the one SSRI that generally does not elevate prolactin)

Potential Disadvantages

- Initiating treatment in anxious patients with some insomnia
- Patients with comorbid irritable bowel syndrome
- Can require dosage titration

Primary Target Symptoms

- Depressed mood
- Anxiety
- Sleep disturbance, both insomnia and hypersomnia (eventually, but may actually cause insomnia, especially short-term)
- Panic attacks, avoidant behavior, reexperiencing, hyperarousal

Pearls

✻ May be a type of "dual action" agent with both potent serotonin reuptake inhibition and less potent dopamine reuptake inhibition, but the clinical significance of this is unknown
- Cognitive and affective "flattening" may theoretically be diminished in some patients by sertraline's dopamine reuptake blocking properties

✻ May be a first-line choice for atypical depression (e.g., hypersomnia, hyperphagia, low energy, mood reactivity)
- Best documented cardiovascular safety of any antidepressant, proven safe for depressed patients with recent myocardial infarction or angina
- May block sigma 1 receptors, enhancing sertraline's anxiolytic actions
- Can have more gastrointestinal effects, particularly diarrhea, than some other antidepressants
- May be more effective treatment for women with PTSD or depression than for men with PTSD or depression, but the clinical significance of this is unknown
- SSRIs may be less effective in women over 50, especially if they are not taking estrogen
- SSRIs may be useful for hot flushes in perimenopausal women
- For sexual dysfunction, can augment with bupropion, sildenafil, vardenafil, tadalafil, or switch to a non-SSRI such as bupropion or mirtazapine
- Some postmenopausal women's depression will respond better to sertraline plus estrogen augmentation than to sertraline alone
- Nonresponse to sertraline in elderly may require consideration of mild cognitive impairment or Alzheimer disease
- Not as well tolerated as some SSRIs for panic, especially when dosing is initiated, unless given with co-therapies such as benzodiazepines or trazodone
- Relative lack of effect on prolactin may make it a preferred agent for some children, adolescents, and women
- Some evidence suggests that sertraline treatment during only the luteal phase may be more effective than continuous treatment for patients with PMDD

Suggested Reading

DeVane CL, Liston HL, Markowitz JS. Clinical pharmacokinetics of sertraline. Clin Pharmacokinet 2002;41:1247–66.

Flament MF, Lane RM, Zhu R, Ying Z. Predictors of an acute antidepressant response to fluoxetine and sertraline. International Clin Psychopharmacol 1999;14:259–75.

Khouzam HR, Emes R, Gill T, Raroque R. The antidepressant sertraline: a review of its uses in a range of psychiatric and medical conditions. Compr Ther 2003;29:47–53.

McRae AL, Brady KT. Review of sertraline and its clinical applications in psychiatric disorders. Expert Opin Pharmacother 2001;2:883–92.

THERAPEUTICS

Brands • Dolmatil

see index for additional brand names

Generic? Yes

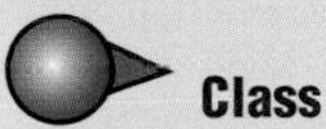

Class

- Conventional antipsychotic (neuroleptic, benzamide, dopamine 2 antagonist)

Commonly Prescribed for

(bold for FDA approved)

- Schizophrenia
- Depression

How the Drug Works

- Blocks dopamine 2 receptors, reducing positive symptoms of psychosis
- Blocks dopamine 3 and 4 receptors, which may contribute to sulpiride's actions

✻ Possibly blocks presynaptic dopamine 2 autoreceptors more potently at low doses, which could theoretically contribute to improving negative symptoms of schizophrenia as well as depression

How Long Until It Works

- Psychotic symptoms can improve within 1 week, but it may take several weeks for full effect on behavior

If It Works

- Most often reduces positive symptoms in schizophrenia but does not eliminate them
- Most schizophrenic patients do not have a total remission of symptoms but rather a reduction of symptoms by about a third
- Continue treatment in schizophrenia until reaching a plateau of improvement
- After reaching a satisfactory plateau, continue treatment for at least a year after first episode of psychosis in schizophrenia
- For second and subsequent episodes of psychosis in schizophrenia, treatment may need to be indefinite

If It Doesn't Work

- Consider trying one of the first-line atypical antipsychotics (risperidone, olanzapine, quetiapine, ziprasidone, aripiprazole, paliperidone, amisulpride)
- Consider trying another conventional antipsychotic
- If 2 or more antipsychotic monotherapies do not work, consider clozapine

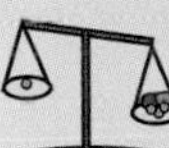

Best Augmenting Combos for Partial Response or Treatment Resistance

- Augmentation of conventional antipsychotics has not been systematically studied
- Addition of a mood-stabilizing anticonvulsant such as valproate, carbamazepine, or lamotrigine may be helpful in both schizophrenia and bipolar mania
- Augmentation with lithium in bipolar mania may be helpful
- Addition of a benzodiazepine, especially short-term for agitation

Tests

✻ Since conventional antipsychotics are frequently associated with weight gain, before starting treatment, weigh all patients and determine if the patient is already overweight (BMI 25.0–29.9) or obese (BMI ≥30)

- Before giving a drug that can cause weight gain to an overweight or obese patient, consider determining whether the patient already has pre-diabetes (fasting plasma glucose 100–25 mg/dL), diabetes (fasting plasma glucose >126 mg/dL), or dyslipidemia (increased total cholesterol, LDL cholesterol and triglycerides; decreased HDL cholesterol), and treat or refer such patients for treatment, including nutrition and weight management, physical activity counseling, smoking cessation, and medical management

✻ Consider monitoring fasting triglycerides monthly for several months in patients at high risk for metabolic complications and when initiating or switching antipsychotics

✻ Monitor weight and BMI during treatment

✻ While giving a drug to a patient who has gained >5% of initial weight, consider evaluating for the presence of pre-diabetes, diabetes, or dyslipidemia, or consider switching to a different antipsychotic

- Monitoring elevated prolactin levels of dubious clinical benefit

SIDE EFFECTS

How Drug Causes Side Effects

- By blocking dopamine 2 receptors in the striatum, it can cause motor side effects
- By blocking dopamine 2 receptors in the pituitary, it can cause elevations in prolactin
- By blocking dopamine 2 receptors excessively in the mesocortical and mesolimbic dopamine pathways, especially at high doses, it can cause worsening of negative and cognitive symptoms (neuroleptic-induced deficit syndrome)
- Anticholinergic actions may cause sedation, blurred vision, constipation, dry mouth
- Antihistaminic actions may cause sedation, weight gain
- By blocking alpha 1 adrenergic receptors, it can cause dizziness, sedation, and hypotension
- Mechanism of weight gain and any possible increased incidence of diabetes or dyslipidemia with conventional antipsychotics is unknown

Notable Side Effects

✱ Extrapyramidal symptoms, akathisia
✱ Prolactin elevation, galactorrhea, amenorrhea
- Sedation, dizziness, sleep disturbance, headache, impaired concentration
- Dry mouth, nausea, vomiting, constipation, anorexia
- Impotence
- Rare tardive dyskinesia
- Rare hypomania
- Palpitations, hypertension
- Weight gain

Life-Threatening or Dangerous Side Effects

- Rare neuroleptic malignant syndrome
- Rare seizures
- Increased risk of death and cerebrovascular events in elderly patients with dementia-related psychosis

Weight Gain

unusual | not unusual | **common** | problematic

- Many experience and/or can be significant in amount

Sedation

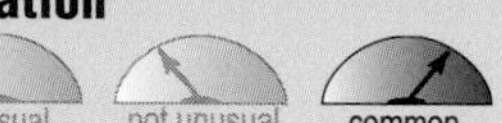
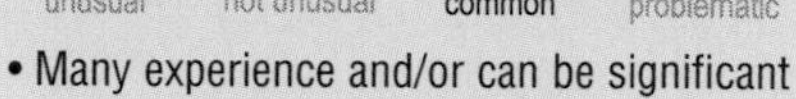

- Many experience and/or can be significant in amount, especially at high doses

What to Do About Side Effects

- Wait
- Wait
- Wait
- For motor symptoms, add an anticholinergic agent
- Reduce the dose
- For sedation, give at night
- Switch to an atypical antipsychotic
- Weight loss, exercise programs, and medical management for high BMIs, diabetes, dyslipidemia

Best Augmenting Agents for Side Effects

- Benztropine or trihexyphenidyl for motor side effects
- Sometimes amantadine can be helpful for motor side effects
- Benzodiazepines may be helpful for akathisia
- Many side effects cannot be improved with an augmenting agent

DOSING AND USE

Usual Dosage Range

- Schizophrenia: 400–800 mg/day in 2 doses (oral)
- Predominantly negative symptoms: 50–300 mg/day (oral)
- Intramuscular injection: 600–800 mg/day
- Depression: 150–300 mg/day (oral)

Dosage Forms

- Different formulations may be available in different markets
- Tablet 200 mg, 400 mg, 500 mg
- Intramuscular injection 50 mg/mL, 100 mg/mL

How To Dose

- Initial 400–800 mg/day in 1–2 doses; may need to increase dose to control positive symptoms; maximum generally 2,400 mg/day

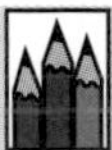

Dosing Tips

- ✻ Low doses of sulpiride may be more effective at reducing negative symptoms than positive symptoms in schizophrenia; high doses may be equally effective at reducing both symptom dimensions
- ✻ Lower doses are more likely to be activating; higher doses are more likely to be sedating
- Some patients receive more than 2,400 mg/day

Overdose

- Can be fatal; vomiting, agitation, hypotension, hallucinations, CNS depression, sinus tachycardia, arrhythmia, dystonia, dysarthria, hyperreflexia

Long-Term Use

- Apparently safe, but not well-studied

Habit Forming

- No

How to Stop

- Recommended to reduce dose over a week
- Slow down-titration (over 6–8 weeks), especially when simultaneously beginning a new antipsychotic while switching (i.e., cross-titration)
- Rapid discontinuation may lead to rebound psychosis and worsening of symptoms
- If antiparkinson agents are being used, they should be continued for a few weeks after sulpiride is discontinued

Pharmacokinetics

- Elimination half-life approximately 6–8 hours
- Excreted largely unchanged

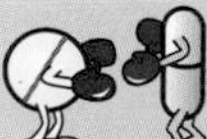

Drug Interactions

- Sulpiride may increase the effects of antihypertensive drugs
- CNS effects may be increased if sulpiride is used with other CNS depressants
- May decrease the effects of levodopa, dopamine agonists
- Antacids or sucralfate may reduce the absorption of sulpiride

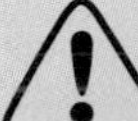

Other Warnings/ Precautions

- If signs of neuroleptic malignant syndrome develop, treatment should be immediately discontinued
- Use cautiously in patients with alcohol withdrawal or convulsive disorders because of possible lowering of seizure threshold
- Antiemetic effect of sulpiride may mask signs of other disorders or overdose; suppression of cough reflex may cause asphyxia
- Use with caution in patients with hypertension, cardiovascular disease, pulmonary disease, hyperthyroidism, urinary retention, glaucoma
- May exacerbate symptoms of mania or hypomania
- Use only with caution if at all in Parkinson's disease or Lewy body dementia

Do Not Use

- If patient has pheochromocytoma
- If patient has prolactin-dependent tumor
- If patient is pregnant or nursing
- In children under age 15
- If there is a proven allergy to sulpiride

SPECIAL POPULATIONS

Renal Impairment

- Use with caution; drug may accumulate
- Sulpiride is eliminated by the renal route; in cases of severe renal insufficiency, the dose should be decreased and intermittent treatment or switching to another antipsychotic should be considered

Heptic Impairment

- Use with caution

Cardiac Impairment

- Use with caution

Elderly

- Some patients may tolerate lower doses better
- Although conventional antipsychotics are commonly used for behavioral disturbances in dementia, no agent has been approved for treatment of elderly patients with dementia-related psychosis

- Elderly patients with dementia-related psychosis treated with antipsychotics are at an increased risk of death compared to placebo, and also have an increased risk of cerebrovascular events

Children and Adolescents

- Not recommended for use in children under age 15
- 14 and older: recommended 3–5 mg/kg per day

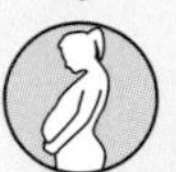

Pregnancy

- Potential risks should be weighed against the potential benefits, and sulpiride should be used only if deemed necessary
- Psychotic symptoms may worsen during pregnancy and some form of treatment may be necessary
- Atypical antipsychotics may be preferable to conventional antipsychotics or anticonvulsant mood stabilizers if treatment is required during pregnancy

Breast Feeding

- Some drug is found in mother's breast milk
- ✻ Recommended either to discontinue drug or bottle feed
- Immediate postpartum period is a high-risk time for relapse of psychosis

THE ART OF PSYCHOPHARMACOLOGY

Potential Advantages

- For negative symptoms in some patients

Potential Disadvantages

- Patients who cannot tolerate sedation at high doses
- Patients with severe renal impairment

Primary Target Symptoms

- Positive symptoms of psychosis
- Negative symptoms of psychosis
- Cognitive functioning
- Depressive symptoms
- Aggressive symptoms

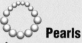

Pearls

- ✻ There is some controversy over whether sulpiride is more effective than older conventionals at treating negative symptoms
- Sulpiride has been used to treat migraine associated with hormonal changes
- ✻ Some patients with inadequate response to clozapine may benefit from augmentation with sulpiride
- Sulpiride is poorly absorbed from the gastrointestinal tract and penetrates the blood-brain barrier poorly, which can lead to highly variable clinical responses, especially at lower doses
- Small studies and clinical anecdotes suggest efficacy in depression and anxiety disorders ("neuroses") at low doses
- Patients have very similar antipsychotic responses to any conventional antipsychotic, which is different from atypical antipsychotics where antipsychotic responses of individual patients can occasionally vary greatly from one atypical antipsychotic to another
- Patients with inadequate responses to atypical antipsychotics may benefit from a trial of augmentation with a conventional antipsychotic such as sulpiride or from switching to a conventional antipsychotic such as sulpiride
- However, long-term polypharmacy with a combination of a conventional antipsychotic with an atypical antipsychotic may combine their side effects without clearly augmenting the efficacy of either
- Although a frequent practice by some prescribers, adding 2 conventional antipsychotics together has little rationale and may reduce tolerability without clearly enhancing efficacy

Suggested Reading

Caley CF, Weber SS. Sulpiride: an antipsychotic with selective dopaminergic antagonist properties. Ann Pharmacother 1995;29(2):152–60.

Mauri MC, Bravin S, Bitetto A, Rudelli R, Invernizzi G. A risk-benefit assessment of sulpiride in the treatment of schizophrenia. Drug Saf 1996;14(5):288–98.

O'Connor SE, Brown RA. The pharmacology of sulpiride—a dopamine receptor antagonist. Gen Pharmacol 1982;13(3):185–93.

Soares BG, Fenton M, Chue P. Sulpiride for schizophrenia. Cochrane Database Syst Rev 2000;(2):CD001162.

THERAPEUTICS

Brands • Restoril

see index for additional brand names

Generic? Yes

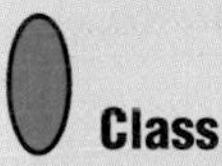

Class

• Benzodiazepine (hypnotic)

Commonly Prescribed for

(bold for FDA approved)

• **Short-term treatment of insomnia**

How the Drug Works

• Binds to benzodiazepine receptors at the GABA-A ligand-gated chloride channel complex
• Enhances the inhibitory effects of GABA
• Boosts chloride conductance through GABA-regulated channels
• Inhibitory actions in sleep centers may provide sedative hypnotic effects

How Long Until It Works

• Generally takes effect in less than an hour, but can take longer in some patients

If It Works

• Improves quality of sleep
• Effects on total wake-time and number of nighttime awakenings may be decreased over time

If It Doesn't Work

• If insomnia does not improve after 7–10 days, it may be a manifestation of a primary psychiatric or physical illness such as obstructive sleep apnea or restless leg syndrome, which requires independent evaluation
• Increase the dose
• Improve sleep hygiene
• Switch to another agent

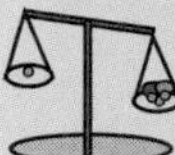

Best Augmenting Combos for Partial Response or Treatment Resistance

• Generally, best to switch to another agent
• Trazodone
• Agents with antihistamine actions (e.g., diphenhydramine, tricyclic antidepressants)

Tests

• In patients with seizure disorders, concomitant medical illness, and/or those with multiple concomitant long-term medications, periodic liver tests and blood counts may be prudent

SIDE EFFECTS

How Drug Causes Side Effects

• Same mechanism for side effects as for therapeutic effects – namely due to excessive actions at benzodiazepine receptors
• Actions at benzodiazepine receptors that carry over to the next day can cause daytime sedation, amnesia, and ataxia
• Long-term adaptations in benzodiazepine receptors may explain the development of dependence, tolerance, and withdrawal

Notable Side Effects

* Sedation, fatigue, depression
* Dizziness, ataxia, slurred speech, weakness
* Forgetfulness, confusion
* Hyperexcitability, nervousness
• Rare hallucinations, mania
• Rare hypotension
• Hypersalivation, dry mouth
• Rebound insomnia when withdrawing from long-term treatment

Life-Threatening or Dangerous Side Effects

• Respiratory depression, especially when taken with CNS depressants in overdose
• Rare hepatic dysfunction, renal dysfunction, blood dyscrasias

Weight Gain

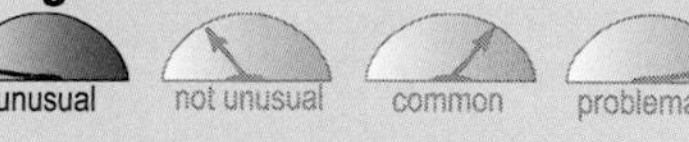

• Reported but not expected

Sedation

unusual not unusual **common** problematic

• Many experience and/or can be significant in amount

What to do About Side Effects

- Wait
- To avoid problems with memory, only take temazepam if planning to have a full night's sleep
- Lower the dose
- Switch to a shorter-acting sedative hypnotic
- Switch to a non-benzodiazepine hypnotic
- Administer flumazenil if side effects are severe or life-threatening

Best Augmenting Agents for Side Effects

- Many side effects cannot be improved with an augmenting agent

DOSING AND USE

Usual Dosage Range

- 15 mg/day at bedtime

Dosage Forms

- Capsule 7.5 mg, 15 mg, 30 mg

How To Dose

- 15 mg/day at bedtime; may increase to 30 mg/day at bedtime if ineffective

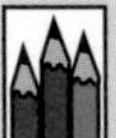

Dosing Tips

- Use lowest possible effective dose and assess need for continued treatment regularly
- Temazepam should generally not be prescribed in quantities greater than a 1-month supply
- Patients with lower body weights may require lower doses

✻ Because temazepam is slowly absorbed, administering the dose 1–2 hours before bedtime may improve onset of action and shorter sleep latency

- Risk of dependence may increase with dose and duration of treatment

Overdose

- Can be fatal in monotherapy; slurred speech, poor coordination, respiratory depression, sedation, confusion, coma

Long-Term Use

- Not generally intended for long-term use

Habit Forming

- Temazepam is a Schedule IV drug
- Some patients may develop dependence and/or tolerance; risk may be greater with higher doses
- History of drug addiction may increase risk of dependence

How to Stop

- If taken for more than a few weeks, taper to reduce chances of withdrawal effects
- Patients with history of seizure may seize upon sudden withdrawal
- Rebound insomnia may occur the first 1–2 nights after stopping
- For patients with severe problems discontinuing a benzodiazepine, dosing may need to be tapered over many months (i.e., reduce dose by 1% every 3 days by crushing tablet and suspending or dissolving in 100 mL of fruit juice and then disposing of 1 mL while drinking the rest; 3–7 days later, dispose of 2 mL, and so on). This is both a form of very slow biological tapering and a form of behavioral desensitization

Pharmacokinetics

- No active metabolites
- Half-life approximately 8–15 hours

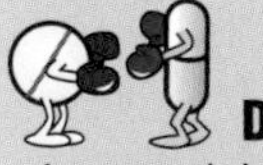

Drug Interactions

- Increased depressive effects when taken with other CNS depressants
- If temazepam is used with kava, clearance of either drug may be affected

Other Warnings/ Precautions

- Insomnia may be a symptom of a primary disorder, rather than a primary disorder itself
- Some patients may exhibit abnormal thinking or behavioral changes similar to those caused by other CNS depressants (i.e., either depressant actions or disinhibiting actions)
- Some depressed patients may experience a worsening of suicidal ideation
- Use only with extreme caution in patients with impaired respiratory function or obstructive sleep apnea

- Temazepam should only be administered at bedtime

Do Not Use
- If patient is pregnant
- If patient has narrow angle-closure glaucoma
- If there is a proven allergy to temazepam or any benzodiazepine

SPECIAL POPULATIONS

Renal Impairment
- Recommended dose: 7.5 mg/day

Hepatic Impairment
- Recommended dose: 7.5 mg/day

Cardiac Impairment
- Dosage adjustment may not be necessary
- Benzodiazepines have been used to treat insomnia associated with acute myocardial infarction

Elderly
- Recommended dose: 7.5 mg/day

Children and Adolescents
- Safety and efficacy have not been established
- Long-term effects of temazepam in children/adolescents are unknown
- Should generally receive lower doses and be more closely monitored

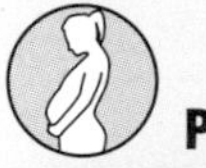

Pregnancy
- Risk Category X [positive evidence of risk to human fetus; contraindicated for use in pregnancy]
- Infants whose mothers received a benzodiazepine late in pregnancy may experience withdrawal effects
- Neonatal flaccidity has been reported in infants whose mothers took a benzodiazepine during pregnancy

Breast Feeding
- Unknown if temazepam is secreted in human breast milk, but all psychotropics assumed to be secreted in breast milk
- ✻ Recommended either to discontinue drug or bottle feed
- Effects on infant have been observed and include feeding difficulties, sedation, and weight loss

THE ART OF PSYCHOPHARMACOLOGY

Potential Advantages
- Patients with middle insomnia (nocturnal awakening)

Potential Disadvantages
- Patients with early insomnia (problems falling asleep)

Primary Target Symptoms
- Time to sleep onset
- Total sleep time
- Nighttime awakenings

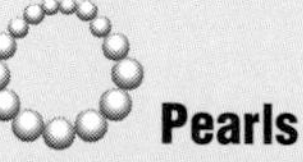

Pearls
- If tolerance develops, it may result in increased anxiety during the day and/or increased wakefulness during the latter part of the night
- ✻ Slow gastrointestinal absorption compared to other sedative benzodiazepines, so may be more effective for nocturnal awakening than for initial insomnia unless dosed 1–2 hours prior to bedtime
- ✻ Notable for delayed onset of action compared to some other sedative hypnotics

Suggested Reading

Ashton H. Guidelines for the rational use of benzodiazepines. When and what to use. Drugs 1994;48:25–40.

Fraschini F, Stankov B. Temazepam: pharmacological profile of a benzodiazepine and new trends in its clinical application. Pharmacol Res 1993;27:97–113.

Heel RC, Brogden RN, Speight TM, Avery GS. Temazepam: a review of its pharmacological properties and therapeutic efficacy as an hypnotic. Drugs 1981;21:321–40.

McElnay JC, Jones ME, Alexander B. Temazepam (Restoril, Sandoz Pharmaceuticals). Drug Intell Clin Pharm 1982;16:650–6.

THERAPEUTICS

Brands • Mellaril

see index for additional brand names

Generic? Yes

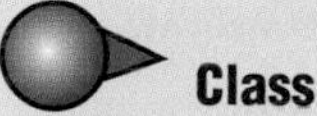

Class

- Conventional antipsychotic (neuroleptic, phenothiazine, dopamine 2 antagonist)

Commonly Prescribed for

(bold for FDA approved)

- **Schizophrenic patients who fail to respond to treatment with other antipsychotic drugs**

How the Drug Works

- Blocks dopamine 2 receptors, reducing positive symptoms of psychosis

How Long Until It Works

- Psychotic symptoms can improve within 1 week, but it may take several weeks for full effect on behavior

If It Works

- Is a second-line treatment option

❋ Should evaluate for switching to an antipsychotic with a better risk/benefit ratio

If It Doesn't Work

- Consider trying one of the first-line atypical antipsychotics (risperidone, olanzapine, quetiapine, ziprasidone, aripiprazole, paliperidone, amisulpride)
- Consider trying another conventional antipsychotic
- If 2 or more antipsychotic monotherapies do not work, consider clozapine

Best Augmenting Combos for Partial Response or Treatment Resistance

❋ Augmentation of thioridazine has not been systematically studied and can be dangerous, especially with drugs that can either prolong QTc interval or raise thioridazine plasma levels

Tests

❋ Baseline EKG and serum potassium levels should be determined

❋ Periodic evaluation of EKG and serum potassium levels

- Serum magnesium levels may also need to be monitored

❋ Since conventional antipsychotics are frequently associated with weight gain, before starting treatment, weigh all patients and determine if the patient is already overweight (BMI 25.0–29.9) or obese (BMI ≥30)

- Before giving a drug that can cause weight gain to an overweight or obese patient, consider determining whether the patient already has pre-diabetes (fasting plasma glucose 100–25 mg/dL), diabetes (fasting plasma glucose >126 mg/dL), or dyslipidemia (increased total cholesterol, LDL cholesterol and triglycerides; decreased HDL cholesterol), and treat or refer such patients for treatment, including nutrition and weight management, physical activity counseling, smoking cessation, and medical management

❋ Monitor weight and BMI during treatment

❋ Consider monitoring fasting triglycerides monthly for several months in patients at high risk for metabolic complications and when initiating or switching antipsychotics

❋ While giving a drug to a patient who has gained >5% of initial weight, consider evaluating for the presence of pre-diabetes, diabetes, or dyslipidemia, or consider switching to a different antipsychotic

- Should check blood pressure in the elderly before starting and for the first few weeks of treatment
- Monitoring elevated prolactin levels of dubious clinical benefit
- Phenothiazines may cause false-positive phenylketonuria results

SIDE EFFECTS

How Drug Causes Side Effects

- By blocking dopamine 2 receptors in the striatum, it can cause motor side effects
- By blocking dopamine 2 receptors in the pituitary, it can cause elevations in prolactin
- By blocking dopamine 2 receptors excessively in the mesocortical and mesolimbic dopamine pathways, especially at high doses, it can cause worsening of

negative and cognitive symptoms (neuroleptic-induced deficit syndrome)
- Anticholinergic actions may cause sedation, blurred vision, constipation, dry mouth
- Antihistaminic actions may cause sedation, weight gain
- By blocking alpha 1 adrenergic receptors, it can cause dizziness, sedation, and hypotension
- Mechanism of weight gain and any possible increased incidence of diabetes or dyslipidemia with conventional antipsychotics is unknown

✽ Mechanism of potentially dangerous QTc prolongation may be related to actions at ion channels

Notable Side Effects

✽ Neuroleptic-induced deficit syndrome
✽ Akathisia
✽ Priapism
✽ Extrapyramidal symptoms, Parkinsonism, tardive dyskinesia
✽ Galactorrhea, amenorrhea
✽ Pigmentary retinopathy at high doses
- Dizziness, sedation
- Dry mouth, constipation, blurred vision
- Decreased sweating
- Sexual dysfunction
- Hypotension
- Weight gain

Life-Threatening or Dangerous Side Effects

- Rare neuroleptic malignant syndrome
- Rare jaundice, agranulocytosis
- Rare seizures

✽ Dose-dependent QTc prolongation
- Ventricular arrhythmias and sudden death
- Increased risk of death and cerebrovascular events in elderly patients with dementia-related psychosis

Weight Gain

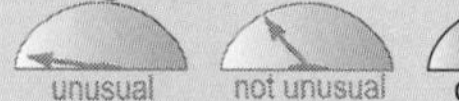
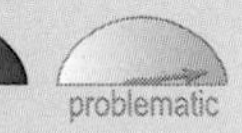

- Many experience and/or can be significant in amount

Sedation

unusual not unusual **common** problematic

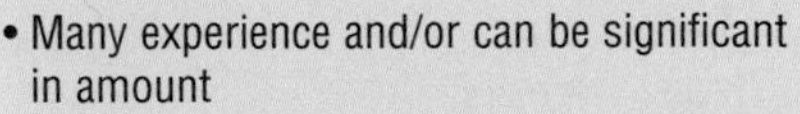

- Many experience and/or can be significant in amount
- Sedation is usually transient

What to do About Side Effects

- Wait
- Wait
- Wait
- For motor symptoms, add an anticholinergic agent
- Reduce the dose
- For sedation, give at night
- Switch to an atypical antipsychotic
- Weight loss, exercise programs, and medical management for high BMIs, diabetes, dyslipidemia

Best Augmenting Agents for Side Effects

✽ Augmentation of thioridazine has not been systematically studied and can be dangerous

DOSING AND USE

Usual Dosage Range

- 200–800 mg/day in divided doses

Dosage Forms

- Tablet 10 mg, 15 mg, 25 mg, 50 mg, 100 mg, 150 mg, 200 mg
- Liquid 30 mg/mL, 100 mg/mL
- Suspension 5 mg/mL, 20 mg/mL

How To Dose

- 50–100 mg 3 times a day; increase gradually; maximum 800 mg/day in divided doses

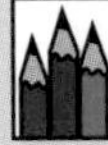

Dosing Tips

✽ Prolongation of the QTc interval is dose-dependent, so start low and go slow while carefully monitoring QTc interval
- Pigmentary retinopathy has been reported in patients taking doses exceeding the recommended range

Overdose

- Sedation, confusion, respiratory depression, cardiac disturbance, hypotension, seizure, coma

Long-Term Use
- Some side effects may be irreversible (e.g., tardive dyskinesia)

Habit Forming
- No

How to Stop
- Slow down-titration (over 6–8 weeks), especially when simultaneously beginning a new antipsychotic while switching (i.e., cross-titration)
- Rapid discontinuation may lead to rebound psychosis and worsening of symptoms
- If antiparkinson agents are being used, they should be continued for a few weeks after thioridazine is discontinued

Pharmacokinetics
- Metabolized by CYP450 2D6

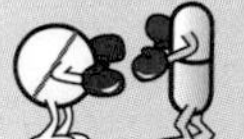

Drug Interactions
- May decrease the effects of levodopa, dopamine agonists
- May increase the effects of antihypertensive drugs
- May enhance QTc prolongation of other drugs capable of prolonging QTc interval

* CYP450 2D6 inhibitors including paroxetine, fluoxetine, duloxetine, bupropion, sertraline, citalopram, and others can raise thioridazine to dangerous levels

* Fluvoxamine, propranolol, and pindolol also inhibit thioridazine metabolism and can raise thioridazine to dangerous levels

- Respiratory depression/arrest may occur if used with a barbiturate
- Additive effects may occur if used with CNS depressants
- Alcohol and diuretics may increase the risk of hypotension; epinephrine may lower blood pressure
- Some patients taking a neuroleptic and lithium have developed an encephalopathic syndrome similar to neuroleptic malignant syndrome

Other Warnings/ Precautions
- If signs of neuroleptic malignant syndrome develop, treatment should be immediately discontinued

* Thioridazine can increase the QTc interval and potentially cause torsades de pointes-type arrhythmia or sudden death, especially in combination with drugs that raise its levels

- Use cautiously in patients with respiratory disorders, glaucoma, or urinary retention
- Avoid extreme heat exposure
- Antiemetic effect can mask signs of other disorders or overdose
- Use cautiously in patients with alcohol withdrawal or convulsive disorders because of possible lowering of seizure threshold
- Do not use epinephrine in event of overdose, as interaction with some pressor agents may lower blood pressure
- Use only with caution if at all in Parkinson's disease or Lewy body dementia
- Observe for signs of pigmentary retinopathy, especially at higher doses
- Because thioridazine may dose-dependently prolong QTc interval, use with caution in patients who have bradycardia or who are taking drugs that can induce bradycardia (e.g., beta blockers, calcium channel blockers, clonidine, digitalis)
- Because thioridazine may dose-dependently prolong QTc interval, use with caution in patients who have hypokalemia and/or hypomagnesemia or who are taking drugs that can induce hypokalemia and/or magnesemia (e.g., diuretics, stimulant laxatives, intravenous amphotericin B, glucocorticoids, tetracosactide)

Do Not Use
- If patient is in a comatose state or has CNS depression
- If patient suffers from extreme hypertension/hypotension

* If QTc interval greater than 450 msec or if taking an agent capable of significantly prolonging QTc interval (e.g., pimozide, selected antiarrhythmics, moxifoxacin, and sparfloxacin)
* If there is a history of QTc prolongation or cardiac arrhythmia, recent acute myocardial infarction, uncompensated heart failure
* If patient is taking drugs that inhibit thioridazine metabolism, including CYP450 inhibitors

✻ If there is reduced CYP450 2D6 function, such as in patients who are 2D6 poor metabolizers
- If there is a proven allergy to thioridazine
- If there is a known sensitivity to any phenothiazine

SPECIAL POPULATIONS

Renal Impairment
- Use with caution

Hepatic Impairment
- Use with caution

Cardiac Impairment
- Thioridazine produces a dose-dependent prolongation of QTc interval, which may be enhanced by the existence of bradycardia, hypokalemia, congenital or acquired long QTc interval, which should be evaluated prior to administering thioridazine
- Use with caution if treating concomitantly with a medication likely to produce prolonged bradycardia, hypokalemia slowing of intracardiac conduction, or prolongation of the QTc interval
- Avoid thioridazine in patients with a known history of QTc prolongation, recent acute myocardial infarction, and uncompensated heart failure

✻ Risk/benefit ratio may not justify use in cardiac impairment

Elderly
- Some patients may tolerate lower doses better
- Elderly patients may be more sensitive to adverse effects, including agranulocytosis and leukopenia
- Although conventional antipsychotics are commonly used for behavioral disturbances in dementia, no agent has been approved for treatment of elderly patients with dementia-related psychosis
- Elderly patients with dementia-related psychosis treated with antipsychotics are at an increased risk of death compared to placebo, and also have an increased risk of cerebrovascular events

Children and Adolescents
- Safety and efficacy not established in children under age 2
- Dose: initial 0.5 mg/kg per day in divided doses; increase gradually; maximum 3 mg/kg/day
- Risk/benefit ratio may not justify use in children or adolescents

Pregnancy
- Risk Category C [some animal studies show adverse effects; no controlled studies in humans]
- Reports of extrapyramidal symptoms, jaundice, hyperreflexia, hyporeflexia in infants whose mothers took a phenothiazine during pregnancy
- Psychotic symptoms may worsen during pregnancy and some form of treatment may be necessary
- Atypical antipsychotic may be preferable to conventional antipsychotics or anticonvulsant mood stabilizers if treatment is required during pregnancy
- Should evaluate for an antipsychotic with a better risk/benefit ratio if treatment is required during pregnancy

Breast Feeding
- Unknown if thioridazine is secreted in human breast milk, but all psychotropics assumed to be secreted in breast milk

✻ Recommended either to discontinue drug or bottle feed

THE ART OF PSYCHOPHARMACOLOGY

Potential Advantages
- Only for patients who respond to this agent and not other antipsychotics

Potential Disadvantages
- Children
- Elderly
- Patients on other drugs
- Those with low CYP450 2D6 metabolism

Primary Target Symptoms
- Positive symptoms of psychosis in patients who fail to respond to treatment with other antipsychotics

- Motor and autonomic hyperactivity in patients who fail to respond to treatment with other antipsychotics
- Violent or aggressive behavior in patients who fail to respond to treatment with other antipsychotics

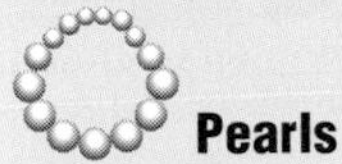

Pearls

* Generally, the benefits of thioridazine do not outweigh its risks for most patients
* Because of its effects on the QTc interval, thioridazine is not intended for use unless other options (at least 2 antipsychotics) have failed
- Thioridazine has not been systematically studied in treatment-refractory schizophrenia
* Phenotypic testing may be necessary in order to detect the 7% of the normal population for whom thioridazine is contraindicated due to a genetic variant leading to reduced activity of CYP450 2D6
- Conventional antipsychotics are much less expensive than atypical antipsychotics
- Thioridazine causes less extrapyramidal symptoms than some other conventional antipsychotics
* Was once a preferred antipsychotic for children and the elderly, and for those whose symptoms benefited from a sedating low potency phenothiazine with a lower incidence of extrapyramidal symptoms
* However, now it is recognized that the dangers of cardiac arrhythmias and drug interactions outweigh the benefits of thioridazine, and it is now considered a second-line treatment if it is considered at all

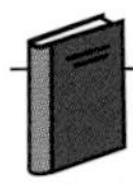

Suggested Reading

Frankenburg FR. Choices in antipsychotic therapy in schizophrenia. Harv Rev Psychiatry 1999;6:241–9.

Gardos G, Tecce JJ, Hartmann E, Bowers P, Cole JO. Treatment with mesoridazine and thioridazine in chronic schizophrenia: II. Potential predictors of drug response. Compr Psychiatry 1978;19:527–32.

Sultana A, Reilly J, Fenton M. Thioridazine for schizophrenia. Cochrane Database Syst Rev 2000;(3):CD001944.

Leucht S, Wahlbeck K, Hamann J, Kissling W. New generation antipsychotics versus low-potency conventional antipsychotics: a systematic review and meta-analysis. The Lancet 2003;361:1581–9.

THERAPEUTICS

Brands • Navane

see index for additional brand names

Generic? Yes

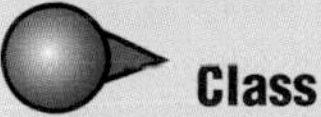

Class

- Conventional antipsychotic (neuroleptic, thioxanthene, dopamine 2 antagonist)

Commonly Prescribed for

(bold for FDA approved)

- **Schizophrenia**
- Other psychotic disorders
- Bipolar disorder

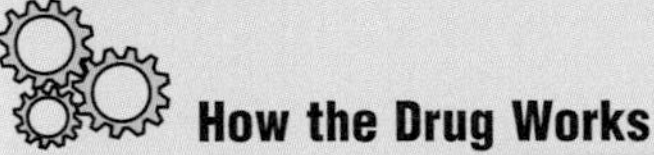

How the Drug Works

- Blocks dopamine 2 receptors, reducing positive symptoms of psychosis

How Long Until It Works

- Psychotic symptoms can improve within 1 week, but it may take several weeks for full effect on behavior

If It Works

- Most often reduces positive symptoms in schizophrenia but does not eliminate them
- Most schizophrenic patients do not have a total remission of symptoms but rather a reduction of symptoms by about a third
- Continue treatment in schizophrenia until reaching a plateau of improvement
- After reaching a satisfactory plateau, continue treatment for at least a year after first episode of psychosis in schizophrenia
- For second and subsequent episodes of psychosis in schizophrenia, treatment may need to be indefinite
- Reduces symptoms of acute psychotic mania but not proven as a mood stabilizer or as an effective maintenance treatment in bipolar disorder
- After reducing acute psychotic symptoms in mania, switch to a mood stabilizer and/or an atypical antipsychotic for mood stabilization and maintenance

If It Doesn't Work

- Consider trying one of the first-line atypical antipsychotics (risperidone, olanzapine, quetiapine, ziprasidone, aripiprazole, paliperidone, amisulpride)
- Consider trying another conventional antipsychotic
- If 2 or more antipsychotic monotherapies do not work, consider clozapine

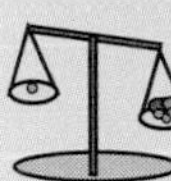

Best Augmenting Combos for Partial Response or Treatment Resistance

- Augmentation of conventional antipsychotics has not been systematically studied
- Addition of a mood-stabilizing anticonvulsant such as valproate, carbamazepine, or lamotrigine may be helpful in both schizophrenia and bipolar mania
- Augmentation with lithium in bipolar mania may be helpful
- Addition of a benzodiazepine, especially short-term for agitation

Tests

❋ Since conventional antipsychotics are frequently associated with weight gain, before starting treatment, weigh all patients and determine if the patient is already overweight (BMI 25.0–29.9) or obese (BMI ≥30)

- Before giving a drug that can cause weight gain to an overweight or obese patient, consider determining whether the patient already has pre-diabetes (fasting plasma glucose 100–25 mg/dL), diabetes (fasting plasma glucose >126 mg/dlL), or dyslipidemia (increased total cholesterol, LDL cholesterol and triglycerides; decreased HDL cholesterol), and treat or refer such patients for treatment, including nutrition and weight management, physical activity counseling, smoking cessation, and medical management

❋ Monitor weight and BMI during treatment

❋ Consider monitoring fasting triglycerides monthly for several months in patients at high risk for metabolic complications and when initiating or switching antipsychotics

❋ While giving a drug to a patient who has gained >5% of initial weight, consider evaluating for the presence of pre-diabetes, diabetes, or dyslipidemia, or consider switching to a different antipsychotic

- Monitoring elevated prolactin levels of dubious clinical benefit

SIDE EFFECTS

How Drug Causes Side Effects

- By blocking dopamine 2 receptors in the striatum, it can cause motor side effects
- By blocking dopamine 2 receptors in the pituitary, it can cause elevations in prolactin
- By blocking dopamine 2 receptors excessively in the mesocortical and mesolimbic dopamine pathways, especially at high doses, it can cause worsening of negative and cognitive symptoms (neuroleptic-induced deficit syndrome)
- Anticholinergic actions may cause sedation, blurred vision, constipation, dry mouth
- Antihistaminic actions may cause sedation, weight gain
- By blocking alpha 1 adrenergic receptors, it can cause dizziness, sedation, and hypotension
- Mechanism of weight gain and any possible increased incidence of diabetes or dyslipidemia with conventional antipsychotics is unknown

Notable Side Effects

✻ Neuroleptic-induced deficit syndrome
✻ Akathisia
✻ Extrapyramidal symptoms, Parkinsonism, tardive dyskinesia
✻ Galactorrhea, amenorrhea
- Sedation
- Dry mouth, constipation, vision disturbance, urninary retention
- Hypotension, tachycardia
- Rare fine lenticular pigmentation

Life-Threatening or Dangerous Side Effects

- Rare neuroleptic malignant syndrome
- Rare seizures
- Rare blood dyscrasias
- Rare hepatic toxicity
- Increased risk of death and cerebrovascular events in elderly patients with dementia-related psychosis

Weight Gain

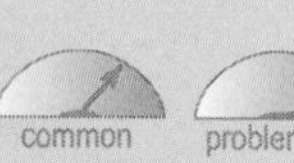

unusual | not unusual | common | problematic

✻ Reported but not expected

Sedation

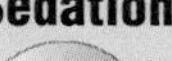

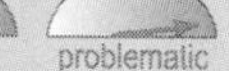

unusual | not unusual | common | problematic

- Occurs in significant minority

What to do About Side Effects

- Wait
- Wait
- Wait
- For motor symptoms, add an anticholinergic agent
- For sedation, take at night
- Reduce the dose
- Switch to an atypical antipsychotic
- Weight loss, exercise programs, and medical management for high BMIs, diabetes, dyslipidemia

Best Augmenting Agents for Side Effects

- Benztropine or trihexyphenidyl for motor side effects
- Sometimes amantadine can be helpful for motor side effects
- Benzodiazepines may be helpful for akathisia
- Many side effects cannot be improved with an augmenting agent

DOSING AND USE

Usual Dosage Range

- 15–30 mg/day

Dosage Forms

- Capsule 2 mg, 5 mg, 10 mg

How To Dose

- Initial 5–10 mg/day; maximum dose generally 60 mg/day; higher doses may be given in divided doses

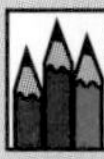

Dosing Tips

- When thiothixene is dosed too high, it can induce or worsen negative symptoms of schizophrenia
- Lower doses may provide the best benefit with fewest side effects in patients who respond to low doses

Overdose
- Muscle twitching, sedation, dizziness, CNS depression, rigidity, weakness, torticollis, dysphagia, hypotension, coma

Long-Term Use
- Some side effects may be irreversible (e.g., tardive dyskinesia)

Habit Forming
- No

How to Stop
- Slow down-titration (over 6–8 weeks), especially when simultaneously beginning a new antipsychotic while switching (i.e., cross-titration)
- Rapid discontinuation may lead to rebound psychosis and worsening of symptoms
- If antiparkinson agents are being used, they should be continued for a few weeks after thiothixene is discontinued

Pharmacokinetics
- Initial elimination half-life approximately 3.4 hours
- Terminal elimination half-life approximately 34 hours

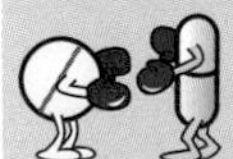

Drug Interactions
- Respiratory depression may occur when thiothixene is combined with lorazepam
- Additive effects may occur if used with CNS depressants
- May decrease the effects of levodopa, dopamine agonists
- Some patients taking a neuroleptic and lithium have developed an encephalopathic syndrome similar to neuroleptic malignant syndrome
- Combined use with epinephrine may lower blood pressure
- May increase the effects of antihypertensive drugs except for guanethidine, whose antihypertensive actions thiothixene may antagonize

Other Warnings/ Precautions
- If signs of neuroleptic malignant syndrome develop, treatment should be immediately discontinued
- Use cautiously in patients with alcohol withdrawal or convulsive disorders because of possible lowering of seizure threshold
- Antiemetic effect can mask signs of other disorders or overdose
- Do not use epinephrine in event of overdose, as interaction with some pressor agents may lower blood pressure
- Use cautiously in patients with glaucoma, urinary retention
- Observe for signs of ocular toxicity (pigmentary retinopathy, lenticular pigmentation)
- Avoid extreme heat exposure
- Use only with caution if at all in Parkinson's disease or Lewy body dementia

Do Not Use
- If patient has CNS depression, is in a comatose state, has circulatory collapse, or there is presence of blood dyscrasias
- If there is a proven allergy to thiothixene

SPECIAL POPULATIONS

Renal Impairment
- Use with caution

Hepatic Impairment
- Use with caution

Cardiac Impairment
- Thiothixene may cause or aggravate EKG changes

Elderly
- Some patients may tolerate lower doses better
- Although conventional antipsychotics are commonly used for behavioral disturbances in dementia, no agent has been approved for treatment of elderly patients with dementia-related psychosis
- Elderly patients with dementia-related psychosis treated with antipsychotics are at an increased risk ofdeath compared to placebo, and also have an increased risk of cerebrovascular events

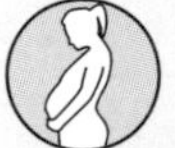

Children and Adolescents

- Safety and efficacy have not been established in children under age 12
- Generally consider second-line after atypical antipsychotics

Pregnancy

- Use of thiothixene has not been studied in pregnant women
- Reports of extrapyramidal symptoms, jaundice, hyperreflexia, hyporeflexia in infants whose mothers took a phenothiazine during pregnancy
- Psychotic symptoms may worsen during pregnancy and some form of treatment may be necessary
- Atypical antipsychotics may be preferable to conventional antipsychotics or anticonvulsant mood stabilizers if treatment is required during pregnancy
- Thiothixene should generally not be used during the first trimester
- Thiothixene should be used during pregnancy only if clearly needed

Breast Feeding

- Unknown if thiothixene is secreted in human breast milk, but all psychotropics assumed to be secreted in breast milk

✻ Recommended either to discontinue drug or bottle feed

THE ART OF PSYCHOPHARMACOLOGY

Potential Advantages

- For patients who do not respond to other antipsychotics

Potential Disadvantages

- Patients with tardive dyskinesia
- Children
- Elderly

Primary Target Symptoms

- Positive symptoms of psychosis
- Negative symptoms of psychosis

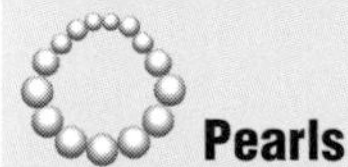

Pearls

✻ Although not systematically studied, may cause less weight gain than other antipsychotics

- Conventional antipsychotics are less expensive than atypical antipsychotics
- Patients have very similar antipsychotic responses to any conventional antipsychotic, which is different from atypical antipsychotics where antipsychotic responses of individual patients can occasionally vary greatly from one atypical antipsychotic to another
- Patients with inadequate responses to atypical antipsychotics may benefit from a trial of augmentation with a conventional antipsychotic such as thiothixene or from switching to a conventional antipsychotic such as thiothixene
- However, long-term polypharmacy with a combination of a conventional antipsychotic such as thiothixene with an atypical antipsychotic may combine their side effects without clearly augmenting the efficacy of either
- Although a frequent practice by some prescribers, adding 2 conventional antipsychotics together has little rationale and may reduce tolerability without clearly enhancing efficacy

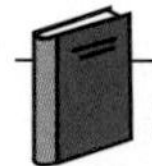

Suggested Reading

Huang CC, Gerhardstein RP, Kim DY, Hollister L. Treatment-resistant schizophrenia: controlled study of moderate- and high-dose thiothixene. Int Clin Psychopharmacol 1987;2:69–75.

Sterlin C, Ban TA, Jarrold L. The place of thiothixene among the thioxanthenes. Curr Ther Res Clin Exp 1972;14:205–14.

THERAPEUTICS

Brands • Cabitril

see index for additional brand names

Generic? No

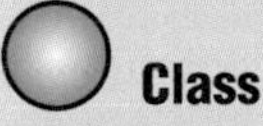

Class

- Anticonvulsant; selective GABA reuptake inhibitor (SGRI)

Commonly Prescribed for

(bold for FDA approved)

- **Partial seizures (adjunctive; adults and children 12 years and older)**
- Anxiety disorders
- Neuropathic pain/chronic pain

How the Drug Works

- Selectively blocks reuptake of gamma-aminobutyric acid (GABA) by presynaptic and glial GABA transporters

How Long Until It Works

- Should reduce seizures by 2 weeks
- Not clear that it works in anxiety disorders or chronic pain but some patients may respond, and if they do, therapeutic actions can be seen by 2 weeks

If It Works

- The goal of treatment is complete remission of symptoms (e.g., seizures, anxiety)
- The goal of treatment of chronic neuropathic pain is to reduce symptoms as much as possible, especially in combination with other treatments
- Treatment of chronic neuropathic pain most often reduces but does not eliminate symptoms and is not a cure since symptoms usually recur after medicine stopped
- Continue treatment until all symptoms are gone or until improvement is stable and then continue treating indefinitely as long as improvement persists

If It Doesn't Work (for neuropathic pain or anxiety disorders)

- Many patients have only a partial response where some symptoms are improved but others persist
- Other patients may be nonresponders, sometimes called treatment-resistant or treatment-refractory
- May only be effective in a subset of patients with neuropathic pain or anxiety disorders, in some patients who fail to respond to other treatments, or it may not work at all
- Consider increasing dose, switching to another agent or adding an appropriate augmenting agent
- Consider biofeedback or hypnosis for pain
- Consider evaluation for another diagnosis or for a comorbid condition (e.g., medical illness, substance abuse, etc.)
- Switch to another agent with fewer side effects
- Consider evaluation for another diagnosis or for a comorbid condition (e.g., medical illness, substance abuse, etc.)

Best Augmenting Combos for Partial Response or Treatment Resistance

- Tiagabine is itself an augmenting agent for numerous other anticonvulsants in treating epilepsy
- ✻ For neuropathic pain, tiagabine can augment tricyclic antidepressants and SNRIs as well as gabapentin, other anticonvulsants, and even opiates if done by experts while carefully monitoring in difficult cases
- For anxiety, tiagabine is a second-line treatment to augment SSRIs, SNRIs, or benzodiazepines

Tests

- None for healthy individuals
- Tiagabine may bind to tissue that contains melanin, so for long-term treatment opthalmological checks may be considered

SIDE EFFECTS

How Drug Causes Side Effects

- CNS side effects may be due to excessive actions of GABA

Notable Side Effects

- ✻ Sedation, dizziness, asthenia, nervousness, difficulty concentrating,

speech/language problems, confusion, tremor
- Diarrhea, vomiting, nausea
- Ecchymosis, depression

Life-Threatening or Dangerous Side Effects

- Exacerbation of EEG abnormalities in epilepsy
- Status epilepticus in epilepsy (unknown if associated with tiagabine use)
- Sudden unexplained deaths have occurred in epilepsy (unknown if related to tiagabine use)
- New onset seizures and status epilepticus have been reported in patients without epilepsy
- Rare activation of suicidal ideation and behavior (suicidality)

Weight Gain

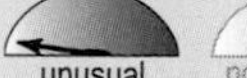

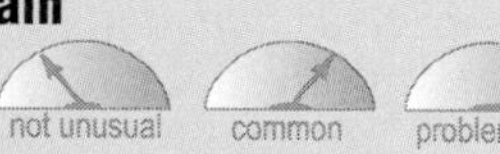

- Reported but not expected
- Some patients experience increased appetite

Sedation

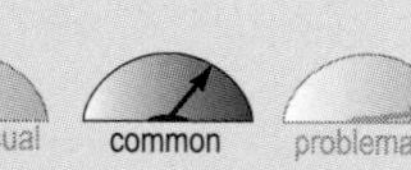

- Many experience and/or can be significant in amount

What to do About Side Effects

- Wait
- Wait
- Wait
- Take more of the dose at night or all of the dose at night to reduce daytime sedation
- Lower the dose
- Switch to another agent

Best Augmenting Agents for Side Effects

- Many side effects cannot be improved with an augmenting agent

DOSING AND USE

Usual Dosage Range

- 32–56 mg/day in 2–4 divided doses for adjunctive treatment of epilepsy
- 2–12 mg/day for adjunctive treatment of chronic pain and anxiety disorders

Dosage Forms

- Tablet 2 mg, 4 mg, 12 mg, 16 mg, 20 mg

How To Dose

- Adjunct to enzyme-inducing antiepileptic drugs: initial 4 mg once daily; after 1 week can increase dose by 4–8 mg/day each week; maximum dose generally 56 mg/day in 2–4 divided doses
- Dosing for chronic pain or anxiety disorders not well established, but start as low as 2 mg at night, increasing by 2 mg increments every few days as tolerated to 8–12 mg/day
- Exercise particular caution when prescribing in uninduced patients

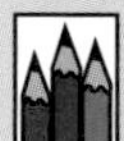

Dosing Tips

- Usually administered as adjunctive medication to other anticonvulsants in the treatment of epilepsy

✻ Dosing recommendations are based on studies of adjunctive use with enzyme-inducing antiepileptic drugs, which lower plasma levels of tiagabine by half; thus, when tiagabine is used without enzyme-inducing antiepileptic drugs the dose may need to be significantly reduced and may require a much slower titration rate

✻ Also administered as adjunctive medication to benzodiazepines, SSRIs, and/or SNRIs in the treatment of anxiety disorders; and to SNRIs, gabapentin, other anticonvulsants, and even opiates in the treatment of chronic pain

✻ Dosing varies considerably among individual patients but is definitely at the lower end of the dosing spectrum for patients with chronic neuropathic pain or anxiety disorders (i.e., 2–12 mg either as a split dose or all at night)

✻ Patients with chronic neuropathic pain and anxiety disorders are far less tolerant of CNS side effects, so they require a much slower dosage titration as well as a lower maintenance dose

- Gastrointestinal absorption is markedly slowed by the concomitant intake of food, which also lessens the peak plasma concentrations

* Thus, for improved tolerability and consistent clinical actions, instruct patients to always take with food
- Side effects may increase with dose

Overdose
- No fatalities have been reported; sedation, agitation, confusion, speech difficulty, hostility, depression, weakness, myoclonus, seizures, status epilepticus

Long-Term Use
- Safe

Habit Forming
- No

How to Stop
- Taper
- Epilepsy patients may seize upon withdrawal, especially if withdrawal is abrupt
- Discontinuation symptoms uncommon

Pharmacokinetics
- Primarily metabolized by CYP450 3A4
- Steady state concentrations tend to be lower in the evening than in the morning
- Half-life approximately 7–9 hours
- Renally excreted

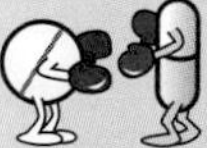

Drug Interactions
- Clearance of tiagabine may be reduced and thus plasma levels increased if taken with a non-enzyme inducing antiepileptic drug (e.g., valproate, gabapentin, lamotrigine), so tiagabine dose may need to be reduced
- CYP450 3A4 inducers such as carbamazepine can lower the plasma levels of tiagabine
- CYP450 3A4 inhibitors such as nefazodone, fluvoxamine, and fluoxetine could theoretically increase the plasma levels of tiagabine
- Clearance of tiagabine is increased if taken with an enzyme-inducing antiepileptic drug (e.g., carbamazepine, phenobarbital, phenytoin, primidone) and thus plasma levels are reduced; however, no dose adjustments are necessary for treatment of epilepsy as the dosing recommendations for epilepsy are based on adjunctive treatment with an enzyme-inducing antiepileptic drug
- Despite common actions upon GABA, no pharmacodynamic or pharmacokinetic interations have been shown when tiagabine is combined with the benzodiazepine triazolam or with alcohol
- However, sedating actions of any two sedative drugs given in combination can be additive

Other Warnings/ Precautions
- Seizures have occurred in individuals without epilepsy who took tiagabine
- Risk of seizure may be dose-related; when tiagabine is used in the absence of enzyme-inducing antiepileptic drugs, which lower plasma levels of tiagabine, the dose may need to be reduced
- Depressive effects may be increased by other CNS depressants (alcohol, MAOIs, other anticonvulsants, etc.)
- Tiagabine may bind to melanin, raising the possibility of long-term ophthalmologic effects
- Warn patients and their caregivers about the possibility of activation of suicidal ideation and advise them to report such side effects immediately

Do Not Use
- If there is a proven allergy to tiagabine

SPECIAL POPULATIONS

Renal Impairment
- Although tiagabine is renally excreted, the pharmacokinetics of tiagabine in healthy patients and in those with impaired renal function are similar and no dose adjustment is recommended

Hepatic Impairment
- Clearance is decreased
- May require lower dose

Cardiac Impairment
- No dose adjustment recommended

Elderly
- Some patients may tolerate lower doses better

Children and Adolescents

- Safety and efficacy not established under age 12
- Maximum recommended dose generally 32 mg/day in 2–4 divided doses

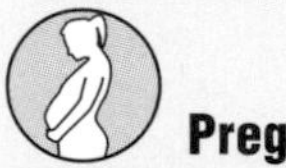

Pregnancy

- Risk Category C [some animal studies show adverse effects; no controlled studies in humans]
- Use in women of childbearing potential requires weighing potential benefits to the mother against the risks to the fetus
- Antiepileptic Drug Pregnancy Registry: (888) 233-2334
- Taper drug if discontinuing
- Seizures, even mild seizures, may cause harm to the embryo/fetus
- ✽ Lack of definitive evidence of efficacy for chronic neuropathic pain or anxiety disorders suggests risk/benefit ratio is in favor of discontinuing tiagabine during pregnancy for those indications

Breast Feeding

- Some drug is found in mother's breast milk
- ✽ Recommended either to discontinue drug or bottle fee
- If drug is continued while breast feeding, infant should be monitored for possible adverse effects
- If infant shows signs of irritability or sedation, drug may need to be discontinued

THE ART OF PSYCHOPHARMACOLOGY

Potential Advantages

- Treatment-resistant chronic neuropathic pain
- Treatment-resistant anxiety disorders

Potential Disadvantages

- May require 2–4 times a day dosing
- Needs to be taken with food

Primary Target Symptoms

- Incidence of seizures
- Pain
- Anxiety

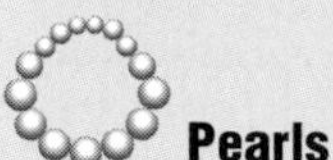

Pearls

- Well studied in epilepsy
- Much use is off-label
- ✽ Off-label use second-line and as an augmenting agent may be justified for treatment resistant anxiety disorders and neuropathic pain and also for fibromyalgia
- ✽ Off-label use for bipolar disorder may <u>not</u> be justified
- ✽ One of the few agents that enhances slow-wave delta sleep, which may be helpful in chronic neuropathic pain syndromes
- Can be difficult to dose in patients who are not taking enzyme-inducing anticonvulsant drugs as the doses in uninduced patients have not been well studied, are generally much lower, and titration is much slower than in induced patients
- Can cause seizures even in patients without epilepsy, especially in patients taking other agents (antidepressants, antipsychotics, stimulants, narcotics) that are thought to lower the seizure threshold

Suggested Reading

Backonja NM. Use of anticonvulsants for treatment of neuropathic pain. Neurology 2002 10;59(Suppl 2):S14–7.

Carta MG, Hardoy MC, Grunze H, Carpiniello B. The use of tiagabine in affective disorders. Pharmacopsychiatry 2002;35:33–4.

Evans EA. Efficacy of newer anticonvulsant medications in bipolar spectrum mood disorders. J Clin Psychiatry 2003;64(Suppl 8):9–14.

Lydiard RB. The role of GABA in anxiety disorders. J Clin Psychiatry 2003;64(Suppl 3):21–7.

Schmidt D, Gram L, Brodie M, Kramer G, Perucca E, Kalviainen R, Elger CE. Tiagabine in the treatment of epilepsy—a clinical review with a guide for the prescribing physician. Epilepsy Res 2000; 41: 245–51.

Stahl SM. Psychopharmacology of anticonvulsants: do all anticonvulsants have the same mechanism of action? J Clin Psychiatry 2004;65:149–50.

Stahl SM. Anticonvulsants as anxiolytics, part 1: tiagabine and other anticonvulsants with actions on GABA. J Clin Psychiatry 2004;65:291–2.

THERAPEUTICS

Brands
- Coaxil
- Stablon
- Tatinol

see index for additional brand names

Generic? No

Class

- Glutamatergic modulator
- Often classified as a tricyclic antidepressant, but pharmacologically distinct
- Serotonin reuptake enhancer

Commonly Prescribed for

(bold for FDA approved)
- Major depressive disorder
- Dysthymia
- Anxiety associated with depression, alcohol dependence

How the Drug Works

✻ Modulates glutamatergic neurotransmission, perhaps through potentiation of AMPA (alpha-amino-3-hydroxy-5-methyl-4-isoxazolepropioninc acid) receptor function
- Possibly increases serotonin uptake, but could also act similarly to agents that block serotonin reuptake

How Long Until It Works

- Onset of therapeutic actions usually not immediate, but often delayed 2–4 weeks
- If it is not working within 6–8 weeks for depression, it may require a dosage increase or it may not work at all
- May continue to work for many years to prevent relapse of symptoms

If It Works

- The goal of treatment is complete remission of current symptoms as well as prevention of future relapses
- Treatment most often reduces or even eliminates symptoms, but not a cure since symptoms can recur after medicine stopped
- Continue treatment until all symptoms are gone (remission)
- Once symptoms gone, continue treating for 1 year for the first episode of depression
- For second and subsequent episodes of depression, treatment may need to be indefinite

If It Doesn't Work

- Many patients only have a partial response where some symptoms are improved but others persist (especially insomnia, fatigue, and problems concentrating)
- Other patients may be nonresponders, sometimes called treatment-resistant or treatment-refractory
- Consider increasing dose, switching to another agent or adding an appropriate augmenting agent
- Consider psychotherapy
- Consider evaluation for another diagnosis or for a comorbid condition (e.g., medical illness, substance abuse, etc.)

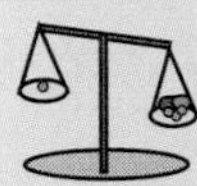

Best Augmenting Combos for Partial Response or Treatment Resistance

- Augmentation has not been systematically studied with tianeptine

Tests

✻ May have less weight gain than classical tricyclic antidepressants
- None for healthy individuals
- Since tricyclic and tetracyclic antidepressants are frequently associated with weight gain, it is possible that this may also be the case for tianeptine; thus, before starting treatment, weigh all patients and determine if the patient is already overweight (BMI 25.0–29.9) or obese (BMI ≥30)
- Before giving a drug that can cause weight gain to an overweight or obese patient, consider determining whether the patient already has pre-diabetes (fasting plasma glucose 100–25 mg/dL), diabetes (fasting plasma glucose >126 mg/dL), or dyslipidemia (increased total cholesterol, LDL cholesterol and triglycerides; decreased HDL cholesterol), and treat or refer such patients for treatment, including nutrition and weight management, physical activity counseling, smoking cessation, and medical management
- Monitor weight and BMI during treatment
- While giving a drug to a patient who has gained >5% of initial weight, consider evaluating for the presence of pre-diabetes,

diabetes, or dyslipidemia, or consider switching to a different antidepressant
- Theoretically, by analogy with TCAs, EKGs may be useful for selected patients (e.g., those with personal or family history of QTc prolongation; cardiac arrhythmia; recent myocardial infarction; uncompensated heart failure; or taking agents that prolong QTc interval such as pimozide, thioridazine, selected antiarrhythmics, moxifloxacin, sparfloxacin, etc.)
- On a theoretical basis and by analogy with TCAs, patients at risk for electrolyte disturbances (e.g., patients on diuretic therapy) should have baseline and periodic serum potassium and magnesium measurements

SIDE EFFECTS

How Drug Causes Side Effects

❊ Mild anticholinergic activity (less than some other tricyclic antidepressants) could possibly lead to sedative effects, dry mouth, constipation, and blurred vision
- Most side effects are immediate but often go away with time

❊ Pharmacologic studies indicate tianeptine may not be a potent alpha 1antagonist or H1 antihistamine
- Theoretically, cardiac arrhythmias and seizures, especially in overdose, may be caused by blockade of ion channels

Notable Side Effects

- Headache, dizziness, insomnia, sedation
- Nausea, constipation, abdominal pain, dry mouth
- Abnormal dreams
- Rare hepatotoxicity
- Tachycardia

Life-Threatening or Dangerous Side Effects

- Theoretically, lowered seizure threshold and rare seizures
- Theoretically, rare induction of mania and activation of suicidal ideation or behavior
- Short-term studies did not show an increase in the risk of suicidality with antidepressants compared to placebo beyond age 24
- Theoretically, could prolong QTc interval, but not well-studied

Weight Gain

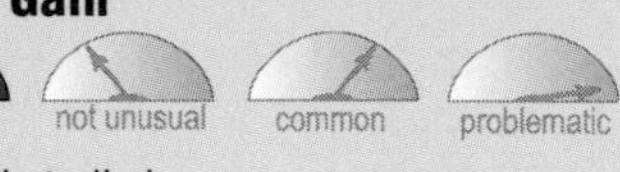

- Not well studied

Sedation

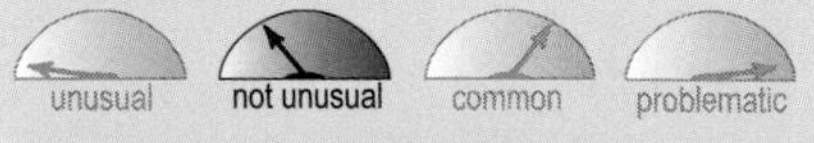

- Occurs in significant minority

What to do About Side Effects

- Wait
- Wait
- Wait
- Lower the dose
- In a few weeks, switch or add other drugs

Best Augmenting Agents for Side Effects

- Augmentation for side effects of tianeptine has not been systematically studied

DOSING AND USE

Usual Dosage Range

- 25–50 mg/day

Dosage Forms

- Tablet 12.5 mg

How To Dose

- 12.5 mg 3 times/day

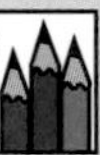

Dosing Tips

- Tianeptine's rapid elimination necessitates strict adherence to the dosing schedule

❊ Short half-life means multiple daily doses

❊ Although tianeptine has a tricyclic structure, it is dosed lower than usual TCA dosing

Overdose

- Effects are generally mild and nonfatal; unlikely to cause cardiovascular effects

Long-Term Use

- Safe

Habit Forming
- No

How to Stop
- Taper to avoid withdrawal symptoms
- Many patients tolerate 50% dose reduction for 3 days, then another 50% reduction for 3 days, then discontinuation
- If withdrawal symptoms emerge during discontinuation, raise dose to stop symptoms and then restart withdrawal much more slowly

Pharmacokinetics
- Not primarily metabolized by CYP 450 enzyme system
- Tianeptine is rapidly eliminated
- Half-life approximately 2.5 hours

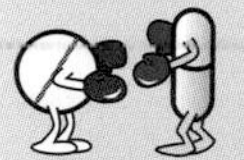

Drug Interactions
- Tramadol increases the risk of seizures in patients taking TCAs
- Activation and agitation, especially following switching or adding antidepressants, may represent the induction of a bipolar state, especially a mixed dysphoric bipolar II condition sometimes associated with suicidal ideation, and require the addition of lithium, a mood stabilizer or an atypical antipsychotic, and/or discontinuation of tianeptine
- Other drug interactions not well-studied

Other Warnings/ Precautions
- Add or initiate other antidepressants with caution for up to 2 weeks after discontinuing tianeptine
- For elective surgery, tianeptine should be stopped 24–48 hours before general anesthesia is administered
- Generally, use only with extreme caution with MAO inhibitors; do not use until 14 days after MAOIs are stopped; do not start an MAOI until 2 weeks after discontinuing tianeptine
- Although not well studied for tianeptine, TCAs can prolong QTc interval, especially at toxic doses, potentially causing torsade de pointes-type arrhythmia or sudden death; this has not been reported specifically for tianeptine
- Because TCAs can prolong QTc interval, use with caution in patients who have bradycardia or who are taking drugs that can induce bradycardia (e.g., beta blockers, calcium channel blockers, clonidine, digitalis)
- Because TCAs can prolong QTc interval, use with caution in patients who have hypokalemia and/or hypomagnesemia or who are taking drugs that can induce hypokalemia and/or magnesemia (e.g., diuretics, stimulant laxatives, intravenous amphotericin B, glucocorticoids, tetracosactide)
- When treating children, carefully weigh the risks and benefits of pharmacological treatment against the risks and benefits of nontreatment with antidepressants and make sure to document this in the patient's chart
- Warn patients and their caregivers about the possibility of activating side effects and advise them to report such symptoms immediately
- Monitor patients for activation of suicidal ideation, especially children and adolescents

Do Not Use
- If patient is taking an MAO inhibitor
- If patient is pregnant or nursing
- On a theoretical basis, if patient is taking agents capable of significantly prolonging QTc interval (e.g., pimozide, thioridazine, selected antiarrhythmics, moxifloxacin, sparfloxacin)
- On a theoretical basis, if there is a history of QTc prolongation or cardiac arrhythmia, recent acute myocardial infarction, uncompensated heart failure
- If there is a proven allergy to tianeptine

SPECIAL POPULATIONS

Renal Impairment
- Dose should be reduced for severe impairment to 25 mg/day
- Dose reduction not necessary for patients on hemodialysis

Hepatic Impairment
- No dose adjustment necessary

Cardiac Impairment
- No dose adjustment necessary
- Safety of tianeptine in patients with cardiac impairment has not been specifically demonstrated
- TCAs have been reported to cause arrhythmias, prolongation of conduction time, orthostatic hypotension, sinus tachycardia, and heart failure, especially in the diseased heart
- Myocardial infarction and stroke have been reported with TCAs
- TCAs produce QTc prolongation, which may be enhanced by the existence of bradycardia, hypokalemia, congenital or acquired long QTc interval, which should be evaluated prior to administering tianeptine
- Avoid TCAs in patients with a known history of QTc prolongation, recent acute myocardial infarction, and uncompensated heart failure
- TCAs may cause a sustained increase in heart rate in patients with ischemic heart disease and may worsen (decrease) heart rate variability, an independent risk of mortality in cardiac populations

✻ Risk/benefit ratio may not justify use of TCAs in cardiac impairment

Elderly
- Dose should be reduced to 25 mg/day
- Reduction in risk of suicidality with antidepressants compared to placebo in adults age 65 and older

Children and Adolescents
- Carefully weigh the risks and benefits of pharmacological treatment against the risks and benefits of nontreatment with antidepressants and make sure to document this in the patient's chart
- Monitor patients face-to-face regularly, particularly during the first several weeks of treatment
- Use with caution, observing for activation of known or unknown bipolar disorder and/or suicidal ideation, and inform parents or guardian of this risk so they can help observe child or adolescent patients
- Has been used successfully to treat asthmatic symptoms in children
- Not recommended for use in children under age 15

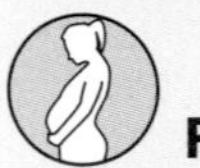

Pregnancy
- Risk Category not formally assessed by the US FDA
- Not recommended for use during pregnancy

Breast Feeding
- Some drug is found in mother's breast milk

✻ Not recommended for use during pregnancy

- Immediate postpartum period is a high-risk time for depression, especially in women who have had prior depressive episodes, so drug may need to be reinstituted late in the third trimester or shortly after childbirth to prevent a recurrence during the postpartum period
- Must weigh benefits of breast feeding with risks and benefits of antidepressant treatment versus nontreatment to both the infant and the mother
- For many patients, this may mean continuing treatment during breast feeding

THE ART OF PSYCHOPHARMACOLOGY

Potential Advantages
- Elderly patients
- Alcohol withdrawal

Potential Disadvantages
- Patients who have difficulty being compliant with multiple daily dosing

Primary Target Symptoms
- Depressed mood
- Symptoms of anxiety

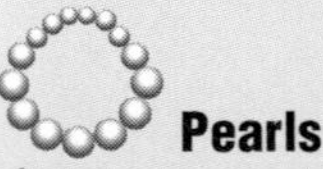

Pearls
✻ Possibly a unique mechanism of action

- However, mechanism of action not well understood
- Not marketed widely throughout the world, but mostly in France

✻ Effects on QTc prolongation not systematically studied

Suggested Reading

Brink CB, Harvey BH, Brand L. Tianeptine: a novel atypical antidepressant that may provide new insights into the biomolecular basis of depression. Recent Patents CNS Drug Discov 2006;1(1):29–41.

Kasper S, McEwen BS. Neurobiological and clinical effects of the antidepressant tianeptine. CNS Drugs 2008;22(1):15–26.

Svenningsson P, Bateup H, Qi H, et al. Involvement of AMPA receptor phosphorylation in antidepressant actions with special reference to tianeptine. Eur J Neurosci 2007;26:3509–17.

Wagstaff AJ, Ormrod D, Spencer CM. Tianeptine: a review of its use in depressive disorders. CNS Drugs 2001;15(3):231–59.

Wilde MI, Benfield P. Tianeptine. A review of its pharmacodynamic and pharmacokinetic properties, and therapeutic efficacy in depression and coexisting anxiety and depression. Drugs 1995;49(3):411–39.

THERAPEUTICS

Brands
- Topamax
- Epitomax
- Topamac
- Topimax

see index for additional brand names

Generic? No

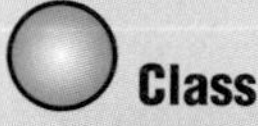

Class
- Anticonvulsant, voltage-sensitive sodium channel modulator

Commonly Prescribed for

(bold for FDA approved)
- **Partial onset seizures (adjunctive; adults and pediatric patients 2–16 years of age)**
- **Primary generalized tonic-clonic seizures (adjunctive; adults and pediatric patients 2–16 years of age)**
- **Seizures associated with Lennox-Gastaut Syndrome (2 years of age or older)**
- **Migraine prophylaxis**
- Bipolar disorder (adjunctive; no longer in development)
- Psychotropic drug-induced weight gain
- Binge-eating disorder

How the Drug Works

- * Blocks voltage-sensitive sodium channels by an unknown mechanism
- Inhibits release of glutamate
- Potentiates activity of gamma-aminobutyric acid (GABA)
- Carbonic anhydrase inhibitor

How Long Until It Works

- Should reduce seizures by 2 weeks
- Not clear that it has mood-stabilizing properties, but some bipolar patients may respond and if so, it may take several weeks to months to optimize an effect on mood stabilization

If It Works

- The goal of treatment is complete remission of symptoms (e.g., mania, seizures, migraine)
- Continue treatment until all symptoms are gone or until improvement is stable and then continue treating indefinitely as long as improvement persists
- Continue treatment indefinitely to avoid recurrence of mania, seizures, and headaches

If It Doesn't Work (for bipolar disorder)

- * May be effective only in a subset of bipolar patients, in some patients who fail to respond to other mood stabilizers, or it may not work at all
- * Consider increasing dose or switching to another agent with better demonstrated efficacy in bipolar disorder

Best Augmenting Combos for Partial Response or Treatment Resistance

- Topiramate is itself a second-line augmenting agent for numerous other anticonvulsants, lithium, and antipsychotics in treating bipolar disorder

Tests

- * Baseline and periodic serum bicarbonate levels to monitor for hyperchloremic, non-anion gap metabolic acidosis (i.e., decreased serum bicarbonate below the normal reference range in the absence of chronic respiratory alkalosis)

SIDE EFFECTS

How Drug Causes Side Effects

- CNS side effects theoretically due to excessive actions at voltage-sensitive sodium channels
- Weak inhibition of carbonic anhydrase may lead to kidney stones and paresthesias
- Inhibition of carbonic anhydrase may also lead to metabolic acidosis

Notable Side Effects

- * Sedation, asthenia, dizziness, ataxia, parasthesia, nervousness, nystagmus, tremor
- * Nausea, appetite loss, weight loss
- Blurred or double vision, mood problems, problems concentrating, confusion, memory problems, psychomotor retardation, language problems, speech problems, fatigue, taste perversion

Life-Threatening or Dangerous Side Effects

- ✽ Metabolic acidosis
- ✽ Kidney stones
- Secondary narrow angle-closure glaucoma
- Oligohidrosis and hyperthermia (more common in children)
- Sudden unexplained deaths have occurred in epilepsy (unknown if related to topiramate use)
- Rare activation of suicidal ideation and behavior (suicidality)

Weight Gain

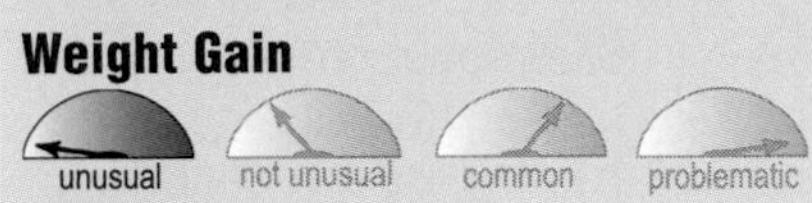

- Reported but not expected
- ✽ Patients may experience weight loss

Sedation

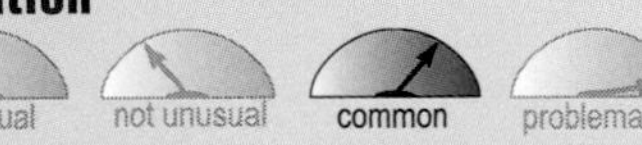

- Many experience and/or can be significant in amount

What to do About Side Effects

- Wait
- Wait
- Wait
- Take at night to reduce daytime sedation
- Increase fluid intake to reduce the risk of kidney stones
- Switch to another agent

Best Augmenting Agents for Side Effects

- Many side effects cannot be improved with an augmenting agent

DOSING AND USE

Usual Dosage Range

- Adults: 200–400 mg/day in 2 divided doses for epilepsy; 50–300 mg/day for adjunctive treatment of bipolar disorder

Dosage Forms

- Tablet 25 mg, 100 mg, 200 mg
- Sprinkle capsule 15 mg, 25 mg

How To Dose

- Adults: initial 25–50 mg/day; increase each week by 50 mg/day; administer in 2 divided doses; maximum dose generally 1,600 mg/day
- Seizures (ages 2–16): see Children and Adolescents

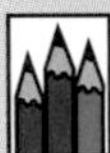

Dosing Tips

- Adverse effects may increase as dose increases
- Topiramate is available in a sprinkle capsule formulation, which can be swallowed whole or sprinkled over approximately a teaspoon of soft food (e.g., applesauce); the mixture should be consumed immediately
- Bipolar patients are generally administered doses at the lower end of the dosing range
- Slow upward titration from doses as low as 25 mg/day can reduce the incidence of unacceptable sedation
- Many bipolar patients do not tolerate more than 200 mg/day
- ✽ Weight loss is dose-related but most patients treated for weight gain receive doses at the lower end of the dosing range

Overdose

- No fatalities have been reported in monotherapy; convulsions, sedation, speech disturbance, blurred or double vision, metabolic acidosis, impaired coordination, hypotension, abdominal pain, agitation, dizziness

Long-Term Use

- Probably safe
- Periodic monitoring of serum bicarbonate levels may be required

Habit Forming

- No

How to Stop

- Taper
- Epilepsy patients may seize upon withdrawal, especially if withdrawal is abrupt
- ✽ Rapid discontinuation may increase the risk of relapse in bipolar patients
- ✽ Discontinuation symptoms uncommon

Pharmacokinetics

- Elimination half-life approximately 21 hours
- Renally excreted

Drug Interactions

- Carbamazepine, phenytoin, and valproate may increase the clearance of topiramate, and thus decrease topiramate levels, possibly requiring a higher dose of topiramate
- Topiramate may increase the clearance of phenytoin and thus decrease phenytoin levels, possibly requiring a higher dose of phenytoin
- Topiramate may increase the clearance of valproate and thus decrease valproate levels, possibly requiring a higher dose of valproate
- Topiramate may increase plasma levels of metformin; also, metformin may reduce clearance of topiramate and increase topiramate levels
- Topiramate may interact with carbonic anhydrase inhibitors to increase the risk of kidney stones
- Topiramate may reduce the effectiveness of oral contraceptives
- Reports of hyperammonemia with or without encephalopthay in patients taking topiramate combined with valproate, though this is not due to a pharmacokinetic interaction; in patients who develop unexplained lethargy, vomiting, or change in mental status, an ammonia level should be measured

Other Warnings/ Precautions

✻ If symptoms of metabolic acidosis develop (hyperventilation, fatigue, anorexia, cardiac arrhythmias, stupor), then dose may need to be reduced or treatment may need to be discontinued

- Depressive effects may be increased by other CNS depressants (alcohol, MAOIs, other anticonvulsants, etc.)
- Use with caution when combining with other drugs that predispose patients to heat-related disorders, including carbonic anhydrase inhibitors and anticholinergics
- Warn patients and their caregivers about the possibility of activation of suicidal ideation and advise them to report such side effects immediately

Do Not Use

- If there is a proven allergy to topiramate

SPECIAL POPULATIONS

Renal Impairment

- Topiramate is renally excreted, so the dose should be lowered by half
- Can be removed by hemodialysis; patients receiving hemodialysis may require supplemental doses of topiramate

Hepatic Impairment

- Drug should be used with caution

Cardiac Impairment

- Drug should be used with caution

Elderly

- Elderly patients may be more susceptible to adverse effects

Children and Adolescents

- Approved for use in children age 2 and older for treatment of seizures
- Clearance is increased in pediatric patients
- Seizures (ages 2–16): initial 1–3 mg/kg per day at night; after 1 week increase by 1–3 mg/kg per day every 1–2 weeks with total daily dose administered in 2 divided doses; recommended dose generally 5–9 mg/kg per day in 2 divided doses

Pregnancy

- Risk Category C [some animal studies show adverse effects; no controlled studies in humans]
- Use in women of childbearing potential requires weighing potential benefits to the mother against the risks to the fetus
- Hypospadia has occurred in some male infants whose mothers took topiramate during pregnancy

✻ Lack of convincing efficacy for treatment of bipolar disorder suggests risk/benefit ratio is in favor of discontinuing topiramate in bipolar patients during pregnancy

* For bipolar patients, topiramate should generally be discontinued before anticipated pregnancies
- Antiepileptic Drug Pregnancy Registry: (888) 233-2334
- Taper drug if discontinuing
* For bipolar patients, given the risk of relapse in the postpartum period, mood stabilizer treatment, especially with agents with better evidence of efficacy than topiramate, should generally be restarted immediately after delivery if patient is unmedicated during pregnancy
* Atypical antipsychotics may be preferable to topiramate if treatment of bipolar disorder is required during pregnancy
- Bipolar symptoms may recur or worsen during pregnancy and some form of treatment may be necessary
- Seizures, even mild seizures, may cause harm to the embryo/fetus

Breast Feeding

- Some drug is found in mother's breast milk
* Recommended either to discontinue drug or bottle feed
- If drug is continued while breast feeding, infant should be monitored for possible adverse effects
- If infant shows signs of irritability or sedation, drug may need to be discontinued
* Bipolar disorder may recur during the postpartum period, particularly if there is a history of prior postpartum episodes of either depression or psychosis
* Relapse rates may be lower in women who receive prophylactic treatment for postpartum episodes of bipolar disorder
- Atypical antipsychotics and anticonvulsants such as valproate may be safer and more effective than topiramate during the postpartum period when treating nursing mother with bipolar disorder

THE ART OF PSYCHOPHARMACOLOGY

Potential Advantages

- Treatment-resistant bipolar disorder
- Patients who wish to avoid weight gain

Potential Disadvantages

- Efficacy in bipolar disorder uncertain
- Patients with a history of kidney stones or risks for metabolic acidosis

Primary Target Symptoms

- Incidence of seizures
- Unstable mood

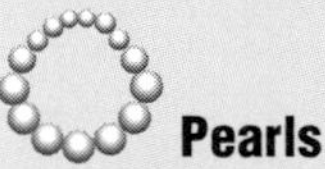

Pearls

- Side effects may actually occur less often in pediatric patients
- Has been studied in a wide range of psychiatric disorders, including bipolar disorder, posttraumatic stress disorder, binge-eating disorder, obesity and others
- Some anecdotes, case series, and open-label studies have been published and are widely known suggesting efficacy in bipolar disorder
* However, randomized clinical trials do not suggest efficacy in bipolar disorder; unfortunately these important studies have not been published by the manufacturer, who has dropped topiramate from further development as a mood stabilizer, though this is not widely known
* Misperceptions about topiramate's efficacy in bipolar disorder have led to its use in more patients than other agents with proven efficacy, such as lamotrigine
* Due to reported weight loss in some patients in trials with epilepsy, topiramate is commonly used to treat weight gain, especially in patients with psychotropic drug-induced weight gain
* Weight loss in epilepsy patients is dose related with more weight loss at high doses (mean 6.5 kg or 7.3% decline) and less weight loss at lower doses (mean 1.6 kg or 2.2% decline)
* Changes in weight were greatest in epilepsy patients who weighed the most at baseline (>100 kg), with mean loss of 9.6 kg or 8.4% decline, while those weighing <60 kg had only a mean loss of 1.3 kg or 2.5% decline
* Long-term studies demonstrate that weight losses in epilepsy patients were seen within the first 3 months of treatment and peaked at a mean of 6 kg after 12–18 months of treatment; however, weight tended to return to pretreatment levels after 18 months

* Some patients with psychotropic drug-induced weight gain may experience significant weight loss (>7% of body weight) with topiramate up to 200 mg/day for 3 months, but this is not typical, is not often sustained, and has not been systemically studied
- Early studies suggest potential efficacy in binge-eating disorder

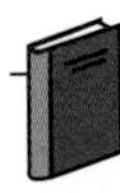

Suggested Reading

Chengappa KR, Gershon S, Levine J. The evolving role of topiramate among other mood stabilizers in the management of bipolar disorder. Bipolar Disord 2001;3:215–232.

Ormrod D, McClellan K. Topiramate: a review of its use in childhood epilepsy. Paediatr Drugs 2001;3:293–319.

MacDonald KJ, Young LT. Newer antiepileptic drugs in bipolar disorder. CNS Drugs 2002;16:549–62.

Shank RP, Gardocki JF, Streeter AJ, Maryanoff BE. An overview of the preclinical aspects of topiramate: pharmacology, pharmacokinetics, and mechanism of action. Epilepsia 2000; 41 (Suppl 1):S3–9.

Suppes T. Review of the use of topiramate for treatment of bipolar disorders. J Clin Psychopharmacol 2002;22:599–609.

THERAPEUTICS

Brands • Parnate
see index for additional brand names

Generic? Yes

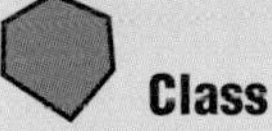

Class
- Monoamine oxidase inhibitor (MAOI)

Commonly Prescribed for
(bold for FDA approved)
- **Major depressive episode without melancholia**
- Treatment-resistant depression
- Treatment-resistant panic disorder
- Treatment-resistant social anxiety disorder

How the Drug Works
- Irreversibly blocks monoamine oxidase (MAO) from breaking down norepinephrine, serotonin, and dopamine
- This presumably boosts noradrenergic, serotonergic, and dopaminergic neurotransmission

✻ As the drug is structurally related to amphetamine, it may have some stimulant-like actions due to monoamine release and reuptake inhibition

How Long Until It Works
- Some patients may experience stimulant-like actions early in dosing
- Onset of therapeutic actions usually not immediate, but often delayed 2–4 weeks
- If it is not working within 6–8 weeks, it may require a dosage increase or it may not work at all
- May continue to work for many years to prevent relapse of symptoms

If It Works
- The goal of treatment is complete remission of current symptoms as well as prevention of future relapses
- Treatment most often reduces or even eliminates symptoms, but not a cure since symptoms can recur after medicine stopped
- Continue treatment until all symptoms are gone (remission)
- Once symptoms gone, continue treating for 1 year for the first episode of depression
- For second and subsequent episodes of depression, treatment may need to be indefinite
- Use in anxiety disorders may also need to be indefinite

If It Doesn't Work
- Many patients only have a partial response where some symptoms are improved but others persist (especially insomnia, fatigue, and problems concentrating)
- Other patients may be nonresponders, sometimes called treatment-resistant or treatment-refractory
- Some patients who have an initial response may relapse even though they continue treatment, sometimes called "poop-out"
- Consider increasing dose, switching to another agent or adding an appropriate augmenting agent
- Consider psychotherapy
- Consider evaluation for another diagnosis or for a comorbid condition (e.g., medical illness, substance abuse, etc.)
- Some patients may experience apparent lack of consistent efficacy due to activation of latent or underlying bipolar disorder, and require antidepressant discontinuation and a switch to a mood stabilizer

Best Augmenting Combos for Partial Response or Treatment Resistance

✻ Augmentation of MAOIs has not been systematically studied, and this is something for the expert, to be done with caution and with careful monitoring

✻ A stimulant such as d-amphetamine or methylphenidate (with caution; may activate bipolar disorder and suicidal ideation; may elevate blood pressure)

- Lithium
- Mood-stabilizing anticonvulsants
- Atypical antipsychotics (with special caution for those agents with monoamine reuptake blocking properties, such as ziprasidone and zotepine)

Tests
- Patients should be monitored for changes in blood pressure
- Patients receiving high doses or long-term treatment should have hepatic function evaluated periodically

SIDE EFFECTS

How Drug Causes Side Effects

- Theoretically due to increases in monoamines in parts of the brain and body and at receptors other than those that cause therapeutic actions (e.g., unwanted actions of serotonin in sleep centers causing insomnia, unwanted actions of norepinephrine on vascular smooth muscle causing hypertension, etc.)
- Side effects are generally immediate, but immediate side effects often disappear in time

Notable Side Effects

- Agitation, anxiety, insomnia, weakness, sedation, dizziness
- Constipation, dry mouth, nausea, diarrhea, change in appetite, weight gain
- Sexual dysfunction
- Orthostatic hypotension (dose-related); syncope may develop at high doses

Life-Threatening or Dangerous Side Effects

- Hypertensive crisis (especially when MAOIs are used with certain tyramine-containing foods or prohibited drugs)
- Induction of mania
- Rare activation of suicidal ideation and behavior (suicidality) (short-term studies did not show an increase in the risk of suicidality with antidepressants compared to placebo beyond age 24)
- Seizures
- Hepatotoxicity

Weight Gain

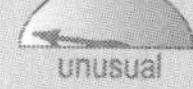
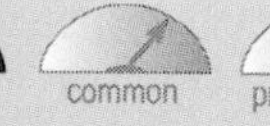

- Occurs in significant minority

Sedation

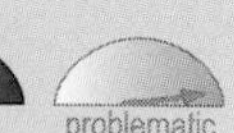

- Many experience and/or can be significant in amount
- Can also cause activation

What to do About Side Effects

- Wait
- Wait
- Wait
- Lower the dose
- Take at night if daytime sedation; take in daytime if overstimulated at night
- Switch after appropriate washout to an SSRI or newer antidepressant

Best Augmenting Agents for Side Effects

- Trazodone (with caution) for insomnia
- Benzodiazepines for insomnia
- ✻ Single oral or sublingual dose of a calcium channel blocker (e.g., nifedipine) for urgent treatment of hypertension due to drug interaction or dietary tyramine
- Many side effects cannot be improved with an augmenting agent

DOSING AND USE

Usual Dosage Range

- 30 mg/day in divided doses

Dosage Forms

- Tablet 10 mg

How To Dose

- Initial 30 mg/day in divided doses; after 2 weeks increase by 10 mg/day each 1–3 weeks; maximum 60 mg/day

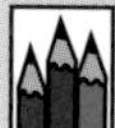

Dosing Tips

- Orthostatic hypotension, especially at high doses, may require splitting into 3–4 daily doses
- Patients receiving high doses may need to be evaluated periodically for effects on the liver

Overdose

- Dizziness, sedation, ataxia, headache, insomnia, restlessness, anxiety, irritability; cardiovascular effects, confusion, respiratory depression, or coma may also occur

Long-Term Use

- May require periodic evaluation of hepatic function
- MAOIs may lose efficacy long-term

Habit Forming

- Some patients have developed dependence to MAOIs

How to Stop

- Generally no need to taper, as the drug wears off slowly over 2–3 weeks

Pharmacokinetics

- Clinical duration of action may be up to 21 days due to irreversible enzyme inhibition

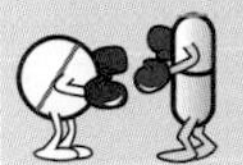

Drug Interactions

- Tramadol may increase the risk of seizures in patients taking an MAO inhibitor
- Can cause a fatal "serotonin syndrome" when combined with drugs that block serotonin reuptake (e.g., SSRIs, SNRIs, sibutramine, tramadol, etc.), so do not use with a serotonin reuptake inhibitor or for up to 5 weeks after stopping the serotonin reuptake inhibitor
- Hypertensive crisis with headache, intracranial bleeding, and death may result from combining MAO inhibitors with sympathomimetic drugs (e.g., amphetamines, methylphenidate, cocaine, dopamine, epinephrine, norepinephrine, and related compounds methyldopa, levodopa, L-tryptophan, L-tyrosine, and phenylalanine
- Excitation, seizures, delirium, hyperpyrexia, circulatory collapse, coma, and death may result from combining MAO inhibitors with mepiridine or dextromethorphan
- Do not combine with another MAO inhibitor, alcohol, buspirone, bupropion, or guanethidine
- Adverse drug reactions can result from combining MAO inhibitors with tricyclic/tetracyclic antidepressants and related compounds, including carbamazepine, cyclobenzaprine, and mirtazapine, and should be avoided except by experts to treat difficult cases
- MAO inhibitors in combination with spinal anesthesia may cause combined hypotensive effects
- Combination of MAOIs and CNS depressants may enhance sedation and hypotension

Other Warnings/ Precautions

- Use requires low-tyramine diet
- Patients taking MAO inhibitors should avoid high protein food that has undergone protein breakdown by aging, fermentation, pickling, smoking, or bacterial contamination
- Patients taking MAO inhibitors should avoid cheeses (especially aged varieties), pickled herring, beer, wine, liver, yeast extract, dry sausage, hard salami, pepperoni, Lebanon bologna, pods of broad beans (fava beans), yogurt, and excessive use of caffeine and chocolate
- Patient and prescriber must be vigilant to potential interactions with any drug, including antihypertensives and over-the-counter cough/cold preparations
- Over-the-counter medications to avoid include cough and cold preparations, including those containing dextromethorphan, nasal decongestants (tablets, drops, or spray), hay-fever medications, sinus medications, asthma inhalant medications, anti-appetite medications, weight reducing preparations, "pep" pills
- Hypoglycemia may occur in diabetic patients receiving insulin or oral antidiabetic agents
- Use cautiously in patients receiving reserpine, anesthetics, disulfiram, metrizamide, anticholinergic agents
- Tranylcypromine is not recommended for use in patients who cannot be monitored closely
- When treating children, carefully weigh the risks and benefits of pharmacological treatment against the risks and benefits of nontreatment with antidepressants and make sure to document this in the patient's chart
- Distribute the brochures provided by the FDA and the drug companies
- Warn patients and their caregivers about the possibility of activating side effects and advise them to report such symptoms immediately
- Monitor patients for activation of suicidal ideation, especially children and adolescents

Do Not Use

- If patient is taking meperidine (pethidine)
- If patient is taking a sympathomimetic agent or taking guanethidine
- If patient is taking another MAOI
- If patient is taking any agent that can inhibit serotonin reuptake (e.g., SSRIs,

sibutramine, tramadol, milnacipran, duloxetine, venlafaxine, clomipramine, etc.)
- If patient is taking diuretics, dextromethorphan, buspirone, bupropion
- If patient has pheochromocytoma
- If patient has cardiovascular or cerebrovascular disease
- If patient has frequent or severe headaches
- If patient is undergoing elective surgery and requires general anesthesia
- If patient has a history of liver disease or abnormal liver function tests
- If patient is taking a prohibited drug
- If patient is not compliant with a low-tyramine diet
- If there is a proven allergy to tranylcypromine

SPECIAL POPULATIONS

Renal Impairment
- Use with caution – drug may accumulate in plasma
- May require lower than usual adult dose

Hepatic Impairment
- Tranylcypromine should not be used in patients with history of hepatic impairment or in patients with abnormal liver function tests

Cardiac Impairment
- Contraindicated in patients with any cardiac impairment

Elderly
- Initial dose lower than usual adult dose
- Elderly patients may have greater sensitivity to adverse effects
- Reduction in risk of suicidality with antidepressants compared to placebo in adults age 65 and older

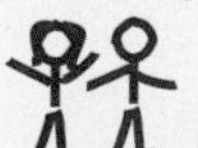

Children and Adolescents
- Not generally recommended for use in children under age 18
- Carefully weigh the risks and benefits of pharmacological treatment against the risks and benefits of nontreatment with antidepressants and make sure to document this in the patient's chart
- Monitor patients face-to-face regularly, particularly during the first several weeks of treatment
- Use with caution, observing for activation of known or unknown bipolar disorder and/or suicidal ideation, and inform parents or guardian of this risk so they can help observe child or adolescent patients

Pregnancy
- Risk Category C [some animal studies show adverse effects; no controlled studies in humans]
- Not generally recommended for use during pregnancy, especially during first trimester
- Should evaluate patient for treatment with an antidepressant with a better risk/benefit ratio

Breast Feeding
- Some drug is found in mother's breast milk
- Effects on infant unknown
- Immediate postpartum period is a high-risk time for depression, especially in women who have had prior depressive episodes, so drug may need to be reinstituted late in the third trimester or shortly after childbirth to prevent a recurrence during the postpartum period
- Should evaluate patient for treatment with an antidepressant with a better risk/benefit ratio

THE ART OF PSYCHOPHARMACOLOGY

Potential Advantages
- Atypical depression
- Severe depression
- Treatment-resistant depression or anxiety disorders

Potential Disadvantages
- Requires compliance to dietary restrictions, concomitant drug restrictions
- Patients with cardiac problems or hypertension
- Multiple daily doses

Primary Target Symptoms
- Depressed mood
- Somatic symptoms
- Sleep and eating disturbances

- Psychomotor retardation
- Morbid preoccupation

Pearls

- MAOIs are generally reserved for second-line use after SSRIs, SNRIs, and combinations of newer antidepressants have failed
- Patient should be advised not to take any prescription or over-the-counter drugs without consulting their doctor because of possible drug interactions with the MAOI
- Headache is often the first symptom of hypertensive crisis
- Foods generally to avoid as they are usually high in tyramine content: dry sausage, pickled herring, liver, broad bean pods, sauerkraut, cheese, yogurt, alcoholic beverages, nonalcoholic beer and wine, chocolate, caffeine, meat and fish
- The rigid dietary restrictions may reduce compliance
- Mood disorders can be associated with eating disorders (especially in adolescent females), and tranylcypromine can be used to treat both depression and bulimia
- MAOIs are a viable second-line treatment option in depression, but are not frequently used

✱ Myths about the danger of dietary tyramine can be exaggerated, but prohibitions against concomitant drugs often not followed closely enough

- Orthostatic hypotension, insomnia, and sexual dysfunction are often the most troublesome common side effects

✱ MAOIs should be for the expert, especially if combining with agents of potential risk (e.g., stimulants, trazodone, TCAs)

✱ MAOIs should not be neglected as therapeutic agents for the treatment-resistant

- Although generally prohibited, a heroic but potentially dangerous treatment for severely treatment-resistant patients is for an expert to give a tricyclic/tetracyclic antidepressant other than clomipramine simultaneously with an MAO inhibitor for patients who fail to respond to numerous other antidepressants
- Use of MAOIs with clomipramine is always prohibited because of the risk of serotonin syndrome and death
- Amoxapine may be the preferred trycyclic/tetracyclic antidepressant to combine with an MAOI in heroic cases due to its theoretically protective 5HT2A antagonist properties
- If this option is elected, start the MAOI with the tricyclic/tetracyclic antidepressant simultaneously at low doses after appropriate drug washout, then alternately increase doses of these agents every few days to a week as tolerated
- Although very strict dietary and concomitant drug restrictions must be observed to prevent hypertensive crises and serotonin syndrome, the most common side effects of MAOI and tricyclic/tetracyclic combinations may be weight gain and orthostatic hypotension

Suggested Reading

Baker GB, Coutts RT, McKenna KF, Sherry-McKenna RL. Insights into the mechanisms of action of the MAO inhibitors phenelzine and tranylcypromine: a review. J Psychiatry Neurosci 1992;17:206–14.

Kennedy SH. Continuation and maintenance treatments in major depression: the neglected role of monoamine oxidase inhibitors. J Psychiatry Neurosci 1997;22:127–31.

Lippman SB, Nash K. Monoamine oxidase inhibitor update. Potential adverse food and drug interactions. Drug Saf 1990;5:195–204.

Thase ME, Triyedi MH, Rush AJ. MAOIs in the contemporary treatment of depression. Neuropsychopharmacology 1995;12:185–219.

THERAPEUTICS

Brands • Desyrel

see index for additional brand names

Generic? Yes

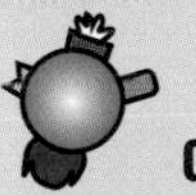

Class

- SARI (serotonin 2 antagonist/reuptake inhibitor); antidepressant; hypnotic

Commonly Prescribed for

(bold for FDA approved)

- **Depression**
- Insomnia (primary and secondary)
- Anxiety

How the Drug Works

- Blocks serotonin 2A receptors potently
- Blocks serotonin reuptake pump (serotonin transporter) less potently

How Long Until It Works

✻ Onset of therapeutic actions in insomnia are immediate if dosing is correct

- Onset of therapeutic actions in depression usually not immediate, but often delayed 2–4 weeks whether given as an adjunct to another antidepressant or as a monotherapy
- If it is not working within 6–8 weeks for depression, it may require a dosage increase or it may not work at all
- May continue to work for many years to prevent relapse of symptoms in depression and to reduce symptoms of chronic insomnia

If It Works

✻ For insomnia, use possibly can be indefinite as there is no reliable evidence of tolerance, dependence, or withdrawal, but few long-term studies

- For secondary insomnia, if underlying condition (e.g., depression, anxiety disorder) is in remission, trazodone treatment may be discontinued if insomnia does not reemerge
- The goal of treatment for depression is complete remission of current symptoms of depression as well as prevention of future relapses
- Treatment most often reduces or even eliminates symptoms of depression, but is not a cure since symptoms can recur after medicine stopped
- Continue treatment until all symptoms of depression are gone (remission)
- Once symptoms of depression are gone, continue treating for 1 year for the first episode of depression
- For second and subsequent episodes of depression, treatment may need to be indefinite

If It Doesn't Work

- For insomnia, try escalating doses or switch to another agent
- Many patients have only a partial antidepressant response where some symptoms are improved but others persist (especially insomnia, fatigue, and problems concentrating)
- Other patients may be nonresponders, sometimes called treatment-resistant or treatment-refractory
- Consider increasing dose, switching to another agent or adding an appropriate augmenting agent for treatment of depression
- Consider psychotherapy
- Consider evaluation for another diagnosis or for a comorbid condition (e.g., medical illness, substance abuse, etc.)
- Some patients may experience apparent lack of consistent efficacy due to activation of latent or underlying bipolar disorder, and require antidepressant discontinuation and a switch to a mood stabilizer

Best Augmenting Combos for Partial Response or Treatment Resistance

- Trazodone is not frequently used as a monotherapy for insomnia, but can be combined with sedative hypnotic benzodiazepines in difficult cases
- Trazodone is most frequently used in depression as an augmenting agent to numerous psychotropic drugs
- Trazodone can not only improve insomnia in depressed patients treated with antidepressants, but can also be an effective booster of antidepressant actions of other antidepressants (use combinations of antidepressants with caution as this may

activate bipolar disorder and suicidal ideation)
- Trazodone can also improve insomnia in numerous other psychiatric conditions (e.g., bipolar disorder, schizophrenia, alcohol withdrawal) and be added to numerous other psychotropic drugs (e.g., lithium, mood stabilizers, antipsychotics)

Tests
- None for healthy individuals

SIDE EFFECTS

How Drug Causes Side Effects
- Sedative effects may be due to antihistamine properties
- Blockade of alpha adrenergic 1 receptors may explain dizziness, sedation, and hypotension
- Most side effects are immediate but often go away with time

Notable Side Effects
- Nausea, vomiting, edema, blurred vision, constipation, dry mouth
- Dizziness, sedation, fatigue, headache, incoordination, tremor
- Hypotension, syncope
- Occasional sinus bradycardia (long-term)
- Rare rash

Life-Threatening or Dangerous Side Effects
- Rare priapism
- Rare seizures
- Rare induction of mania
- Rare activation of suicidal ideation and behavior (suicidality) (short-term studies did not show an increase in the risk of suicidality with antidepressants compared to placebo beyond age 24)

Weight Gain

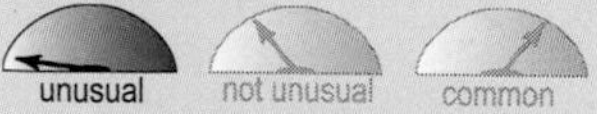

- Reported but not expected

Sedation

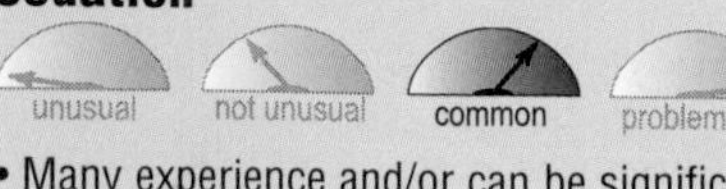

- Many experience and/or can be significant in amount

What to do About Side Effects
- Wait
- Wait
- Wait
- Take larger dose at night to prevent daytime sedation
- Switch to another agent

Best Augmenting Agents for Side Effects
- Most side effects cannot be improved with an augmenting agent
- Activation and agitation may represent the induction of a bipolar state, especially a mixed dysphoric bipolar II condition sometimes associated with suicidal ideation, and require the addition of lithium, a mood stabilizer or an atypical antipsychotic, and/or discontinuation of trazodone

DOSING AND USE

Usual Dosage Range
- 150–600 mg/day

Dosage Forms
- Tablet 50 mg scored, 100 mg scored, 150 mg, 150 mg with pividone scored, 300 mg with pividone scored

How To Dose
- For depression as a monotherapy, initial 150 mg/day in divided doses; can increase every 3–4 days by 50 mg/day as needed; maximum 400 mg/day (outpatient) or 600 mg/day (inpatient), split into 2 daily doses
- For insomnia, initial 25–50 mg at bedtime; increase as tolerated, usually to 50–100 mg/day, but some patients may require up to full antidepressant dose range
- For augmentation of other antidepressants in the treatment of depression, dose as recommended for insomnia

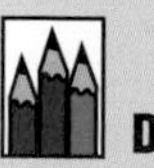

Dosing Tips
- Start low and go slow

* Patients can have carryover sedation, ataxia, and intoxicated-like feeling if dosed too aggressively, particularly when initiating dosing

✻ Do not discontinue trials if ineffective at low doses (<50 mg) as many patients with difficult cases may respond to higher doses (150–300 mg, even up to 600 mg in some cases)
- For relief of daytime anxiety, can give part of the dose in the daytime if not too sedating
- Although use as a monotherapy for depression is usually in divided doses due to its short half-life, use as an adjunct is often effective and best tolerated once daily at bedtime

Overdose
- Rarely lethal; sedation, vomiting, priapism, respiratory arrest, seizure, EKG changes

Long-Term Use
- Safe

Habit Forming
- No

How to Stop
- Taper is prudent to avoid withdrawal effects, but tolerance, dependence, and withdrawal effects have not been reliably demonstrated

Pharmacokinetics
- Metabolized by CYP450 3A4
- Half-life is biphasic; first phase is approximately 3–6 hours; second phase is approximately 5–9 hours

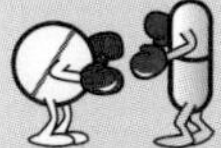

Drug Interactions
- Tramadol increases the risk of seizures in patients taking an antidepressant
- Fluoxetine and other SSRIs may raise trazodone plasma levels
- Trazodone may block the hypotensive effects of some antihypertensive drugs
- Trazodone may increase digoxin or phenytoin concentrations
- Trazodone may interfere with the antihypertensive effects of clonidine
- Generally, do not use with MAO inhibitors, including 14 days after MAOIs are stopped
- Reports of increased and decreased prothrombin time in patients taking warfarin and trazodone

Other Warnings/ Precautions
- Possibility of additive effects if trazodone is used with other CNS depressants
- Treatment should be discontinued if prolonged penile erection occurs because of the risk of permanent erectile dysfunction
- Advise patients to seek medical attention immediately if painful erections occur lasting more than one hour
- Generally, priapism reverses spontaneously, while penile blood flow and other signs being monitored, but in urgent cases, local phenylephrine injections or even surgery may be indicated
- Use with caution in patients with history of seizures
- Use with caution in patients with bipolar disorder unless treated with concomitant mood stabilizing agent
- When treating children, carefully weigh the risks and benefits of pharmacological treatment against the risks and benefits of nontreatment with antidepressants and make sure to document this in the patient's chart
- Distribute the brochures provided by the FDA and the drug companies
- Warn patients and their caregivers about the possibility of activating side effects and advise them to report such symptoms immediately
- Monitor patients for activation of suicidal ideation, especially children and adolescents

Do Not Use
- If patient is taking an MAO inhibitor, but see Pearls
- If there is a proven allergy to trazodone

SPECIAL POPULATIONS

Renal Impairment
- No dose adjustment necessary

Hepatic Impairment
- Drug should be used with caution

Cardiac Impairment
- Trazodone may be arrhythmogenic
- Monitor patients closely

- Not recommended for use during recovery from myocardial infarction

Elderly

- Elderly patients may be more sensitive to adverse effects and may require lower doses
- Reduction in risk of suicidality with antidepressants compared to placebo in adults age 65 and older

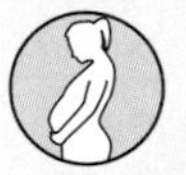

Children and Adolescents

- Carefully weigh the risks and benefits of pharmacological treatment against the risks and benefits of nontreatment with antidepressants and make sure to document this in the patient's chart
- Monitor patients face-to-face regularly, particularly during the first several weeks of treatment
- Use with caution, observing for activation of known or unknown bipolar disorder and/or suicidal ideation, and inform parents or guardian of this risk so they can help observe child or adolescent patients
- Safety and efficacy have not been established, but trazodone has been used for behavioral disturbances, depression, and night terrors
- Children require lower initial dose and slow titration
- Boys may be even more sensitive to having prolonged erections than adult men

Pregnancy

- Risk Category C [some animal studies show adverse effects; no controlled studies in humans]
- Avoid use during first trimester
- Must weigh the risk of treatment (first trimester fetal development, third trimester newborn delivery) to the child against the risk of no treatment (recurrence of depression, maternal health, infant bonding) to the mother and child
- For many patients this may mean continuing treatment during pregnancy

Breast Feeding

- Some drug is found in mother's breast milk
- If child becomes irritable or sedated, breast feeding or drug may need to be discontinued
- Immediate postpartum period is a high-risk time for depression, especially in women who have had prior depressive episodes, so drug may need to be reinstituted late in the third trimester or shortly after childbirth to prevent a recurrence during the postpartum period
- Must weigh benefits of breast feeding with risks and benefits of antidepressant treatment versus nontreatment to both the infant and the mother
- For many patients, this may mean continuing treatment during breast feeding

THE ART OF PSYCHOPHARMACOLOGY

Potential Advantages

- For insomnia when it is preferred to avoid the use of dependence-forming agents
- As an adjunct to the treatment of residual anxiety and insomnia with other antidepressants
- Depressed patients with anxiety
- Patients concerned about sexual side effects or weight gain

Potential Disadvantages

- For patients with fatigue, hypersomnia
- For patients intolerant to sedating effects

Primary Target Symptoms

- Depression
- Anxiety
- Sleep disturbances

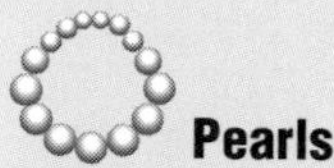

Pearls

- May be less likely than some antidepressants to precipitate hypomania or mania
- Preliminary data suggest that trazodone may be effective treatment for drug-induced dyskinesias, perhaps in part because it reduces accompanying anxiety
- Trazodone may have some efficacy in treating agitation and aggression associated with dementia
- ✻ May cause sexual dysfunction only infrequently
- Can cause carryover sedation, sometimes severe, if dosed too high

- Often not tolerated as a monotherapy for moderate to severe cases of depression, as many patients cannot tolerate high doses (>150 mg)
- Do not forget to try at high doses, up to 600 mg/day, if lower doses well tolerated but ineffective
- ✻ For the expert psychopharmacologist, trazodone can be used cautiously for insomnia associated with MAO inhibitors, despite the warning – must be attempted only if patients closely monitored and by experts experienced in the use of MAOIs
- Priapism may occur in one in 8,000 men
- Early indications of impending priapism may be slow penile detumescence when awakening from REM sleep
- When using to treat insomnia, remember that insomnia may be a symptom of some other primary disorder, and not a primary disorder itself, and thus warrant evaluation for comorbid psychiatric and/or medical conditions
- Rarely, patients may complain of visual "trails" or after-images on trazodone

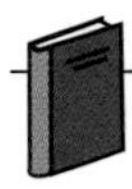

Suggested Reading

DeVane CL. Differential pharmacology of newer antidepressants. J Clin Psychiatry 1998;59 Suppl 20:85–93.

Haria M, Fitton A, McTavish D. Trazodone. A review of its pharmacology, therapeutic use in depression and therapeutic potential in other disorders. Drugs Aging 1994;4:331–55.

Rotzinger S, Bourin M, Akimoto Y, Coutts RT, Baker GB. Metabolism of some "second"- and "fourth"-generation antidepressants: iprindole, viloxazine, bupropion, mianserin, maprotiline, trazodone, nefazodone, and venlafaxine. Cell Mol Neurobiol 1999;19:427–42.

THERAPEUTICS

Brands • Halcion

see index for additional brand names

Generic? Yes

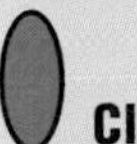

Class

- Benzodiazepine (hypnotic)

Commonly Prescribed for

(bold for FDA approved)

- **Short-term treatment of insomnia**

How the Drug Works

- Binds to benzodiazepine receptors at the GABA-A ligand-gated chloride channel complex
- Enhances the inhibitory effects of GABA
- Boosts chloride conductance through GABA-regulated channels
- Inhibitory actions in sleep centers may provide sedative hypnotic effects

How Long Until It Works

- Generally takes effect in less than an hour

If It Works

- Improves quality of sleep
- Effects on total wake-time and number of nighttime awakenings may be decreased over time

If It Doesn't Work

- If insomnia does not improve after 7–10 days, it may be a manifestation of a primary psychiatric or physical illness such as obstructive sleep apnea or restless leg syndrome, which requires independent evaluation
- Increase the dose
- Improve sleep hygiene
- Switch to another agent

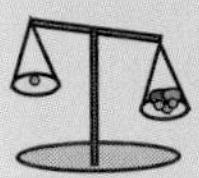

Best Augmenting Combos for Partial Response or Treatment Resistance

- Generally, best to switch to another agent
- Trazodone
- Agents with antihistamine actions (e.g., diphenhydramine, tricyclic antidepressants)

Tests

- In patients with seizure disorders, concomitant medical illness, and/or those with multiple concomitant long-term medications, periodic liver tests and blood counts may be prudent

SIDE EFFECTS

How Drug Causes Side Effects

- Same mechanism for side effects as for therapeutic effects – namely due to excessive actions at benzodiazepine receptors
- Actions at benzodiazepine receptors that carry over to the next day can cause daytime sedation, amnesia, and ataxia
- Long-term adaptations in benzodiazepine receptors may explain the development of dependence, tolerance, and withdrawal

Notable Side Effects

* Sedation, fatigue, depression
* Dizziness, ataxia, slurred speech, weakness
* Forgetfulness, confusion
* Hyperexcitability, nervousness
* Anterograde amnesia
- Rare hallucinations, mania
- Rare hypotension
- Hypersalivation, dry mouth
- Rebound insomnia when withdrawing from long-term treatment

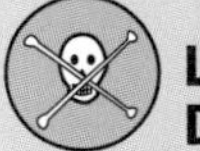

Life-Threatening or Dangerous Side Effects

- Respiratory depression, especially when taken with CNS depressants in overdose
- Rare hepatic dysfunction, renal dysfunction, blood dyscrasias

Weight Gain

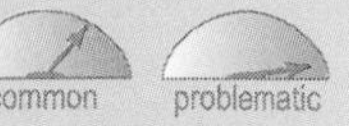

- Reported but not expected

Sedation

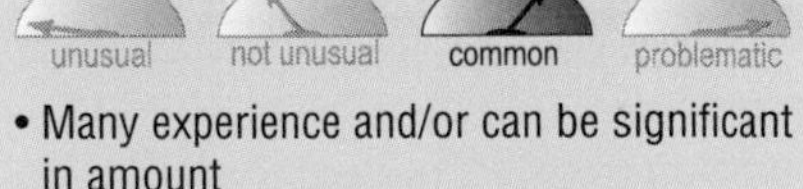

- Many experience and/or can be significant in amount

What to do About Side Effects
- Wait
- To avoid problems with memory, take triazolam only if planning to have a full night's sleep
- Lower the dose
- Switch to a shorter-acting sedative hypnotic
- Switch to a non-benzodiazepine hypnotic
- Administer flumazenil if side effects are severe or life-threatening

Best Augmenting Agents for Side Effects
- Many side effects cannot be improved with an augmenting agent

DOSING AND USE

Usual Dosage Range
- 0.125–0.25 mg/day at bedtime for 7–10 days

Dosage Forms
- Tablet 0.125 mg, 0.25 mg

How To Dose
- Initial 0.125 or 0.25 mg/day at bedtime; may increase cautiously to 0.5 mg/day if ineffective; maximum dose generally 0.5 mg/day

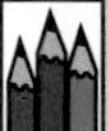

Dosing Tips
- Use lowest possible effective dose and assess need for continued treatment regularly
- ✻ Many patients cannot tolerate 0.5 mg dose (e.g., developing anterograde amnesia)
- Triazolam should generally not be prescribed in quantities greater than a 1-month supply
- Some side effects (sedation, dizziness, lightheadedness, amnesia) seem to increase with dose
- Patients with lower weights may require only a 0.125 mg dose
- Risk of dependence may increase with dose and duration of treatment
- ✻ Higher doses associated with more behavioral problems and anterograde amnesia

Overdose
- Can be fatal in monotherapy; poor coordination, confusion, seizure, slurred speech, sedation, coma, respiratory depression

Long-Term Use
- Not generally intended for long-term use
- Increased wakefulness during the latter part of night (wearing off) or an increase in daytime anxiety (rebound) may occur because of short half-life

Habit Forming
- Triazolam is a Schedule IV drug
- Some patients may develop dependence and/or tolerance; risk may be greater with higher doses
- History of drug addiction may increase risk of dependence

How to Stop
- If taken for more than a few weeks, taper to reduce chances of withdrawal effects
- Patients with seizure history may seize upon sudden withdrawal
- Rebound insomnia may occur the first 1–2 nights after stopping
- For patients with severe problems discontinuing a benzodiazepine, dosing may need to be tapered over many months (i.e., reduce dose by 1% every 3 days by crushing tablet and suspending or dissolving in 100 mL of fruit juice and then disposing of 1 mL while drinking the rest; 3–7 days later, dispose of 2 mL, and so on). This is both a form of very slow biological tapering and a form of behavioral desensitization

Pharmacokinetics
- Half-life 1.5–5.5 hours
- Inactive metabolites

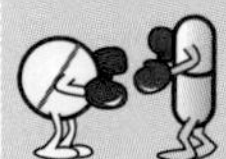

Drug Interactions
- CYP450 3A inhibitors such as nefazodone, fluoxetine, and fluvoxamine may decrease clearance of triazolam and raise triazolam levels significantly
- Ranitidine may increase plasma concentrations of triazolam
- Increased depressive effects when taken with other CNS depressants

Other Warnings/ Precautions

- Insomnia may be a symptom of a primary disorder, rather than a primary disorder itself
- Some patients may exhibit abnormal thinking or behavioral changes similar to those caused by other CNS depressants (i.e., either depressant actions or disinhibiting actions)
- Some depressed patients may experience a worsening of suicidal ideation
- Use only with extreme caution in patients with impaired respiratory function or obstructive sleep apnea
- Triazolam should be administered only at bedtime
- Grapefruit juice could increase triazolam levels

Do Not Use

- If patient is pregnant
- If patient has narrow angle-closure glaucoma
- If patient is taking ketoconazole, itraconazole, nefazodone, or other potent CYP450 3A4 inhibitors
- If there is a proven allergy to triazolam or any benzodiazepine

SPECIAL POPULATIONS

Renal Impairment

- Drug should be used with caution

Hepatic Impairment

- Drug should be used with caution

Cardiac Impairment

- Benzodiazepines have been used to treat insomnia associated with acute myocardial infarction

Elderly

- Recommended initial dose: 0.125 mg
- May be more sensitive to adverse effects

Children and Adolescents

- Safety and efficacy have not been established
- Long-term effects of triazolam in children/adolescents are unknown
- Should generally receive lower doses and be more closely monitored

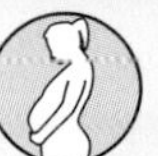

Pregnancy

- Risk Category X [positive evidence of risk to human fetus; contraindicated for use in pregnancy]
- Infants whose mothers received a benzodiazepine late in pregnancy may experience withdrawal effects
- Neonatal flaccidity has been reported in infants whose mothers took a benzodiazepine during pregnancy

Breast Feeding

- Unknown if triazolam is secreted in human breast milk, but all psychotropics assumed to be secreted in breast milk
- ✻ Recommended either to discontinue drug or bottle feed
- Effects on infant have been observed and include feeding difficulties, sedation, and weight loss

THE ART OF PSYCHOPHARMACOLOGY

Potential Advantages

- Short-acting

Potential Disadvantages

- Patients on concomitant CYP450 3A4 inhibitors
- Patients with terminal insomnia (early morning awakenings)

Primary Target Symptoms

- Time to sleep onset
- Total sleep time
- Nighttime awakenings

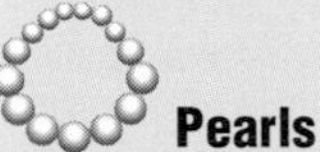

Pearls

- ✻ The shorter half-life should prevent impairments in cognitive and motor performance during the day as well as daytime sedation
- ✻ If tolerance develops, the short half-life of elimination may result in increased anxiety during the day and/or increased wakefulness during the latter part of the night

- The short half-life may minimize the risk of drug interactions with agents taken during the day (e.g., alcohol)

✻ However, the risk of drug interactions with alcohol taken at night may be greater than for some other sedative hypnotics, especially for anterograde amnesia

✻ Anterograde amnesia may be more likely with triazolam than with other sedative benzodiazepines

- Because of its short half-life and inactive metabolites, triazolam may be preferred over some benzodiazepines for patients with liver disease

✻ The risk of unusual behaviors or hallucinations may be greater with triazolam than with other sedative benzodiazepines

- Clearance of triazolam may be slightly faster in women than in men
- Women taking oral progesterone may be more sensitive to the effects of triazolam

Suggested Reading

Jonas JM, Coleman BS, Sheridan AQ, Kalinske RW. Comparative clinical profiles of triazolam versus other shorter-acting hypnotics. J Clin Psychiatry 1992;53(Suppl):19–31.

Lobo BL, Greene WL. Zolpidem: distinct from triazolam? Ann Pharmacother 1997; 31:625–32.

Rothschild AJ. Disinhibition, amnestic reactions, and other adverse reactions secondary to triazolam: a review of the literature. J Clin Psychiatry 1992; 53(Suppl):69–79.

Yuan R, Flockhart DA, Balian JD. Pharmacokinetic and pharmacodynamic consequences of metabolism-based drug interactions with alprazolam, midazolam, and triazolam. J Clin Pharmacol 1999;39:1109–25.

TRIFLUOPERAZINE

THERAPEUTICS

Brands • Stelazine

see index for additional brand names

Generic? Yes

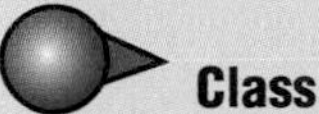

Class

- Conventional antipsychotic (neuroleptic, phenothiazine, dopamine 2 antagonist)

Commonly Prescribed For

(bold for FDA approved)

- **Schizophrenia (oral, intramuscular)**
- **Nonpsychotic anxiety (short-term, second-line)**
- Other psychotic disorders
- Bipolar disorder

How the Drug Works

- Blocks dopamine 2 receptors, reducing positive symptoms of psychosis

How Long Until It Works

- Psychotic symptoms can improve within 1 week, but it may take several weeks for full effect on behavior

If It Works

- Most often reduces positive symptoms in schizophrenia but does not eliminate them
- Most schizophrenic patients do not have a total remission of symptoms but rather a reduction of symptoms by about a third
- Continue treatment in schizophrenia until reaching a plateau of improvement
- After reaching a satisfactory plateau, continue treatment for at least a year after first episode of psychosis in schizophrenia
- For second and subsequent episodes of psychosis in schizophrenia, treatment may need to be indefinite
- Reduces symptoms of acute psychotic mania but not proven as a mood stabilizer or as an effective maintenance treatment in bipolar disorder
- After reducing acute psychotic symptoms in mania, switch to a mood stabilizer and/or an atypical antipsychotic for mood stabilization and maintenance

If It Doesn't Work

- Consider trying one of the first-line atypical antipsychotics (risperidone, olanzapine, quetiapine, ziprasidone, aripiprazole, paliperidone, amisulpride)
- Consider trying another conventional antipsychotic
- If 2 or more antipsychotic monotherapies do not work, consider clozapine

Best Augmenting Combos for Partial Response or Treatment Resistance

- Augmentation of conventional antipsychotics has not been systematically studied
- Addition of a mood-stabilizing anticonvulsant such as valproate, carbamazepine, or lamotrigine may be helpful in both schizophrenia and bipolar mania
- Augmentation with lithium in bipolar mania may be helpful
- Addition of a benzodiazepine, especially short-term for agitation

Tests

- ✽ Since conventional antipsychotics are frequently associated with weight gain, before starting treatment, weigh all patients and determine if the patient is already overweight (BMI 25.0–29.9) or obese (BMI ≥30)
- Before giving a drug that can cause weight gain to an overweight or obese patient, consider determining whether the patient already has pre-diabetes (fasting plasma glucose 100–25 mg/dL), diabetes (fasting plasma glucose >126 mg/dL), or dyslipidemia (increased total cholesterol, LDL cholesterol and triglycerides; decreased HDL cholesterol), and treat or refer such patients for treatment, including nutrition and weight management, physical activity counseling, smoking cessation, and medical management
- ✽ Monitor weight and BMI during treatment
- ✽ Consider monitoring fasting triglycerides monthly for several months in patients at high risk for metabolic complications and when initiating or switching antipsychotics
- ✽ While giving a drug to a patient who has gained >5% of initial weight, consider evaluating for the presence of pre-diabetes, diabetes, or dyslipidemia, or consider switching to a different antipsychotic
- Should check blood pressure in the elderly before starting and for the first few weeks

of treatment
- Monitoring elevated prolactin levels of dubious clinical benefit
- Phenothiazines may cause false-positive phenylketonuria results

SIDE EFFECTS

How Drug Causes Side Effects
- By blocking dopamine 2 receptors in the striatum, it can cause motor side effects
- By blocking dopamine 2 receptors in the pituitary, it can cause elevations in prolactin
- By blocking dopamine 2 receptors excessively in the mesocortical and mesolimbic dopamine pathways, especially at high doses, it can cause worsening of negative and cognitive symptoms (neuroleptic-induced deficit syndrome)
- Anticholinergic actions may cause sedation, blurred vision, constipation, dry mouth
- Antihistaminic actions may cause sedation, weight gain
- By blocking alpha 1 adrenergic receptors, it can cause dizziness, sedation, and hypotension
- Mechanism of weight gain and any possible increased incidence of diabetes or dyslipidemia with conventional antipsychotics is unknown

Notable Side Effects
✻ Neuroleptic-induced deficit syndrome
✻ Akathisia
✻ Rash
✻ Priapism
✻ Extrapyramidal symptoms, Parkinsonism, tardive dyskinesia, tardive dystonia
✻ Galactorrhea, amenorrhea
- Dizziness, sedation
- Dry mouth, constipation, blurred vision, urinary retention
- Decreased sweating
- Sexual dysfunction
- Hypotension

Life-Threatening or Dangerous Side Effects
- Rare neuroleptic malignant syndrome
- Rare jaundice, agranulocytosis
- Rare seizures
- Increased risk of death and cerebrovascular events in elderly patients with dementia-related psychosis

Weight Gain
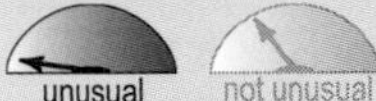
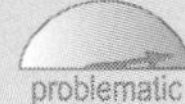

✻ Reported but not expected

Sedation
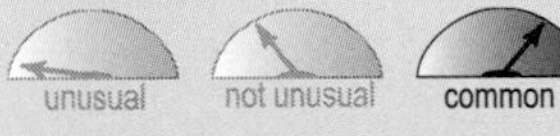

- Many experience and/or can be significant in amount
- Sedation is usually transient

What to do About Side Effects
- Wait
- Wait
- Wait
- For motor symptoms, add an anticholinergic agent
- Reduce the dose
- For sedation, give at night
- Switch to an atypical antipsychotic
- Weight loss, exercise programs, and medical management for high BMIs, diabetes, dyslipidemia

Best Augmenting Agents for Side Effects
- Benztropine or trihexyphenidyl for motor side effects
- Sometimes amantadine can be helpful for motor side effects
- Benzodiazepines may be helpful for akathisia
- Many side effects cannot be improved with an augmenting agent

DOSING AND USE

Usual Dosage Range
- Oral: Psychosis: 15–20 mg/day

Dosage Forms
- Tablet 1 mg, 2 mg, 5 mg, 10 mg
- Vial 2 mg/mL
- Concentrate 10 mg/mL

How To Dose
- Psychosis: oral: initial 2–5 mg twice a day; increase gradually over 2–3 weeks

- Psychosis: intramuscular: 1–2 mg every 4–6 hours; generally do not exceed 6 mg/day
- Anxiety: initial 1–2 mg/day; maximum 6 mg/day

Dosing Tips

* Use only low doses and short-term for anxiety because trifluoperazine is now a second-line treatment and has the risk of tardive dyskinesia
- Concentrate contains sulfites that may cause allergic reactions, particularly in patients with asthma
- Many patients can be dosed once a day

Overdose

- Extrapyramidal symptoms, sedation, seizures, coma, hypotension, respiratory depression

Long-Term Use

- Some side effects may be irreversible (e.g., tardive dyskinesia)
- Not intended to treat anxiety long-term (i.e., longer than 12 weeks)

Habit Forming

- No

How to Stop

- Slow down-titration of oral formulation (over 6–8 weeks), especially when simultaneously beginning a new antipsychotic while switching (i.e., cross-titration)
- Rapid oral discontinuation may lead to rebound psychosis and worsening of symptoms
- If antiparkinson agents are being used, they should be continued for a few weeks after trifluoperazine is discontinued

Pharmacokinetics

- Mean elimination half-life approximately 12.5 hours

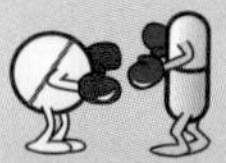

Drug Interactions

- May decrease the effects of levodopa, dopamine agonists
- May increase the effects of antihypertensive drugs except for guanethidine, whose antihypertensive actions trifluoperazine may antagonize
- Additive effects may occur if used with CNS depressants
- Alcohol and diuretics may increase the risk of hypotension; epinephrine may lower blood pressure
- Phenothiazines may reduce effects of anticoagulants
- Some patients taking a neuroleptic and lithium have developed an encephalopathic syndrome similar to neuroleptic malignant syndrome
- If used with propranolol, plasma levels of both drugs may rise

Other Warnings/ Precautions

- If signs of neuroleptic malignant syndrome develop, treatment should be immediately discontinued
- Use cautiously in patients with alcohol withdrawal or convulsive disorders because of possible lowering of seizure threshold
- Use with caution in patients with respiratory disorders, glaucoma, or urinary retention
- Avoid undue exposure to sunlight
- Avoid extreme heat exposure
- Antiemetic effect may mask signs of other disorders or overdose; suppression of cough reflex may cause asphyxia
- Do not use epinephrine in event of overdose as interaction with some pressor agents may lower blood pressure
- Use only with caution if at all in Parkinson's disease or Lewy body dementia

Do Not Use

- If patient is in a comatose state or has CNS depression
- If there is the presence of blood dyscrasias, bone marrow depression, or liver disease
- If there is a proven allergy to trifluoperazine
- If there is a known sensitivity to any phenothiazine

SPECIAL POPULATIONS

Renal Impairment
- Use with caution

Hepatic Impairment
- Not recommended for use

Cardiac Impairment
- Dose should be lowered
- Do not use parenteral administration unless necessary

Elderly
- Lower doses should be used and patient should be monitored closely
- Although conventional antipsychotics are commonly used for behavioral disturbances in dementia, no agent has been approved for treatment of elderly patients with dementia-related psychosis
- Elderly patients with dementia-related psychosis treated with antipsychotics are at an increased risk of death compared to placebo, and also have an increased risk of cerebrovascular events

Children and Adolescents
- Not recommended for use in children under age 6
- Children should be closely monitored when taking trifluoperazine
- Oral: initial 1 mg; increase gradually; maximum 15 mg/day except in older children with severe symptoms
- Intramuscular: 1 mg once or twice a day
- Generally consider second-line after atypical antipsychotics

Pregnancy
- Risk Category C [some animal studies show adverse effects; no controlled studies in humans]
- Reports of extrapyramidal symptoms, jaundice, hyperreflexia, hyporeflexia in infants whose mothers took a phenothiazine during pregnancy
- Trifluoperazine should only be used during pregnancy if clearly needed
- Psychotic symptoms may worsen during pregnancy and some form of treatment may be necessary
- Atypical antipsychotics may be preferable to conventional antipsychotics or anticonvulsant mood stabilizers if treatment is required during pregnancy

Breast Feeding
- Some drug is found in mother's breast milk.
- ✽ Recommended either to discontinue drug or bottle feed

THE ART OF PSYCHOPHARMACOLOGY

Potential Advantages
- Intramuscular formulation for emergency use

Potential Disadvantages
- Patients with tardive dyskinesia
- Children
- Elderly

Primary Target Symptoms
- Positive symptoms of psychosis
- Motor and autonomic hyperactivity
- Violent or aggressive behavior

Pearls
- Trifluoperazine is a higher potency phenothiazine
- ✽ Although not systematically studied, may cause less weight gain than other antipsychotics
- Less risk of sedation and orthostatic hypotension but greater extrapyramidal symptoms than with low potency phenothiazines
- Conventional antipsychotics are much less expensive than atypical antipsychotics
- Patients have very similar antipsychotic responses to any conventional antipsychotic, which is different from atypical antipsychotics where antipsychotic responses of individual patients can occasionally vary greatly from one atypical antipsychotic to another
- Patients with inadequate responses to atypical antipsychotics may benefit from a trial of augmentation with a conventional antipsychotic such as trifluoperazine or from switching to a conventional antipsychotic such as trifluoperazine

- However, long-term polypharmacy with a combination of a conventional antipsychotic such as trifluoperazine with an atypical antipsychotic may combine their side effects without clearly augmenting the efficacy of either
- Although a frequent practice by some prescribers, adding 2 conventional antipsychotics together has little rationale and may reduce tolerability without clearly enhancing efficacy

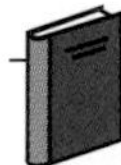

Suggested Reading

Doongaji DR, Satoskar RS, Sheth AS, Apte JS, Desai AB, Shah BR. Centbutindole vs trifluoperazine: a double-blind controlled clinical study in acute schizophrenia. J Postgrad Med 1989;35:3–8.

Frankenburg FR. Choices in antipsychotic therapy in schizophrenia. Harv Rev Psychiatry 1999;6:241–9.

Kiloh LG, Williams SE, Grant DA, Whetton PS. A double-blind comparative trial of loxapine and trifluoperazine in acute and chronic schizophrenic patients. J Int Med Res 1976;4:441–8.

THERAPEUTICS

Brands • Surmontil

see index for additional brand names

Generic? Yes

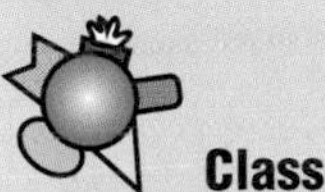

Class

- Tricyclic antidepressant (TCA)
- Serotonin and norepinephrine/noradrenaline reuptake inhibitor

Commonly Prescribed For

(bold for FDA approved)

- **Depression**
- **Endogenous depression**
- Anxiety
- Insomnia
- Neuropathic pain/chronic pain
- Treatment-resistant depression

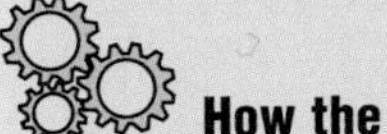

How the Drug Works

- Boosts neurotransmitters serotonin and norepinephrine/noradrenaline
- Blocks serotonin reuptake pump (serotonin transporter), presumably increasing serotonergic neurotransmission
- Blocks norepinephrine reuptake pump (norepinephrine transporter), presumably increasing noradrenergic neurotransmission
- Presumably desensitizes both serotonin 1A receptors and beta adrenergic receptors
- Since dopamine is inactivated by norepinephrine reuptake in frontal cortex, which largely lacks dopamine transporters, trimipramine can increase dopamine neurotransmission in this part of the brain

How Long Until It Works

- May have immediate effects in treating insomnia, agitation, or anxiety
- Onset of therapeutic actions usually not immediate, but often delayed 2–4 weeks
- If it is not working within 6–8 weeks for depression, it may require a dosage increase or it may not work at all
- May continue to work for many years to prevent relapse of symptoms

If It Works

- The goal of treatment of depression is complete remission of current symptoms as well as prevention of future relapses
- The goal of treatment of chronic neuropathic pain is to reduce symptoms as much as possible, especially in combination with other treatments
- Treatment of depression most often reduces or even eliminates symptoms, but not a cure since symptoms can recur after medicine stopped
- Treatment of chronic neuropathic pain may reduce symptoms, but rarely eliminates them completely, and is not a cure since symptoms can recur after medicine is stopped
- Continue treatment of depression until all symptoms are gone (remission)
- Once symptoms of depression are gone, continue treating for 1 year for the first episode of depression
- For second and subsequent episodes of depression, treatment may need to be indefinite
- Use in anxiety disorders and chronic pain may also need to be indefinite, but long-term treatment is not well studied in these conditions

If It Doesn't Work

- Many depressed patients only have a partial response where some symptoms are improved but others persist (especially insomnia, fatigue, and problems concentrating)
- Other depressed patients may be nonresponders, sometimes called treatment-resistant or treatment-refractory
- Consider increasing dose, switching to another agent or adding an appropriate augmenting agent
- Consider psychotherapy
- Consider evaluation for another diagnosis or for a comorbid condition (e.g., medical illness, substance abuse, etc.)
- Some patients may experience apparent lack of consistent efficacy due to activation of latent or underlying bipolar disorder, and require antidepressant discontinuation and a switch to a mood stabilizer

Best Augmenting Combos for Partial Response or Treatment Resistance

- Lithium, buspirone, thyroid hormone (for depression)
- Gabapentin, tiagabine, other anticonvulsants, even opiates if done by experts while monitoring carefully in difficult cases (for chronic pain)

Tests

- None for healthy individuals
- ✻ Since tricyclic and tetracyclic antidepressants are frequently associated with weight gain, before starting treatment, weigh all patients and determine if the patient is already overweight (BMI 25.0–29.9) or obese (BMI ≥30)
- Before giving a drug that can cause weight gain to an overweight or obese patient, consider determining whether the patient already has pre-diabetes (fasting plasma glucose 100–25 mg/dL), diabetes (fasting plasma glucose >126 mg/dL), or dyslipidemia (increased total cholesterol, LDL cholesterol and triglycerides; decreased HDL cholesterol), and treat or refer such patients for treatment, including nutrition and weight management, physical activity counseling, smoking cessation, and medical management
- ✻ Monitor weight and BMI during treatment
- ✻ While giving a drug to a patient who has gained >5% of initial weight, consider evaluating for the presence of pre-diabetes, diabetes, or dyslipidemia, or consider switching to a different antipsychotic
- EKGs may be useful for selected patients (e.g., those with personal or family history of QTc prolongation; cardiac arrhythmia; recent myocardial infarction; uncompensated heart failure; or taking agents that prolong QTc interval such as pimozide, thioridazine, selected antiarrhythmics, moxifloxacin, sparfloxacin, etc.)
- Patients at risk for electrolyte disturbances (e.g., patients on diuretic therapy) should have baseline and periodic serum potassium and magnesium measurements

SIDE EFFECTS

How Drug Causes Side Effects

- Anticholinergic activity may explain sedative effects, dry mouth, constipation, and blurred vision
- Sedative effects and weight gain may be due to antihistamine properties
- Blockade of alpha adrenergic 1 receptors may explain dizziness, sedation, and hypotension
- Cardiac arrhythmias and seizures, especially in overdose, may be caused by blockade of ion channels

Notable Side Effects

- Blurred vision, constipation, urinary retention, increased appetite, dry mouth, nausea, diarrhea, heartburn, unusual taste in mouth, weight gain
- Fatigue, weakness, dizziness, sedation, headache, anxiety, nervousness, restlessness
- Sexual dysfunction (impotence, change in libido)
- Sweating, rash, itching

Life-Threatening or Dangerous Side Effects

- Paralytic ileus, hyperthermia (TCAs + anticholinergic agents)
- Lowered seizure threshold and rare seizures
- Orthostatic hypotension, sudden death, arrhythmias, tachycardia
- QTc prolongation
- Hepatic failure, extrapyramidal symptoms
- Increased intraocular pressure
- Rare induction of mania
- Rare activation of suicidal ideation and behavior (suicidality) (short-term studies did not show an increase in the risk of suicidality with antidepressants compared to placebo beyond age 24)

Weight Gain

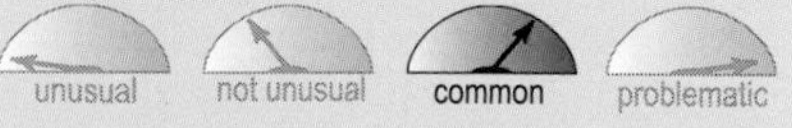

- Many experience and/or can be significant in amount
- Can increase appetite and carbohydrate craving

Sedation

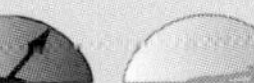

- Many experience and/or can be significant in amount
- Tolerance to sedative effects may develop with long-term use

What to do About Side Effects

- Wait
- Wait
- Wait
- Lower the dose
- Switch to an SSRI or newer antidepressant

Best Augmenting Agents for Side Effects

- Many side effects cannot be improved with an augmenting agent

DOSING AND USE

Usual Dosage Range

- 50–150 mg/day

Dosage Forms

- Capsule 25 mg, 50 mg, 100 mg

How To Dose

- Initial 25 mg/day at bedtime; increase by 75 mg every 3–7 days
- 75 mg/day in divided doses; increase to 150 mg/day; maximum 200 mg/day; hospitalized patients may receive doses up to 300 mg/day

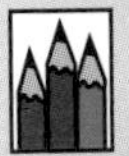

Dosing Tips

- If given in a single dose, should generally be administered at bedtime because of its sedative properties
- If given in split doses, largest dose should generally be given at bedtime because of its sedative properties
- If patients experience nightmares, split dose and do not give large dose at bedtime
- Patients treated for chronic pain may only require lower doses
- If intolerable anxiety, insomnia, agitation, akathisia, or activation occur either upon dosing initiation or discontinuation, consider the possibility of activated bipolar disorder, and switch to a mood stabilizer or an atypical antipsychotic

Overdose

- Death may occur; CNS depression, convulsions, cardiac dysrhythmias, severe hypotension, EKG changes, coma

Long-Term Use

- Safe

Habit Forming

- No

How to Stop

- Taper to avoid withdrawal effects
- Even with gradual dose reduction some withdrawal symptoms may appear within the first 2 weeks
- Many patients tolerate 50% dose reduction for 3 days, then another 50% reduction for 3 days, then discontinuation
- If withdrawal symptoms emerge during discontinuation, raise dose to stop symptoms and then restart withdrawal much more slowly

Pharmacokinetics

- Substrate for CYP450 2D6, 2C19, and 2C9
- Half-life approximately 7–23 hours

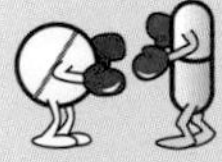

Drug Interactions

- Tramadol increases the risk of seizures in patients taking TCAs
- Use of TCAs with anticholinergic drugs may result in paralytic ileus or hyperthermia
- Fluoxetine, paroxetine, bupropion, duloxetine, and other CYP450 2D6 inhibitors may increase TCA concentrations
- Cimetidine may increase plasma concentrations of TCAs and cause anticholinergic symptoms
- Phenothiazines or haloperidol may raise TCA blood concentrations
- May alter effects of antihypertensive drugs; may inhibit hypotensive effects of clonidine
- Use with sympathomimetic agents may increase sympathetic activity
- Methylphenidate may inhibit metabolism of TCAs
- Activation and agitation, especially following switching or adding antidepressants, may represent the

induction of a bipolar state, especially a mixed dysphoric bipolar II condition sometimes associated with suicidal ideation, and require the addition of lithium, a mood stabilizer or an atypical antipsychotic, and/or discontinuation of trimipramine

Other Warnings/ Precautions

- Add or initiate other antidepressants with caution for up to 2 weeks after discontinuing trimipramine
- Generally, do not use with MAO inhibitors, including 14 days after MAOIs are stopped; do not start an MAOI until 2 weeks after discontinuing trimipramine, but see Pearls
- Use with caution in patients with history of seizures, urinary retention, narrow angle-closure glaucoma, hyperthyroidism
- TCAs can increase QTc interval, especially at toxic doses which can be attained not only by overdose but also by combining with drugs that inhibit TCA metabolism via CYP450 2D6, potentially causing torsade de pointes-type arrhythmia or sudden death
- Because TCAs can prolong QTc interval, use with caution in patients who have bradycardia or who are taking drugs that can induce bradycardia (e.g., beta blockers, calcium channel blockers, clonidine, digitalis)
- Because TCAs can prolong QTc interval, use with caution in patients who have hypokalemia and/or hypomagnesemia or who are taking drugs that can induce hypokalemia and/or magnesemia (e.g., diuretics, stimulant laxatives, intravenous amphotericin B, glucocorticoids, tetracosactide)
- When treating children, carefully weigh the risks and benefits of pharmacological treatment against the risks and benefits of nontreatment with antidepressants and make sure to document this in the patient's chart
- Distribute the brochures provided by the FDA and the drug companies
- Warn patients and their caregivers about the possibility of activating side effects and advise them to report such symptoms immediately
- Monitor patients for activation of suicidal ideation, especially children and adolescents

Do Not Use

- If patient is recovering from myocardial infarction
- If patient is taking agents capable of significantly prolonging QTc interval (e.g., pimozide, thioridazine, selected antiarrhythmics, moxifloxacin, sparfloxacin)
- If there is a history of QTc prolongation or cardiac arrhythmia, recent acute myocardial infarction, uncompensated heart failure
- If patient is taking drugs that inhibit TCA metabolism, including CYP450 2D6 inhibitors, except by an expert
- If there is reduced CYP450 2D6 function, such as patients who are poor 2D6 metabolizers, except by an expert and at low doses
- If there is a proven allergy to trimipramine

SPECIAL POPULATIONS

Renal Impairment

- Use with caution; may need to lower dose

Hepatic Impairment

- Use with caution; may need to lower dose

Cardiac Impairment

- TCAs have been reported to cause arrhythmias, prolongation of conduction time, orthostatic hypotension, sinus tachycardia, and heart failure, especially in the diseased heart
- Myocardial infarction and stroke have been reported with TCAs
- TCAs produce QTc prolongation, which may be enhanced by the existence of bradycardia, hypokalemia, congenital or acquired long QTc interval, which should be evaluated prior to administering trimipramine
- Use with caution if treating concomitantly with a medication likely to produce prolonged bradycardia, hypokalemia, slowing of intracardiac conduction, or prolongation of the QTc interval
- Avoid TCAs in patients with a known history of QTc prolongation, recent acute

myocardial infarction, and uncompensated heart failure
- TCAs may cause a sustained increase in heart rate in patients with ischemic heart disease and may worsen (decrease) heart rate variability, an independent risk of mortality in cardiac populations
- Since SSRIs may improve (increase) heart rate variability in patients following a myocardial infarct and may improve survival as well as mood in patients with acute angina or following a myocardial infarction, these are more appropriate agents for cardiac population than tricyclic/tetracyclic antidepressants

✻ Risk/benefit ratio may not justify use of TCAs in cardiac impairment

Elderly
- May be more sensitive to anticholinergic, cardiovascular, hypotensive, and sedative effects
- Initial dose 50 mg/day; increase gradually up to 100 mg/day
- Reduction in risk of suicidality with antidepressants compared to placebo in adults age 65 and older

Children and Adolescents
- Carefully weigh the risks and benefits of pharmacological treatment against the risks and benefits of nontreatment with antidepressants and make sure to document this in the patient's chart
- Monitor patients face-to-face regularly, particularly during the first several weeks of treatment
- Use with caution, observing for activation of known or unknown bipolar disorder and/or suicidal ideation, and inform parents or guardian of this risk so they can help observe child or adolescent patients
- Not recommended for use in children under age 12
- Several studies show lack of efficacy of TCAs for depression
- May be used to treat enuresis or hyperactive/impulsive behaviors
- Some cases of sudden death have occurred in children taking TCAs
- Adolescents: initial dose 50 mg/day; increase gradually up to 100 mg/day

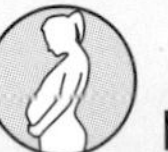

Pregnancy
- Risk Category C [some animal studies show adverse effects; no controlled studies in humans]
- Crosses the placenta
- Adverse effects have been reported in infants whose mothers took a TCA (lethargy, withdrawal symptoms, fetal malformations)
- Must weigh the risk of treatment (first trimester fetal development, third trimester newborn delivery) to the child against the risk of no treatment (recurrence of depression, maternal health, infant bonding) to the mother and child
- For many patients this may mean continuing treatment during pregnancy

Breast Feeding
- Some drug is found in mother's breast milk

✻ Recommended either to discontinue drug or bottle feed

- Immediate postpartum period is a high-risk time for depression, especially in women who have had prior depressive episodes, so drug may need to be reinstituted late in the third trimester or shortly after childbirth to prevent a recurrence during the postpartum period
- Must weigh the risk of treatment (first trimester fetal development, third trimester newborn delivery) to the child against the risk of no treatment (recurrence of depression, maternal health, infant bonding) to the mother and child
- For many patients this may mean continuing treatment during breast feeding

THE ART OF PSYCHOPHARMACOLOGY

Potential Advantages
- Patients with insomnia, anxiety
- Severe or treatment-resistant depression

Potential Disadvantages
- Pediatric and geriatric patients
- Patients concerned with weight gain and sedation

Primary Target Symptoms
- Depressed mood
- Symptoms of anxiety
- Somatic symptoms

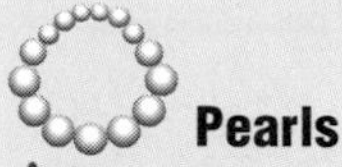

Pearls

- ✻ May be more useful than some other TCAs for patients with anxiety, sleep disturbance, and depression with physical illness
- ✻ May be more sedating than some other TCAs
- Tricyclic antidepressants are often a first-line treatment option for chronic pain
- Tricyclic antidepressants are no longer generally considered a first-line option for depression because of their side effect profile
- Tricyclic antidepressants continue to be useful for severe or treatment-resistant depression
- TCAs may aggravate psychotic symptoms
- Alcohol should be avoided because of additive CNS effects
- Underweight patients may be more susceptible to adverse cardiovascular effects
- Children, patients with inadequate hydration, and patients with cardiac disease may be more susceptible to TCA-induced cardiotoxicity than healthy adults
- For the expert only: although generally prohibited, a heroic but potentially dangerous treatment for severely treatment-resistant patients is for an expert to give a tricyclic/tetracyclic antidepressant other than clomipramine simultaneously with an MAO inhibitor for patients who fail to respond to numerous other antidepressants
- If this option is elected, start the MAOI with the tricyclic/tetracyclic antidepressant simultaneously at low doses after appropriate drug washout, then alternately increase doses of these agents every few days to a week as tolerated
- Although very strict dietary and concomitant drug restrictions must be observed to prevent hypertensive crises and serotonin syndrome, the most common side effects of MAOI and tricyclic/tetracyclic antidepressant combinations may be weight gain and orthostatic hypotension
- Patients on tricyclics should be aware that they may experience symptoms such as photosensitivity or blue-green urine
- SSRIs may be more effective than TCAs in women, and TCAs may be more effective than SSRIs in men
- Since tricyclic/tetracyclic antidepressants are substrates for CYP450 2D6, and 7% of the population (especially Caucasians) may have a genetic variant leading to reduced activity of 2D6, such patients may not safely tolerate normal doses of tricyclic/tetracyclic antidepressants and may require dose reduction
- Phenotypic testing may be necessary to detect this genetic variant prior to dosing with a tricyclic/tetracyclic antidepressant, especially in vulnerable populations such as children, elderly, cardiac populations, and those on concomitant medications
- Patients who seem to have extraordinarily severe side effects at normal or low doses may have this phenotypic CYP450 2D6 variant and require low doses or switching to another antidepressant not metabolized by 2D6

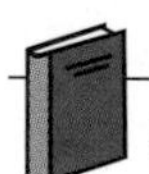

Suggested Reading

Anderson IM. Meta-analytical studies on new antidepressants. Br Med Bull 2001;57:161–78.

Anderson IM. Selective serotonin reuptake inhibitors versus tricyclic antidepressants: a meta-analysis of efficacy and tolerability. J Aff Disorders 2000;58:19–36.

Berger M, Gastpar M. Trimipramine: a challenge to current concepts on antidepressives. Eur Arch Psychiatry Clin Neurosci 1996;246:235–9.

Lapierre YD. A review of trimipramine. 30 years of clinical use. Drugs 1989;38 (Suppl 1):17–24;discussion 49–50.

THERAPEUTICS

Brands
- Depakene
- Depacon
- Depakote, Depakote ER
- Stavzor

see index for additional brand names

Generic? Yes (not for Depakote, Depakote ER, or Stavzor)

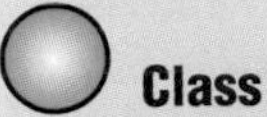

Class
- Anticonvulsant, mood stabilizer, migraine prophylaxis, voltage-sensitive sodium channel modulator

Commonly Prescribed For
(bold for FDA approved)
- **Acute mania (divalproex) and mixed episodes (divalproex, divalproex ER, valproic acid delayed-release)**
- **Complex partial seizures that occur either in isolation or in association with other types of seizures (monotherapy and adjunctive)**
- **Simple and complex absence seizures (monotherapy and adjunctive)**
- **Multiple seizure types which include absence seizures (adjunctive)**
- **Migraine prophylaxis (divalproex, divalproex ER, valproic acid delayed-release)**
- Maintenance treatment of bipolar disorder
- Bipolar depression
- Psychosis, schizophrenia (adjunctive)

How the Drug Works
✻ Blocks voltage-sensitive sodium channels by an unknown mechanism
- Increases brain concentrations of gamma-aminobutyric acid (GABA) by an unknown mechanism

How Long Until It Works
- For acute mania, effects should occur within a few days depending on the formulation of the drug
- May take several weeks to months to optimize an effect on mood stabilization
- Should also reduce seizures and improve migraine within a few weeks

If It Works
- The goal of treatment is complete remission of symptoms (e.g., mania, seizures, migraine)
- Continue treatment until all symptoms are gone or until improvement is stable and then continue treating indefinitely as long as improvement persists
- Continue treatment indefinitely to avoid recurrence of mania, depression, seizures, and headaches

If It Doesn't Work (for bipolar disorder)
✻ Many patients only have a partial response where some symptoms are improved but others persist or continue to wax and wane without stabilization of mood
- Other patients may be nonresponders, sometimes called treatment-resistant or treatment-refractory
- Consider checking plasma drug level, increasing dose, switching to another agent or adding an appropriate augmenting agent
- Consider adding psychotherapy
- Consider the presence of noncompliance and counsel patient
- Switch to another mood stabilizer with fewer side effects
- Consider evaluation for another diagnosis or for a comorbid condition (e.g., medical illness, substance abuse, etc.)

Best Augmenting Combos for Partial Response or Treatment Resistance (for bipolar disorder)
- Lithium
- Atypical antipsychotics (especially risperidone, olanzapine, quetiapine, ziprasidone, and aripiprazole)

✻ Lamotrigine (with caution and at half the dose in the presence of valproate because valproate can double lamotrigine levels)

✻ Antidepressants (with caution because antidepressants can destabilize mood in some patients, including induction of rapid cycling or suicidal ideation; in particular consider bupropion; also SSRIs, SNRIs, others; generally avoid TCAs, MAOIs)

Tests
✻ Before starting treatment, platelet counts and liver function tests

- Consider coagulation tests prior to planned surgery or if there is a history of bleeding
- During the first few months of treatment, regular liver function tests and platelet counts; this can be shifted to once or twice a year for the remainder of treatment
- Plasma drug levels can assist monitoring of efficacy, side effects, and compliance

✽ Since valproate is frequently associated with weight gain, before starting treatment, weigh all patients and determine if the patient is already overweight (BMI 25.0–29.9) or obese (BMI ≥30)

- Before giving a drug that can cause weight gain to an overweight or obese patient, consider determining whether the patient already has pre-diabetes (fasting plasma glucose 100–25 mg/dL), diabetes (fasting plasma glucose >126 mg/dL), or dyslipidemia (increased total cholesterol, LDL cholesterol and triglycerides; decreased HDL cholesterol), and treat or refer such patients for treatment, including nutrition and weight management, physical activity counseling, smoking cessation, and medical management

✽ Monitor weight and BMI during treatment

✽ While giving a drug to a patient who has gained >5% of initial weight, consider evaluating for the presence of pre-diabetes, diabetes, or dyslipidemia, or consider switching to a different agent

SIDE EFFECTS

How Drug Causes Side Effects

- CNS side effects theoretically due to excessive actions at voltage-sensitive sodium channels

Notable Side Effects

✽ Sedation, tremor, dizziness, ataxia, asthenia, headache

✽ Abdominal pain, nausea, vomiting, diarrhea, reduced appetite, constipation, dyspepsia, weight gain

✽ Alopecia (unusual)

- Polycystic ovaries (controversial)
- Hyperandrogenism, hyperinsulinemia, lipid dysregulation (controversial)
- Decreased bone mineral density (controversial)

Life-Threatening or Dangerous Side Effects

- Rare hepatotoxicity with liver failure sometimes severe and fatal, particularly in children under 2
- Rare pancreatitis, sometimes fatal
- Rare activation of suicidal ideation and behavior (suicidality)

Weight Gain

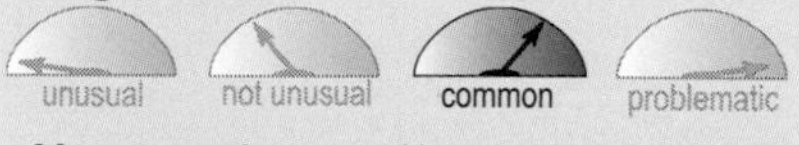

- Many experience and/or can be significant in amount
- Can become a health problem in some

Sedation

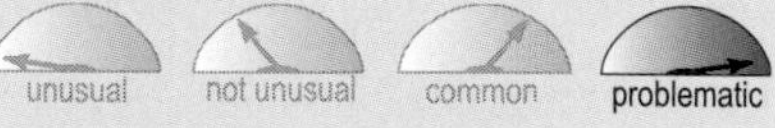

- Frequent and can be significant in amount
- Some patients may not tolerate it
- Can wear off over time
- Can reemerge as dose increases and then wear off again over time

What to do About Side Effects

- Wait
- Wait
- Wait
- Take at night to reduce daytime sedation, especially with divalproex ER
- Lower the dose
- Switch to another agent

Best Augmenting Agents for Side Effects

✽ Propranolol 20–30 mg 2–3 times/day may reduce tremor

✽ Multivitamins fortified with zinc and selenium may help reduce alopecia

- Many side effects cannot be improved with an augmenting agent

DOSING AND USE

Usual Dosage Range

- Mania: 1,200–1,500 mg/day
- Migraine: 500–1,000 mg/day
- Epilepsy: 10–60 mg/kg per day

Dosage Forms

- Tablet [delayed-release, as divalproex sodium (Depakote)] 125 mg, 250 mg, 500 mg
- Tablet [extended-release, as divalproex sodium (Depakote ER)] 250 mg, 500 mg
- Capsule [sprinkle, as divalproex sodium (Depakote Sprinkle)] 125 mg
- Capsule [as valproic acid (Depakene)] 250 mg
- Capsule [delayed-release, as valproic acid (Stavzor)] 125 mg, 250 mg, 500 mg
- Injection [as sodium valproate (Depacon)] 100 mg/mL (5 mL)
- Syrup [as sodium valproate (Depakene)] 250 mg/5 mL (5 mL, 50 mL, 480 mL)

How To Dose

- Usual starting dose for mania or epilepsy is 15 mg/kg in 2 divided doses (once daily for extended-release valproate)
- Acute mania (adults): initial 1,000 mg/day; increase dose rapidly; maximum dose generally 60 mg/kg per day
- For less acute mania, may begin at 250–500 mg the first day, and then titrate upward as tolerated
- Migraine (adults): initial 500 mg/day, maximum recommended dose 1,000 mg/day
- Epilepsy (adults): initial 10–15 mg/kg per day; increase by 5–10 mg/kg per week; maximum dose generally 60 mg/kg per day

Dosing Tips

✽ Oral loading with 20–30 mg/kg per day may reduce onset of action to 5 days or less and may be especially useful for treatment of acute mania in inpatient settings

- Given the half-life of immediate-release valproate (e.g., Depakene, Depakote), twice daily dosing is probably ideal
- Extended-release valproate (e.g., Depakote ER) can be given once daily
- However, extended-release valproate is only about 80% as bioavailable as immediate-release valproate, producing plasma drug levels 10–20% lower than with immediate-release valproate

✽ Thus, extended-release valproate is dosed approximately 8–20% higher when converting patients to the ER formulation

- Depakote (divalproex sodium) is an enteric-coated stable compound containing both valproic acid and sodium valproate

✽ Divalproex immediate-release formulation reduces gastrointestinal side effects compared to generic valproate

✽ Divalproex ER improves gastrointestinal side effects and alopecia compared to immediate-release divalproex or generic valproate

- The amide of valproic acid is available in Europe [valpromide (Depamide)]
- Trough plasma drug levels >45 μg/mL may be required for either antimanic effects or anticonvulsant actions
- Trough plasma drug levels up to 100 μg/mL are generally well tolerated
- Trough plasma drug levels up to 125 μg/mL may be required in some acutely manic patients
- Dosages to achieve therapeutic plasma levels vary widely, often between 750–3,000 mg/day

Overdose

- Fatalities have been reported; coma, restlessness, hallucinations, sedation, heart block

Long-Term Use

- Requires regular liver function tests and platelet counts

Habit Forming

- No

How to Stop

- Taper; may need to adjust dosage of concurrent medications as valproate is being discontinued
- Patients may seize upon withdrawal, especially if withdrawal is abrupt

✽ Rapid discontinuation increases the risk of relapse in bipolar disorder

- Discontinuation symptoms uncommon

Pharmacokinetics

- Mean terminal half-life 9–16 hours
- Metabolized primarily by the liver, approximately 25% dependent upon CYP450 system

Drug Interactions

- ✻ Lamotrigine dose should be reduced by perhaps 50% if used with valproate, as valproate inhibits metabolism of lamotrigine and raises lamotrigine plasma levels, theoretically increasing the risk of rash
- Plasma levels of valproate may be lowered by carbamazepine, phenytoin, ethosuximide, phenobarbital, rifampin
- Aspirin may inhibit metabolism of valproate and increase valproate plasma levels
- Plasma levels of valproate may also be increased by felbamate, chlorpromazine, fluoxetine, fluvoxamine, topiramate, cimetidine, erythromycin, and ibuprofen
- Valproate inhibits metabolism of ethosuximide, phenobarbital, and phenytoin, and can thus increase their plasma levels
- No likely pharmacokinetic interactions of valproate with lithium or atypical antipsychotics
- Use of valproate with clonazepam may cause absence status
- Reports of hyperammonemia with or without encephalopthay in patients taking topiramate combined with valproate, though this is not due to a pharmacokinetic interaction; in patients who develop unexplained lethargy, vomiting, or change in mental status, an ammonia level should be measured

Other Warnings/ Precautions

- ✻ Be alert to the following symptoms of hepatotoxicity that require immediate attention: malaise, weakness, lethargy, facial edema, anorexia, vomiting, yellowing of the skin and eyes
- ✻ Be alert to the following symptoms of pancreatitis that require immediate attention: abdominal pain, nausea, vomiting, anorexia
- ✻ Teratogenic effects in developing fetuses such as neural tube defects may occur with valproate use
- ✻ Somnolence may be more common in the elderly and may be associated with dehydration, reduced nutritional intake, and weight loss, requiring slower dosage increases, lower doses, and monitoring of fluid and nutritional intake
- Use in patients with thrombocytopenia is not recommended; patients should report easy bruising or bleeding
- Evaluate for urea cycle disorders, as hyperammonemic encephalopathy, sometimes fatal, has been associated with valproate administration in these uncommon disorders; urea cycle disorders, such as ormithine transcarbamylase deficiency, are associated with unexplained encephalopathy, mental retardation, elevated plasma ammonia, cyclical vomiting, and lethargy
- Warn patients and their caregivers about the possibility of activation of suicidal ideation and advise them to report such side effects immediately

Do Not Use

- If patient has pancreatitis
- If patient has serious liver disease
- If patient has urea cycle disorder
- If there is a proven allergy to valproic acid, valproate, or divalproex

SPECIAL POPULATIONS

Renal Impairment

- No dose adjustment necessary

Hepatic Impairment

- Contraindicated

Cardiac Impairment

- No dose adjustment necessary

Elderly

- Reduce starting dose and titrate slowly; dosing is generally lower than in healthy adults
- ✻ Sedation in the elderly may be more common and associated with dehydration, reduced nutritional intake, and weight loss
- Monitor fluid and nutritional intake

Children and Adolescents

- ✻ Not generally recommended for use in children under age 10 for bipolar disorder except by experts and when other options have been considered

- Children under age 2 have significantly increased risk of hepatotoxicity, as they have a markedly decreased ability to eliminate valproate compared to older children and adults
- Use requires close medical supervision

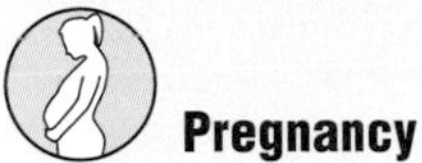

Pregnancy

- Risk Category D [positive evidence of risk to human fetus; potential benefits may still justify its use during pregnancy]
- ✻ Use during first trimester may raise risk of neural tube defects (e.g., spina bifida) or other congenital anomalies
- Use in women of childbearing potential requires weighing potential benefits to the mother against the risks to the fetus
- ✻ If drug is continued, monitor clotting parameters and perform tests to detect birth defects
- ✻ If drug is continued, start on folate 1 mg/day early in pregnancy to reduce risk of neural tube defects
- ✻ If drug is continued, consider vitamin K during the last 6 weeks of pregnancy to reduce risks of bleeding
- Antiepileptic Drug Pregnancy Registry: (888) 233-2334
- Taper drug if discontinuing
- Seizures, even mild seizures, may cause harm to the embryo/fetus
- ✻ For bipolar patients, valproate should generally be discontinued before anticipated pregnancies
- Recurrent bipolar illness during pregnancy can be quite disruptive
- ✻ For bipolar patients, given the risk of relapse in the postpartum period, mood stabilizer treatment such as valproate should generally be restarted immediately after delivery if patient is unmedicated during pregnancy
- ✻ Atypical antipsychotics may be preferable to lithium or anticonvulsants such as valproate if treatment of bipolar disorder is required during pregnancy
- Bipolar symptoms may recur or worsen during pregnancy and some form of treatment may be necessary

Breast Feeding

- Some drug is found in mother's breast milk
- ✻ Generally considered safe to breast feed while taking valproate
- If drug is continued while breast feeding, infant should be monitored for possible adverse effects
- If infant shows signs of irritability or sedation, drug may need to be discontinued
- ✻ Bipolar disorder may recur during the postpartum period, particularly if there is a history of prior postpartum episodes of either depression or psychosis
- ✻ Relapse rates may be lower in women who receive prophylactic treatment for postpartum episodes of bipolar disorder
- Atypical antipsychotics and anticonvulsants such as valproate may be safer than lithium during the postpartum period when breast feeding

THE ART OF PSYCHOPHARMACOLOGY

Potential Advantages

- Manic phase of bipolar disorder
- Works well in combination with lithium and/or atypical antipsychotics
- Patients for whom therapeutic drug monitoring is desirable

Potential Disadvantages

- Depressed phase of bipolar disorder
- Patients unable to tolerate sedation or weight gain
- Multiple drug interactions
- Multiple side effect risks
- Pregnant patients

Primary Target Symptoms

- Unstable mood
- Incidence of migraine
- Incidence of partial complex seizures

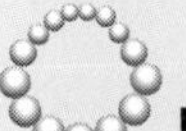

Pearls (for bipolar disorder)

- ✻ Valproate is a first-line treatment option that may be best for patients with mixed states of bipolar disorder or for patients with rapid-cycling bipolar disorder
- ✻ Seems to be more effective in treating manic episodes than depressive episodes in bipolar disorder (treats from above better than it treats from below)
- ✻ May also be more effective in preventing manic relapses than in preventing depressive episodes (stabilizes from above better than it stabilizes from below)

- Only a third of bipolar patients experience adequate relief with a monotherapy, so most patients need multiple medications for best control
- Useful in combination with atypical antipsychotics and/or lithium for acute mania
- ✻ May also be useful for bipolar disorder in combination with lamotrigine, but must reduce lamotrigine dose by half when combined with valproate
- Usefulness for bipolar disorder in combination with anticonvulsants other than lamotrigine is not well demonstrated; such combinations can be expensive and are possibly ineffective or even irrational
- ✻ May be useful as an adjunct to atypical antipsychotics for rapid onset of action in schizophrenia
- ✻ Used to treat aggression, agitation, and impulsivity not only in bipolar disorder and schizophrenia but also in many other disorders, including dementia, personality disorders, and brain injury
- Patients with acute mania tend to tolerate side effects better than patients with hypomania or depression
- Multivitamins fortified with zinc and selenium may help reduce alopecia
- Association of valproate with polycystic ovaries is controversial and may be related to weight gain, obesity, or epilepsy
- Nevertheless, may wish to be cautious in administering valproate to women of child bearing potential, especially adolescent female bipolar patients, and carefully monitor weight, endocrine status, and ovarian size and function
- ✻ In women of child bearing potential who are or are likely to become sexually active, should inform about risk of harm to the fetus and monitor contraceptive status
- Association of valproate with decreased bone mass is controversial and may be related to activity levels, exposure to sunlight, and epilepsy, and might be prevented by supplemental vitamin D 2,000 IU/day and calcium 600–1,000 mg/day
- New delayed-release capsule of valproic acid (Stavzor) may be easier to swallow than other formulations
- A prodrug of valproic acid, valpromide, is available in several European countries
- Although valpromide is rapidly transformed to valproic acid, it has some unique characteristics that can affect drug interactions
- In particular, valpromide is a potent inhibitor of liver microsomal epoxide hydrolase and thus causes clinically significant increases in the plasma levels of carbamazepine-10,11-epoxide (the active metabolite of carbamazepine)

Suggested Reading

Bowden CL. Valproate. Bipolar Disorders 2003;5:189–202.

Landy SH, McGinnis J. Divalproex sodium—review of prophylactic migraine efficacy, safety and dosage, with recommendations. Tenn Med 1999;92:135–6.

Macritchie KA, Geddes JR, Scott J, Haslam DR, Goodwin GM. Valproic acid, valproate and divalproex in the maintenance treatment of bipolar disorder. Cochrane Database Syst Rev 2001;(3):CD003196.

Smith LA, Cornelius V, Warnock A, Tacchi MJ, Taylor D. Pharmacological interventions for acute bipolar mania: a systematic review of randomized placebo-controlled trials. Bipolar Disord 2007;9(6):551–60.

THERAPEUTICS

Brands
- Chantix
- Champix

see index for additional brand names

Generic? No

Class
- Smoking cessation treatment; alpha 4 beta 2 partial agonist at nicotinic acetylcholine receptors

Commonly Prescribed For
(bold for FDA approved)
- **Nicotine addiction/dependence**

How the Drug Works
- Causes sustained but small amounts of dopamine release (less than with nicotine)
- Specifically, as a partial agonist at alpha 4 beta 2 nicotinic acetylcholine receptors, varenicline activates these receptors to a lesser extent than the full agonist nicotine and also prevents nicotine from binding to these receptors
- Most prominent actions are on mesolimbic dopaminergic neurons in the ventral tegmental area

How Long Until It Works
- Recommended initial treatment trial is 12 weeks; an additional 12-week trial in individuals who stop smoking after 12 weeks may increase likelihood of long-term abstinence

If It Works
- Reduces withdrawal symptoms and the urge to smoke; increases abstinence

If It Doesn't Work
- Evaluate for and address contributing factors, then reattempt treatment
- Consider switching to another agent

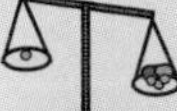

Best Augmenting Combos for Partial Response or Treatment Resistance
- Best to attempt other monotherapies

Tests
- None for healthy individuals

SIDE EFFECTS

How Drug Causes Side Effects
- Theoretically due to increases in dopamine concentrations at receptors in parts of the brain and body other than those that cause therapeutic actions

Notable Side Effects
- Dose-dependent nausea, vomiting, constipation, flatulence
- Insomnia, headache, abnormal dreams

Life-Threatening or Dangerous Side Effects
- Rare activation of agitation, depressed mood, suicidal ideation, suicidal behavior

Weight Gain

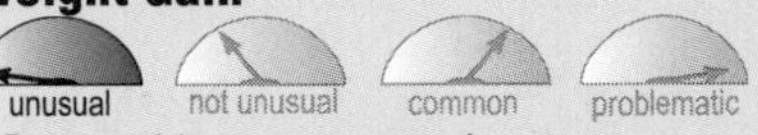

- Reported but not expected
- Some patients report weight loss

Sedation

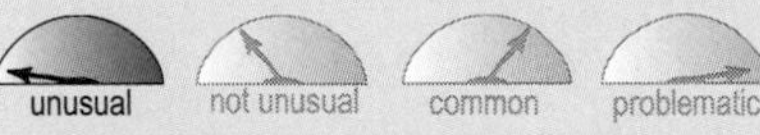

- Reported but not expected
- Some patients report activation and insomnia

What to do About Side Effects
- Wait
- Adjust dose
- If side effects persist, discontinue use

Best Augmenting Agents for Side Effects
- Dose reduction or switching to another agent may be more effective since most side effects cannot be improved with an augmenting agent

DOSING AND USE

Usual Dosage Range
- 1 mg twice daily

Dosage Forms
- Tablet 0.5 mg, 1 mg

How To Dose
- Patient should set a quit date and begin varenicline one week before the quit date
- Initial 0.5 mg/day; after three days increase to 1 mg/day in two divided doses; after 4 days can increase to 2 mg/day in two divided doses

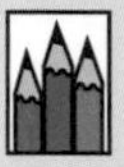

Dosing Tips
- Varenicline should be taken following a meal and with a full glass of water
- Providing educational materials and counseling in combination with varenicline treatment can increase the chances of success
- Initial recommended treatment duration is 12 weeks; for individuals who have stopped smoking after 12 weeks continued treatment for an additional 12 weeks can increase the likelihood of long-term abstinence
- For patients who are unsuccessful in their attempt to quit following 12 weeks of treatment or those who relapse following treatment, it is best to attempt to address factors contributing to the failed attempt and then reintroduce treatment

Overdose
- Limited available data

Long Term Use
- Treatment for up to 24 weeks has been found effective

Habit Forming
- No

How to Stop
- Taper to avoid withdrawal effects, but no well-documented tolerance, dependence, or withdrawal reactions

Pharmacokinetics
- Elimination half-life 24 hours

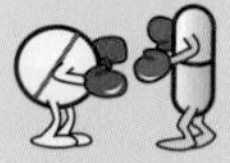

Drug Interactions
- Does not inhibit hepatic enzymes or renal transport proteins, and thus is unlikely to affect plasma concentrations of other drugs
- Is not hepatically metabolized and thus is unlikely to be affected by other drugs
- Side effects may be increased if varenicline is taken with nicotine replacement therapy

Other Warnings/Precautions
- Monitor patients for changes in behavior, agitation, depressed mood, worsening of preexisting psychiatric illness, and suicidality
- Use cautiously in individuals with known psychiatric illness
- Discontinuing smoking may lead to pharmacokinetic or pharmacodynamic changes in other drugs the patient is taking, which could potentially require dose adjustment

Do Not Use
- If there is a proven allergy to varenicline

SPECIAL POPULATIONS

Renal Impairment
- For severe impairment, maximum recommended dose is 0.5 mg twice per day
- For patients with end-stage renal disease undergoing hemodialysis, maximum recommended dose is 0.5 mg once per day
- Removed by hemodialysis

Hepatic Impairment
- Dose adjustment not generally necessary

Cardiac Impairment
- Limited available data

Elderly
- Some patients may tolerate lower doses better

Children and Adolescents
- Safety and efficacy have not been established

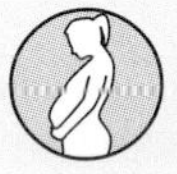

Pregnancy

- Risk Category C [some animal studies show adverse effects; no controlled studies in humans]
- Pregnant women wishing to stop smoking may consider behavioral therapy before pharmacotherapy
- Not generally recommended for use during pregnancy, especially during first trimester

Breast Feeding

- Unknown if varenicline is secreted in human breast milk, but all psychotropics assumed to be secreted in breast milk
- Recommended either to discontinue drug or bottle feed

THE ART OF PSYCHOPHARMACOLOGY

Potential Advantages

- More effective than other pharmacotherapies for smoking cessation

Potential Disadvantages

- Not well studied in patients with comorbid psychiatric disorders

Primary Target Symptoms

- Cravings associated with nicotine withdrawal

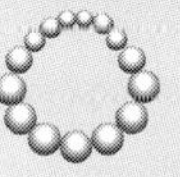

Pearls

- More effective than nicotine or bupropion
- Unlike nicotine or bupropion, the patient cannot "smoke over" varenicline since varenicline, but not the others, will block the effects of additional smoked nicotine if the patient decides to smoke during treatment
- Although tested in the general population excluding psychiatric patients, where smoking rates in the U.S. are about 20–25%, there is great unmet need for smoking cessation treatments in patients with psychiatric disorders, especially attention deficit hyperactivity disorder and schizophrenia, which have smoking rates in the U.S. as high as 50–75%
- However, smoking cessation treatment in patients with comorbid psychiatric disorders is not well studied, should be done by experts, and patients closely monitored in terms of their psychiatric symptoms, especially suicidality

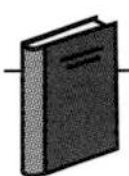

Suggested Reading

Jorenby DE, Hays JT, Rigotti NA. Efficacy of varenicline, an alpha4beta2 nicotinic acetylcholine receptor partial agonist, vs placebo or sustained-release bupropion for smoking cessation: a randomized controlled trial. JAMA 2006;296(1):56–63.

Rollema H, Coe JW, Chambers LK et al. Rationale, pharmacology and clinical efficacy of partial agonists of alpha4beta2 nACh receptors for smoking cessation. Trends Pharmacol Sci 2007;28(7):316–25.

Wu P, Wilson K, Dimoulas P, Mills EJ. Effectiveness of smoking cessation therapies: a systematic review and meta-analysis. BMC Public Health 2006;6:300.

THERAPEUTICS

Brands
- Effexor
- Effexor XR

see index for additional brand names

Generic? Yes

Class

- SNRI (dual serotonin and norepinephrine reuptake inhibitor); often classified as an antidepressant, but it is not just an antidepressant

Commonly Prescribed For

(bold for FDA approved)

- **Depression**
- **Generalized anxiety disorder (GAD)**
- **Social anxiety disorder (social phobia)**
- **Panic disorder**
- Posttraumatic stress disorder (PTSD)
- Premenstrual dysphoric disorder (PMDD)

How the Drug Works

- Boosts neurotransmitters serotonin, norepinephrine/noradrenaline, and dopamine
- Blocks serotonin reuptake pump (serotonin transporter), presumably increasing serotonergic neurotransmission
- Blocks norepinephrine reuptake pump (norepinephrine transporter), presumably increasing noradrenergic neurotransmission
- Presumably desensitizes both serotonin 1A receptors and beta adrenergic receptors
- Since dopamine is inactivated by norepinephrine reuptake in frontal cortex, which largely lacks dopamine transporters, venlafaxine can increase dopamine neurotransmission in this part of the brain
- Weakly blocks dopamine reuptake pump (dopamine transporter), and may increase dopamine neurotransmission

How Long Until It Works

- Onset of therapeutic actions usually not immediate, but often delayed 2–4 weeks
- If it is not working within 6–8 weeks for depression, it may require a dosage increase or it may not work at all
- By contrast, for generalized anxiety, onset of response and increases in remission rates may still occur after 8 weeks, and for up to 6 months after initiating dosing
- May continue to work for many years to prevent relapse of symptoms

If It Works

- The goal of treatment is complete remission of current symptoms as well as prevention of future relapses
- Treatment most often reduces or even eliminates symptoms, but not a cure since symptoms can recur after medicine stopped
- Continue treatment until all symptoms are gone (remission), especially in depression and whenever possible in anxiety disorders
- Once symptoms gone, continue treating for 1 year for the first episode of depression
- For second and subsequent episodes of depression, treatment may need to be indefinite
- Use in anxiety disorders may also need to be indefinite

If It Doesn't Work

- Many patients have only a partial response where some symptoms are improved but others persist (especially insomnia, fatigue, and problems concentrating)
- Other patients may be nonresponders, sometimes called treatment-resistant or treatment-refractory
- Some patients who have an initial response may relapse even though they continue treatment, sometimes called "poop-out"
- Consider increasing dose, switching to another agent or adding an appropriate augmenting agent
- Consider psychotherapy
- Consider evaluation for another diagnosis or for a comorbid condition (e.g., medical illness, substance abuse, etc.)
- Some patients may experience apparent lack of consistent efficacy due to activation of latent or underlying bipolar disorder, and require antidepressant discontinuation and a switch to a mood stabilizer

Best Augmenting Combos for Partial Response or Treatment Resistance

✽ Mirtazapine ("California rocket fuel"; a potentially powerful dual serotonin and norepinephrine combination, but observe

for activation of bipolar disorder and suicidal ideation)
- Bupropion, reboxetine, nortriptyline, desipramine, maprotiline, atomoxetine (all potentially powerful enhancers of noradrenergic action, but observe for activation of bipolar disorder and suicidal ideation)
- Modafinil, especially for fatigue, sleepiness, and lack of concentration
- Mood stabilizers or atypical antipsychotics for bipolar depression, psychotic depression or treatment-resistant depression
- Benzodiazepines
- If all else fails for anxiety disorders, consider gabapentin or tiagabine
- Hypnotics or trazodone for insomnia
- Classically, lithium, buspirone, or thyroid hormone

Tests

- Check blood pressure before initiating treatment and regularly during treatment

SIDE EFFECTS

How Drug Causes Side Effects

- Theoretically due to increases in serotonin and norepinephrine concentrations at receptors in parts of the brain and body other than those that cause therapeutic actions (e.g., unwanted actions of serotonin in sleep centers causing insomnia, unwanted actions of norepinephrine on acetylcholine release causing constipation and dry mouth, etc.)
- Most side effects are immediate but often go away with time

Notable Side Effects

- Most side effects increase with higher doses, at least transiently
- Headache, nervousness, insomnia, sedation
- Nausea, diarrhea, decreased appetite
- Sexual dysfunction (abnormal ejaculation/orgasm, impotence)
- Asthenia, sweating
- SIADH (syndrome of inappropriate antidiuretic hormone secretion)
- Hyponatremia
- Dose-dependent increase in blood pressure

Life-Threatening or Dangerous Side Effects

- Rare seizures
- Rare induction of hypomania
- Rare activation of suicidal ideation and behavior (suicidality) (short-term studies did not show an increase in the risk of suicidality with antidepressants compared to placebo beyond age 24)

Weight Gain

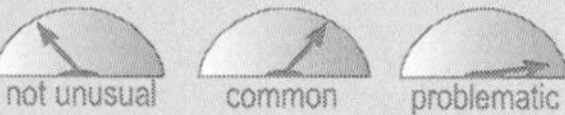

- Reported but not expected
- Possible weight loss, especially short-term

Sedation

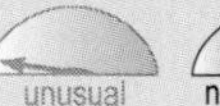

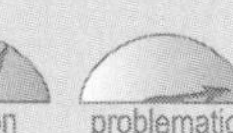

- Occurs in significant minority
- May also be activating in some patients

What to do About Side Effects

- Wait
- Wait
- Wait
- Lower the dose
- In a few weeks, switch or add other drugs

Best Augmenting Agents for Side Effects

- Often best to try another antidepressant monotherapy prior to resorting to augmentation strategies to treat side effects
- Trazodone or a hypnotic for insomnia
- Bupropion, sildenafil, vardenafil, or tadalafil for sexual dysfunction
- Benzodiazepines for jitteriness and anxiety, especially at initiation of treatment and especially for anxious patients
- Mirtazapine for insomnia, agitation, and gastrointestinal side effects
- Many side effects are dose-dependent (i.e., they increase as dose increases, or they reemerge until tolerance redevelops)
- Many side effects are time-dependent (i.e., they start immediately upon dosing and upon each dose increase, but go away with time)
- Activation and agitation may represent the induction of a bipolar state, especially a mixed dysphoric bipolar II condition sometimes associated with suicidal ideation,

and require the addition of lithium, a mood stabilizer or an atypical antipsychotic, and/or discontinuation of venlafaxine

DOSING AND USE

Usual Dosage Range

- Depression: 75–225 mg/day, once daily (extended-release) or divided into 2–3 doses (immediate-release)
- GAD: 150–225 mg/day

Dosage Forms

- Capsule (extended-release) 37.5 mg, 75 mg, 150 mg
- Tablet (extended-release) 37.5 mg, 75 mg, 150 mg, 225 mg
- Tablet 25 mg scored, 37.5 mg scored, 50 mg scored, 75 mg scored, 100 mg scored

How To Dose

- Initial dose 37.5 mg once daily (extended-release) or 25–50 mg divided into 2–3 doses (immediate-release) for a week, if tolerated; increase daily dose generally no faster than 75 mg every 4 days until desired efficacy is reached; maximum dose generally 375 mg/day
- Usually try doses at 75 mg increments for a few weeks prior to incrementing by an additional 75 mg

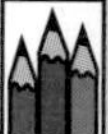

Dosing Tips

- At all doses, potent serotonin reuptake blockade
- 75–225 mg/day may be predominantly serotonergic in some patients, and dual serotonin and norepinephrine acting in other patients
- 225–375 mg/day is dual serotonin and norepinephrine acting in most patients

✻ Thus, nonresponders at lower doses should try higher doses to be assured of the benefits of dual SNRI action

- At very high doses (e.g., >375 mg/day), dopamine reuptake blocked as well in some patients
- Up to 600 mg/day has been given for heroic cases
- Venlafaxine has an active metabolite O-desmethylvenlafaxine (ODV), which is formed as the result of CYP450 2D6
- Thus, CYP450 2D6 inhibition reduces the formation of ODV, but this is of uncertain clinical significance

✻ Consider checking plasma levels of ODV and venlafaxine in nonresponders who tolerate high doses, and if plasma levels are low, experts can prudently prescribe doses above 375 mg/day while monitoring closely

- Do not break or chew venlafaxine XR capsules, as this will alter controlled-release properties

✻ For patients with severe problems discontinuing venlafaxine, dosing may need to be tapered over many months (i.e., reduce dose by 1% every 3 days by crushing tablet and suspending or dissolving in 100 mL of fruit juice, and then disposing of 1 mL while drinking the rest; 3–7 days later, dispose of 2 mL, and so on). This is both a form of very slow biological tapering and a form of behavioral desensitization

- For some patients with severe problems discontinuing venlafaxine, it may be useful to add an SSRI with a long half-life, especially fluoxetine, prior to taper of venlafaxine; while maintaining fluoxetine dosing, first slowly taper venlafaxine and then taper fluoxetine
- Be sure to differentiate between reemergence of symptoms requiring reinstitution of treatment and withdrawal symptoms

Overdose

- Can be lethal; may cause no symptoms; possible symptoms include sedation, convulsions, rapid heartbeat
- Fatal toxicity index data from the U.K. suggest a higher rate of deaths from overdose with venlafaxine than with SSRIs
- Unknown whether this is related to differences in patients who receive venlafaxine or to potential cardiovascular toxicity of venlafaxine

Long-Term Use

- See doctor regularly to monitor blood pressure, especially at doses >225 mg/day

Habit Forming

- No

How to Stop
- Taper to avoid withdrawal effects (dizziness, nausea, stomach cramps, sweating, tingling, dysesthesias)
- Many patients tolerate 50% dose reduction for 3 days, then another 50% reduction for 3 days, then discontinuation
- If withdrawal symptoms emerge during discontinuation, raise dose to stop symptoms and then restart withdrawal much more slowly

✻ Withdrawal effects can be more common or more severe with venlafaxine than with some other antidepressants

Pharmacokinetics
- Parent drug has 3–7 hour half-life
- Active metabolite has 9–13 hour half-life

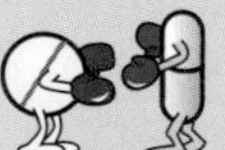

Drug Interactions
- Tramadol increases the risk of seizures in patients taking an antidepressant
- Can cause a fatal "serotonin syndrome" when combined with MAO inhibitors, so do not use with MAO inhibitors or for at least 14 days after MAOIs are stopped
- Do not start an MAO inhibitor for at least 2 weeks after discontinuing venlafaxine
- Possible increased risk of bleeding, especially when combined with anticoagulants (e.g., warfarin, NSAIDs)
- Concomitant use with cimetidine may reduce clearance of venlafaxine and raise venlafaxine levels
- Could theoretically interfere with the analgesic actions of codeine or possibly with other triptans
- Few known adverse drug interactions

Other Warnings/ Precautions
- Use with caution in patients with history of seizures
- Use with caution in patients with heart disease
- Use with caution in patients with bipolar disorder unless treated with concomitant mood stabilizing agent
- When treating children, carefully weigh the risks and benefits of pharmacological treatment against the risks and benefits of nontreatment with antidepressants and make sure to document this in the patient's chart
- Distribute the brochures provided by the FDA and the drug companies
- Warn patients and their caregivers about the possibility of activating side effects and advise them to report such symptoms immediately
- Monitor patients for activation of suicidal ideation, especially children and adolescents

Do Not Use
- If patient has uncontrolled narrow angle-closure glaucoma
- If patient is taking an MAO inhibitor
- If there is a proven allergy to venlafaxine

SPECIAL POPULATIONS

Renal Impairment
- Lower dose by 25–50%
- Patients on dialysis should not receive subsequent dose until dialysis is completed

Hepatic Impairment
- Lower dose by 50%

Cardiac Impairment
- Drug should be used with caution
- Hypertension should be controlled prior to initiation of venlafaxine and should be monitored regularly during treatment
- Venlafaxine has a dose-dependent effect on increasing blood pressure
- Venlafaxine is contraindicated in patients with heart disease in the U.K.
- Venlafaxine can block cardiac ion channels in vitro
- Venlafaxine worsens (i.e., reduces) heart rate variability in depression, perhaps due to norepinephrine reuptake inhibition

Elderly
- Some patients may tolerate lower doses better
- Reduction in risk of suicidality with antidepressants compared to placebo in adults age 65 and older

Children and Adolescents
- Carefully weigh the risks and benefits of pharmacological treatment against the

risks and benefits of nontreatment with antidepressants and make sure to document this in the patient's chart
- Monitor patients face-to-face regularly, particularly during the first several weeks of treatment
- Use with caution, observing for activation of known or unknown bipolar disorder and/or suicidal ideation, and inform parents or guardian of this risk so they can help observe child or adolescent patients
- Not specifically approved, but preliminary data suggest that venlafaxine is effective in children and adolescents with depression, anxiety disorders, and ADHD

Pregnancy

- Risk Category C [some animal studies show adverse effects; no controlled studies in humans]
- Not generally recommended for use during pregnancy, especially during first trimester
- Nonetheless, continuous treatment during pregnancy may be necessary and has not been proven to be harmful to the fetus
- Must weigh the risk of treatment (first trimester fetal development, third trimester newborn delivery) to the child against the risk of no treatment (recurrence of depression, maternal health, infant bonding) to the mother and child
- For many patients this may mean continuing treatment during pregnancy
- Neonates exposed to SSRIs or SNRIs late in the third trimester have developed complications requiring prolonged hospitalization, respiratory support, and tube feeding; reported symptoms are consistent with either a direct toxic effect of SSRIs and SNRIs or, possibly, a drug discontinuation syndrome, and include respiratory distress, cyanosis, apnea, seizures, temperature instability, feeding difficulty, vomiting, hypoglycemia, hypotonia, hypertonia, hyperreflexia, tremor, jitteriness, irritability, and constant crying

Breast Feeding

- Some drug is found in mother's breast milk
- Trace amounts may be present in nursing children whose mothers are on venlafaxine
- If child becomes irritable or sedated, breast feeding or drug may need to be discontinued
- Immediate postpartum period is a high-risk time for depression, especially in women who have had prior depressive episodes, so drug may need to be reinstituted late in the third trimester or shortly after childbirth to prevent a recurrence during the postpartum period
- Must weigh benefits of breast feeding with risks and benefits of antidepressant treatment versus nontreatment to both the infant and the mother
- For many patients, this may mean continuing treatment during breast feeding

THE ART OF PSYCHOPHARMACOLOGY

Potential Advantages

- Patients with retarded depression
- Patients with atypical depression
- Patients with comorbid anxiety
- Patients with depression may have higher remission rates on SNRIs than on SSRIs
- Depressed patients with somatic symptoms, fatigue, and pain
- Patients who do not respond or remit on treatment with SSRIs

Potential Disadvantages

- Patients sensitive to nausea
- Patients with borderline or uncontrolled hypertension
- Patients with cardiac disease

Primary Target Symptoms

- Depressed mood
- Energy, motivation, and interest
- Sleep disturbance
- Anxiety

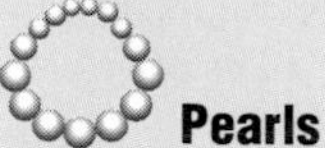

Pearls

✽ May be effective in patients who fail to respond to SSRIs, and may be one of the preferred treatments for treatment-resistant depression

✽ May be used in combination with other antidepressants for treatment-refractory cases

- XR formulation improves tolerability, reduces nausea, and requires only once-daily dosing

- May be effective in a broad array of anxiety disorders
- May be effective in adult ADHD
- Not studied in stress urinary incontinence

✻ Has greater potency for serotonin reuptake blockade than for norepinephrine reuptake blockade, but this is of unclear clinical significance as a differentiating feature from other SNRIs

✻ In vitro binding studies tend to underestimate in vivo potency for reuptake blockade, as they do not factor in the presence of high concentrations of an active metabolite, higher oral mg dosing, or the lower protein binding which can increase functional drug levels at receptor sites

- Effective dose range is broad (i.e., 75–375 mg in many difficult cases, and up to 600 mg or more in heroic cases)

✻ Preliminary studies in neuropathic pain and fibromyalgia suggest potential efficacy

- Efficacy as well as side effects (especially nausea and increased blood pressure) are dose-dependent
- Blood pressure increases rare for XR formulation in doses up to 225 mg
- More withdrawal reactions reported upon discontinuation than for some other antidepressants
- May be helpful for hot flushes in perimenopausal women
- May be associated with higher depression remission rates than SSRIs

✻ Because of recent studies from the U.K. that suggest a higher rate of deaths from overdose with venlafaxine than with SSRIs, and because of its potential to affect heart function, venlafaxine can only be prescribed in the U.K. by specialist doctors and is contraindicated there in patients with heart disease

- Overdose data are from fatal toxicity index studies, which do not take into account patient characteristics or whether drug use was first- or second-line
- Venlafaxine's toxicity in overdose is less than that for tricyclic antidepressants

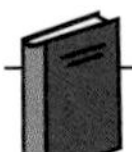

Suggested Reading

Buckley NA, McManus PR, Fatal toxicity of serotonergic and other antidepressant drugs: analysis of United Kingdom mortality data. BMJ 2002;325:1332–3.

Cheeta S, Schifano F, An Oyefeso A, Webb L, Ghodse AH. Antidepressant-related deaths and antidepressant prescriptions in England and Wales, 1998–2000. Br J Psychiatry 2004;184:41–7

Davidson J, Watkins L, Owens M, Krulewicz S, Connor K, Carpenter D, et al. Effects of paroxetine and venlafaxine XR on heart rate variability in depression. J Clin Psychopharmacol 2005;25:480–4.

Hackett D. Venlafaxine XR in the treatment of anxiety. Acta Psychiatrica Scand 2000; 406[Suppl]:30–35.

Sheehan DV. Attaining remission in generalized anxiety disorder: venlafaxine extended-release comparative data. J Clin Psychiatry 2001;62 Suppl 19:26–31.

Smith D, Dempster C, Glanville J, Freemantle N, Anderson I. Efficacy and tolerability of venlafaxine compared with selective serotonin reuptake inhibitors and other antidepressants: a meta-analysis. Br J Psychiatry 2002; 180:396–404.

Wellington K, Perry CM. Venlafaxine extended-release: a review of its use in the management of major depression. CNS Drugs 2001; 15:643–69.

ZALEPLON

THERAPEUTICS

Brands • Sonata

see index for additional brand names

Generic? No

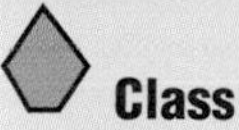

Class

• Non-benzodiazepine hypnotic; alpha 1 isoform agonist of GABA-A/benzodiazepine receptors

Commonly Prescribed For

(bold for FDA approved)

• **Short-term treatment of insomnia**

How the Drug Works

• Binds selectively to a subtype of the benzodiazepine receptor, the alpha 1 isoform
• May enhance GABA inhibitory actions that provide sedative hypnotic effects more selectively than other actions of GABA
• Boosts chloride conductance through GABA-regulated channels
• Inhibitory actions in sleep centers may provide sedative hypnotic effects

How Long Until It Works

• Generally takes effect in less than an hour

If It Works

• Improves quality of sleep
• Effects on total wake-time and number of nighttime awakenings may be decreased over time

If It Doesn't Work

• If insomnia does not improve after 7–10 days, it may be a manifestation of a primary psychiatric or physical illness such as obstructive sleep apnea or restless leg syndrome, which requires independent evaluation
• Increase the dose
• Improve sleep hygiene
• Switch to another agent

Best Augmenting Combos for Partial Response or Treatment Resistance

• Generally, best to switch to another agent
• Trazodone
• Agents with antihistamine actions (e.g., diphenhydramine, tricyclic antidepressants)

Tests

• None for healthy individuals

SIDE EFFECTS

How Drug Causes Side Effects

• Actions at benzodiazepine receptors that carry over to the next day can cause daytime sedation, amnesia, and ataxia
• Long-term adaptations of zaleplon not well studied, but chronic studies of other alpha 1 selective non-benzodiazepine hypnotics suggest lack of notable tolerance or dependence developing over time

Notable Side Effects

✻ Sedation
✻ Dizziness, ataxia
✻ Dose-dependent amnesia
✻ Hyper-excitability, nervousness
• Rare hallucinations
• Headache
• Decreased appetite

Life-Threatening or Dangerous Side Effects

• Respiratory depression, especially when taken with other CNS depressants in overdose
• Rare angioedema

Weight Gain

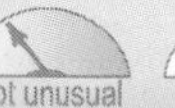
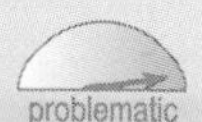

• Reported but not expected

Sedation

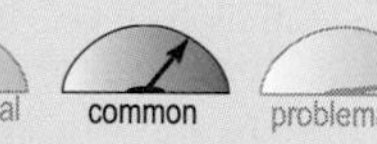

• Many experience and/or can be significant in amount

What to do About Side Effects

• Wait
• To avoid problems with memory, do not take zaleplon if planning to sleep for less than 4 hours
• Lower the dose
• Administer flumazenil if side effects are severe or life-threatening

Best Augmenting Agents for Side Effects

- Many side effects cannot be improved with an augmenting agent

DOSING AND USE

Usual Dosage Range

- 10 mg/day at bedtime for 7–10 days

Dosage Forms

- Capsule 5 mg, 10 mg

How To Dose

- Initial 10 mg/day at bedtime; may increase to 20 mg/day at bedtime if ineffective; maximum dose generally 20 mg/day

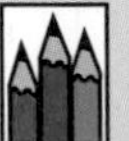

Dosing Tips

- Patients with lower body weights may require only a 5 mg dose
- Zaleplon should generally not be prescribed in quantities greater than a 1-month supply
- Risk of dependence may increase with dose and duration of treatment

✻ However, treatment with alpha 1 selective non-benzodiazepine hypnotics may cause less tolerance or dependence than benzodiazepine hypnotics

Overdose

- No fatalities reported with zaleplon; fatalities have occurred with other sedative hypnotics; sedation, confusion, ataxia, hypotension, respiratory depression, coma

Long-Term Use

- Not generally intended for long-term use
- Increased wakefulness during the latter part of night (wearing off) or an increase in daytime anxiety (rebound) may occur because of short half-life

Habit Forming

- Zaleplon is a Schedule IV drug
- Some patients may develop dependence and/or tolerance; risk may be greater with higher doses
- History of drug addiction may increase risk of dependence

How to Stop

- Rebound insomnia may occur the first night after stopping
- If taken for more than a few weeks, taper to reduce chances of withdrawal effects

Pharmacokinetics

- Terminal phase elimination half-life approximately 1 hour (ultra-short half-life)

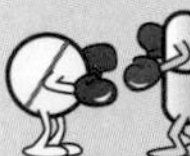

Drug Interactions

- Increased depressive effects when taken with other CNS depressants
- Cimetidine may increase plasma concentrations of zaleplon, requiring a lower initial dose of zaleplon (5 mg/day)
- CYP450 3A4 inducers such as carbamazepine may reduce the effectiveness of zaleplon

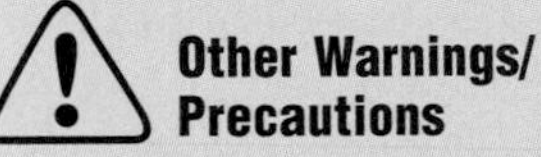

Other Warnings/ Precautions

- Insomnia may be a symptom of a primary disorder, rather than a primary disorder itself
- Some patients may exhibit abnormal thinking or behavioral changes similar to those caused by other CNS depressants (i.e., either depressant actions or disinhibiting actions)
- Some depressed patients may experience a worsening of suicidal ideation
- Use only with extreme caution in patients with impaired respiratory function or obstructive sleep apnea
- Zaleplon should be administered only at bedtime
- Rare angioedema has occurred with sedative hypnotic use and could potentially cause fatal airway obstruction if it involves the throat, glottis, or larynx; thus if angioedema occurs treatment should be discontinued
- Sleep driving and other complex behaviors, such as eating and preparing food and making phone calls, have been reported in patients taking sedative hypnotics

Do Not Use

- If there is a proven allergy to zaleplon

SPECIAL POPULATIONS

Renal Impairment
- No dose adjustment necessary
- Use with caution in patients with severe impairment

Hepatic Impairment
- Mild to moderate impairment: recommended dose 5 mg
- Not recommended for use in patients with severe impairment

Cardiac Impairment
- Zaleplon has not been studied in patients with cardiac impairment, but dose adjustment may not be necessary

Elderly
- Recommended dose: 5 mg

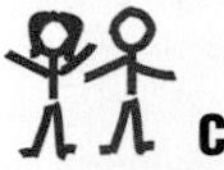

Children and Adolescents
- Safety and efficacy have not been established
- Long-term effects of zaleplon in children/adolescents are unknown
- Should generally receive lower doses and be more closely monitored

Pregnancy
- Risk Category C [some animal studies show adverse effects; no controlled studies in humans]
- Infants whose mothers took sedative hypnotics during pregnancy may experience some withdrawal symptoms
- Neonatal flaccidity has been reported in infants whose mothers took sedative hypnotics during pregnancy

Breast Feeding
- Some drug is found in mother's breast milk
- ✻ Recommended either to discontinue drug or bottle feed

THE ART OF PSYCHOPHARMACOLOGY

Potential Advantages
- Those needing short duration of action

Potential Disadvantages
- Those needing longer duration of action
- More expensive than some other sedative hypnotics

Primary Target Symptoms
- Time to sleep onset
- Total sleep time
- Nighttime awakenings

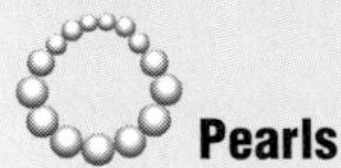

Pearls
- Zaleplon has not been shown to increase the total time asleep or to decrease the number of awakenings
- ✻ May be preferred over benzodiazepines because of its rapid onset of action, short duration of effect, and safety profile
- ✻ Popular for uses requiring short half-life (e.g., dosing in the middle of the night, sleeping on airplanes, jet lag)
- ✻ May not be ideal for patients who desire immediate hypnotic onset and eat just prior to bedtime
- Not a benzodiazepine itself, but binds to benzodiazepine receptors
- May have fewer carryover side effects than some other sedative hypnotics
- May not have sufficient efficacy in patients with severe chronic insomnia resistant to some other sedative hypnotics
- May cause less dependence than some other sedative hypnotics, especially in those without a history of substance abuse
- ✻ Zaleplon is not absorbed as quickly if taken with high-fat foods, which may reduce onset of action

Suggested Reading

Dooley M, Plosker GL. Zaleplon: a review of its use in the treatment of insomnia. Drugs 2000; 60:413–45.

Heydorn WE. Zaleplon – a review of a novel sedative hypnotic used in the treatment of insomnia. Expert Opin Invest Drugs 2000; 9:841–58.

Mangano RM. Efficacy and safety of zaleplon at peak plasma levels. Int J Clin Pract Suppl 2001;116:9–13.

Weitzel KW, Wickman JM, Augustin SG, Strom JG. Zaleplon: a pyrazolopyrimidine sedative-hypnotic agent for the treatment of insomnia. Clin Ther 2000;22:1254–67.

ZIPRASIDONE

THERAPEUTICS

Brands • Geodon
see index for additional brand names

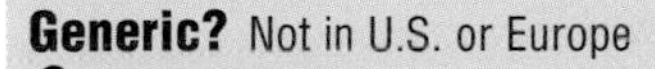

Generic? Not in U.S. or Europe

Class

- Atypical antipsychotic (serotonin-dopamine antagonist; second generation antipsychotic; also a mood stabilizer)

Commonly Prescribed For

(bold for FDA approved)

- **Schizophrenia**
- **Delaying relapse in schizophrenia**
- **Acute agitation in schizophrenia (intramuscular)**
- **Acute mania/mixed mania**
- Other psychotic disorders
- Bipolar maintenance
- Bipolar depression
- Behavioral disturbances in dementias
- Behavioral disturbances in children and adolescents
- Disorders associated with problems with impulse control

How the Drug Works

- Blocks dopamine 2 receptors, reducing positive symptoms of psychosis and stabilizing affective symptoms
- Blocks serotonin 2A receptors, causing enhancement of dopamine release in certain brain regions and thus reducing motor side effects and possibly improving cognitive and affective symptoms
- Interactions at a myriad of other neurotransmitter receptors may contribute to ziprasidone's efficacy

✻ Specifically, interactions at 5HT2C and 5HT1A receptors may contribute to efficacy for cognitive and affective symptoms in some patients

✻ Specifically, interactions at 5HT1D receptors and at serotonin, norepinephrine, and dopamine transporters (especially at high doses) may contribute to efficacy for affective symptoms in some patients

How Long Until It Works

- Psychotic and manic symptoms can improve within 1 week, but it may take several weeks for full effect on behavior as well as on cognition and affective stabilization
- Classically recommended to wait at least 4–6 weeks to determine efficacy of drug, but in practice some patients require up to 16–20 weeks to show a good response, especially on cognitive symptoms
- IM formulation can reduce agitation in 15 minutes

If It Works

- Most often reduces positive symptoms in schizophrenia but does not eliminate them
- Can improve negative symptoms, as well as aggressive, cognitive, and affective symptoms in schizophrenia
- Most schizophrenic patients do not have a total remission of symptoms but rather a reduction of symptoms by about a third
- Perhaps 5–15% of schizophrenic patients can experience an overall improvement of greater than 50–60%, especially when receiving stable treatment for more than a year
- Such patients are considered super-responders or "awakeners" since they may be well enough to be employed, live independently, and sustain long-term relationships
- Many bipolar patients may experience a reduction of symptoms by half or more
- Continue treatment until reaching a plateau of improvement
- After reaching a satisfactory plateau, continue treatment for at least a year after first episode of psychosis
- For second and subsequent episodes of psychosis, treatment may need to be indefinite
- Even for first episodes of psychosis, it may be preferable to continue treatment indefinitely to avoid subsequent episodes
- Treatment may not only reduce mania but also prevent recurrences of mania in bipolar disorder

If It Doesn't Work

- Try one of the other atypical antipsychotics (risperidone, olanzapine, quetiapine, aripiprazole, paliperidone, amisulpride)
- If 2 or more antipsychotic monotherapies do not work, consider clozapine

- If no first-line atypical antipsychotic is effective, consider higher doses or augmentation with valproate or lamotrigine
- Some patients may require treatment with a conventional antipsychotic
- Consider noncompliance and switch to another antipsychotic with fewer side effects or to an antipsychotic that can be given by depot injection
- Consider initiating rehabilitation and psychotherapy
- Consider presence of concomitant drug abuse

Best Augmenting Combos for Partial Response or Treatment Resistance

- Valproic acid (valproate, divalproex, divalproex ER)
- Other mood-stabilizing anticonvulsants (carbamazepine, oxcarbazepine, lamotrigine)
- Lithium
- Benzodiazepines

Tests

Before starting an atypical antipsychotic

✻ Weigh all patients and track BMI during treatment
- Get baseline personal and family history of diabetes, obesity, dyslipidemia, hypertension, and cardiovascular disease

✻ Get waist circumference (at umbilicus), blood pressure, fasting plasma glucose, and fasting lipid profile
- Determine if the patient is
  - overweight (BMI 25.0–29.9)
  - obese (BMI ≥30)
  - has pre-diabetes (fasting plasma glucose 100–25 mg/dL)
  - has diabetes (fasting plasma glucose >126 mg/dL)
  - has hypertension (BP >140/90 mm Hg)
  - has dyslipidemia (increased total cholesterol, LDL cholesterol, and triglycerides; decreased HDL cholesterol)
- Treat or refer such patients for treatment, including nutrition and weight management, physical activity counseling, smoking cessation, and medical management

Monitoring after starting an atypical antipsychotic

✻ BMI monthly for 3 months, then quarterly

✻ Consider monitoring fasting triglycerides monthly for several months in patients at high risk for metabolic complications and when initiating or switching antipsychotics

✻ Blood pressure, fasting plasma glucose, fasting lipids within 3 months and then annually, but earlier and more frequently for patients with diabetes or who have gained >5% of initial weight
- Treat or refer for treatment and consider switching to another atypical antipsychotic for patients who become overweight, obese, pre-diabetic, diabetic, hypertensive, or dyslipidemic while receiving an atypical antipsychotic

✻ Even in patients without known diabetes, be vigilant for the rare but life threatening onset of diabetic ketoacidosis, which always requires immediate treatment, by monitoring for the rapid onset of polyuria, polydipsia, weight loss, nausea, vomiting, dehydration, rapid respiration, weakness and clouding of sensorium, even coma
- Routine EKGs for screening or monitoring of dubious clinical value
- EKGs may be useful for selected patients (e.g., those with personal or family history of QTc prolongation; cardiac arrhythmia; recent myocardial infarction; uncompensated heart failure; or those taking agents that prolong QTc interval such as pimozide, thioridazine, selected antiarrhythmics, moxifloxacin, sparfloxacin, etc.)
- Patients at risk for electrolyte disturbances (e.g., patients on diuretic therapy) should have baseline and periodic serum potassium and magnesium measurements

SIDE EFFECTS

How Drug Causes Side Effects

- By blocking alpha 1 adrenergic receptors, it can cause dizziness, sedation, and hypotension, especially at high doses
- By blocking dopamine 2 receptors in the striatum, it can cause motor side effects (unusual)

✻ Mechanism of any possible weight gain is unknown; weight gain is not common with ziprasidone and may thus have a different mechanism from atypical antipsychotics for which weight gain is common or problematic

✻ Mechanism of any possible increased incidence of diabetes or dyslipidemia is unknown; early experience suggests these complications are not clearly associated with ziprasidone and if present may therefore have a different mechanism from that of atypical antipsychotics associated with an increased incidence of diabetes and dyslipidemia

Notable Side Effects

✻ Some patients may experience activating side effects at very low to low doses
- Dizziness, extrapyramidal symptoms, sedation, dystonia at high doses
- Nausea, dry mouth
- Asthenia, skin rash
- Rare tardive dyskinesia (much reduced risk compared to conventional antipsychotics)
- Orthostatic hypotension

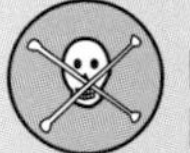

Life-Threatening or Dangerous Side Effects

- Rare neuroleptic malignant syndrome (much reduced risk compared to conventional antipsychotics)
- Rare seizures
- Increased risk of death and cerebrovascular events in elderly patients with dementia-related psychosis

Weight Gain

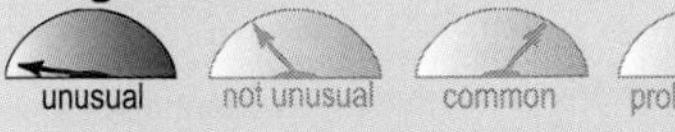

- Reported in a few patients, especially those with low BMIs, but not expected
- Less frequent and less severe than for most other antipsychotics

Sedation

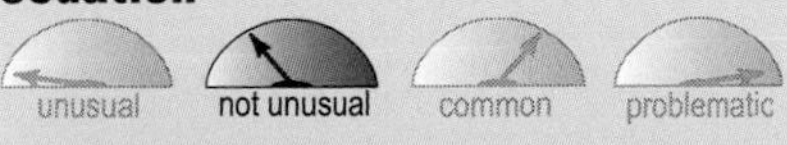

- Some patients experience, especially at high doses
- May be less than for some antipsychotics, more than for others
- Usually transient and at higher doses
- Can be activating at low doses

What to do About Side Effects

- Wait
- Wait
- Wait
- Usually dosed twice daily, so take more of the total daily dose at bedtime to help reduce daytime sedation
- Anticholinergics may reduce motor side effects when present
- Weight loss, exercise programs, and medical management for high BMIs, diabetes, dyslipidemia

✻ For activating side effects at low doses, raise the dose

✻ For sedating side effects at high doses, lower the dose
- Switch to another atypical antipsychotic

Best Augmenting Agents for Side Effects

- Benztropine or trihexyphenidyl for motor side effects
- Many side effects cannot be improved with an augmenting agent

DOSING AND USE

Usual Dosage Range

- Schizophrenia: 40–200 mg/day (in divided doses) orally
- Bipolar disorder: 80–160 mg/day (in divided doses) orally
- 10–20 mg intramuscularly

Dosage Forms

- Capsules 20 mg, 40 mg, 60 mg, 80 mg
- Injection 20 mg/mL

How To Dose

- Schizophrenia (according to manufacturer): initial oral dose 20 mg twice a day; however, 40 mg twice a day or 60 mg twice a day may be better tolerated in many patients (less activation); maximum approved dose 100 mg twice a day
- Biplar disorder (according to manufacturer): initial oral dose 40 mg twice a day; on day 2 increase to 60 or 80 mg twice a day
- For intramuscular formulation, recommended dose is 10–20 mg given as required; doses of 10 mg may be administered every 2 hours; doses of 20 mg may be administered every 4 hours; maximum daily dose 40 mg intramuscularly; should not be administered for more than 3 consecutive days

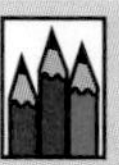

Dosing Tips

✽ **More may be much more:** clinical practice suggests ziprasidone often under-dosed, then switched prior to adequate trials, perhaps due to unjustified fears of QTc prolongation

✽ Dosing many patients at 20–40 mg twice a day is too low and in fact activating, perhaps due to potent 5HT2C antagonist properties

✽ Paradoxically, such activation is often reduced by increasing the dose to 60–80 mg twice a day, perhaps due to increasing amounts of dopamine 2 receptor antagonism

✽ Best efficacy in schizophrenia and bipolar disorder is at doses >120 mg/day, but only a minority of patients are adequately dosed in clinical practice

- Doses up to 80 mg twice a day may have a lower cost than some other atypical antipsychotics
- Intramuscular formulation costs about the same as haloperidol injections

✽ Recommended to be taken with food because food can double bioavailability by increasing absorption and thus increasing plasma drug levels

- Meals of a few hundred calories (e.g., turkey sandwich and a piece of fruit) or more necessary to enhance the absorption of ziprasidone
- Some patients respond better to doses >160 mg/day and up to 320 mg/day in 2 divided doses (i.e., 80–160 mg twice a day)
- Many patients do well with a single daily oral dose, usually at bedtime
- Although studies suggest patients switching to ziprasidone from another antipsychotic can do well with rapid cross-titration, clinical experience suggests many patients do best by building up a full dose of ziprasidone (>120 mg/day) added to the maintenance dose of the first antipsychotic for up to 3 weeks prior to slow down-titration of the first antipsychotic
- QTc prolongation at 320 mg/day not significantly greater than at 160 mg/day
- Rather than raise the dose above these levels in acutely agitated patients requiring acute antipsychotic actions, consider augmentation with a benzodiazepine or conventional antipsychotic, either orally or intramuscularly
- Rather than raise the dose above these levels in partial responders, consider augmentation with a mood stabilizing anticonvulsant, such as valproate or lamotrigine
- Children and elderly should generally be dosed at the lower end of the dosage spectrum
- Ziprasidone intramuscular can be given short-term, both to initiate dosing with oral ziprasidone or another oral antipsychotic and to treat breakthrough agitation in patients maintained on oral antipsychotics
- QTc prolongation of intramuscular ziprasidone is the same or less than with intramuscular haloperidol

Overdose

- Rarely lethal in monotherapy overdose; sedation, slurred speech, transitory hypertension

Long-Term Use

- Approved to delay relapse in long-term treatment of schizophrenia
- Often used for long-term maintenance in bipolar disorder and various behavioral disorders

Habit Forming

- No

How to Stop

- Slow down-titration of oral formulation (over 6–8 weeks), especially when simultaneously beginning a new antipsychotic while switching (i.e., cross-titration)
- Rapid oral discontinuation may lead to rebound psychosis and worsening of symptoms

Pharmacokinetics

- Mean half-life 6.6 hours
- Protein binding >99%
- Metabolized by CYP450 3A4

Drug Interactions

- Neither CYP450 3A4 nor CYP450 2D6 inhibitors significantly affect ziprasidone plasma levels

- Little potential to affect metabolism of drugs cleared by CYP450 enzymes
- May enhance the effects of antihypertensive drugs
- May antagonize levodopa, dopamine agonists
- May enhance QTc prolongation of other drugs capable of prolonging QTc interval

Other Warnings/ Precautions

- Ziprasidone prolongs QTc interval more than some other antipsychotics
- Use with caution in patients with conditions that predispose to hypotension (dehydration, overheating)
- Priapism has been reported
- Dysphagia has been associated with antipsychotic use, and ziprasidone should be used cautiously in patients at risk for aspiration pneumonia

Do Not Use

- If patient is taking agents capable of significantly prolonging QTc interval (e.g., pimozide, thioridazine, selected antiarrhythmics, moxifloxacin, sparfloxacin)
- If there is a history of QTc prolongation or cardiac arrhythmia, recent acute myocardial infarction, uncompensated heart failure
- If there is a proven allergy to ziprasidone

SPECIAL POPULATIONS

Renal Impairment

- No dose adjustment necessary
- Not removed by hemodialysis
- Intramuscular formulation should be used with caution

Hepatic Impairment

- No dose adjustment necessary

Cardiac Impairment

- Ziprasidone is contraindicated in patients with a known history of QTc prolongation, recent acute myocardial infarction, and uncompensated heart failure
- Should be used with caution in other cases of cardiac impairment because of risk of orthostatic hypotension

Elderly

- Some patients may tolerate lower doses better
- Although atypical antipsychotics are commonly used for behavioral disturbances in dementia, no agent has been approved for treatment of elderly patients with dementia-related psychosis
- Elderly patients with dementia-related psychosis treated with atypical antipsychotics are at an increased risk of death compared to placebo, and also have an increased risk of cerebrovascular events

Children and Adolescents

- Not officially recommended for patients under age 18
- Clinical experience and early data suggest ziprasidone may be safe and effective for behavioral disturbances in children and adolescents
- Children and adolescents using ziprasidone may need to be monitored more often than adults and may tolerate lower doses better

Pregnancy

- Risk Category C [some animal studies show adverse effects; no controlled studies in humans]
- Psychotic symptoms may worsen during pregnancy and some form of treatment may be necessary
- Ziprasidone may be preferable to anticonvulsant mood stabilizers if treatment is required during pregnancy

Breast Feeding

- Unknown if ziprasidone is secreted in human breast milk, but all psychotropics assumed to be secreted in breast milk

✻ Recommended either to discontinue drug or bottle feed

- Infants of women who choose to breast feed while on ziprasidone should be monitored for possible adverse effects

THE ART OF PSYCHOPHARMACOLOGY

Potential Advantages

- Some cases of psychosis and bipolar disorder refractory to treatment with other antipsychotics
- * Patients concerned about gaining weight and patients who are already obese or overweight
- * Patients with diabetes
- * Patients with dyslipidemia (especially elevated triglycerides)
- Patients requiring rapid relief of symptoms (intramuscular injection)
- Patients switching from intramuscular ziprasidone to an oral preparation

Potential Disadvantages

- Patients noncompliant with twice daily dosing
- * Patients noncompliant with dosing with food

Primary Target Symptoms

- Positive symptoms of psychosis
- Negative symptoms of psychosis
- Cognitive symptoms
- Unstable mood (both depression and mania)
- Aggressive symptoms

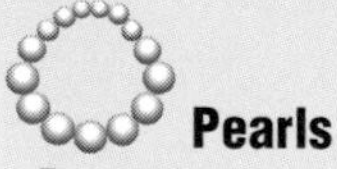

Pearls

- Recent landmark head to head study in schizophrenia suggests lower metabolic side effects and comparable efficacy compared to some other atypical and conventional antipsychotics
- * When given to patients with obesity and dyslipidemia associated with prior treatment with another atypical antipsychotic, many experience weight loss and decrease in fasting triglycerides
- * QTc prolongation fears are often exaggerated and not justified since QTc prolongation with ziprasidone is not dose-related and few drugs have any potential to increase ziprasidone's plasma levels
- * Efficacy may be underestimated since ziprasidone is mostly under-dosed (<120 mg/day) in clinical practice
- * Well-accepted in clinical practice when wanting to avoid weight gain because less weight gain than most other atypical antipsychotics
- * May not have diabetes or dyslipidemia risk, but monitoring is still indicated
- Less sedation than some antipsychotics, more than others (at moderate to high doses)
- * More activating than some other antipsychotics at low doses
- One of the least expensive atypical antipsychotics within recommended therapeutic dosing range
- Anecdotal reports of utility in treatment-resistant cases, especially when adequately dosed
- * One of only 2 atypical antipsychotics with a short-acting intramuscular dosage formulation

Suggested Reading

Greenberg WM, Citrome L. Ziprasidone for schizophrenia and bipolar disorder: a review of the clinical trials. CNS Drug Rev 2007;13(2):137–77.

Lieberman JA, Stroup TS, McEvoy JP, Swartz MS, Rosenheck RA, Perkins DO, et al. Effectiveness of antipsychotic drugs in patients with chronic schizophrenia. N Engl J Med 2005;353(12):1209–23.

Nasrallah HA. Atypical antipsychotic-induced metabolic side effects: insights from receptor-binding profiles. Mol Psychiatry 2008;13(1):27–35.

Smith LA, Cornelius V, Warnock A, Tacchi MJ, Taylor D. Pharmacological interventions for acute bipolar mania: a systematic review of randomized placebo-controlled trials. Bipolar Disord 2007;9(6):551–60.

Taylor D. Ziprasidone in the management of schizophrenia : the QT interval issue in context. CNS Drugs 2003;17:423–30.

THERAPEUTICS

Brands • Ambien, Ambien CR
see index for additional brand names

Generic? Yes

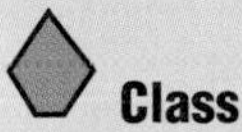

Class

- Non-benzodiazepine hypnotic; alpha 1 isoform selective agonist of GABA-A/ benzodiazepine receptors

Commonly Prescribed For

(bold for FDA approved)

- **Short-term treatment of insomnia (controlled-release indication is not restricted to short-term)**

How the Drug Works

- Binds selectively to a subtype of the benzodiazepine receptor, the alpha 1 isoform
- May enhance GABA inhibitory actions that provide sedative hypnotic effects more selectively than other actions of GABA
- Boosts chloride conductance through GABA-regulated channels
- Inhibitory actions in sleep centers may provide sedative hypnotic effects
- CR formulation may allow sufficient drug to persist at receptors to improve total sleep time and to prevent early morning awakenings that can be associated with the immediate-release formulation of zolpidem

How Long Until It Works

- Generally takes effect in less than an hour

If It Works

- Improves quality of sleep
- Effects on total wake-time and number of nighttime awakenings may be decreased over time

If It Doesn't Work

- If insomnia does not improve after 7–10 days, it may be a manifestation of a primary psychiatric or physical illness such as obstructive sleep apnea or restless leg syndrome, which requires independent evaluation
- Increase the dose
- Improve sleep hygiene
- Switch to another agent

Best Augmenting Combos for Partial Response or Treatment Resistance

- Generally, best to switch to another agent
- Trazodone
- Agents with antihistamine actions (e.g., diphenhydramine, tricyclic antidepressants)

Tests

- None for healthy individuals

SIDE EFFECTS

How Drug Causes Side Effects

- Actions at benzodiazepine receptors that carry over to the next day can cause daytime sedation, amnesia, and ataxia
- Long-term adaptations of zolpidem immediate-release not well studied, but chronic studies of zolpidem CR and other alpha 1 selective non-benzodiazepine hypnotics suggest lack of notable tolerance or dependence developing over time

Notable Side Effects

✱ Sedation
✱ Dizziness, ataxia
✱ Dose-dependent amnesia
✱ Hyper-excitability, nervousness
- Rare hallucinations
- Diarrhea, nausea
- Headache

Life-Threatening or Dangerous Side Effects

- Respiratory depression, especially when taken with other CNS depressants in overdose
- Rare angioedema

Weight Gain

unusual
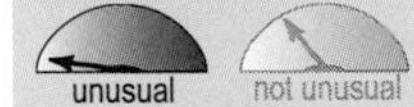

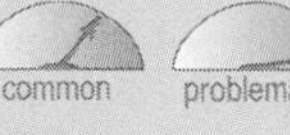

- Reported but not expected

Sedation

unusual | not unusual | **common** | problematic

- Many experience and/or can be significant in amount

What to do About Side Effects
- Wait
- To avoid problems with memory, take zolpidem or zolpidem CR only if planning to have a full night's sleep
- Lower the dose
- Switch to a shorter-acting sedative hypnotic
- Administer flumazenil if side effects are severe or life-threatening

Best Augmenting Agents for Side Effects
- Many side effects cannot be improved with an augmenting agent

DOSING AND USE

Usual Dosage Range
- 10 mg/day at bedtime for 7–10 days (immediate-release)
- 12.5 mg/day at bedtime (controlled-release)

Dosage Forms
- Immediate-release tablet 5 mg
- Controlled-release tablet 6.25 mg

How To Dose
- 10 mg/day at bedtime (immediate-release)
- 12.5 mg/day at bedtime (controlled-release)

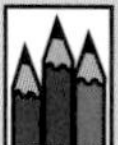

Dosing Tips
✻ Zolpidem is not absorbed as quickly if taken with food, which could reduce onset of action
- Patients with lower body weights may require only a 5-mg dose immediate-release or 6.25 mg controlled-release
- Zolpidem should generally not be prescribed in quantities greater than a 1-month supply; however, zolpidem CR is not restricted to short-term use
- Risk of dependence may increase with dose and duration of treatment

✻ However, treatment with alpha 1 selective non-benzodiazepine hypnotics may cause less tolerance or dependence than benzodiazepine hypnotics
- Controlled-release tablets should be swallowed whole and should not be divided, crushed, or chewed

Overdose
- No fatalities reported with zolpidem monotherapy; sedation, ataxia, confusion, hypotension, respiratory depression, coma

Long-Term Use
- Original studies with zolpidem immediate-release did not assess long-term use
- Zolpidem CR is not restricted to short-term use
- Increased wakefulness during the latter part of night (wearing off) or an increase in daytime anxiety (rebound) may occur with immediate-release and be less common with controlled-release

Habit Forming
- Zolpidem is a Schedule IV drug
- Some patients may develop dependence and/or tolerance; risk may be greater with higher doses
- History of drug addiction may increase risk of dependence

How to Stop
- Although rebound insomnia could occur, this effect has not generally been seen with therapeutic doses of zolpidem or zolpidem CR
- If taken for more than a few weeks, taper to reduce chances of withdrawal effects

Pharmacokinetics
- Short elimination half-life (approximately 2.5 hours)

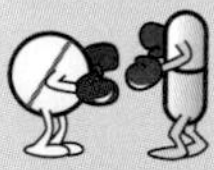

Drug Interactions
- Increased depressive effects when taken with other CNS depressants
- Sertraline may increase plasma levels of zolpidem
- Rifampin may decrease plasma levels of zolpidem

Other Warnings/ Precautions
- Insomnia may be a symptom of a primary disorder, rather than a primary disorder itself
- Some patients may exhibit abnormal thinking or behavioral changes similar to those caused by other CNS depressants

(i.e., either depressant actions or disinhibiting actions)
- Some depressed patients may experience a worsening of suicidal ideation
- Use only with extreme caution in patients with impaired respiratory function or obstructive sleep apnea
- Zolpidem and zolpidem CR should only be administered at bedtime
- Temporary memory loss may occur at doses above 10 mg/night
- Rare angioedema has occurred with sedative hypnotic use and could potentially cause fatal airway obstruction if it involves the throat, glottis, or larynx; thus if angioedema occurs treatment should be discontinued
- Sleep driving and other complex behaviors, such as eating and preparing food and making phone calls, have been reported in patients taking sedative hypnotics

Do Not Use
- If there is a proven allergy to zolpidem

SPECIAL POPULATIONS

Renal Impairment
- No dose adjustment necessary
- Patients should be monitored

Hepatic Impairment
- Recommended dose 5 mg (immediate-release) or 6.25 mg (controlled-release)
- Patients should be monitored

Cardiac Impairment
- No available data

Elderly
- Recommended initial dose: 5 mg (immediate-release) or 6.25 mg (controlled-release)
- Elderly may have increased risk for falls, confusion

Children and Adolescents
- Safety and efficacy have not been established
- Long-term effects of zolpidem or zolpidem CR in children/adolescents are unknown
- Should generally receive lower doses and be more closely monitored
- Hallucinations in children ages 6-17 have been reported

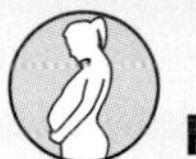

Pregnancy
- Risk category B [animal studies do not show adverse effects; no controlled studies in humans]
- Infants whose mothers took sedative hypnotics during pregnancy may experience some withdrawal symptoms
- Neonatal flaccidity has been reported in infants whose mothers took sedative hypnotics during pregnancy

Breast Feeding
- Some drug is found in mother's breast milk

✻ Recommended either to discontinue drug or bottle feed

THE ART OF PSYCHOPHARMACOLOGY

Potential Advantages
- Patients who require long-term treatment, especially CR formulation

Potential Disadvantages
- More expensive than some other sedative hypnotics

Primary Target Symptoms
- Time to sleep onset
- Total sleep time
- Nighttime awakenings

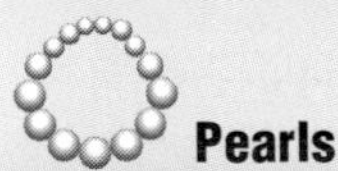

Pearls
✻ One of the most popular sedative hypnotic agents in psychopharmacology
- Zolpidem has been shown to increase the total time asleep and to reduce the amount of nighttime awakenings
- Zolpidem CR may be even more effective on these sleep parameters than immediate-release zolpidem due to prolonged drug delivery

✻ May be preferred over benzodiazepines because of its rapid onset of action, short duration of effect, and safety profile
- Clearance of zolpidem may be slightly slower in women than in men
- May not be ideal for patients who desire immediate hypnotic onset and eat just prior to bedtime

- Not a benzodiazepine itself, but binds to benzodiazepine receptors
- May have fewer carryover side effects than some other sedative hypnotics
- May cause less dependence than some other sedative hypnotics, especially in those without a history of substance abuse

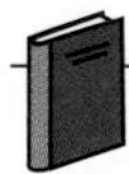

Suggested Reading

Holm KJ, Goa KL. Zolpidem: an update of its pharmacology, therapeutic efficacy and tolerability in the treatment of insomnia. Drugs 2000;59:865–89.

Rush CR. Behavioral pharmacology of zolpidem relative to benzodiazepines: a review. Pharmacol Biochem Behav 1998;61:253–69.

Soyka M, Bottlender R, Moller HJ. Epidemiological evidence for a low abuse potential of zolpidem. Pharmacopsychiatry 2000;33:138–41.

Toner LC, Tsambiras BM, Catalano G, Catalano MC, Cooper DS. Central nervous system side effects associated with zolpidem treatment. Clin Neuropharmacol 2000;23:54–8.

THERAPEUTICS

Brands • Zonegran
• Excegran

see index for additional brand names

Generic? Not in U.S.

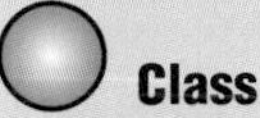

Class

- Anticonvulsant, voltage-sensitive sodium channel modulator; T-type calcium channel modulator; structurally a sulfonamide

Commonly Prescribed For

(bold for FDA approved)

- **Adjunct therapy for partial seizures in adults with epilepsy**
- Bipolar disorder
- Chronic neuropathic pain
- Migraine
- Parkinson's disease
- Psychotropic drug-induced weight gain
- Binge-eating disorder

How the Drug Works

- Unknown
- Modulates voltage-sensitive sodium channels by an unknown mechanism
- Also modulates T-type calcium channels
- Facilitates dopamine and serotonin release
- Inhibits carbonic anhydrase

How Long Until It Works

- Should reduce seizures by 2 weeks
- Onset of action as well as convincing therapeutic efficacy have not been demonstrated for uses other than adjunctive treatment of partial seizures

If It Works

- The goal of treatment is complete remission of symptoms (e.g., seizures, pain, mania, migraine)
- Would currently only be expected to work in a subset of patients for conditions other than epilepsy as an adjunctive treatment to agents with better demonstration of efficacy

If It Doesn't Work (for conditions other than epilepsy)

- May be effective only in patients who fail to respond to agents with proven efficacy, or it may not work at all
- Consider increasing dose or switching to another agent with better demonstrated efficacy

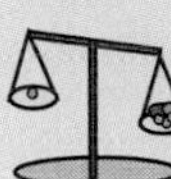

Best Augmenting Combos for Partial Response or Treatment Resistance

- Zonisamide is itself a second-line augmenting agent to numerous other agents in treating conditions other than epilepsy, such as bipolar disorder, chronic neuropathic pain, and migraine

Tests

- Consider baseline and periodic monitoring of renal function

SIDE EFFECTS

How Drug Causes Side Effects

- CNS side effects theoretically due to excessive actions at voltage-sensitive ion channels
- Weak inhibition of carbonic anhydrase may lead to kidney stones
- Serious rash theoretically an allergic reaction

Notable Side Effects

✻ Sedation, depression, difficulty concentrating, agitation, irritability, psychomotor slowing, dizziness, ataxia
- Headache
- Nausea, anorexia, abdominal pain, vomiting
- Kidney stones
- Elevated serum creatinine and blood urea nitrogen

Life-Threatening or Dangerous Side Effects

- Rare serious rash (Stevens-Johnson syndrome, toxic epidermal necrolysis) (sulfonamide)
- Rare oligohidrosis and hyperthermia (pediatric patients)
- Rare blood dyscrasias (aplastic anemia; agranulocytosis)
- Sudden hepatic necrosis
- Sudden unexplained deaths have occurred (unknown if related to zonisamide use)
- Rare activation of suicidal ideation and behavior (suicidality)

Weight Gain

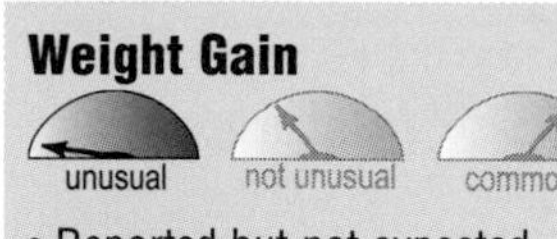

- Reported but not expected

✻ Patients may experience weight loss

Sedation

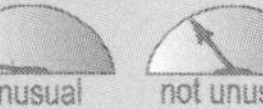
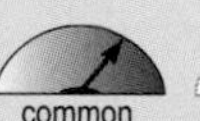

- Many experience and/or can be significant in amount
- Dose-related
- Can wear off with time but may not wear off at high doses

What to do About Side Effects

- Wait
- Wait
- Wait
- Take more of the dose at night to reduce daytime sedation
- Lower the dose
- Switch to another agent

Best Augmenting Agents for Side Effects

- Many side effects cannot be improved with an augmenting agent

DOSING AND USE

Usual Dosage Range

- 100–600 mg/day in 1–2 doses

Dosage Forms

- Capsule 25 mg, 50 mg, 100 mg

How To Dose

- Initial 100 mg/day; after 2 weeks can increase to 200 mg/day; dose can be increased by 100 mg/day every 2 weeks if necessary and tolerated; maximum dose generally 600 mg/day; maintain stable dose for at least 2 weeks before increasing dose

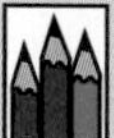

Dosing Tips

✻ Most clinical experience is at doses up to 400 mg/day

- No evidence from controlled trials of increasing response over 400 mg/day
- However, some patients may tolerate and respond to doses up to 600 mg/day
- Little experience with doses greater than 600 mg/day
- Side effects may increase notably at doses greater than 300 mg/day
- For intolerable sedation, can give most of the dose at night and less during the day

Overdose

- Can cause bradycardia, hypotension, respiratory depression

Long-Term Use

- Safe
- Consider periodic monitoring of blood urea nitrogen and creatinine

Habit Forming

- No

How to Stop

- Taper
- Epilepsy patients may seize upon withdrawal, especially if withdrawal is abrupt
- Rapid discontinuation may increase the risk of relapse in bipolar patients
- Discontinuation symptoms uncommon

Pharmacokinetics

- Plasma elimination half-life approximately 63 hours
- Metabolized in part by CYP450 3A4
- Partially eliminated renally

Drug Interactions

- Agents that inhibit CYP450 3A4 (such as nefazodone, fluvoxamine, and fluoxetine) may decrease the clearance of zonisamide, and increase plasma zonisamide levels, possibly requiring lower doses of zonisamide
- Agents that induce CYP450 3A4 (such as carbamazepine) may increase the clearance of zonisamide and decrease plasma zonisamide levels, possibly requiring higher doses of zonisamide
- Enzyme-inducing antiepileptic drugs (carbamazepine, phenytoin, phenobarbital, and primidone) may decrease plasma levels of zonisamide
- Theoretically, zonisamide may interact with carbonic anhydrase inhibitors to increase the risk of kidney stones

Other Warnings/ Precautions

- Depressive effects may be increased by other CNS depressants (alcohol, MAOIs, other anticonvulsants, etc.)
- Use with caution when combining with other drugs that predispose patients to heat-related disorders, including carbonic anhydrase inhibitors and anticholinergics
- ✻ Life-threatening rashes have developed in association with zonisamide use; zonisamide should generally be discontinued at the first sign of serious rash
- Patient should be instructed to report any symptoms of hypersensitivity immediately (fever; flu-like symptoms; rash; blisters on skin or in eyes, mouth, ears, nose, or genital areas; swelling of eyelids, conjunctivitis, lymphadenopathy)
- Patients should be monitored for signs of unusual bleeding or bruising, mouth sores, infections, fever, and sore throat, as there may be an increased risk of aplastic anemia and agranulocytosis with zonisamide
- Warn patients and their caregivers about the possibility of activation of suicidal ideation and advise them to report such side effects immediately

Do Not Use

- If there is a proven allergy to zonisamide or sulfonamides

SPECIAL POPULATIONS

Renal Impairment

- Zonisamide is primarily renally excreted
- Use with caution
- May require slower titration

Hepatic Impairment

- Use with caution
- May require slower titration

Cardiac Impairment

- No specific recommendations

Elderly

- Some patients may tolerate lower doses better
- Elderly patients may be more susceptible to adverse effects

Children and Adolescents

- Cases of oligohidrosis and hyperthermia have been reported
- Not approved for use in children under age 16
- Use in children for the expert only, with close monitoring, after other options have failed

Pregnancy

- Risk Category C [some animal studies show adverse effects; no controlled studies in humans]
- Use in women of childbearing potential requires weighing potential benefits to the mother against the risks to the fetus
- Antiepileptic Drug Pregnancy Registry: (888) 233-2334
- Taper drug if discontinuing
- Seizures, even mild seizures, may cause harm to the embryo/fetus
- Lack of convincing efficacy for treatment of conditions other than epilepsy suggests risk/benefit ratio is in favor of discontinuing zonisamide during pregnancy for these indications

Breast Feeding

- Unknown if zonisamide is secreted in human breast milk, but all psychotropics assumed to be secreted in breast milk
- ✻ Recommended either to discontinue drug or bottle feed
- If drug is continued while breast feeding, infant should be monitored for possible adverse effects
- If child becomes irritable or sedated, breast feeding or drug may need to be discontinued

THE ART OF PSYCHOPHARMACOLOGY

Potential Advantages

- Treatment-resistant conditions
- Patients who wish to avoid weight gain

Potential Disadvantages

- Poor documentation of efficacy for off-label uses
- Patients noncompliant with twice daily dosing

Primary Target Symptoms

- Seizures
- Numerous other symptoms for off-label uses
- Patients with a history of kidney stones

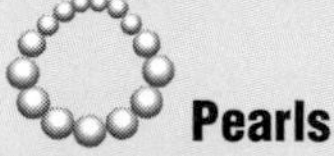

Pearls

- Well studied in epilepsy
- ✻ Much off-label use is based upon theoretical considerations rather than clinical experience or compelling efficacy studies
- Early studies suggest efficacy in binge-eating disorder
- Early studies suggest possible efficacy in migraine
- Early studies suggest possible utility in Parkinson's disease
- Early studies suggest possible utility in neuropathic pain
- Early studies suggest some therapeutic potential for mood stabilizing
- Chronic intake of caffeine may lower brain zonisamide concentrations and attenuate its anticonvulsant effects (based on animal studies)
- ✻ Due to reported weight loss in some patients in trials with epilepsy, some patients with psychotropic-induced weight gain are treated with zonisamide
- Utility for this indication is not clear nor has it been systematically studied

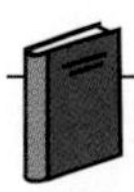

Suggested Reading

Chadwick DW, Marson AG. Zonisamide add-on for drug-resistant partial epilepsy. Cochrane Database Syst Rev 2002;(2):CD001416.

Glauser TA, Pellock JM. Zonisamide in pediatric epilepsy: review of the Japanese experience. J Child Neurol 2002;17:87–96.

Jain KK. An assessment of zonisamide as an anti-epileptic drug. Expert Opin Pharmacother 2000;1:1245–60.

Leppik IE. Three new drugs for epilepsy: levetiracetam, oxcarbazepine, and zonisamide. J Child Neurol 2002;17 Suppl 1:S53–7.

THERAPEUTICS

Brands • Imovane

see index for additional brand names

Generic? No

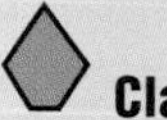

Class

- Non-benzodiazepine hypnotic; alpha 1 isoform selective agonist of GABA-A/benzodiazepine receptors

Commonly Prescribed For

(bold for FDA approved)

- Short-term treatment of insomnia

How the Drug Works

- May bind selectively to a subtype of the benzodiazepine receptor, the alpha 1 isoform
- May enhance GABA inhibitory actions that provide sedative hypnotic effects more selectively than other actions of GABA
- Boosts chloride conductance through GABA-regulated channels
- Inhibitory actions in sleep centers may provide sedative hypnotic effects

How Long Until It Works

- Generally takes effect in less than an hour

If It Works

- Improves quality of sleep
- Effects on total wake-time and number of nighttime awakenings may be decreased over time

If It Doesn't Work

- If insomnia does not improve after 7–10 days, it may be a manifestation of a primary psychiatric or physical illness such as obstructive sleep apnea or restless leg syndrome, which requires independent evaluation
- Increase the dose
- Improve sleep hygiene
- Switch to another agent

Best Augmenting Combos for Partial Response or Treatment Resistance

- Generally, best to switch to another agent
- Trazodone
- Agents with antihistamine actions (e.g., diphenhydramine, tricyclic antidepressants)

Tests

- None for healthy individuals

SIDE EFFECTS

How Drug Causes Side Effects

- Actions at benzodiazepine receptors that carry over to the next day can cause daytime sedation, amnesia, and ataxia
- ✻ Long-term adaptations of zopiclone, a mixture of an active S enantiomer and an inactive R enantiomer, have not been well studied, but chronic studies of the active isomer eszopiclone suggest lack of notable tolerance or dependence developing over time

Notable Side Effects

- ✻ Sedation
- ✻ Dizziness, ataxia
- ✻ Dose-dependent amnesia
- ✻ Hyperexcitability, nervousness
- Dry mouth, loss of appetite, constipation, bitter taste
- Impaired vision

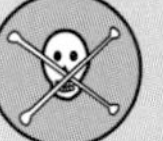

Life-Threatening or Dangerous Side Effects

- Respiratory depression, especially when taken with other CNS depressants in overdose
- Rare angioedema

Weight Gain

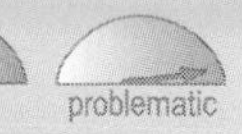

- Reported but not expected

Sedation

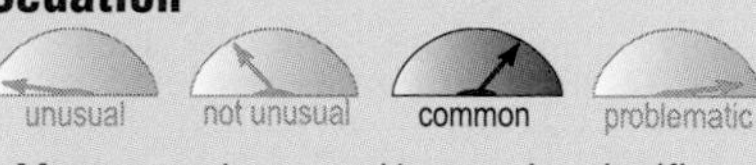

- Many experience and/or can be significant in amount

What to do About Side Effects

- Wait
- To avoid problems with memory, only take zopiclone if planning to have a full night's sleep
- Lower the dose

- Switch to a shorter-acting sedative hypnotic
- Administer flumazenil if side effects are severe or life-threatening

Best Augmenting Agents for Side Effects

- Many side effects cannot be improved with an augmenting agent

DOSING AND USE

Usual Dosage Range

- 7.5 mg at bedtime

Dosage Forms

- Tablet 7.5 mg scored

How To Dose

- No titration, take dose at bedtime

Dosing Tips

- Zopiclone should generally not be prescribed in quantities greater than a 1-month supply
- Risk of dependence may increase with dose and duration of treatment
- However, chronic treatment with alpha 1 selective non-benzodiazepine hypnotics may cause less tolerance or dependence than benzodiazepine hypnotics

Overdose

- Can be fatal; clumsiness, mood changes, sedation, weakness, breathing trouble, unconsciousness

Long-Term Use

- Not generally intended for use past 4 weeks

Habit Forming

- Some patients may develop dependence and/or tolerance; risk may be greater with higher doses
- History of drug addiction may increase risk of dependence

How to Stop

- Rebound insomnia may occur the first night after stopping
- If taken for more than a few weeks, taper to reduce chances of withdrawal effects

Pharmacokinetics

- Metabolized by CYP450 3A4
- Terminal elimination half-life approximately 3.5–6.5 hours

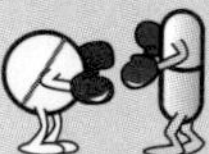

Drug Interactions

- Increased depressive effects when taken with other CNS depressants
- Theoretically, inhibitors of CYP450 3A4, such as nefazodone and fluvoxamine, could increase plasma levels of zopiclone

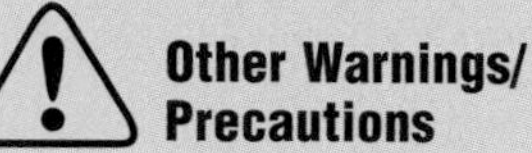

Other Warnings/ Precautions

- Insomnia may be a symptom of a primary disorder, rather than a primary disorder itself
- Some patients may exhibit abnormal thinking or behavioral changes similar to those caused by other CNS depressants (i.e., either depressant actions or disinhibiting actions)
- Some depressed patients may experience a worsening of suicidal ideation
- Use only with extreme caution in patients with impaired respiratory function or obstructive sleep apnea
- Zopiclone should be administered only at bedtime
- Rare angioedema has occurred with sedative hypnotic use and could potentially cause fatal airway obstruction if it involves the throat, glottis, or larynx; thus if angioedema occurs treatment should be discontinued
- Sleep driving and other complex behaviors, such as eating and preparing food and making phone calls, have been reported in patients taking sedative hypnotics

Do Not Use

- If patient has myasthenia gravis
- If patient has severe respiratory impairment
- If patient has had a stroke
- If there is a proven allergy to zopiclone

SPECIAL POPULATIONS

Renal Impairment

- Increased plasma levels
- May need to lower dose

Hepatic Impairment
- Increased plasma levels
- Recommended dose 3.75 mg

Cardiac Impairment
- Dosage adjustment may not be necessary

Elderly
- May be more susceptible to adverse effects
- Initial dose 3.75 mg at bedtime; can increase to usual adult dose if necessary and tolerated

Children and Adolescents
- Safety and efficacy have not been established
- Long-term effects of zopiclone in children/adolescents are unknown
- Should generally receive lower doses and be more closely monitored

Pregnancy
- Risk Category C [some animal studies show adverse effects; no controlled studies in humans]
- Infants whose mothers took sedative hypnotics during pregnancy may experience some withdrawal symptoms
- Neonatal flaccidity has been reported in infants whose mothers took sedative hypnotics during pregnancy

Breast Feeding
- Some drug is found in mother's breast milk

✽ Recommended either to discontinue drug or bottle feed

THE ART OF PSYCHOPHARMACOLOGY

Potential Advantages
- Those who require long-term treatment

Potential Disadvantages
- More expensive than some other sedative hypnotics

Primary Target Symptoms
- Time to sleep onset
- Nighttime awakenings
- Total sleep time

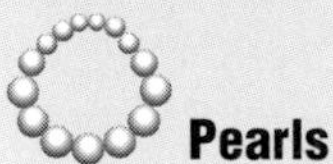

Pearls

✽ May be preferred over benzodiazepines because of its rapid onset of action, short duration of effect, and safety profile
- Zopiclone does not appear to be a highly dependence-causing drug, at least not in patients with no history of drug abuse
- Rebound insomnia does not appear to be common
- Not a benzodiazepine itself, but binds to benzodiazepine receptors
- May have fewer carryover side effects than some other sedative hypnotics
- The active enantiomer of zopiclone, eszopiclone, has received an approvable letter from the United States Food and Drug Administration

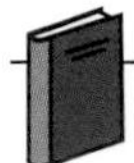

Suggested Reading

Fernandez C, Martin C, Gimenez F, Farinotti R. Clinical pharmacokinetics of zopiclone. Clin Pharmacokinet 1995;29:431–41.

Hajak G. A comparative assessment of the risks and benefits of zopiclone: a review of 15 years' clinical experience. Drug Saf 1999; 21:457–69.

Noble S, Langtry HD, Lamb HM. Zopiclone. An update of its pharmacology, clinical efficacy and tolerability in the treatment of insomnia. Drugs 1998;55:277–302.

THERAPEUTICS

Brands • Lodopin
• Zoleptil

see index for additional brand names

Generic? No

Class

- Atypical antipsychotic (serotonin-dopamine antagonist)

Commonly Prescribed For

(bold for FDA approved)

- Schizophrenia
- Other psychotic disorders
- Mania

How the Drug Works

- Blocks dopamine 2 receptors, reducing positive symptoms of psychosis
- Blocks serotonin 2A receptors, causing enhancement of dopamine release in certain brain regions and thus reducing motor side effects and possibly improving cognitive and affective symptoms
- Interactions at a myriad of other neurotransmitter receptors may contribute to zotepine's efficacy

* Specifically inhibits norepinephrine uptake

How Long Until It Works

- Psychotic and manic symptoms can improve within 1 week, but it may take several weeks for full effect on behavior as well as on cognition and affective stabilization
- Classically recommended to wait at least 4–6 weeks to determine efficacy of drug, but in practice some patients require up to 16–20 weeks to show a good response, especially on cognitive symptoms

If It Works

- Most often reduces positive symptoms in schizophrenia but does not eliminate them
- Can improve negative symptoms, as well as aggressive, cognitive, and affective symptoms in schizophrenia
- Most schizophrenic patients do not have a total remission of symptoms but rather a reduction of symptoms by about a third
- Perhaps 5–15% of schizophrenic patients can experience an overall improvement of greater than 50–60%, especially when receiving stable treatment for more than a year
- Such patients are considered super-responders or "awakeners" since they may be well enough to be employed, live independently, and sustain long-term relationships
- Many bipolar patients may experience a reduction of symptoms by half or more
- Continue treatment until reaching a plateau of improvement
- After reaching a satisfactory plateau, continue treatment for at least a year after first episode of psychosis
- For second and subsequent episodes of psychosis, treatment may need to be indefinite
- Even for first episodes of psychosis, it may be preferable to continue treatment indefinitely to avoid subsequent episodes
- Treatment may not only reduce mania but also prevent recurrences of mania in bipolar disorder

If It Doesn't Work

- Consider trying one of the first-line atypical antipsychotics (risperidone, olanzapine, quetiapine, ziprasidone, aripiprazole, paliperidone, amisulpride)
- If 2 or more antipsychotic monotherapies do not work, consider clozapine
- If no first-line atypical antipsychotic is effective, consider higher doses or augmentation with valproate or lamotrigine
- Some patients may require treatment with a conventional antipsychotic
- Consider noncompliance and switch to another antipsychotic with fewer side effects or to an antipsychotic that can be given by depot injection
- Consider initiating rehabilitation and psychotherapy
- Consider presence of concomitant drug abuse

Best Augmenting Combos for Partial Response or Treatment Resistance

- Augmentation of zotepine has not been systematically studied
- Valproic acid (valproate, divalproex, divalproex ER)

- Other mood-stabilizing anticonvulsants (carbamazepine, oxcarbazepine, lamotrigine)
- Lithium
- Benzodiazepines

Tests

❋ Although risk of diabetes and dyslipidemia with zotepine has not been systematically studied, monitoring as for all other atypical antipsychotics is suggested

Before starting an atypical antipsychotic

❋ Weigh all patients and track BMI during treatment
- Get baseline personal and family history of diabetes, obesity, dyslipidemia, hypertension, and cardiovascular disease

❋ Get waist circumference (at umbilicus), blood pressure, fasting plasma glucose, and fasting lipid profile
- Determine if the patient is
  - overweight (BMI 25.0–29.9)
  - obese (BMI ≥30)
  - has pre-diabetes (fasting plasma glucose 100–25 mg/dL)
  - has diabetes (fasting plasma glucose >126 mg/dL)
  - has hypertension (BP >140/90 mm Hg)
  - has dyslipidemia (increased total cholesterol, LDL cholesterol, and triglycerides; decreased HDL cholesterol)
- Treat or refer such patients for treatment, including nutrition and weight management, physical activity counseling, smoking cessation, and medical management

Monitoring after starting an atypical antipsychotic

❋ BMI monthly for 3 months, then quarterly

❋ Consider monitoring fasting triglycerides monthly for several months in patients at high risk for metabolic complications and when initiating or switching antipsychotics

❋ Blood pressure, fasting plasma glucose, fasting lipids within 3 months and then annually, but earlier and more frequently for patients with diabetes or who have gained >5% of initial weight
- Treat or refer for treatment and consider switching to another atypical antipsychotic for patients who become overweight, obese, pre-diabetic, diabetic, hypertensive, or dyslipidemic while receiving an atypical antipsychotic

❋ Even in patients without known diabetes, be vigilant for the rare but life threatening onset of diabetic ketoacidosis, which always requires immediate treatment, by monitoring for the rapid onset of polyuria, polydipsia, weight loss, nausea, vomiting, dehydration, rapid respiration, weakness and clouding of sensorium, even coma
- EKGs may be useful for selected patients (e.g., those with personal or family history of QTc prolongation; cardiac arrhythmia; recent myocardial infarction; uncompensated heart failure; or those taking agents that prolong QTc interval such as pimozide, thioridazine, selected antiarrhythmics, moxifloxacin, sparfloxacin, etc.)
- Patients at risk for electrolyte disturbances (e.g., patients on diuretic therapy) should have baseline and periodic serum potassium and magnesium measurements
- Patients with suspected hematologic abnormalities may require a white blood cell count before initiating treatment
- Monitor liver function tests in patients with established liver disease
- Should check blood pressure in the elderly before starting and for the first few weeks of treatment

SIDE EFFECTS

How Drug Causes Side Effects

- By blocking alpha 1 adrenergic receptors, it can cause dizziness, sedation, and hypotension
- By blocking histamine 1 receptors in the brain, it can cause sedation and weight gain
- By blocking dopamine 2 receptors in the striatum, it can cause motor side effects
- By blocking dopamine 2 receptors in the pituitary, it can cause elevations in prolactin
- Mechanism of weight gain and possible increased incidence of dyslipidemia and diabetes of atypical antipsychotics is unknown

Notable Side Effects

- Atypical antipsychotics may increase the risk for diabetes and dyslipidemia, although the specific risks associated with zotepine are unknown

- Agitation, anxiety, depression, asthenia, headache, insomnia, sedation, hypo/hyperthermia
- Constipation, dry mouth, dyspepsia, weight gain
- Tachycardia, hypotension, sweating, blurred vision
- Rare tardive dyskinesia
- Dose-related hyperprolactinemia

Life-Threatening or Dangerous Side Effects

- Rare neuroleptic malignant syndrome
- Rare seizures (risk increases with dose, especially over 300 mg/day)
- Blood dyscrasias
- Dose-dependent QTc prolongation
- Increased risk of death and cerebrovascular events in elderly patients with dementia-related psychosis

Weight Gain

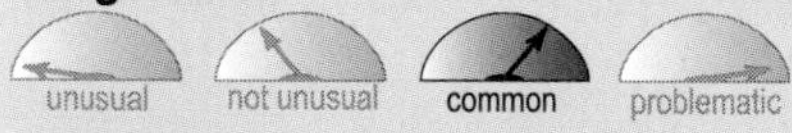

- Many experience and/or can be significant in amount

Sedation

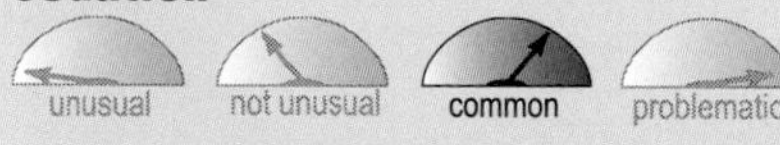

- Many experience and/or can be significant in amount

What to do About Side Effects

- Wait
- Wait
- Wait
- For motor symptoms, add an anticholinergic agent
- Take more of the dose at bedtime to help reduce daytime sedation
- Weight loss, exercise programs, and medical management for high BMIs, diabetes, dyslipidemia
- Reduce the dose
- Switch to a first-line atypical antipsychotic

Best Augmenting Agents for Side Effects

- Benztropine or trihexyphenidyl for motor side effects
- Sometimes amantadine can be helpful for motor side effects
- Benzodiazepines may be helpful for akathisia
- Many side effects cannot be improved with an augmenting agent

DOSING AND USE

Usual Dosage Range

- 75–300 mg/day in 3 divided doses

Dosage Forms

- Tablet 25 mg, 50 mg, 100 mg

How To Dose

- Initial 75 mg/day in 3 doses; can increase every 4 days; maximum 300 mg/day in 3 doses

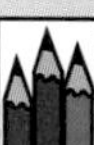

Dosing Tips

- Slow initial titration can minimize hypotension
- No formal studies, but some patients may do well on twice daily dosing rather than 3 times daily dosing

✱ Dose-related QTc prolongation, so use with caution, especially at high doses

Overdose

- Can be fatal, especially in mixed overdoses; seizures, coma

Long-Term Use

- Can be used to delay relapse in long-term treatment of schizophrenia

Habit Forming

- No

How to Stop

- Slow down-titration (over 6 to 8 weeks), especially when simultaneously beginning a new antipsychotic while switching (i.e., cross-titration)
- Rapid discontinuation may lead to rebound psychosis and worsening of symptoms
- If antiparkinson agents are being used, they should be continued for a few weeks after zotepine is discontinued

Pharmacokinetics

- Metabolized by CYP450 3A4 and CYP450 1A2
- Active metabolite norzotepine

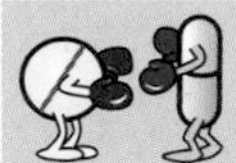

Drug Interactions

- Combined use with phenothiazines may increase risk of seizures
- Can decrease the effects of levodopa, dopamine agonists
- Epinephrine may lower blood pressure
- May interact with hypotensive agents due to alpha 1 adrenergic blockade
- May enhance QTc prolongation of other drugs capable of prolonging QTc interval
- Plasma concentrations increased by diazepam, fluoxetine
- Zotepine may increase plasma levels of phenytoin
- May increase risk of bleeding if used with anticoagulants
- Theoretically, dose may need to be raised if given in conjunction with CYP450 1A2 inducers (e.g., cigarette smoke)
- Theoretically, dose may need to be lowered if given in conjunction with CYP450 1A2 inhibitors (e.g., fluvoxamine) in order to prevent dangers of dose-dependent QTc prolongation
- Theoretically, dose may need to be lowered if given in conjunction with CYP450 3A4 inhibitors (e.g., fluvoxamine, nefazodone, fluoxetine) in order to prevent dangers of dose-dependent QTc prolongation

Other Warnings/ Precautions

- Not recommended for use with sibutramine
- Use cautiously in patients with alcohol withdrawal or convulsive disorders because of possible lowering of seizure threshold
- If signs of neuroleptic malignant syndrome develop, treatment should be immediately discontinued
- Because zotepine may dose-dependently prolong QTc interval, use with caution in patients who have bradycardia or who are taking drugs that can induce bradycardia (e.g., beta blockers, calcium channel blockers, clonidine, digitalis)
- Because zotepine may dose-dependently prolong QTc interval, use with caution in patients who have hypokalemia and or hypomagnesemia or who are taking drugs than can induce hypokalemia and/or magnesemia (e.g., diuretics, stimulant laxatives, intravenous amphotericin B, glucocorticoids, tetracosactide)
- Because zotepine dose-dependently prolongs QTc interval, use with caution in patients taking any agent capable of increasing zotepine plasma levels (e.g., diazepam, CYP450 1A2 inhibitors and CYP450 3A4 inhibitors)

Do Not Use

- If patient has epilepsy or family history of epilepsy
- If patient has gout or history of nephrolithiasis
- If patient is taking other CNS depressants
- If patient is taking high doses of other antipsychotics
- If patient is taking agents capable of significantly prolonging QTc interval (e.g., pimozide; thioridazine; selected antiarrhythmics such as quinidine, disopyramide, amiodarone, and sotalol; selected antibiotics such as moxifloxacin and sparfloxacin)
- If there is a history of QTc prolongation or cardiac arrhythmia, recent acute myocardial infarction, uncompensated heart failure
- If patient is pregnant or breast feeding
- If there is a proven allergy to zotepine

SPECIAL POPULATIONS

Renal Impairment

- Recommended starting dose 25 mg twice a day; recommended maximum dose generally 75 mg twice a day

Hepatic Impairment

- Recommended starting dose 25 mg twice a day; recommended maximum dose generally 75 mg twice a day
- May require weekly monitoring of liver function during the first few months of treatment

Cardiac Impairment

- Drug should be used with caution
- Zotepine produces a dose-dependent prolongation of QTc interval, which may be enhanced by the existence of bradycardia, hypokalemia, congenital or acquired long QTc interval, which should be evaluated prior to administering zotepine

- Use with caution if treating concomitantly with a medication likely to produce prolonged bradycardia, hypokalemia, slowing of intracardiac conduction, or prolongation of the QTc interval
- Avoid zotepine in patients with a known history of QTc prolongation, recent acute myocardial infraction, and uncompensated heart failure

Elderly

- Recommended starting dose 25 mg twice a day; recommended maximum dose generally 75 mg twice a day
- Although atypical antipsychotics are commonly used for behavioral disturbances in dementia, no agent has been approved for treatment of elderly patients with dementia-related psychosis
- Elderly patients with dementia-related psychosis treated with atypical antipsychotics are at an increased risk of death compared to placebo, and also have an increased risk of cerebrovascular events

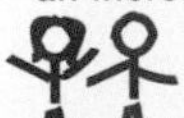

Children and Adolescents

- Not recommended in children under age 18

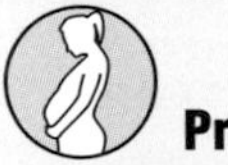

Pregnancy

- Insufficient data in humans to determine risk
- Zotepine is not recommended during pregnancy

Breast Feeding

- Zotepine is not recommended during breast feeding
- Immediate postpartum period is a high-risk time for relapse of psychosis, so may consider treatment with another antipsychotic

THE ART OF PSYCHOPHARMACOLOGY

Potential Advantages

- Norepinephrine reuptake blocking actions have theoretical benefits for cognition (attention) and for depression

Potential Disadvantages

- Patients not compliant with 3 times daily dosing
- Patients requiring rapid onset of antipsychotic action
- Patients with uncontrolled seizures

Primary Target Symptoms

- Positive symptoms of psychosis
- Negative symptoms of psychosis
- Cognitive functioning
- Depressive symptoms

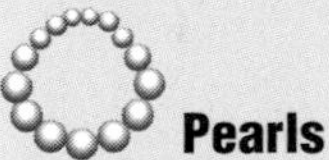

Pearls

* Zotepine inhibits norepinephrine reuptake, which may have implications for treatment of depression, as well as for cognitive symptoms of schizophrenia
- Risks of diabetes and dyslipidemia not well-studied for zotepine, but known significant weight gain suggests the need for careful monitoring during zotepine treatment
- Not as well investigated in bipolar disorder, but its mechanism of action suggests efficacy in acute bipolar mania

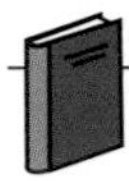

Suggested Reading

Ackenheil M. [The biochemical effect profile of zotepine in comparison with other neuroleptics]. Fortschr Neurol Psychiatr 1991; 59 Suppl1:2–9.

Fenton M, Morris S, De-Silva P, Bagnall A, Cooper SJ, Gammelin G, Leitner M. Zotepine for schizophrenia. Cochrane Database Syst Rev 2000;(2):CD001948.

Stanniland C, Taylor D. Tolerability of atypical antipsychotics. Drug Saf 2000;22(3):195–214.

ZUCLOPENTHIXOL

THERAPEUTICS

Brands • Clopixol
• Clopixol-Acuphase

see index for additional brand names

Generic? No

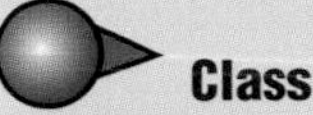

Class

- Conventional antipsychotic (neuroleptic, thioxanthene, dopamine 2 antagonist)

Commonly Prescribed For

(bold for FDA approved)

- Acute schizophrenia (oral, acetate injection)
- Maintenance treatment of schizophrenia (oral, decanoate injection)
- Bipolar disorder
- Aggression

How the Drug Works

- Blocks dopamine 2 receptors, reducing positive symptoms of psychosis

How Long Until It Works

- For injection, psychotic symptoms can improve within a few days, but it may take 1–2 weeks for notable improvement
- For oral formulation, psychotic symptoms can improve within 1 week, but may take several weeks for full effect on behavior

If It Works

- Most often reduces positive symptoms in schizophrenia but does not eliminate them
- Most schizophrenic patients do not have a total remission of symptoms but rather a reduction of symptoms by about a third
- Continue treatment in schizophrenia until reaching a plateau of improvement
- After reaching a satisfactory plateau, continue treatment for at least a year after first episode of psychosis in schizophrenia
- For second and subsequent episodes of psychosis in schizophrenia, treatment may need to be indefinite
- Reduces symptoms of acute psychotic mania but not proven as a mood stabilizer or as an effective maintenance treatment in bipolar disorder
- After reducing acute psychotic symptoms in mania, switch to a mood stabilizer and/or an atypical antipsychotic for mood stabilization and maintenance

If It Doesn't Work

- Consider trying one of the first-line atypical antipsychotics (risperidone, olanzapine, quetiapine, ziprasidone, aripiprazole, paliperidone, amisulpride)
- Consider trying another conventional antipsychotic
- If 2 or more antipsychotic monotherapies do not work, consider clozapine

Best Augmenting Combos for Partial Response or Treatment Resistance

- Augmentation of conventional antipsychotics has not been systematically studied
- Addition of a mood stabilizing anticonvulsant such as valproate, carbamazepine, or lamotrigine may be helpful in both schizophrenia and bipolar mania
- Augmentation with lithium in bipolar mania may be helpful
- Addition of a benzodiazepine, especially short-term for agitation

Tests

- ✻ Since conventional antipsychotics are frequently associated with weight gain, before starting treatment, weigh all patients and determine if the patient is already overweight (BMI 25.0–29.9) or obese (BMI ≥30)
- Before giving a drug that can cause weight gain to an overweight or obese patient, consider determining whether the patient already has pre-diabetes (fasting plasma glucose 100–25 mg/dL), diabetes (fasting plasma glucose >126 mg/dL), or dyslipidemia (increased total cholesterol, LDL cholesterol and triglycerides; decreased HDL cholesterol), and treat or refer such patients for treatment, including nutrition and weight management, physical activity counseling, smoking cessation, and medical management
- ✻ Monitor weight and BMI during treatment
- ✻ Consider monitoring fasting triglycerides monthly for several months in patients at high risk for metabolic complications and when initiating or switching antipsychotics
- ✻ While giving a drug to a patient who has gained >5% of initial weight, consider evaluating for the presence of pre-diabetes,

diabetes, or dyslipidemia, or consider switching to a different antipsychotic
- Should check blood pressure in the elderly before starting and for the first few weeks of treatment
- Monitoring elevated prolactin levels of dubious clinical benefit

SIDE EFFECTS

How Drug Causes Side Effects

- By blocking dopamine 2 receptors in the striatum, it can cause motor side effects
- By blocking dopamine 2 receptors in the pituitary, it can cause elevations in prolactin
- By blocking dopamine 2 receptors excessively in the mesocortical and mesolimbic dopamine pathways, especially at high doses, it can cause worsening of negative and cognitive symptoms (neuroleptic-induced deficit syndrome)
- Anticholinergic actions may cause sedation, blurred vision, constipation, dry mouth
- Antihistaminic actions may cause sedation, weight gain
- By blocking alpha 1 adrenergic receptors, it can cause dizziness, sedation, and hypotension
- Mechanism of weight gain and any possible increased incidence of diabetes or dyslipidemia with conventional antipsychotics is unknown

Notable Side Effects

✻ Extrapyramidal symptoms
✻ Tardive dyskinesia (risk increases with duration of treatment and with dose)
✻ Priapism
✻ Galactorrhea, amenorrhea
- Rare lens opacity
- Sedation, dizziness
- Dry mouth, constipation, vision problems
- Hypotension
- Weight gain

Life-Threatening or Dangerous Side Effects

- Rare neuroleptic malignant syndrome
- Rare neutropenia
- Rare respiratory depression
- Rare agranulocytosis
- Rare seizures
- Increased risk of death and cerebrovascular events in elderly patients with dementia-related psychosis

Weight Gain

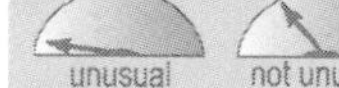

- Many experience and/or can be significant in amount
- Some people may lose weight

Sedation

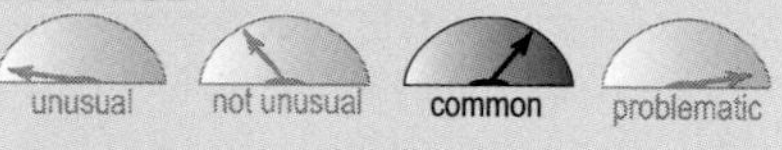

- Many experience and/or can be significant in amount
- Acetate formulation may be associated with an initial sedative response

What to do About Side Effects

- Wait
- Wait
- Wait
- For motor symptoms, add an anticholinergic agent
- Reduce the dose
- For sedation, take at night
- Switch to an atypical antipsychotic
- Weight loss, exercise programs, and medical management for high BMIs, diabetes dyslipidemia

Best Augmenting Agents for Side Effects

- Benztropine or trihexyphenidyl for motor side effects
- Sometimes amantadine can be helpful for motor side effects
- Benzodiazepines may be helpful for akathisia
- Many side effects cannot be improved with an augmenting agent

DOSING AND USE

Usual Dosage Range

- Oral 20–60 mg/day
- Acetate 50–150 mg every 2–3 days
- Decanoate 150–300 mg every 2–4 weeks

Dosage Forms

- Tablet 10 mg, 25 mg, 40 mg

- Acetate 50 mg/mL (equivalent to zuclopenthixol 45.25 mg/mL), 100 mg/2 mL (equivalent to zuclopenthixol 45.25 mg/mL)
- Decanoate 200 mg/mL (equivalent to zuclopenthixol 144.4 mg/mL), 500 mg/mL (equivalent to zuclopenthixol 361.1 mg/mL)

How To Dose

- Oral: initial 10–5 mg/day in divided doses; can increase by 10–20 mg/day every 2–3 days; maintenance dose can be administered as a single nighttime dose; maximum dose generally 100 mg/day
- Injection should be administered intramuscularly in the gluteal region in the morning
- Acetate generally should be administered every 2–3 days; some patients may require a second dose 24–48 hours after the first injection; duration of treatment should not exceed 2 weeks; maximum cumulative dosage should not exceed 400 mg; maximum number of injections should not exceed 4
- Decanoate: initial dose 100 mg; after 1–4 weeks administer a second injection of 100–200 mg; maintenance treatment is generally 100–600 mg every 1–4 weeks

Dosing Tips

- Onset of action of the intramuscular acetate formulation following a single injection is generally 2–4 hours; duration of action is generally 2–3 days
- Zuclopenthixol acetate is not intended for long-term use, and should not generally be used for longer than 2 weeks; patients requiring treatment longer than 2 weeks should be switched to a depot or oral formulation of zuclopenthixol or another antipsychotic
- When changing from zuclopenthixol acetate to maintenance treatment with zuclopenthixol decanoate, administer the last injection of acetate concomitantly with the initial injection of decanoate
- The peak of action for the decanoate is usually 4–9 days, and doses generally have to be administered every 2–3 weeks

Overdose

- Sedation, convulsions, extrapyramidal symptoms, coma, hypotension, shock, hypo/hyperthermia

Long-Term Use

- Zuclopenthixol decanoate is intended for maintenance treatment
- Some side effects may be irreversible (e.g., tardive dyskinesia)

Habit Forming

- No

How to Stop

- Slow down-titration of oral formulation (over 6–8 weeks), especially when simultaneously beginning a new antipsychotic while switching (i.e., cross-titration)
- Rapid oral discontinuation may lead to rebound psychosis and worsening of symptoms
- If antiparkinson agents are being used, they should be continued for a few weeks after zuclopenthixol is discontinued

Pharmacokinetics

- Metabolized by CYP450 2D6
- For oral formulation, elimination half-life approximately 20 hours
- For acetate, rate-limiting half-life approximately 32 hours
- For decanoate, rate-limiting half-life approximately 17–21 days with multiple doses

Drug Interactions

- Theoretically, concomitant use with CYP450 2D6 inhibitors (such as paroxetine and fluoxetine) could raise zuclopenthixol plasma levels and require dosage reduction
- CNS effects may be increased if used with other CNS depressants
- If used with anticholinergic agents, may potentiate their effects
- Combined use with epinephrine may lower blood pressure
- Zuclopenthixol may block the antihypertensive effects of drugs such as guanethidine, but may enhance the actions of other antihypertensive drugs
- Using zuclopenthixol with metoclopramide

or piperazine may increase the risk of extrapyramidal symptoms
- Zuclopenthixol may antagonize the effects of levodopa and dopamine agonists
- Some patients taking a neuroleptic and lithium have developed an encephalopathic syndrome similar to neuroleptic malignant syndrome

Other Warnings/ Precautions
- If signs of neuroleptic malignant syndrome develop, treatment should be immediately discontinued
- Use with caution in patients with epilepsy, glaucoma, urinary retention
- Decanoate should not be used with clozapine because it cannot be withdrawn quickly in the event of serious adverse effects such as neutropenia
- Possible antiemetic effect of zuclopenthixol may mask signs of other disorders or overdose; suppression of cough reflex may cause asphyxia
- Use only with great caution if at all in Parkinson's disease or Lewy body dementia
- Observe for signs of ocular toxicity (pigmentary retinopathy and lenticular and corneal deposits)
- Avoid undue exposure to sunlight
- Avoid extreme heat exposure
- Do not use epinephrine in event of overdose as interaction with some pressor agents may lower blood pressure

Do Not Use
- If patient is taking a large concomitant dose of a sedative hypnotic
- If patient is taking guanethidine or a similar acting compound
- If patient has CNS depression, is comatose, or has subcortical brain damage
- If patient has acute alcohol, barbiturate, or opiate intoxication
- If patient has narrow angle-closure glaucoma
- If patient has pheochromocytoma, circulatory collapse, or blood dyscrasias
- In case of pregnancy
- If there is a proven allergy to zuclopenthixol

SPECIAL POPULATIONS

Renal Impairment
- Use with caution

Hepatic Impairment
- Use with caution

Cardiac Impairment
- Use with caution

Elderly
- Some patients may tolerate lower doses better
- Maximum acetate dose 100 mg
- Although conventional antipsychotics are commonly used for behavioral disturbances in dementia, no agent has been approved for treatment of elderly patients with dementia-related psychosis
- Elderly patients with dementia-related psychosis treated with antipsychotics are at an increased risk of death compared to placebo, and also have an increased risk of cerebrovascular events

Children and Adolescents
- Safety and efficacy have not been established in children under age 18
- Preliminary open-label data show that oral zuclopenthixol may be effective in reducing aggression in mentally impaired children

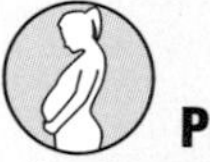

Pregnancy
- Not recommended for use during pregnancy
- Psychotic symptoms may worsen during pregnancy and some form of treatment may be necessary
- Atypical antipsychotics may be preferable to conventional antipsychotics or anticonvulsant mood stabilizers if treatment is required during pregnancy

Breast Feeding
- Some drug is found in mother's breast milk
- ✽ Recommended either to discontinue drug or bottle feed
- Infants of women who choose to breast feed should be monitored for possible adverse effects

THE ART OF PSYCHOPHARMACOLOGY

Potential Advantages

- Noncompliant patients (decanoate)
- Emergency use (acute injection)

Potential Disadvantages

- Children
- Elderly
- Patients with tardive dyskinesia

Primary Target Symptoms

- Positive symptoms of psychosis
- Negative symptoms of psychosis
- Aggressive symptoms

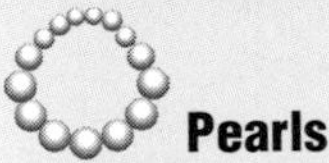

Pearls

- Zuclopenthixol depot may reduce risk of relapse more than some other depot conventional antipsychotics, but it may also be associated with more adverse effects
- Can combine acute injection with depot injection in the same syringe for rapid onset and long duration effects when initiating treatment
- Zuclopenthixol may have serotonin 2A antagonist properties, but these have never been systematically investigated for atypical antipsychotic properties at low doses
- Patients have very similar antipsychotic responses to any conventional antipsychotic, which is different from atypical antipsychotics where antipsychotic responses of individual patients can occasionally vary greatly from one atypical antipsychotic to another
- Patients with inadequate responses to atypical antipsychotics may benefit from a trial of augmentation with a conventional antipsychotic such as zuclopenthixol or from switching to a conventional antipsychotic such as zuclopenthixol
- However, long-term polypharmacy with a combination of a conventional antipsychotic such as zuclopenthixol with an atypical antipsychotic may combine their side effects without clearly augmenting the efficacy of either
- Although a frequent practice by some prescribers, adding 2 conventional antipsychotics together has little rationale and may reduce tolerability without clearly enhancing efficacy

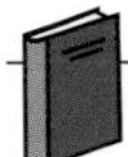

Suggested Reading

Coutinho E, Fenton M, Adams C, Campbell C. Zuclopenthixol acetate in psychiatric emergencies: looking for evidence from clinical trials. Schizophr Res 2000;46:111–8.

Coutinho E, Fenton M, Quraishi S. Zuclopenthixol decanoate for schizophrenia and other serious mental illnesses. Cochrane Database Syst Rev 2000;(2):CD001164.

Fenton M, Coutinho ES, Campbell C. Zuclopenthixol acetate in the treatment of acute schizophrenia and similar serious mental illnesses. Cochrane Database Syst Rev 2000;(2):CD000525.

Index by Drug Name

Apo-Diazepam (diazepam), *139*
Apo-Doxepin (doxepin), *157*
Apo-Fluoxetine (fluoxetine), *193*
Apo-Fluphenazine (fluphenazine), *205*
Apo-Haloperidol (haloperidol), *237*
Apoh-Hydroxyzine (hydroxyzine), *243*
Apo-Imipramine (imipramine), *253*
Apollonset (diazepam), *139*
Apo-Lorazem (lorazepam), *301*
Aponal (doxepin), *157*
Apo-Oxepam (oxazepam), *397*
Apo-Perphenazine (perphenazine), *421*
Apo-Selegiline (selegiline), *489*
Apo-Thioridazine (thioridazine), *519*
Apo-Trazodone (trazodone), *547*
Apo-Triazo (triazolam), *557*
Apo-Trifluoperazine (trifluoperazine), *563*
Apo-Trimip (trimipramine), *569*
Apozepam (diazepam), *139*
Aremis (sertraline), *497*
Aricept (donepezil), *145*
Arima (moclobemide), *353*
Aripax (lorazepam), *295*
aripiprazole, *45*
Arminol (sulpiride), *503*
Arol (moclobemide), *353*
Aropax (paroxetine), *409*
Asendin (amoxapine), *25*
Asendis (amoxapine), *25*
Asepin (triazolam), *553*
Aspam (diazepam), *139*
Atarax (hydroxyzine), *243*
Atarviton (diazepam), *139*
Atensine (diazepam), *139*
Aterax (hydroxyzine), *243*
Ativan (lorazepam), *295*
atomoxetine, *51*
Atretol (carbamazepine), *67*
Audilex (clorazepate), *109*
Audium (diazepam), *139*
Aurorix (moclobemide), *353*
Avant (haloperidol), *237*
Aventyl (nortriptyline), *379*
Avoxin (fluvoxamine), *215*
Axoren (buspirone), *63*
Azene (clorazepate), *109*
Azepa (carbamazepine), *67*
Azepal (carbamazepine), *67*
Azona (trazodone), *547*
Azor (alprazolam), *5*
Azutranquil (oxazepam), *393*
Barclyd (clonidine), *103*
Beconerv neu (flurazepam), *211*
Belivon (risperidone), *475*
Belpax (amitriptyline), *17*
Belseren (clorazepate), *109*
Benpon (nortriptyline), *379*
Bentapam (diazepam), *139*
Benzopin (diazepam), *139*
Benzotran (oxazepam), *393*
Berk-Dothiepin (dothiepin), *151*
Besitran (sertraline), *497*
Bespar (buspirone), *63*
Betamaks (sulpiride), *503*
Betamed (diazepam), *139*
Betapam (diazepam), *139*
Bialzepam (diazepam), *139*
Bikalm (zolpidem), *595*
Bioperidolo (haloperidol), *237*
Bioxetin (fluoxetine), *193*
Biron (buspirone), *63*
Biscasil (chlorpromazine), *77*
Biston (see carbamazepine), *67*
Bortalium (diazepam), *139*
bupropion, *57*
bupropion SR, *57*
bupropion XL, *57*
Buscalm (buspirone), *63*
Buspar (buspirone), *63*
BuSpar (buspirone), *63*
Buspimen (buspirone), *63*
buspirone, *63*
Buspisal (buspirone), *63*
Buteridol (haloperidol), *237*
Calmoflorine (sulpiride), *503*
Camcolit (lithium), *277*
Campral (acamprosate), *1*
Caprysin (clonidine), *103*
Carbabeta (carbamazepine), *67*
Carbagamma (carbamazepine), *67*
carbamazepine, *67*
Carbapin (carbamazepine), *67*
Carbium (carbamazepine), *67*
Carbolith (lithium), *277*
Carbolithium (lithium), *277*
Carbymal (carbamazepine), *67*
Cardilac (fluphenazine), *205*
Carpaz (carbamazepine), *67*
Cassadan (alprazolam), *5*
Catanidin (clonidine), *103*
Catapres (clonidine), *103*
Catapres-TTS (clonidine), *103*
Cedrol (zolpidem), *595*
Celexa (citalopram), *83*
Cenilene (fluphenazine), *205*
Centedrin (d,l-methylphenidate), *329*
Cereen (haloperidol), *237*
Championyl (sulpiride), *503*
Champix (varenicline), *575*
Chantix (varenicline), *575*
Chlorazin (chlorpromazine), *77*
chlordiazepoxide, *73*
Chlorpromazin (chlorpromazine), *77*
Chlorpromazina HCl (chlorpromazine), *77*

chlorpromazine, *109*
Cibalith S-Lithonate (lithium), *277*
Cidoxepin (doxepin), *157*
Cipram (citalopram), *83*
Cipramil (citalopram), *83*
Cisordinol (zuclopenthixol), *613*
citalopram, *83*
clomipramine, *89*
clonazepam, *97*
Clonazepamum (clonazepam), *97*
clonidine, *103*
Clonisin (clonidine), *103*
Clonistada (clonidine), *103*
Clopixol (zuclopenthixol), *613*
Clopixol Acuphase (zuclopenthixol), *613*
Clopixol Conc (zuclopenthixol), *613*
Clopress (clomipramine), *89*
clorazepate, *109*
Clordezalin (chlorpromazine), *77*
Clorpres (clonidine), *103*
clozapine, *113*
Clozaril (clozapine), *113*
Coaxil (tianeptine), *529*
Cognitiv (selegiline), *489*
Combipres (clonidine), *103*
Complutine (diazepam), *139*
Concerta (d,l-methylphenidate), *329*
Concordin (protriptyline), *449*
Concordine (protriptyline), *449*
Contemnol (lithium), *277*
Control (lorazepam), *295*
Convulex (valproate), *569*
Convulsofin (valproate), *569*
Cosmopril (selegiline), *489*
cyamemazine, *119*
Cymbalta (duloxetine), *165*
Dalcipran (milnacipran), *341*
Dalmadorm (flurazepam), *211*
Dalmane (flurazepam), *211*
Dalparan (zolpidem), *595*
Dapotum (fluphenazine), *205*
Dapotum Acutum (fluphenazine), *205*
Dapotum D (fluphenazine), *205*
Dapotum Depot (fluphenazine), *205*
Daprimen (amitriptyline), *17*
Darkene (flunitrazepam), *189*
Darleton (sulpiride), *503*
Decafen (fluphenazine), *205*
Decanoate (haloperidol), *237*
Decazate (fluphenazine), *205*
Decentan (fluphenazine), *205*
Decentan (perphenazine), *237*
Decentan-Depot (perphenazine), *421*
Defanyl (amoxapine), *25*
Defobin (chlordiazepoxide), *73*
Deftan (lofepramine), *283*
Degranol (carbamazepine), *67*
Delepsine (valproate), *569*
Delgian (maprotiline), *307*
Demolox (amoxapine), *25*
Deniban (amisulpride), *11*
Denion (diazepam), *139*
Depacon (valproate), *569*
Depakene (valproate), *569*
Depakine (LA) (valproate), *569*
Depakine Chrono (valproate), *569*
Depakine Zuur (valproate), *569*
Depakote (valproate), *569*
Depakote sprinkle (valproate), *569*
Depamide (valproate), *569*
Deparkin (valproate), *569*
Depex (sulpiride), *503*
Depixol (flupenthixol), *199*
Depixol-Conc (flupenthixol), *199*
Deprakine (valproate), *569*
Depral (sulpiride), *503*
Depramine (imipramine), *247*
Deprax (trazodone), *547*
Deprenon (fluoxetine), *193*
Deprenyl (selegiline), *489*
Depressase (maprotiline), *307*
Deprex (fluoxetine), *193*
Deprilan (selegiline), *489*
Deprilept (maprotiline), *307*
Deprimyl (lofepramine), *283*
Deprinocte (estazolam), *177*
Deprinol (imipramine), *247*
Deptran (doxepin), *157*
Deroxat (paroxetine), *409*
Desconex (loxapine), *301*
Desidox (doxepin), *157*
desipramine, *125*
Desisulpid (sulpiride), *503*
Desitriptylin (amitriptyline), *17*
desvenlafaxine, *133*
Desyrel (trazodone), *547*
Devidon (trazodone), *547*
Dexamphetamine (d-amphetamine), *33*
Dexamphetamine sulfate (d-amphetamine), *33*
Dexedrine (d-amphetamine), *33*
Dexmethylphenidate (d-methylphenidate), *323*
Dextro Stat (d-amphetamine), *33*
Diaceplex (diazepam), *139*
Diaceplex simple (diazepam), *139*
Diapam (diazepam), *139*
Diaquel (diazepam), *139*
Diastat (diazepam), *139*
Diazemuls (diazepam), *139*
diazepam, *139*
Dicepin B6 (diazepam), *139*
Digton (sulpiride), *503*
Diligan (hydroxyzine), *243*
Dinalexin (fluoxetine), *193*
Dipromal (valproate), *569*

Discimer (trifluoperazine), *557*
Distedon (diazepam), *139*
divalproex (valproate), *569*
Divial (lorazepam), *295*
Dixarit (clonidine), *103*
Dixibon (sulpiride), *503*
Dizac (diazepam), *139*
d-methylphenidate, *323*
Dobren (sulpiride), *503*
Dobupal (venlafaxine), *579*
Dogmatil (sulpiride), *503*
Dogmatyl (sulpiride), *503*
Dolmatil (sulpiride), *503*
Domical (amitriptyline), *17*
Dominans (nortriptyline), *379*
Domnamid (estazolam), *177*
DOM-trazodone (trazodone), *547*
donepezil, *145*
Doneurin (doxepin), *157*
Donix (lorazepam), *295*
Dopress (dothiepin), *151*
Doral (quazepam), *455*
Dorken (clorazepate), *109*
Dorm (lorazepam), *295*
Dormalin (quazepam), *455*
Dormapam (temazepam), *509*
Dorme (quazepam), *455*
Dormicum (midazolam), *337*
Dormodor (flurazepam), *211*
Dothep (dothiepin), *151*
dothiepin, *151*
Doxal (doxepin), *157*
Doxedyn (doxepin), *157*
doxepin, *157*
Dozic (haloperidol), *237*
D-Pam (diazepam), *139*
Drenian (diazepam), *139*
Dresent (sulpiride), *503*
Ducene (diazepam), *139*
duloxetine, *165*
Dumirox (fluvoxamine), *215*
Dumozolam (triazolam), *553*
Dumyrox (fluvoxamine), *215*
Duraclon (clonidine), *103*
Duradiazepam (diazepam), *139*
Duralith (lithium), *277*
Duraperidol (haloperidol), *237*
Durazepam (oxazepam), *393*
Durazolam (lorazepam), *295*
Dutonin (nefazodone), *373*
Eclorion (sulpiride), *503*
Edronax (reboxetine), *469*
Efectin (venlafaxine), *579*
Efexir (venlafaxine), *579*
Efexor (venlafaxine), *579*
Efexor XL (venlafaxine), *579*
Effexor (venlafaxine), *579*
Effexor XR (venlafaxine), *579*
Effiplen (buspirone), *63*
Egibren (selegiline), *489*
Eglonyl (sulpiride), *503*
Elavil (amitriptyline), *17*
Elavil Plus (amitriptyline), *17*
Eldepryl (selegiline), *489*
Elenium (chlordiazepoxide), *73*
Eliwel (amitriptyline), *17*
Elmendos (lamotrigine), *259*
Elopram (citalopram), *83*
Elperil (thioridazine), *513*
Elroquil N (hydroxyzine), *243*
Emdalen (lofepramine), *283*
Endep (amitriptyline), *17*
Enimon (sulpiride), *503*
Epial (carbamazepine), *67*
Epilim (valproate), *569*
Epitol (carbamazepine), *67*
Epitomax (topiramate), *535*
Equilid (sulpiride), *503*
Equitam (lorazepam), *295*
Ergenyl (valproate), *569*
Ergocalm (lorazepam), *295*
Eridan (diazepam), *139*
Erocap (fluoxetine), *193*
escitalopram, *171*
Esculid (diazepam), *139*
Esilgan (estazolam), *177*
Esipride (sulpiride), *503*
Eskalith (lithium), *277*
Eskazine (trifluoperazine), *559*
Esparon (alprazolam), *5*
estazolam, *177*
eszopiclone, *181*
Ethipam (diazepam), *139*
Ethipramine (imipramine), *247*
Euhypnos (temazepam), *509*
Euipnos (temazepam), *509*
Eurosan (diazepam), *139*
Eutimil (paroxetine), *409*
Eutimox (fluphenazine), *205*
Evacalm (diazepam), *139*
Everiden (valproate), *569*
Exan (buspirone), *57*
Excegran (zonisamide), *599*
Exelon (rivastigmine), *483*
Exogran (zonisamide), *599*
Exostrept (fluoxetine), *193*
Fardalan (sulpiride), *503*
Fargenor (chlordiazepoxide), *73*
Faustan (diazepam), *139*
Faverin (fluvoxamine), *215*
Felicium (fluoxetine), *193*
Felison (flurazepam), *211*
Fenactil (chlorpromazine), *77*
Fentazin (perphenazine), *421*

Fevarin (fluvoxamine), *215*
Fidelan (sulpiride), *503*
Finlepsin (carbamazepine), *67*
Flaracantyl (thioridazine), *513*
Flonital (fluoxetine), *193*
Floxyfral (fluvoxamine), *215*
Fluanxol (flupenthixol), *199*
Fluanxol Depot (flupenthixol), *199*
Fluanxol Depot 10% (flupenthixol), *199*
Fluanxol Depot 2% (flupenthixol), *199*
Fluanxol LP 100 mg/mL (flupenthixol), *199*
Fluanxol LP 20 mg/mL (flupenthixol), *199*
Fluanxol Retard (flupenthixol), *199*
Fluctin (fluoxetine), *193*
Fluctine (fluoxetine), *193*
Fludecate (fluphenazine), *205*
Flufenazin (fluphenazine), *205*
Flufenazin dekanoat (fluphenazine), *205*
Flufenazin Enantat (fluphenazine), *205*
flumazenil, *185*
Fluni OPT (flunitrazepam), *189*
Flunimerck (flunitrazepam), *189*
Fluninoc (flunitrazepam), *189*
Flunipam (flunitrazepam), *189*
Flunitrax (flunitrazepam), *189*
flunitrazepam, *189*
Flunox (flurazepam), *211*
Fluocim (fluoxetine), *193*
Fluoxeren (fluoxetine), *193*
fluoxetine, *193*
Fluoxifar (fluoxetine), *193*
Fluoxin (fluoxetine), *193*
Flupam (flunitrazepam), *189*
flupenthixol, *199*
fluphenazine, *205*
flurazepam, *211*
Fluscand (flunitrazepam), *189*
Flutepam (flurazepam), *211*
Flutin (fluoxetine), *193*
Flutraz (flunitrazepam), *189*
Fluval (fluoxetine), *193*
fluvoxamine, *215*
Fluxadir (fluoxetine), *193*
Fluxonil (fluoxetine), *193*
Focalin (d-methylphenidate), *323*
Foille (trifluoperazine), *557*
Fokalepsin (carbamazepine), *67*
Fondur (fluoxetine), *193*
Fontex (fluoxetine), *193*
Fonzac (fluoxetine), *193*
Fortunan (haloperidol), *237*
Frontal (alprazolam), *5*
Frosinor (paroxetine), *409*
Frosnor (paroxetine), *409*
gabapentin, *221*
Gabitril (tiagabine), *523*
galantamine, *227*
Gamanil (lofepramine), *283*
Gamibetal Plus (diazepam), *139*
Gamonil (lofepramine), *283*
Gen-Alprazolam (alprazolam), *5*
Gen-Clomipramine (clomipramine), *89*
Gen-Triazolam (triazolam), *553*
Gen-Valproic (valproate), *569*
Geodon (ziprasidone), *589*
Gewakalm (diazepam), *139*
Gladem (sertraline), *497*
Gnostorid (oxazepam), *393*
Gobanal (diazepam), *139*
guanfacine, *233*
Haemiton (clonidine), *103*
Halcion (triazolam), *553*
Haldol (haloperidol), *237*
Haldol decanoas (haloperidol), *237*
Haldol Decanoat (haloperidol), *237*
Haldol Decanoate (haloperidol), *237*
Haldol Decanoato (haloperidol), *237*
Haldol Depot (haloperidol), *237*
Haldol L.A. (haloperidol), *237*
Haloneural (haloperidol), *237*
Haloper (haloperidol), *237*
haloperidol, *237*
Haloperidol Decanoat (haloperidol), *237*
Haloperidol decanoato (haloperidol), *237*
Haloperin (haloperidol), *237*
Haloperin depotinjektio (haloperidol), *237*
Harmomed (dothiepin), *151*
Harmoned (diazepam), *139*
Helex (alprazolam), *5*
Helogaphen (chlordiazepoxide), *73*
Hermolepsin (carbamazepine), *67*
Herphonal (trimipramine), *563*
Hexafene (hydroxyzine), *243*
Hexalid (diazepam), *139*
Hibanil (chlorpromazine), *77*
Hibernal (chlorpromazine), *77*
Hipnodane (quazepam), *455*
Hipnosedon (flunitrazepam), *189*
Histilos (hydroxyzine), *243*
Huberplex (chlordiazepoxide), *73*
Hydoic acid (valproate), *569*
Hydophen (clomipramine), *89*
Hydroxyzin (hydroxyzine), *243*
hydroxyzine, *243*
Hydroxyzinum (hydroxyzine), *243*
Hypam (triazolam), *553*
Hypnocalm (flunitrazepam), *189*
Hypnodorm (flunitrazepam), *189*
Hypnor (flunitrazepam), *189*
Hypnorex retard (lithium), *277*
Hypnovel (midazolam), *337*
Idom (dothiepine), *151*
Iktoviril (clonazepam), *97*
Ilman (flunitrazepam), *189*

Imavate (imipramine), *247*
Imipramiin (imipramine), *247*
Imipramin (imipramine), *247*
imipramine, *247*
Inadalprem (lorazepam), *295*
Insom (flunitrazepam), *189*
Intuniv (guanfacine), *233*
INVEGA (paliperidone), *403*
Ipnovel (midazolam), *337*
Iremo Sedofren (trifluoperazine), *557*
Iremofar (hydroxyzine), *243*
isocarboxazid, *253*
Ivadal (zolpidem), *595*
Ixel (milnacipran), *341*
Janimine (imipramine), *247*
Januar (oxazepam), *393*
Jardin (dothiepin), *151*
Jatroneural (trifluoperazine), *557*
Jatrosom (tranylcypromine), *541*
Jatrosom N (tranylcypromine), *541*
Jatrosom N (trifluoperazine), *557*
Julap (selegiline), *489*
Jumex (selegiline), *489*
Jumexal (selegiline), *489*
Kainever (estazolam), *117*
Kalma (alprazolam), *5*
Kanopan 75 (maprotiline), *307*
Karbazin (carbamazepine), *67*
Keppra (levetiracetam), *267*
Kinabide (selegiline), *489*
Klarium (diazepam), *139*
Klofelins (clonidine), *103*
Klonipin (clonazepam), *97*
Klopoxid (chlordiazepoxide), *73*
Kloproman (chlorpromazine), *77*
Klorproman (chlorpromazine), *77*
Klotriptyl (chlordiazepoxide), *73*
Klozapol (clozapine), *113*
Labileno (lamotrigine), *259*
Ladose (fluoxetine), *193*
Lambipol (lamotrigine), *259*
Lamictal (lamotrigine), *259*
Lamictin (lamotrigine), *259*
lamotrigine, *259*
Lamra (diazepam), *139*
Lanexat (flumazenil), *185*
Largactil (chlorpromazine), *77*
Largatrex (chlorpromazine), *77*
Laroxyl (amitriptyline), *17*
Laubeel (lorazepam), *295*
Lauracalm (lorazepam), *295*
Lebopride (sulpiride), *503*
Lelptilan (valproate), *569*
Lelptilanil (valproate), *569*
Lentizol (amitriptyline), *17*
Lentolith (lithium), *277*
Lentotran (chlordiazepoxide), *73*
Leponex (clozapine), *113*
Leptilin (valproate), *569*
Leukominerase (lithium), *277*
Levanxol (temazepam), *509*
levetiracetam, *267*
Lexapro (escitalopram), *171*
Li-450 (lithium), *277*
Librax (chlordiazepoxide), *73*
Libraxin (chlordiazepoxide), *73*
Librium (chlordiazepoxide), *73*
Lidanil (mesoridazine), *317*
Lidone (molindone), *365*
Li-Liquid (lithium), *277*
Lilly Fluoxetine (fluoxetine), *193*
Limbatril (chlordiazepoxide), *73*
Limbatril F (chlordiazepoxide), *73*
Limbitrol (chlordiazepoxide), *73*
Limbitrol F (chlordiazepoxide), *73*
Limbitryl (chlordiazepoxide), *73*
Limbitryl Plus (chlordiazepoxide), *73*
lisdexamfetamine, *271*
Liskonum (lithium), *277*
Litarex (lithium), *277*
Lithane (lithium), *277*
Lithiofor (lithium), *277*
Lithionit (lithium), *277*
Lithiucarb (lithium), *277*
lithium, *277*
Lithium carbonicum (lithium), *277*
Lithium-aspartat (lithium), *277*
Lithium-Duriles (lithium), *277*
Lithiumkarbonat (lithium), *277*
Lithiumorotat (lithium), *277*
Lithizine (lithium), *277*
Lithobid (lithium), *277*
Lithonate (lithium), *277*
Lito (lithium), *277*
Litoduron (lithium), *277*
Lodopin (zotepine), *607*
lofepramine, *283*
loflazepate, *289*
Lomesta (lorazepam), *295*
Lonseren (pipothiazine), *439*
Lorabenz (lorazepam), *295*
Lorafen (lorazepam), *295*
Loram (lorazepam), *295*
Lorans (lorazepam), *295*
Lorapam (lorazepam), *295*
lorazepam, *295*
Lorenin (lorazepam), *295*
Loridem (lorazepam), *295*
Lorien (fluoxetine), *193*
Lorivan (lorazepam), *295*
Lorsedal (lorazepam), *295*
Lorsifar (lorazepam), *295*
Lorsilan (lorazepam), *295*
Lorzem (lorazepam), *295*

Ozodeprin (sulpiride), *503*
Paceum (diazepam), *139*
Pacinol (fluphenazine), *205*
Pacium (diazepam), *139*
paliperidone, *403*
Pamelor (nortriptyline), *379*
Panix (alprazolam), *5*
Pantrop Retard (chlordiazepoxide), *73*
Paracefan (clonidine), *103*
Paratil (sulpiride), *503*
Parkinyl (selegiline), *489*
Parmodalin (tranylcypromine), *541*
Parmodalin (trifluoperazine), *557*
Parnate (tranylcypromine), *541*
paroxetine, *409*
paroxetine CR, *409*
Parstelin (tranylcypromine), *541*
Parstelin (trifluoperazine), *557*
Pasrin (buspirone), *63*
Pax (diazepam), *139*
Paxal (alprazolam), *5*
Paxam (clonazepam), *97*
Paxil (paroxetine), *409*
Paxil CR (paroxetine CR), *409*
Paxium (chlordiazepoxide), *73*
Paxtibi (nortriptyline), *379*
Pazolan (alprazolam), *5*
Pefanium / Pefanic (chlordiazepoxide), *73*
Peratsin (perphenazine), *421*
Peratsin Dekanoaatti (perphenazine), *421*
Peratsin Enantaati (perphenazine), *421*
Perfenazin (perphenazine), *421*
Peridol (haloperidol), *237*
Permitil (fluphenazine), *205*
perospirone, *417*
perphenazine, *421*
Pertofrane (desipramine), *125*
Pertofrin (desipramine), *125*
Phasal (lithium), *277*
phenelzine, *427*
Piefol (trifluoperazine), *557*
pimozide, *433*
Piportil (pipothiazine), *439*
Piportil Depot (pipothiazine), *439*
Piportil L4 (pipothiazine), *439*
Piportil Longum-4 (pipothiazine), *439*
Piportil palmitate (pipothiazine), *439*
Piportyl palmitat (pipothiazine), *439*
pipothiazine, *439*
Pipotiazine (pipothiazine), *439*
Pirium (pimozide), *433*
Placidia (lorazepam), *295*
Placil (clomipramine), *89*
Placinoral (lorazepam), *295*
Planum (temazepam), *509*
Plegomazin (chlorpromazine), *77*
Plenur (lithium), *277*
Plurimen (selegiline), *489*
PMS-carbamazepine (carbamazepine), *67*
PMS-Clonazepam (clonazepam), *97*
PMS-Desipramine (desipramine), *125*
PMS-Fluoxetine (fluoxetine), *193*
PMS-fluphenazine (fluphenazine), *205*
PMS-Fluphenazine Decanoate (fluphenazine), *205*
PMS-Haloperidol (haloperidol), *237*
PMS-Hydroxyzine (hydroxyzine), *243*
PMS-Lithium (lithium), *277*
PMS-Methylphenidate (d,l-methylphenidate), *329*
PMS-Trazodone (trazodone), *547*
Podium (diazepam), *139*
Poldoxin (doxepin), *157*
Polysal (amitriptyline), *17*
Portal (fluoxetine), *193*
Pragmarel (trazodone), *547*
Praxiten (oxazepam), *393*
pregabalin, *445*
Priadel (lithium), *277*
Prisdal (citalopram), *83*
Pristiq (desvenlafaxine), *133*
Pro Dorm (lorazepam), *295*
Procythol (selegiline), *489*
Prolixin (fluphenazine), *205*
Prolixin Decanoate (fluphenazine), *205*
Prolixin enanthate (fluphenazine), *205*
Prolongatum (fluphenazine), *205*
Pronervon T (temazepam), *509*
Propam (diazepam), *139*
Propaphenin (chlorpromazine), *77*
Propymal (valproate), *569*
Prosedar (quazepam), *455*
ProSom (estazolam), *177*
Prosulpin (sulpiride), *503*
Prothiaden (dothiepin), *151*
Protiaden (dothiepin), *151*
protriptyline, *449*
Provigil (modafinil), *359*
Proxam (oxazepam), *393*
Prozac (fluoxetine), *193*
Prozil (chlorpromazine), *77*
Prozin (chlorpromazine), *77*
Prozyn (fluoxetine), *193*
Pryleugan (imipramine), *247*
Psicocen (sulpiride), *503*
Psicofar (chlordiazepoxide), *73*
Psiquiwas (oxazepam), *393*
Psychopax (diazepam), *139*
Psymoin (maprotiline), *307*
Punktyl (lorazepam), *295*
Purata (oxazepam), *393*
Q-Med Hydroxyzine (hydroxyzine), *243*
Quait (lorazepam), *295*
Quastil (sulpiride), *503*

quazepam, *455*
Quazium (quazepam), *455*
quetiapine, *459*
Quiedorm (quazepam), *455*
Quilibrex (oxazepam), *393*
Quilonum (lithium), *277*
Quilonum Retard (lithium), *277*
Quinolorm (lithium), *277*
Quinolorm Retard (lithium), *277*
Quiridil (sulpiride), *503*
Quitaxon (doxepin), *157*
Radepur (chlordiazepoxide), *73*
ramelteon, *465*
Razadyne (galantamine), *227*
Razadyne ER (galantamine), *227*
Razolam (alprazolam), *5*
reboxetine, *469*
Redomex (amitriptyline), *17*
RedomexDiffucaps (amitriptyline), *17*
Regepar (selegiline), *489*
Relanium (diazepam), *139*
Relax Sedans (chlordiazepoxide), *73*
Relaxedans (chlordiazepoxide), *73*
Reliberan (chlordiazepoxide), *73*
Remdue (flurazepam), *211*
Remergil (mirtazapine), *347*
Remeron (mirtazapine), *347*
Remestan (temazepam), *509*
Reminyl (galantamine), *227*
Reneuron (fluoxetine), *193*
Repazine (chlorpromazine), *77*
Reposium (temazepam), *509*
Reseril (nefazodone), *379*
Restful (sulpiride), *503*
Restoril (temazepam), *509*
Retinyl (maprotiline), *307*
Reval (diazepam), *139*
Revia (naltrexone), *369*
Rexer (mirtazapine), *347*
Rho-Doxepin (doxepin), *157*
RHO-Fluphenazine Decanoate (fluphenazine), *205*
Rho-Haloperidol (haloperidol), *237*
Rho-Trimine (trimipramine), *563*
Ridazine (thioridazine), *513*
Rilamir (triazolam), *553*
Rimarix (moclobemide), *353*
Riminyl (galantamine), *227*
Risolid (chlordiazepoxide), *73*
Risperdal (risperidone), *475*
risperidone, *475*
Risperin (risperidone), *475*
Rispolept (risperidone), *475*
Rispolin (risperidone), *475*
Ritalin (d,l-methylphenidate), *329*
Ritalin SR (d,l-methylphenidate), *329*
Ritaline (d,l-methylphenidate), *329*
rivastigmine, *483*
Rivatril (clonazepam), *97*
Rivotril (clonazepam), *97*
Rocam (midazolam), *337*
Rohipnol (flunitrazepam), *189*
Rohypnol (flunitrazepam), *189*
Roipnol (flunitrazepam), *189*
Romazicon (flumazenil), *185*
Ronal (flunitrazepam), *189*
Ropan (flunitrazepam), *189*
Rozerem (ramelteon), *465*
Rubifen (d,l-methylphenidate), *329*
Rulivan (nefazodone), *373*
Sanval (zolpidem), *595*
Sanzur (fluoxetine), *193*
Sapilent (trimipramine), *563*
Saroten (amitriptyline), *17*
Saroten Retard (amitriptyline), *17*
Sarotex (amitriptyline), *17*
Sartuzin (fluoxetine), *193*
Sebor (lorazepam), *295*
Securit (lorazepam), *295*
Sedacoroxen (imipramine), *247*
Sedans (chlordiazepoxide), *73*
Sedapon (lorazepam), *295*
Sedazin (lorazepam), *295*
Sedex (flunitrazepam), *189*
Sedizepan (lorazepam), *295*
Seduxen (chlordiazepoxide), *73*
Seduxen (diazepam), *139*
Seledat (selegiline), *489*
Selegam (selegiline), *489*
selegiline, *489*
Selepam (quazepam), *455*
Selepar (selegiline), *489*
Selepark (selegiline), *489*
Seletop 5 (selegiline), *489*
Selgene (selegiline), *489*
Selpar (selegiline), *489*
Sensaval (nortriptyline), *379*
Sensival (nortriptyline), *379*
Sepatrem (selegiline), *489*
Serad (sertraline), *497*
Serafem (fluoxetine), *193*
Seralgan (citalopram), *83*
Serax (oxazepam), *393*
Seren (chlordiazepoxide), *73*
Serenace (haloperidol), *237*
Serenase (haloperidol), *237*
Serenase (lorazepam), *295*
Serenase Decanoat (haloperidol), *237*
Serenase Depot (haloperidol), *237*
Serenelfi (haloperidol), *237*
Serentil (mesoridazine), *317*
Serepax (oxazepam), *393*
Seresta (oxazepam), *393*
Sereupin (paroxetine), *409*

Tensopam (diazepam), *139*
Tenso-Timelets (clonidine), *103*
Tepavil (sulpiride), *503*
Tepazepam (diazepam), *139*
Tepazepam (sulpiride), *503*
Teperin (amitriptyline), *17*
Teralithe (lithium), *277*
Tercian (cyamemazine), *119*
Terfluoperazine (perphenazine), *421*
Terflurazine (trifluoperazine), *557*
Terfluzin (trifluoperazine), *557*
Teril (carbamazepine), *67*
Texapam (temazepam), *509*
Thaden (dothiepin), *151*
thioridazine, *513*
thiothixene, *519*
Thombran (trazodone), *547*
Thorazine (chlorpromazine), *77*
Thymal (lorazepam), *295*
tiagabine, *523*
tianeptine, *529*
Timelit (lofepramine), *283*
Timonil (carbamazepine), *67*
Tingus (fluoxetine), *193*
Tirodil (thioridazine), *513*
Titus (lorazepam), *295*
Tofranil (imipramine), *247*
Tofranil pamoata (imipramine), *247*
Tofranil-PM (imipramine), *247*
Tolid (lorazepam), *295*
Tonirem (temazepam), *509*
Topamac (topiramate), *535*
Topamax (topiramate), *535*
Topimax (topiramate), *535*
topiramate, *535*
T-Pam (temazepam), *295*
Tramensan (trazodone), *547*
Trankilium (lorazepam), *295*
Trankimazin (alprazolam), *5*
Tranquase (diazepam), *139*
Tran-Quil (lorazepam), *295*
Tranquipam (lorazepam), *295*
Tranquirit (diazepam), *139*
Tranquo (oxazepam), *393*
Tranquo/Tablinen (diazepam), *139*
Transene (clorazepate), *109*
Tranxene (clorazepate), *109*
Tranxilen (clorazepate), *109*
Tranxilium (clorazepate), *109*
tranylcypromine, *541*
Tranzen (clorazepate), *109*
Travin (buspirone), *63*
Trazepam (oxazepam), *393*
trazodone, *547*
Trazolan (trazodone), *547*
Tremorex (selegiline), *489*
Trepiline (amitriptyline), *17*
Tresleen (sertraline), *497*
Trevilor (venlafaxine), *579*
Trewilor (venlafaxine), *579*
triazolam, *553*
Triazoral (triazolam), *553*
Trifluo perazin (trifluoperazine), *557*
trifluoperazine, *557*
Trilafon (perphenazine), *421*
Trilafon decanoaat (perphenazine), *421*
Trilafon dekanoat (perphenazine), *421*
Trilafon Depot (perphenazine), *421*
Trilafon enantat(e), (perphenazine), *421*
Trilafon enantato (perphenazine), *421*
Trilafon enenthaat (perphenazine), *421*
Trileptal (oxcarbazepine), *397*
Trilifan (perphenazine), *421*
Trilifan retard (perphenazine), *421*
trimipramine, *563*
Trimonil (carbamazepine), *67*
Trimonil Retard (carbamazepine), *67*
Trion (triazolam), *553*
Tripamine Surmontil (trimipramine), *563*
Triptafen (perphenazine), *421*
Triptil (protriptyline), *449*
Triptyl (amitriptyline), *17*
Triptyl Depot (amitriptyline), *17*
Trisedyl (trifluoperazine), *557*
Trittico (trazodone), *547*
Tropargal (nortriptyline), *379*
Tropium (chlordiazepoxide), *73*
Trycam (triazolam), *553*
Tryptanol (amitriptyline), *17*
Tryptine (amitriptyline), *17*
Tryptizol (amitriptyline), *17*
Tydamine (trimipramine), *563*
Tymelyt (lofepramine), *283*
Ucerax (hydroxyzine), *243*
Umbrium (diazepam), *139*
Unilan (alprazolam), *5*
Unisedil (diazepam), *139*
Unitranxene (clorazepate), *109*
U-Pan (lorazepam), *295*
Uskan (oxazepam), *393*
Valaxona (diazepam), *139*
Valclair (chlordiazepoxide), *73*
Valclair (diazepam), *139*
Valcote 250 (valproate), *569*
Valdorm (flurazepam), *211*
Valeans (alprazolam), *5*
Valinil (diazepam), *139*
Valiquid (diazepam), *139*
Valiquid o.3 (diazepam), *139*
Valirem (sulpiride), *503*
Valium (diazepam), *139*
Valocordin Diazepam (diazepam), *139*
Valparine (valproate), *569*
Valpro (valproate), *569*

valproate, *569*
valproic acid (valproate), *569*
valpromide (valproate), *569*
Valsera (flunitrazepam), *189*
Vandral (venlafaxine), *579*
varenicline, *575*
Vatran (diazepam), *139*
Venefon (imipramine), *247*
venlafaxine, *579*
venlafaxine XR, *579*
Versed (midazolam), *337*
Vertigo (sulpiride), *503*
Vesadol (haloperidol), *237*
Vesalium (haloperidol), *237*
Vesparax (hydroxyzine), *243*
Vesparax mite (hydroxyzine), *243*
Vesparax Novum (hydroxyzine), *243*
Vigiten (lorazepam), *295*
Vincosedan (diazepam), *139*
Visergil (thioridazine), *513*
Vistaril (hydroxyzine), *243*
Vivacti (protriptyline), *449*
Vival (diazepam), *139*
Vivapryl (selegiline), *489*
Vividyl (nortriptyline), *379*
Vivitrol (naltrexone), *369*
Vivol (diazepam), *139*
Vulbegal (flunitrazepam), *189*
Vulpral (valproate), *569*
Vyvanse (lisdexamfetamine), *271*
Wellbatrin (bupropion), *57*
Wellbutrin (bupropion), *57*
Wellbutrin SR (bupropion SR), *57*
Wellbutrin XL (bupropion XL), *57*
Xanax (alprazolam), *5*
Xanax XR (alprazolam XR), *5*
Xanor (alprazolam), *5*
Xepin (doxepin), *157*
Zactin (fluoxetine), *193*
Zafrionil (haloperidol), *237*
zelapon (selegiline), *489*
Zemorcon (sulpiride), *503*
Zeptol (carbamazepine), *67*
Zerenal (dothiepin), *151*
ziprasidone, *589*
Ziprexa (olanzapine), *387*
Zispin (mirtazapine), *347*
Zoleptil (zotepine), *607*
Zoloft (sertraline), *497*
zolpidem, *595*
Zonalon (doxepin), *157*
Zonegran (zonisamide), *599*
zonisamide, 599
Zopax (alprazolam), *5*
zopiclone, *603*
Zopite (zotepine), *607*
zotepine, *607*
Z-Pam (temazepam), *509*
zuclopenthixol, *613*
Zuledin (chlorpromazine), *77*
Zulex (acamprosate), *1*
Zyban (bupropion), *57*
Zymocomb (sulpiride), *503*
Zyprexa (olanzapine), *387*

Index by Use

Bold for FDA approved

Index by Class

Abbreviations

5HT	serotonin
ACH	acetylcholine
ACHE	acetylcholinesterase
ADHD	attention deficit hyperactivity disorder
ALT	alanine aminotransferase
ALPT	total serum alkaline phosphatase
AST	aspartate aminotransferase
bid	twice a day
BMI	body mass index
BuChE	butyrylcholinesterase
CMI	clomipramine
CNS	central nervous system
CYP450	cytochrome P450
De-CMI	desmethyl-clomipramine
DA	dopamine
dL	deciliter
DLB	dementia with Lewy bodies
DPNP	diabetic peripheral neuropathic pain
EEG	electroencephalogram
EKG	electrocardiogram
EPS	extrapyramidal side effects
ERT	estrogen replacement therapy
FDA	Food and Drug Administration
FSH	follicle-stimulating hormone
GAD	generalized anxiety disorder
GI	gastrointestinal
HDL	high-density lipoprotein
HMG CoA	beta-hydroxy-beta-methylglutaryl coenzyme A
HRT	hormone replacement therapy
IM	intramuscular
IV	intravenous
LDL	low-density lipoprotein
LH	luteinizing hormone
lb	pound
MAO	monoamine oxidase
MAOI	monoamine oxidase inhibitor
mCPP	*meta*-chloro-phenyl-piperazine
MDD	major depressive disorder
mg	milligram
mL	milliliter
mm Hg	millimeters of mercury

NE	norepinephrine
NMDA	*N*-methyl-D-aspartate
OCD	obsessive-compulsive disorder
ODV	*O*-desmethylvenlafaxine
PET	positron emission tomography
PK	pharmacokinetic
PMDD	premenstrual dysphoric disorder
PMS	premenstrual syndrome
PTSD	posttraumatic stress disorder
qd	once a day
qhs	once a day at bedtime
qid	four times a day
RIMA	reversible inhibitor of monoamine oxidase A
SNRI	dual serotonin and norepinephrine reuptake inhibitor
SSRI	selective serotonin reuptake inhibitor
TCA	tricyclic antidepressant
tid	three times a day
TSH	thyroid stimulating hormone

FDA Use-In-Pregnancy Ratings

Category A: Controlled studies show no risk: adequate, well-controlled studies in pregnant women have failed to demonstrate risk to the fetus

Category B: No evidence of risk in humans: either animal findings show risk, but human findings do not; or, if no adequate human studies have been performed, animal findings are negative

Category C: Risk cannot be ruled out: human studies are lacking, and animal studies are either positive for fetal risk or lacking as well. However, potential benefits may outweigh risks

Category D: Positive evidence of risk: investigational or postmarketing data show risk to the fetus. Nevertheless, potential benefits may outweigh risks

Category X: Contraindicated in pregnancy: studies in animals or humans, or investigational or postmarketing reports, have shown fetal risk that clearly outweighs any possible benefit to the patient

Being White

FINDING OUR PLACE IN A MULTIETHNIC WORLD

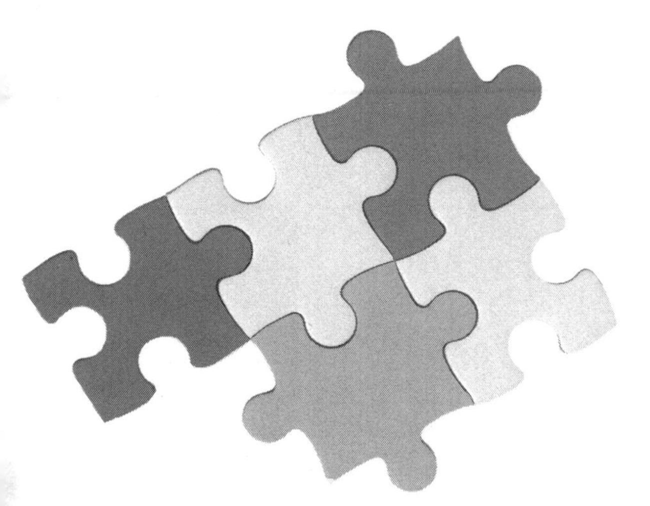

PAULA HARRIS & DOUG SCHAUPP

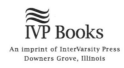

An imprint of InterVarsity Press
Downers Grove, Illinois

InterVarsity Press
P.O. Box 1400, Downers Grove, IL 60515-1426
World Wide Web: www.ivpress.com
E-mail: mail@ivpress.com

InterVarsity Press® is the book-publishing division of InterVarsity Christian Fellowship/USA®, a student movement active on campus at hundreds of universities, colleges and schools of nursing in the United States of America, and a member movement of the International Fellowship of Evangelical Students. For information about local and regional activities, write Public Relations Dept., InterVarsity Christian Fellowship/USA, 6400 Schroeder Rd., P.O. Box 7895, Madison, WI 53707-7895, or visit the IVCF website at <www.intervarsity.org>.

Design: Cindy Kiple

Cover image: Photodisc/Getty Images

ISBN-10: 0-8308-3247-5
ISBN-13: 978-0-8308-3247-7

Printed in the United States of America ∞

Library of Congress Cataloging-in-Publication Data

Harris, Paula, 1964-
Being white: finding our place in a multiethnic world/Paula Harris and Doug Schaupp.
p. cm.
Includes bibliographical references.
ISBN 0-8308-3247-5 (pbk.: alk. paper)
1. Race relations—Religious aspects—Christianity. 2. Ethnicity—Religious aspects—Christianity. I. Schaupp, Doug, 1967- II. Title.
BT734.2.H27 2004
277.3'083'08909—dc22
2004008462

P 20 19 18 17 16 15 14 13 12 11 10 9 8
Y 21 20 19 18 17 16 15 14 13 12 11

"It has been said that white people are no more conscious of white privilege than fish are conscious of water. It just is! Like fish, we swim in privilege, take it for granted and live in denial of our racial legacy. *Being White* will help the reader understand the nature of this water and its impact upon us." **GLEN KEHREIN**, *Author of* Breaking Down Walls, *Director of Circle Urban Ministries*

"Paula's and Doug's personal stories and practical illustrations challenge us without overwhelming us with unachievable ideals. The authors have presented us white folks with a wonderful resource to help us discover where we 'fit' and how we can grow in the changing ethnic context of our lives." **PAUL BORTHWICK**, *Senior Consultant, Development Associates International*

"Paula Harris and Doug Schaupp are onto something big. Their concept of displacement and how it works is worth the price of the book. I am going to highly recommend this book to all my fellow professors who are teaching any kind of course dealing with crosscultural relationships. This book is a winner. God has shaped me personally as I interacted with it." **J. ROBERT CLINTON**, *Professor of Leadership, School of World Mission, Fuller Theological Seminary*

"To be white means being trusted in a grocery store. It means getting a loan easier. It means understanding the rationale behind a school test. Doug and Paula show us how to renounce unfair advantage. To align with, advocate for and access resources for others. To follow Jesus." **MIRIAM ADENEY**, *Associate Professor of Global and Urban Ministries, Seattle Pacific University*

"This book is an important encounter for any person who wants to be a part of God's global redemptive mission. Flowing from their passionate commitment to Christ and to people different than themselves, the authors call all who would be ambassadors of Christ to live out God's passion for justice in a world defined by power allied with race or color."
PAUL MCKAUGHAN, *President, Evangelical Fellowship of Mission Agencies*

"We desperately need this book. Paula and Doug have done the improbable: they've issued a call to whites that is not only comprehensive and specific and scriptural, it is utterly full of both grace and truth. I am grateful for this book both as a missionary who will use it often on college campuses and as a white man wanting to find my place in this wonderfully multiethnic world." **DON EVERTS**, *Author of* Jesus with Dirty Feet *and* The Smell of Sin

"Paula Harris and Doug Schaupp explain that for whites, it is usually just too uncomfortable to deal with our own privilege and the entrenched prejudice of American society. But they also tell how they faced the pain of becoming an advocate for change and what God taught them through the experience. Don't let the challenge discourage you." **ALEC HILL**, *President, InterVarsity Christian Fellowship*

"I'll use *Being White* because of its honesty, thoughtfulness and practical help in equipping a generation of Euro-American leaders to take their place in pursuit of racial solidarity." **RANDY WHITE**, *IVCF National Coordinator for Urban Projects*

"In *Being White,* we are given a framework with practical steps to develop white identity in a multiethnic world. This book overflows with great insights from God's Word, highlighting Jesus' work in crosscultural relationships and ministry. Whether stumbler or seeker, may we all experience the integrated kingdom identity Harris and Schaupp enjoy, and not the white guilt-trap so many fall into." **JOHN TETER**, *Author of* Get the Word Out *and Coauthor of* Jesus & the Hip-Hop Prophets

"*Being White* provides testimony that is as challenging as it is inspiring. Paula Harris and Douglas Schaupp make themselves vulnerable in telling the stories of their struggles and of the rewards of seeing understanding grow, barriers tumble and trust building to the point that relationships are mutually enriching." **EDDIE GIBBS**, *Professor of Church Growth, School of World Mission, Fuller Theological Seminary*

"Building relationships across ethnic and cultural lines is hard work. This is a really fine book: truthful, humble, practical, authentic, challenging and, above all, biblically faithful. I couldn't put it down. And I couldn't walk away unchanged either." **STEPHEN A. HAYNER**, *Professor of Evangelism, Columbia Theological Seminary*

"Harris and Schaupp have done a superb job of integrating creatively their personal stories with scriptural truths to convey very powerful lessons. This is a practical 'how to' book which deals not only with the pain of the past and challenges of the present but also provides hope and encouragement for the future. I recommend it to all fellow travelers who are interested in following Christ's way to bring shalom into human relations in a fragmented world."
SAMUEL BARKAT, *Provost, Nyack College, Former Vice President and Director of Multiethnic Ministries, InterVarsity Christian Fellowship*

"As I read Paula and Doug's thoughtful and provocative book I discerned the presence of yet a third voice, for the very Spirit of God had begun to speak to me through their personal and deep insights. Few Christian 'issue books' integrate as beautifully and thoughtfully the contemporary with the biblical—and the tightly woven movement back and forth was seamless."
WILLIAM D. TAYLOR, *Executive Director, Missions Commission, World Evangelical Alliance*

"Not only does Doug have a brilliant mind but a profoundly spiritual heart as well. This book captures the essence of God's kingdom and his call to each of us to live 'displaced' lives."
MARK PICKERILL, *Senior Pastor, Christian Assembly Church, Los Angeles, California*

"I am delighted to see how Paula Harris and Doug Schaupp have written a book that presents the white person's journey into a multiethnic community. This book helps all people understand that every group has its own journey into another culture. It presents the perspective that God is working, for it is his heavenly vision, to deliver us from our monocultural world and mold us into multiethnic people." **DIANA E. BARRERA**, *Executive Director, Comhina*

"Doug and Paula's insightful book is a wonderful guide." **SHANE DEIKE**, *National Campus Director, Ethnic Student Ministries, Campus Crusade for Christ*

Doug to Sandy:

My journey is our journey together.

You are the best soul mate I could wish for.

Paula to the next generation:

Michal & Joshua Esealuka, Molly, Emma, Dylan & Jacob Hanson,

Cosette LiPing Eisenhauer, Liliana & Cassidy Martinez,

Mark Lee & David Lee Schaupp,

and all your companions.

Contents

STAGE 4: WHITE IDENTITY

STAGE 5: THE JUST COMMUNITY

Acknowledgments

A number of people could have written this book. Many who responded to our ideas and drafts could have authored a book of their own. Thank you to our friends who gave input when we first floated our outline. Thank you to the following readers, who gave very helpful feedback on our first draft: Bruce Alwood, Paul Borthwick, Cindy Bunch, Greg Campbell, Bobby Clinton, Pete Hammond, Lisa Harper, Rich Lamb, Jon Kubu, Jim Lundgren, Kevin Oro-Hahn, Neil Rendall, Douglas Sharp, Steve Tuttle, Randy White, George Yancey and Jeanette Yep. Though only two of us have our names on the cover, this project has been an incredible group effort.

Doug

I would not have much to say about being white if I were on this journey alone. Several amazing communities have nurtured my growth over the past ten years, and they are the reason I am able to contribute to this book. First I want to thank my InterVarsity community at UCLA. From 1995 to 1999 our community made ethnic reconciliation a top priority. My understanding of myself as a white man was transformed through all of our experiences and conversations together. Our honest yet gracious community times helped me find my place in our multiethnic setting. Our conversations were the greenhouse for my ideas in this book. To all my UCLA friends—you inspired me to go deeper.

From 2000 to 2003 I was part of a tremendous learning community focused on this arena of white ethnic development in Christ. A group of my

InterVarsity staff colleagues gathered regularly to envision and plan conferences for white college students in Greater Los Angeles. We helped each other write talks and explore biblical passages. In the process, we developed an evolving curriculum that has shaped my opinions in this book. Without this team and without these conference experiences, I would never have attempted this project. Thank you to my dear staff friends who have helped shape who I am: Tom Allen, Jon Ball, Elizabeth English, Dianna Hole, Anne Hong, Chris Rattay and Sarah Riggio, to name a few. I especially want to thank Molly Rounds, Jenny Hall, Dianna Hole and Nate Young, who were a bouncing board for my ideas and let me spend writing days with them. They gave me moral support and many excellent ideas for this book. Thank you, Nate, for seeing me all the way through this project.

God planted the seed for this book through a conversation with Bob Fryling, the publisher of InterVarsity Press. Over dinner, I asked him about several ideas I had for book topics. He threw a log on the fire when he told me that IVP was looking for someone to write on the white experience in multiethnic settings. I could only laugh out loud at the idea: "I have never dared to consider writing on that subject." But I was intrigued.

A few months later, I asked my respected colleague Paula for her input on our Greater Los Angeles curriculum for white students. Her feedback was very helpful, and that meeting was the genesis of our partnership on this important topic. About a week later she threw out the idea: "Doug, would you be interested in writing a book together?" The wheels began to spin. Thank you, Paula, for believing in me and for taking the initiative to begin this project together.

My biggest gratitude and appreciation goes to my amazing wife, Sandy. My ability to undertake such a consuming side project was completely dependent on Sandy's willingness to create space in our family life to accommodate my writing days. Sandy is by far my biggest fan in the whole world, and she encourages me to pay attention to the dreams God puts in my heart. Sandy, you are the best!

PAULA

I might not have begun this journey without my father's lifelong commitment to loving people of color and doing justice. I'm grateful to my dad, Dan Harrison. My first family gave me the best "positive white community" I have known. We walk this way together. Thank you to them, and to those who have loved us enough to join our family, especially my new husband, Dragutin Cvetkovic, who supported my passion for ethnic justice even when it turned toward writing books and understanding Gypsies.

How can I thank the many mentors who showed me the path to walk on and taught me what God had to say about race, culture and justice? Mary Fisher, Glandion Carney, Miriam Adeney, Sam Barkat and Craig Keener, your investment was significant in my journey as a white follower of Jesus. Marilyn Stewart, you tended my soul on the way.

Dear friends received me as a sister, loved and challenged me as I took risks on this journey: Dumebi Adigwe, Diana Barrera, Kim (Jacobsen) Davidson, Barney Ford, Lisa Harper, Bob Hunter, Jung-An Kim, Terry LeBlanc, Francis Omondi, Jimmy McGee, Brenda Salter McNeil, Ridley Usherwood and my "family group" who live "table fellowship" with me every week: the Bowling-Dyer family, the Hiratas, Lisa Laird and the Stephens.

Growing into a white woman who is loving, truthful and just is a stretch for me. Thank God for good partners. Doug, you have been an honest and humble writing partner. Al Hsu, you advocated for us, critiqued our work and saw this project to completion as our editor. We needed your help. Thank you.

Why This Book?

A ROAD MAP FOR THE JOURNEY

We hope you're reading this book because you want to understand what it means to be white in a racially diverse environment. Maybe your neighborhood has become integrated or a person of color* joined your department. Maybe you are asking questions about affirmative action. Maybe a professor challenged you about being white. Perhaps you go to church and look around and wonder why it's all white. Maybe you wonder why there are so many crosscultural conflicts in your campus fellowship. Maybe you have been on the journey for a while, and you are tired.

This book is written to help white people who want to figure out how to make a difference in multiethnic contexts. We'd like to give you a vision of a journey toward godly interdependence between white people and people of color.

"White" is a racial category that acknowledges our physical skin color as well as our social status. In white culture, as you may have observed, it's fairly unusual to call attention to the fact that someone is white. In this book we will use a small *w* for white because that is most comfortable. We don't want the way the word is typed to shout *WHITE* at you.

Ethnicity refers to a population or group with a common national or cul-

---

*We will mostly use the terms "people of color" and "ethnic minority" as inclusive ways to describe others of different races from ours, simply because we believe these terms are more respectful than *nonwhite*.

tural origin. Whites also are "ethnic." We can be of many ethnicities, perhaps an Italian or Polish ethnicity. This book will focus on the racial category "white" because it is broadly inclusive of different white ethnicities, and it has significance in North America. But that doesn't mean we are going to focus entirely on race. How many of us long for the day when people are judged "not by the color of their skin but by the content of their character"? We do. Dr. Martin Luther King Jr.'s profound vision has shaped us enormously:

> I have a dream that one day this nation will rise up and live out the true meaning of its creed: "We hold these truths to be self-evident: that all men are created equal." I have a dream that one day on the red hills of Georgia the sons of former slaves and the sons of former slave owners will be able to sit down together at a table of brotherhood. I have a dream that one day even the state of Mississippi, a desert state, sweltering with the heat of injustice and oppression, will be transformed into an oasis of freedom and justice. I have a dream that my four children will one day live in a nation where they will not be judged by the color of their skin but by the content of their character. I have a dream today.[1]

When we read his speech, we think, *Yes, we Americans have done a lot of that. Maybe it's not a dream anymore.* In some ways that future is here. All races can vote, and most of us are represented in Congress. Several black men have run for president, and people of color are increasingly represented at all levels of our government. We are the first legally integrated generation in American history. The Supreme Court repealed the law against interracial marriage in 1967, and the last state finally complied in 2000. Recently InterVarsity Christian Fellowship (IVCF)[2] sponsored a multiethnic training program in which the grandson of a slaveholder sat alongside the grandchildren of former slaves as brothers and sisters in Christ.

If you're a person of color reading this book, first of all, thank you for working to understand the white people around you. Second, an explanation. This book may make you mad. Maybe you'll want to throw it across the room. That's okay. Maybe you'll want to write us an e-mail setting us straight. That's okay too. We have a lot to learn. There may be multiple places where we take "the superficial view" of a situation and then try to help white people go back and see more deeply. Or perhaps we "make it seem too easy" and then go on to challenge whites to work harder.

Honestly, this book isn't written for you. There is a whole lot about race that you learned through a long journey and a community that talked about race and racism. We white people mostly start on our racial journey as adults. Generally our parents, pastors, bosses and teachers didn't or even couldn't talk to us about race, racism and interracial interaction. Most of them—and many of us even today—don't have to think about race, because the system set up around us usually runs smoothly. It's not until you show up that we realize something is not quite right, and often we blame the messenger. So we really need to start at the beginning, with milk, before we are ready for the meat you see at the table of cultural diversity.

We pray that we whites will learn to "rid [ourselves], therefore, of all malice, and all guile, insincerity, envy, and all slander. Like newborn infants, [let us] long for the pure, spiritual milk, so that by it [we] may grow into salvation—if indeed [we] have tasted that the Lord is good" (1 Pet 2:1-3).

Doug's Story

This book is an expression of our life journeys, so you will get to know Paula and me through these pages. I was born in San Francisco in a multiethnic urban context (Chinatown), but my family moved to an upper-middle-class suburb, where I spent fourth through twelfth grade in a majority white context. In May 1986, during my first year at Occidental College, I experienced a spiritual revolution and became a follower of Jesus.

During my college years I received a great biblical foundation through InterVarsity, including a compelling picture of God's multiethnic kingdom. After the 1992 Los Angeles riots, God led me through a transformation from being a person of tolerance to being a man of conviction in this multiethnic arena. My wife and I served in an African American church for a few years, and then we led a small Korean American congregation for a few more years. From 1989 to 1999 I worked with IVCF at UCLA. I now serve as a regional director, supervising the work of InterVarsity in Southern California.

Paula and I will both write in the first person in our respective chapters. You will come to recognize our voices as you read. Hopefully you will enjoy the variety of our two styles. One of the joys of collaborating with Paula on this project has been the profound sense of unity we have experienced. We speak in unison in this book, though our voices and stories are different.

We welcome you to join us on this journey of being white in a multiethnic world. I doubt if there are any experts on this journey; we have never met any. We see ourselves as two white people on a lifelong journey, and both of us are very aware that we have much yet to learn and much room for growth.

And while we are exploring this journey from a Christian perspective, we welcome everyone from all perspectives to join the discussion, and we hope you find something helpful in this book.[3] If you are spiritually unconvinced, here are a few pointers to enhance your reading experience. We have included a fair amount of discussion of the Bible in these pages. You can either skim those parts or get a Bible and follow along. In case you are wondering, our Christian frame of reference presupposes a few basics:

1. We humans are spiritual beings, and we need spiritual solutions to the messiness of life.
2. We are broken people, and we need repeated infusions of the life of God into our souls.
3. We are followers of Jesus, and we find our life in God through Jesus.
4. The Bible is our guidebook, our inspiration, and our way of understanding the invisible Creator and all creation.

Paula's Story

My journey started when the civil rights movement was changing America. I was born in Dallas, Texas, the year after President Kennedy was shot. I was four when Dr. King was murdered.

My family was profoundly shaped by this era. My parents intentionally taught us to be colorblind, to ignore skin color and look for common traits of humanity. My sisters and I had friends from all races. We had a sort of unspoken family rule: you can talk about what people do and say, but not their physical appearance. As missionaries in Papua New Guinea my parents pursued justice for people of color, at some cost to themselves. As a working missionary mother of four daughters—three in diapers—my mother agreed not to have a household servant, so that we didn't learn to associate class differences with race. My father integrated the missionary schools where he worked, inviting indigenous black children to study alongside white missionary children. He worked hard to integrate the pool of missionaries in the organization, initiating both personal and structural changes, including partnering with black New Guineans and African Americans.

Today, my family is remarkably diverse. In my immediate family are African, Chinese, Hispanic, multiracial Native American and white children. Learning to be colorblind, to judge by character and not by color, was a good *beginning* for my sisters and me to this journey into a multicultural future.

Like Doug, I can remember when God transformed me from a "colorblind" woman who befriended people of color to one having real convictions based on what Scripture teaches about justice and shalom. Many people mentored me, and the InterVarsity community has shaped me in this journey. Translating those convictions into practical steps is still challenging. After studying the missionary growth of the Antioch church in the book of Acts, I recruited multiethnic missions teams of staff and students out of conviction that loving one another across cultural boundaries honors God and gives testimony to the power of the gospel. I looked for elders/mentors and peers in each of the communities to become better equipped to lead ethnically diverse American students to minister as missionaries in Europe.

During those years I fell in love with an African graduate student. Shortly after we married, he became verbally and physically abusive, but I was convinced that I could figure out how to make the marriage work. I tried everything I knew—counseling, prayer from Christian leaders, help from his family—but nothing changed. On one level, I thought divorce was wrong. And on another, I was too proud to admit I had been wrong about this relationship. We had two wonderful children together, and I feared that as a white woman, I couldn't raise them well in their biracial, bicultural identity.

After five years, though, my husband became so violent that I feared for our safety, and we fled. The courts protected us with restraining orders, and he was convicted on several counts of domestic abuse.

When I decided to continue on the journey of reconciliation after my experience of marriage and divorce, there was no turning back. God is still showing me how I can walk a straight path between recklessness (not enough caution) and fearfulness (too much caution). I pray that my journey in understanding my own fears about race is helpful to others. Not everyone has an abusive spouse of another race, but for many of us, unaddressed fears lead to failure to connect deeply with people of color.

A Lifelong Journey

This book is neither academic nor theoretical. We are not race scholars, and we won't write abstractly about racial issues for white people. We are both thirty-something people on the journey. We stand on the shoulders of those who paved the way since the '60s, and yet we connect with the postmodern generation. We want to see changed hearts and a changed society. We hope sharing our souls and our personal journeys gives you an idea of what commitments and stages can equip whites to move forward in a healthy interracial journey. A lot of us whites *begin* this journey. We hope more of us can continue it when it gets hard.

"All men are created equal" is written in the Declaration of Independence, as Dr. King observed. But the truth is that the law *meant* "all [white] men [with property] are created equal." At that time white men without property were counted in the census and paid taxes but could not vote. The "Three-fifths Compromise," article 1, section 2 of the U.S. Constitution, determined that a black man would be counted as three-fifths of a white man for determining the Southern states' representation in Congress, but he could not vote. And the rest of us—Asian, Hispanic, Native American men and all women—had no legal rights and could not vote. Married women of all races were not legally persons but the property of their husbands.[4]

Consider the InterVarsity training program we mentioned, where the white grandson of a slave owner sat alongside the grandsons and granddaughters of slaves. This happened, yes, but it was training for whites and blacks, managers and staff who needed help in intercultural communication. Every white person in the room was a manager, supervising black staff. Is America an "oasis of freedom and justice"? Do we judge each other by color or by character? Well, if truth is told, some of both.

Stages on a Journey

We want to help you on your journey as a white person by telling you our stories, by asking questions of Scripture, and by pointing out steps we whites can take toward healthy communities and identities. We think the journey of a white person into multiethnic community has five basic stages.

Encounter usually begins when we first meet a person of color. Most often encounter happens because the nonwhite person has left her comfort zone and has chosen to enter a white context through displacement and to function in our white culture. The key task for us whites to move beyond this stage is choosing to enter into a relationship with a person of color.

Some whites begin the multiethnic journey because they have been personally convicted of wrong through study of interracial history or current events. They may repent and may make an intellectual commitment to racial justice without ever encountering a person of color. A white journey that lasts, though, probably needs to engage the heart as well as the mind, and this is done through loving another person.

When we begin a relationship with a person of color, we enter *friendship*. We learn to listen to his experiences, to see his individuality, to trust and love him as a person. We also learn to repent of particular sins against our friend, especially if he helps us by telling us where we've gone wrong.

Friendship will teach us a lot, and it will help us open our heart. But it won't change society, and it won't correct racism.[5] It may leave us still not understanding how racism functions on a structural level.

To go beyond the friendship stage, the white person chooses to put herself in a context where people of color are dominant in number and culture and whites are in the minority. We call this *displacement*. Maybe she joins an Asian-led campus fellowship; maybe he goes to live and work on a reservation. Maybe a family moves into a neighborhood and school district that are mostly nonwhite. In this stage, the white person can learn to see whites and people of color in groups. He starts to see our respective racial and cultural systems and how they truly function. The key work in displacement is learning to submit and becoming a student of nonwhite cultures. The white person learns the other culture—celebrations, conflict-resolution styles and so on—and begins having productive, healthy conflict. He learns history through books and people's stories. It is a profoundly stretching stage of the white journey. Toward the end he has a healthy place in the nonwhite community and owes a deep debt of gratitude to his teachers.

The active crosscultural growth process a white person experiences in displacement causes her to reconsider her white *identity* in foundational ways. Some psychologists have described this stage as "disintegration" of the identity, as the former identity is questioned and a new identity begins to be formed. In other words, the white person who formerly had an unquestioned white identity, seeing herself as "normal," begins to realize through displacement that white and nonwhite identities are very different, that our experiences are different. The white person begins to form a new white identity, strong enough to face the truth about white history and current reality, and positive enough to experience godly redemption of herself and other white people.

Finally the white person can begin to learn how to become a structural advocate and ally of people of color. Through displacement he has learned to identify his own power and privilege; through identity he has learned to confess his sin and believe God is redeeming him. Now as he begins to use privilege, to spend power on behalf of others, he can become a member of a *just community.* This is a wonderful stage of a positive white identity, freedom from shame, quickness to repent from guilt, and true interdependence between whites and people of color.

This journey is not only a linear model of developmental stages white people go through but also a cyclical model in which we find ourselves at various parts of our life. We can always begin. A few years ago a small group of Native American leaders and pastors attended the Urbana Student Mission Convention.[6] My (Paula's) ministry with InterVarsity is to direct programming for Urbana. I invited these Native American guests out of a naive desire to "integrate" the convention properly, as well as, I trust, a godly desire to remove obstacles so that students of every culture can have a part in what God is doing in crosscultural missions. Two of these leaders befriended me, praying for me, telling me their stories, correcting me and inviting me to Native events where I could learn about their cultures—ah, they have two *different* tribes, two *different* cultures.

So I found myself at the very beginning again, *encountering* Native American people (thanks to their open hearts); developing *friendships* and praying that I would learn well and graciously; *displacing* myself into their worlds and putting myself under their authority and the authority of other Native leaders there; reflecting on the questions these experiences pose for my own *identity* as a white person and as a missionary (missionaries have not brought only good to Native American peoples: they have stolen children from Native families and cooperated with those who wreaked violence); and seeking ways we can each use our power and graciously receive the gifts we bring to each other as we build a *just community* together.

As part of our own growth in Jesus, it is our joy to designate all of our proceeds from the sale of this book for Native American ministry. Money you spent on this book that would ordinarily have gone to authors' royalties is instead being put into a fund for Native American leadership development. Thank you for joining us in investing in Native Americans whom you and we may never meet.

STAGE ONE: **ENCOUNTER**

1

Stumbling into Encounter

Doug Schaupp

In 1986 I went on a road trip with my best friends from high school to spend a week sleeping on the beach in Ensenada, Mexico. The first day in Mexico we woke up to the reality that we weren't in the United States any longer. We went grocery shopping in a local market, and Mat was assigned the task of finding milk. Unable, he asked the stranger next to him for help. As he struggled for the right words, he remembered that the Spanish word for "milk" is spelled *l-e-c-h-e*. He made eye contact with a grandmother, gestured with his hands and asked, "Lesh?"

She looked back at him, puzzled. After a moment her eyes lit up. She pointed down the street: "Bocker-eye."

Now Mat was stumped. He repeated to himself those two odd words until the light bulb went on: "Bakery!" He smiled at her, and we soon were successful in finding our *leche* at the bakery down the street.

This interaction in the store was an encounter moment for all of us. Encounter is coming into contact with a person or situation in a way that makes us feel our differences, where our rules for interaction do not fit and we feel out of our element. Seldom do we plan for encounter. Instead, encounters find us, and we suddenly find ourselves a little out of control.

Chances are that you have had your own encounters. They might be humorous, like searching for milk in Ensenada, or they might be serious and painful. In some parts of the world, cross-ethnic encounters are a normal part of daily life. In other parts of the world, encounter moments are more rare, coming through movies, books or music. When was the last time you remember having an interracial encounter?

3-D Glasses Please

I recently went to a 3-D movie with my wife and two sons. It was the first time in about ten years that I put on those funny-looking 3-D glasses. Even though I knew what to expect, I was again surprised at what a different viewing experience it is to have the movie characters jump up in my face. I wasn't the only one who was surprised. About ten minutes into the movie, my five-year-old was ready to leave. This wasn't the kind of movie experience he wanted to have—too real and too in his face.

For a white person it can be tempting to view the world through a 2-D lens. To make my world more safe and simple, I can consciously or unconsciously remove ethnic, cultural and racial realities from my view of life. I may try to avoid encounter moments because they can be uncomfortable. I may really dislike 3-D jump-up-in-my-face surprises.

We white people have the choice to walk through life with either 3-D or 2-D lenses on, either seeing the world with all its dynamic layers or reducing the world to a simple 2-D format. One of the things I have been working on is to study Scripture while asking, "What are the crosscultural dynamics in this book of the Bible?" As I ask that question, my vision slowly expands from 2-D to 3-D, and unexpected movements jump out at me. It is a delightful thing to see the world and Scripture through the 3-D lens they both require.

We have all had moments where we realize how different we are from someone else. Your story is different from Paula's and mine, but we've all had experiences in the cross-ethnic journey of life. Otherwise I doubt you would have picked up this book.

Stumbler or Seeker?

Jesus tells stories about different types of encounter experiences (see Mt

13:44-46). In one he talks about a guy who happens to be in a field, going about his own business, when he suddenly stumbles over something. On close inspection, he discovers that the thing that has tripped him up is a treasure chest holding riches beyond his wildest imagination. He dashes home to liquidate all his resources and buy the land. He is supremely happy with his accidental discovery. He is our prototype of an unintentional awakening to the excellence of Jesus and his kingdom.

Next we get the story of a collector of fine gems. He loves precious jewels and is on the lookout for the best in the world. When he comes upon a supreme jewel, he gladly hocks his entire collection of gems in order to get this one. He has been hoping for just such a perfect object all his life, and when he sees it, he knows this is what he was made for.

Jesus begins both of these stories by saying "The kingdom of heaven is like . . ." These two parables are excellent for describing the varied ways you and I come to fall in love with Jesus.[1] I also find them helpful for how we come to discover and cherish particular facets of Jesus' kingdom. Sometimes we search intentionally and find what we're looking for, but other times we are not looking at all and yet our eyes are suddenly opened.

Paula and I represent these two distinct paths of discovery. As you will see, Paula has been more of a pearl expert and I have been a stumbler. Paula grew up knowing the value and beauty of crosscultural living. She has long known that this is a key priority of God's, and she has grown steadily in these convictions. I, on the other hand, did not seek out this part of the kingdom of God. Instead God repeatedly nudged me to stumble over it, until I finally woke up and became a proactive seeker.

I stumbled into college. My first day at school was a bit of a shock. Lugging my bags, I found my dorm room and looked at the two names on the door. There was my name, but then there was another name that I could not pronounce. *Encounter!* My stomach tightened slightly.

As it turned out, I really enjoyed being roommates with Khalil Kareem. But if I had had a choice in the matter prior to meeting him, I probably would not have intentionally selected an African American roommate. I stumbled into this experience, and God used it to help stir an awakening in my life.

My stumbling continued. A few months later I joined a thriving InterVarsity chapter that highly valued ethnic reconciliation and the biblical texts about God's heart for all people. This emphasis was not something I was seeking as a freshman. But God knew I needed it, and he guided me to trip over it.

My senior year, I fell in love with Sandy, with whom I co-led a small group Bible study. At the time I had no idea what a profound blessing her Korean American identity would be to me. I had simply stumbled into this cross-ethnic relationship. But during the ensuing years of marriage, Sandy and I have intentionally worked through layer after layer of crosscultural issues in our relationship. God has worked dramatically through Sandy to repeatedly open my eyes and regularly redirect my path. When Sandy and I got married, I did not anticipate how much God would work through her to profoundly shape my life.

The good news is that God is not picky. He will engage with you and me whether we are proactive or reactive about living out his priorities. Have you been a stumbler or a seeker regarding this part of God's heart?

The Book of Acts as Our Lesson Book

God is an expert in the art of nudging people like you and me into encounter moments. How do you help a group of people open their hearts and lives to those who are ethnically different? Let's look at God's work in the first church and learn how God likes to move. The book of Acts is a fabulous book for observing God's values and how he guides his people to grow in these values.

In Acts 1:8 Jesus reiterates the vision he has for his people: "You will be my witnesses in Jerusalem, in all Judea and Samaria, and to the ends of the earth." Opening their hearts to encounter people of other ethnic groups and countries is going to be a normal part of their future. Jesus' kingdom is for everyone, and as the leaders of this Jesus movement, the disciples need to proactively go out of their way for all kinds of people. He wants this vision to be on their mind as they lead his community of followers. It is to be central to their priorities. They will need 3-D glasses to fulfill their mandate.

In Acts 2 Jesus brings his disciples into a profound encounter moment.

An amazingly diverse gathering of Jews "from every nation under heaven" (2:5) is together for a Jewish festival in Jerusalem. God picks this moment to pour out his Spirit so that his Jerusalem community would carry this international flavor. By this genius move, God leads his people to stumble into becoming a community of encounter. The community is off to a brilliant beginning. There is sharing of all their resources, great joy in being together and people wanting to join their community daily (2:43-47; 4:32-37).

Luke's narrative indicates that there are no noteworthy conflicts in the launching of this community. In chapter 2 Luke is very explicit about the community's cultural makeup, making sure we get the point of its diversity. But then Luke is silent on crosscultural issues until chapter 6. Given his silence for three chapters, we could be tempted to assume that cultural and ethnic problems had been magically solved in the Jerusalem community, as if we can "all just get along" if we break some bread together. Since the church leaders have their hands full with the challenges of evangelistic growth on one hand and persecution and deception on the other, it seems that crosscultural dynamics have moved to the back burner for them; 2-D glasses are an easy default mode.

The next encounter moment comes in chapter 6. This time the encounter emerges within the community and does not involve outsiders. The apostles, whom Luke describes as superb leaders throughout the first five chapters of Acts, get surprised by an internal glitch. In chapter 2 the church members spontaneously developed the habit of selling their goods and sharing with those in need (2:45), an activity that did not appear to involve any structured distribution system. But by chapter 4 there is clearly a system in place: "They laid [their gift] at the apostles' feet, and it was distributed to each as any had need" (4:35). By this point the apostles have taken leadership over this very sensitive ministry of receiving large sums of money and distributing resources to the poor of the community; they are responsible to ensure that distribution is fair and just. In a community like theirs, you must use 3-D glasses to discern and anticipate the impact of crosscultural realities.

Unfortunately, the apostles are caught off-guard. "The Hellenists complained against the Hebrews because their widows were being neglected in the daily distribution of food" (6:1). A division arises in the community because cultural outsiders (Hellenists were foreign-born Jews) are being systematically neglected by the insiders (Hebrews were those born in Israel). This is not a one-time mistake but a clear trend over time. Notice that it is not the widows complaining but rather the entire Hellenist population of the church. Is their complaint legitimate?

One confusing dynamic in interpreting chapter 6 is that no one set out to hurt the Hellenists. We could easily attribute the problem to the sheer size of this church community and conclude that it was just an inevitable byproduct of rapid growth. However, Luke's meticulous narrative style forces us to look carefully at each word that he does and does not include in his account. In the wider Jerusalem society, how were Hellenists treated? As second-class citizens. And in the Christian community? Unfortunately, as second-class citizens. Luke makes the point that in this way the community of God resembled the surrounding world. While the community operated by a distinct set of kingdom priorities in all other areas, the leaders did not anticipate how the racism of the Hebrew majority would bias their church in regard to distribution of resources.

After the community gathers and resolves the crisis, Luke tells us that their solution of opening leadership to highly qualified Hellenists is excellent: "What they said pleased the whole community. . . . The word of God continued to spread" (6:5, 7). Because of this solution, it might be tempting to ignore the leadership failure prior to the groundswell of grumbling: the Jewish leaders got caught reverting to 2-D glasses. Their inadequate lenses blinded them to something they could have anticipated if they were looking at their community through the 3-D lenses Jesus had taught them to wear. Luke shows us that once again the apostles are stumblers.

As they open up leadership to qualified Hellenists, God does a whole new work of growth and initiative through these empowered "outsiders." God raises up Stephen as a powerful voice in Jerusalem (6:8—7:60) and works through Philip to help the Jerusalem community stretch to include Samaritans in its vision (8:5-40). Through the persecution of Stephen, God nudges the church to remember its calling back in Acts 1. The Jerusalem church was focused on strengthening ministry in its own backyard. If God had not nudged them through the persecution, would they have ever gotten around to fulfilling the call to love others who weren't like them?

What Does Encounter Feel Like?

There is irony in many encounter moments: what is an encounter for me may be very different for the person I am encountering. I stumbled over this reality in 1992. In the early 1990s, our InterVarsity chapter at UCLA was about half white students and half Asian American students, with a sprinkling of others. God brought us a courageous African American student, Andrea, who became our worship leader during her junior year.

Before inviting Andrea to lead the worship team, our staff team approached this question from a self-focused bent: "How would she as an African American change the flavor of our worship?" To us it felt like a significant step to invite Andrea to become our first black student leader. After praying, we sensed it was the right step for us to take. At the time, I unknowingly had 2-D glasses firmly in place, so it never occurred to me to look at what we were asking Andrea to go through.

Having Andrea as a public leader in our community was an encounter experience for many of us. She did bring a different style and perspective on ministry. It was good for us to stretch, to begin to see things through her eyes. She would occasionally critique dynamics in our community. She had a direct communication style that I was not used to. I was glad for how she was challenging us, but it also made things more complicated. God was slowly expanding our world.

How did I feel about this encounter experience? How did I feel about our stretching to include Andrea as a worship leader? I am embarrassed to admit it, but I was secretly proud of us. I was pleased at how this demonstrated our openness to all kinds of people. Though I would not have admitted it at the time, part of me viewed Andrea as a badge of honor, a sign of how progressive we were. At the time I thought we were far along in the journey of ethnic reconciliation, but in retrospect we were just beginning. Her presence was my proof that we were open to "Hellenists."

The irony in this story comes from looking at the exact same situation through the eyes of Andrea. For us, her leadership was an encounter experience. But just to take part in our community, Andrea was suffering a massive displacement (more on displacement in section three of this book). Andrea had attended InterVarsity meetings occasionally her first year of college, but our group felt strange to her in comparison to her African American church at home. She told me, "Church for me was formal. We were trained to see church as God's house, and you carried yourself with a reverence for God. But InterVarsity was so casual. I remember one time I went to a small group Bible study meeting and someone showed up wearing pajamas. I was shocked."

Unfortunately, with my 2-D glasses on, I did not see what she was experiencing, and I did not go out of my way to know or welcome her. Instead of making her transition smoother, I was clueless to her struggle. So she was not initially able to commit to this alienating community.

In addition to others who invested in Andrea, my wife, Sandy, poured herself into Andrea's life, getting to know her perspective on the world. Andrea knew that Sandy cared about her, and Sandy became a safe person for her. The ways she trusted Sandy and a few others allowed her to increase her trust of the rest of us in InterVarsity, though we were still very different from her home church.

Andrea accepted our invitation to lead worship, but her experience of it and mine were opposite. "I was honored to lead worship," she said, "yet it felt like I was being asked to 'lead the show but don't mess with it. Be a black face up here, but lead it just like we do.'" Though in our eyes we were empowering her to be a leader, Andrea did not sense freedom to shape our community life and our style of worship. It was a difficult season in Andrea's life, as she often felt misunderstood, hurt or treated like a token black person by the rest of us.

I focused on how we were stretching to include Andrea in leadership. I was aware of the impact of this dynamic encounter on the majority of InterVarsity student members, who had never had a close black friend. Because I was focused on my encounter dynamics, I was slow to see that Andrea might be feeling something more intense. I needed 3-D glasses to see the complexity of ethnic dynamics, but I kept wearing my 2-D glasses. I did not want to see how much harder it was on her than on the rest of us.

The good news is that ten years later, Andrea continues to be an important friend to Sandy and me. In fact, Andrea invited Sandy to be an attendant in her wedding party. Andrea has developed into a powerful leader in her own right, and she is free to be the African American woman of God that God made her to be. Praise God that he works in spite of my narrow perspective, and he works to open my eyes.

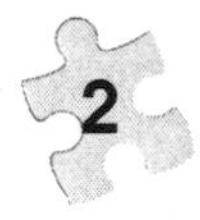
2

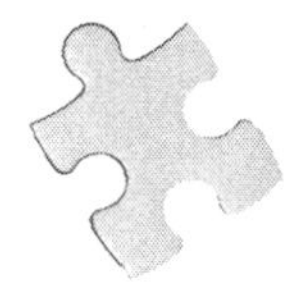

Giving Your Heart Away

Paula Harris

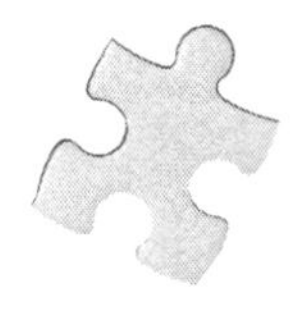

When God sends us crosscultural encounters with people of color, all we have to do is respond. God commands us to be people of encounter. Scripture teaches us to become people who learn to embrace those who are different from us.

When God first chose a unique people for covenant making, he gave their founder, Abram, some very interesting instructions. God told him, "Go from your country and your kindred and your father's house to the land that I will show you" (Gen 12:1). Abram, whom God later renamed Abraham, must have wondered, *Where is that place—"the land that I will show you"?* What was clear was that Abram and his wife Sarai had to go, had to leave their familiar people, their familiar place, and follow God, listen to God's directions to discern the final destination. God's covenantal promise was also clear. If Abram went, if he obeyed, God would bless him, God would make him a nation, God would make his name great, "so that [he would] be a blessing" (Gen 12:2-3).

How were this man and his wife different from others who followed God in the ancient Near East? Genesis 12, which tells the story of Abram's call, doesn't explain why God called him. When we meet him, we don't know anything about Abram except his genealogy. In Hebrews 11 we get the key to the mystery: he was a man of faith and obeyed God. "By faith Abraham obeyed . . . and he set out. . . . By faith he stayed for a time in the land. . . . By faith he received power of procreation" (Heb 11:8-9, 11).

Back in the subsequent chapters of Genesis we can read the details of Abraham and Sarah's journey. God didn't lead them directly to Canaan/Palestine, if we read the story geographically. Both Genesis and Hebrews admit that Abraham and Sarah never reached the physical destination. The point was not the camping trip or the destination. God was leading them on an inner journey of obedience as well as an outer journey to encounter a series of different peoples. Why was crosscultural encounter an intrinsic part of their journey with God? God had promised to bless Abraham so that he would be a blessing. Genesis 12—25 shows God leading Abraham and Sarah through encounters with different nations. God used crosscultural encounter and displacement to grow their faith and obedience as they wandered through the desert.

Jesus too found cultural encounter a necessary part of his journey in ministry. In his inaugural sermon in Luke 4, where he announced to his hometown (and now to us) what would be the shape and result of his ministry, Jesus was intentionally crosscultural. After the reading, Jesus pointed out: "The truth is, there were many widows in Israel in the time of Elijah . . . and there was a severe famine over all the land; yet Elijah was sent to none of them except to a widow at Zarephath in Sidon. There were also many lepers in Israel in the time of the prophet Elisha, and none of them was cleansed except Naaman the Syrian" (Lk 4:25-27). In other words, the good news of God is not simply for the Jews. Jesus seems to be pointing out an intentional model of God's people reaching out to others across cultural boundaries. Jesus also modeled what he preached. He had encounters with everyone from Roman soldiers to Gentile women.

The account of Jesus' encounter with the Samaritan woman (Jn 4) says that Jesus *needed to* go through Samaria on his way to Jerusalem. "He had to" go that way, my translation says. Well, yes, geographically that was true. But Jews in that time frequently went long distances out of their way in terms of the map to stay in familiar territory in terms of the people around. It would be like taking the beltline freeway around a city instead of the direct route through the ghetto. Scripture says it was necessary. Jesus *had to* go that way. Why?

In Luke 10 Jesus makes his point clear about this. A lawyer "stood up to test Jesus," asking, "What must I do to inherit eternal life?" Read the scriptural law, Jesus responded; what does it say? I can hear him teasing: You're the lawyer, what's the answer?

So the lawyer responded, quoting Deuteronomy and Leviticus: Love God, love my neighbor. Then he posed a lawyer's technical question: "Who is my neighbor?"

Jesus responded with the powerful story of the good Samaritan. Who was the man the good Samaritan saved? Everybody else in the story was a Jew. The priest: a Jew. The Levite: a Jew. The original place on the journey: a Jewish city. The destination: a Jewish city. So the victim of the robbers must have been a Jew.

This is a crosscultural encounter. A minority person who is willing to love across cultural boundaries is Jesus' model of faithfulness. Jesus is using a Samaritan loving a Jew as a model of how to get saved.

The question posed when a minority person reaches out to us is, can we love back? Can we respond with welcome and kindness? But Jesus challenges us to a higher standard. Can *we* reach out? Can we find it necessary to go through the ghetto? Can we take a loving minority person, a good Samaritan, as a model?

A few years ago I was at a missionary meeting in Brazil. One evening I joined a Kenyan missionary for dinner. As we began getting to know one another, I started to realize that he was ordering his food in Portuguese.[1] He knew the waitress's name. He taught me how to order my drink, so I got the lemon-lime soda I hoped for instead of lemonade. He helped me tell the waitress my room number in Portuguese, so I could charge my meal.

I asked him, "When did you learn Portuguese? Have you been a missionary in Brazil or Portugal?"

"No," he laughed merrily. "I came here the same day you did."

After I got over being embarrassed, I realized he'd taught me a valuable lesson about good encounters. My Kenyan friend was learning Portuguese by developing relationships with people. Today he is a dear friend and brother to me.

Crosscultural professor Betty Sue Brewster writes about forming new crosscultural relationships. When we enter a new, foreign culture, we "are bombarded by a multitude of new sensations, sights, sounds, and smells, . . . [and we] are able to respond to these new experiences and even enjoy them." At this critical point of beginning, she says, we are "ready to bond—to become a belonger with those to whom [we] are called to be good news. *The timing is critical.* Imprinting occurs at the critical time. Bonding best occurs when the participants are uniquely ready for the experience."[2] If we bond in our crosscultural encounters, if we form a warm, affectionate beginning to our friendship and start by curiously enjoying our differences, we have far less culture shock later on.

But some of us miss the critical time for bonding. Is it still possible later? Of course it is. Developing a relationship in which we belong to people and they belong to us is natural to human beings.

As white people in North America, most of us don't have a chance to start "at the beginning" like missionaries. We have a lot of history in our culture, everything is familiar, and we have expectations that people in our milieu will relate in certain ways and things will function in certain ways. In order to step out into a multiethnic encounter, I need to take a risk. In some ways I'm starting over to create multiethnic relationships. The best place to start is with my own heart and my immediate circumstances. What ethnic minority people are around me, and how can I get to know them as individuals? If a person does things differently from my way, how can I gently ask, "Would you explain this to me?" How can I treat a minority woman as an honored sister in Christ? What can I do to get to know her as a person, an individual?

Similarly, in what ways am I already drawn to ethnic minority cultures? Has God given me a real joy in something that is not from my own culture? It doesn't have to be something profound or difficult. Maybe it's a particular kind of food or music.

If I love reggae music, I could follow that trail. I could begin by really listening to the lyrics, trying to figure out their context. What is "I and I"? Who was Emperor Selassie? Is "the Lion of Judah" from the Bible? I could find a local band and start going to its concerts, preferably ones in tiny venues. At the concerts, out of my context, I need to look around: Are there other fans who reach out to me? Is there a family member or friend of the band selling CDs? It's not hard to start a conversation with someone if I already love the music; I'll be full of questions about the lyrics, the band history, reggae music in general.

After connecting with people, it's important that I keep going back, keep on enjoying the music and the people. One day I'll figure out that reggae music has spiritual bridges as well; it grew out of the Rastafarian religion and poor black Jamaicans' need for justice (they have a very similar history to our own, with slavery and its aftermath). Because I love the music, it doesn't feel too hard to keep going back. Before I realize it, I love the people too.

All I have to do is *go*. Go outside where I usually go. Just talk to somebody—anybody. Be friendly. Ask questions. Become a learner. See them as a unique person. Care about them and what's happening in their life.

A few years ago I went out to lunch with an out-of-town mentor. He is Pakistani, so I chose my favorite Indian buffet, because I love the food and wondered what he would think of it. I figured it might resemble his home cuisine. We were chatting about our families and our work. When the waiter came, my friend started asking him about *his* family and his restaurant. He obviously knew the guy. He knew his wife's name. I realized that my friend had been there before—a lot.

Later, when I asked him about it, I learned that every time he came to Madison, he had lunch at this restaurant. He had chosen it so he could befriend the waiter and proprietor. Soon enough he had learned about their families, the ups and downs of the business, even what was going on back home in India. (India and Pakistan are not friends, as countries go.) My mentor was acting like Jesus. Following him, I learned it's not that hard to choose a favorite ethnic restaurant and get to know the owner.

When I was in graduate school, I enjoyed hanging out sometimes with an African American woman in my fellowship. I really wanted a deeper friendship with Kim but had no idea how to build it or ask for it. How do you go past superficial encounters? Finally I decided to ask her to do something big with me. We talked about it and decided to lead a year-long Bible study together. We decided to study Acts, a crosscultural book. We recruited a diverse group of people for our study.

I think, in retrospect, that when I asked her if she'd lead the study with me, I was really asking her, will you be my friend? Will you commit yourself to a longer-term relationship with me? She did. Pretty soon I knew about her department in the university and some of the struggles of African American students on our campus. I knew about her family, her mother. Later we decided to be roommates. That initial invitation had been the hardest one.

Two things happen every time we develop a crosscultural relationship. The first is that sooner or later we make a mistake. We are fallen, so we sin. But also, in a cultural situation that is new to us, we just can't predict what might happen next. We don't really understand things yet. We don't know why things happen in a certain way. We feel a bit out of control. These are natural parts of culture shock, and they are why we need a friend of that culture to guide us and tell us what's next.

One time I was having dinner with some Middle Eastern friends. My hosts were secular people from Lebanon. I had been to Rana and Ahmed's place several times for dinner; we usually ate together between 10:00 p.m. and midnight. This evening there were other guests, a Palestinian man, some men from Lebanon and some others I couldn't place.

As usual, Rana and I laughed and talked and cooked for hours. We joked with the other guests. When it came time to eat, Rana served the men first, at one corner of the small apartment, and then brought her plate and mine to another corner. *Okay,* I thought, *I'll just follow her lead and eat over here.* But it bothered me. *Why were we eating separately?* I couldn't pay good attention to her. So finally I asked her, "Why are we eating over here? Is it because you have men guests tonight? Are you separating the men and women?"

She looked at me strangely. "No, Paula."

"Then why?" I persisted.

"Because you are American and you eat with a spoon. They want to eat with their hands, and they don't want you to look down on them."

I had made a few mistakes in this situation. I was judgmental about why dinner was so late. It took me a lot of dinners to realize that half the point was the time hanging out in the kitchen first. If dinner were earlier, when would my friend and I get so many hours to talk and laugh? Also, I wasn't brave enough to eat with my hands, if I could eat in the familiar (clean) way using silverware. What was the big deal? There was a sink to wash in afterward. Now it reminds me of art class, being given permission to use fingerpaints instead of a ballpoint pen.

Although it was good that I asked Rana for clarification instead of just assuming, I really didn't ask my question very well. I might have said simply, "Why are we eating differently tonight?" Instead I assumed that these Middle Eastern people must practice strict gender separation—which is often true but wasn't in this situation.

In spite of my mistakes, I persisted, and Rana could see I liked her. I just kept going back to her place and inviting her to mine. I apologized when I made mistakes. When I saw from her face that something wasn't quite right, I asked, "Did I do something to offend you?" But mostly we just hung out and had a good time.

The second thing that happens sooner or later is that we judge people too quickly. As Christians, we know that God is both loving and holy and that we are called to both love people and challenge their sin. This truth is clear throughout Scripture. At the same time, in a crosscultural situation we cannot fully understand what is going on. We must slow down and become learners to truly understand what they do, why they do it and the cultural dynamics behind the behavior.

As I mentioned earlier, I am just beginning to learn about Native American cultures. I am very slowly learning to build friendships. Early on in my encounter with Native American Christian leader Terry LeBlanc, I told him the story of a dream. I had dreamed about some Pacific Island-type sculptures that came to life and frightened me. Recounting my dream, I called the sculptures demonic. Terry responded very gently, "Why do you call them that, Paula? What made you think they were demons?"

It took me several years to absorb the depths of his challenge to me. I had not judged the dream images out of spiritual discernment. I called them demonic because they frightened me. When I was a very small girl, I had attended ceremonies of Papua New Guinean tribes, and the traditional art, fierce costumes and loud drumming had been frightening. As I reflected now on Terry's challenge, I realized that my judgment had come out of fear, not godliness.

Since then I have learned something of how my judgment fits in a broader context of encounters between Native and white people. I have read the history of white missionaries trying to reach out to Native Americans. I have met Native Americans and heard stories of those who were taken from their families by white Christians, put in boarding schools and told not to speak their language or live out their cultural traditions. To my shame, I have learned how often other white people before me have called Native art, music and dance "demonic," how we have suppressed it and told Native Americans that God cannot be worshiped with their cultural traditions. As if Jesus were a white American who spoke English.

Of course Terry knew all this. I was the ignorant one, blundering into the painful place where he and his people had been repeatedly wounded. It is only in retrospect that I realize the depth of his kindness to me with that gentle question. He had reason to judge me, not the other way around. Thank God I answered his question with silence, thinking, *I don't know.*

I've told stories about making mistakes in multiethnic encounters because it happens and that's one way we learn. I have some treasured friendships that developed from the encounters I've described. The lessons and the love made the mistakes worthwhile.

We are not unique in our mistakes. Scripture shows Peter, the rock on whom Christ built the church, making crosscultural mistakes. Sometimes I think "the rock" nickname just meant Peter was hardheaded. In Acts, the Holy Spirit repeatedly corrects Peter's cultural and theological ethnocentrism. Peter was not the apostle to the Gentiles, but God left him no choice but to include them. Struggling but obeying God, Peter goes to Cornelius, a Gentile who is described as "an upright and God-fearing man . . . well spoken of by the whole Jewish nation" (Acts 10:22). But Peter starts with a crosscultural mistake, insulting Cornelius: You know I'm not supposed to associate with you or visit you. But God showed me . . . (see Acts 10:28-29).

Somehow Cornelius forgave Peter, perceived that God was working in him and waited for what he had to offer. Jesus also forgave Peter, seeing his persistence and obedience. The great news is that people of color will often forgive us when we take risks and make mistakes as we follow Jesus. No beginner does things perfectly.

Whether we look at Abraham and Sarah, at Jesus' first sermon in Luke 4 or at his last instruction in Matthew 28, God's message is clear. We are to reach across cultural boundaries to love and bless one another.

Making Encounter Real

We all come to God's multiethnic table in different ways and at different paces. God welcomes you to his table just as you are. God knows who you are and what you can handle. God knows where you feel excited and where you feel intimidated.

Share your heart in prayer as you read this book. How do you feel thinking about this subject and reading this book thus far? Each of us has a unique ethnic journey. God has put key experiences in your life to prepare you to be a person who loves who you are in Christ and who loves those who are different from yourself. Here are some questions for your reflection and for discussion.

1. What has your journey been like? Can you identify a few "light bulb" moments from your past: when you first became aware of race, when you first encountered persons from a different racial/ethnic/cultural context or when you learned to care about another people group? Do you have a story of bonding with another culture? Did you seek that out, or did you stumble upon that experience?
2. How did your family raise you? What are a few positive memories of making friends with people of color?
3. When did you first learn to use "3-D glasses" when reading the Bible? What questions do you ask as you study sections of Scripture in order to grasp the ethnic and cultural elements?
4. How might you take a next step with a cultural group or friend? What cultures are you drawn to? Who has God put in your life?
5. Paula recounted a few examples of being persistent in learning even though she made some mistakes. Mistakes are an inherent part of the journey in our multiethnic world. What mistakes have you made in a multiethnic encounter? Ask God to give you the courage to step through your fears and awkwardness and keep trying.

One of the most important things for you to work on as you finish section one is honesty with yourself, with God and with others. If you cannot be honest in identifying your fears and your questions, your growth will be severely stunted.

Doug recently taught a seminar on a college campus that is about three-quarters white students. In anticipation of the seminar, called "Being White in a Multiethnic World," I asked participants to honestly fill out an anonymous survey about what prevents them from crossing ethnic lines. Here are some of their very honest feelings and questions. What can you relate to here?

"Where do you feel inhibited in extending yourself in love to those of other ethnicities?"

1. I don't know how to put myself in the other people's shoes. I have no convenient social connections with people of other races.
2. I fear feeling misunderstood. I fear being seen as a racist.
3. I do not want to offend. I feel ignorant. I am intimidated.
4. I am hurt.
5. I feel guilty, embarrassed and ashamed.
6. I feel apathetic.
7. I feel isolated and alone.
8. I feel frustrated.
9. I already feel reconciled.

The second question on the survey was "What are your questions?"

1. What are the right questions to ask people of a different race? How do I start?
2. How can I get people of different ethnicities to open up to me? How do I avoid hurting people?
3. How do we solve the problem of people not feeling comfortable in a mostly white setting?
4. How do I deal with my guilt?
5. Does race matter to God? What defines race?

What are your own questions? What are you feeling about extending yourself across ethnic lines? Share these with a friend or two. Bring them to God in prayer.

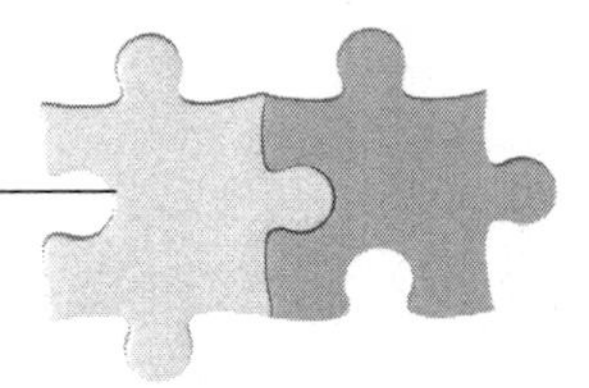

3

Making and Keeping Friendships with People of Color

Paula Harris

My daughter took a bus to school. At the bus stop every day there were two white parents and two black parents, a white boy, a black boy, a black girl and my daughter, who is biracial. Parents and kids chatted about various things—except for one of the black mothers, who stood conspicuously aside. She would smoothly greet the other black mother and then keep to herself while the rest of us parents talked with each other and all the children. She wore her sunglasses like armor. She stood in a cool pose, and her fierceness was tangible. This went on for months.

I started to pray for this woman. Every day I kept trying to make eye contact, say hello and nod at her in greeting. Black women have deep-rooted cultural reasons for not liking white women like me who have biracial kids. I wasn't sure of her perspective; I was figuring out how to respect her boundaries by keeping a polite distance.

One day, this woman, who had never greeted me, never smiled or relaxed in my presence, came over to me and said, "You should try Copa in your daughter's hair." She proceeded to explain how it would help, what it would do and, implicitly, how I could care better for my daughter. I responded politely and talked with her for a short while about hair.

The next day our sons were playing together outside and wandered into my house. I asked the neighbor's son, "Does your mom know where you are?" before letting him stay, and he ran home to tell her. "Mom" turned up on my doorstep, a different person. She was warm, friendly, smiling, talkative.

Since that day, every time we see each other we say hello, and most times we talk—about our lives, struggles with our jobs, our kids, the school, our spiritual journey, you name it. She's helped me watch my pets when I travel. I've helped her with rides and small loans. We keep an eye on each other's kids when they're playing, and we know when they need to be home. Kadisha has become my friend. Not a close friend yet; we don't have a lot of things in common. But we're parents and neighbors, and we like each other.

Miroslav Volf's complex and profound book about reconciliation, *Exclusion and Embrace,* describes how relationships are built between two people of unequal power in a society. He talks about four stages of an embrace.

First, opening the arms, "a sign that I have created space in myself for the other . . . and that I have made a movement out of myself so as to enter the space created by the other."[1] Opening the arms is an invitation. With a morning greeting, a polite hello instead of small talk, I entered the "distant" space Kadisha created.

Next, waiting: "the self has 'postponed' desire and halted at the boundary of the other."[2] I wanted this black woman to be friendly to me, first out of my own racial awkwardness, and later as I learned to see and care for her. But I waited, respecting her boundary. It was up to her whether to accept my quiet daily invitation.

Third, "closing the arms" is the gesture of reciprocity, a mutual embrace in which we both gently hold and are held by the other person. One day she responded and helped me with advice about my daughter's hair. One day I helped her by letting her decide whether her son could play inside my house.

Fourth, opening the arms again: an embrace does not make the two of us one. Our otherness and separate identity remain. But we can begin again, with a new invitation another day.[3]

Wisely, Volf says friendship is like an embrace. Hugs are great, if you love the person hugging you. I have a white friend, Becky, who stops by my desk almost every day to give me a hug. I feel loved and appreciated. Ever so briefly I share her burdens and make them lighter. Her friendship is a gift, as are all friendships. Gifts are wonderful to receive, if you trust the person giving. My friend Becky is a frequent gift giver, the kind of generous person who doesn't wait for your birthday. She notices my likes and dislikes. She gives me beautiful gifts I might not have bought for myself. She listens to me. I feel her love for me, and she tells me the truth. I trust and love Becky.

But if I were afraid, if I had reason to doubt the giver, gifts would be bittersweet and perhaps not welcome at all. If Becky had hurt me, or if her family had hurt my family, or if she lied by saying one thing and doing another, perhaps I would be slower to trust her. Perhaps receiving her embraces and her gifts would be painful for me instead of a pleasure that reinforces our friendship. Perhaps I would need her to wait with her invitations.

Barriers to Embracing

Often in crosscultural situations we have internal and external barriers to internally embracing others. They may be dramatic ones. They may be visible to us. Or they may be invisible to us but profoundly visible to others.

About fifteen years ago I had a traumatic experience with a Chinese man. It left me feeling violated and without personal power. In spite of this, I continued to walk the reconciliation path and take steps of commitment to racial reconciliation because I believe it is what God requires of Christians.

Years later, the Lord suddenly surrounded me with Asian men as ministry partners. I was assigned to a difficult task force with a sympathetic Japanese American man. We supported one another. God gave me a Pakistani man as a mentor. I submitted to him but also spoke the truth to him. A Korean man took a key job on my team. I began to pray that God would help me trust these men and be a good partner to them. Still, I walked into each relationship having all sorts of assumptions about them.

Let me take the Korean. I assumed he wouldn't be able to submit to me as a woman leader. I assumed he would have difficulties working interdependently with the others serving on the teams I led. It took time for me to realize I had this particular man so deeply in a "Korean man" box that I could not see him. It took time to acknowledge my own fears before the

Lord and allow the Holy Spirit to work in and through them. How could I feel any affection for him if I couldn't really see him?

But through God's grace, I was able to bring him my concerns, directly and indirectly. I learned that he was a real servant of his wife and honored her in tangible and intangible ways. I learned he was a patient father, generous with his time and love. I learned that he had a far deeper understanding of interdependence than mine. I learned how he respected me as a leader and how graciously he submitted to my direction. I began to know him and appreciate him. The Holy Spirit began to replace my fears with love, patience, joy and self-control in our interactions.

Sometimes when we reach out across racial boundaries, it puts us outside our own group. A few years ago I worked in an office alongside about a hundred other Christian brothers and sisters. It was a place deeply stuck in racial "encounter," and as a group, we had difficulty developing an interdependent web of relationships. Later an ethnic minority woman told me she spent six months working in our office and I was one of five people who spoke to her the entire time.

What she didn't know was that I was terrified of her. She had a very impressive name and demeanor. She wore a "militant" hairstyle and clothing. She projected authority and personal power. Now I don't remember why we began speaking, and I certainly don't think I did anything special to initiate the relationship. Every time I saw her, I was nervous that she wouldn't remember me *(among all these white people, why should she recognize me?)* or that I would say something offensive *(she has such a clear perspective)* or that I wouldn't understand her. All I did was persist, keep saying hello, keep asking her how her day was, exploring her family and the meaning of her name, her hair, the cultural history of her clothes, the direction of her ministry—fairly superficial questions, but growing deeper. Maybe some of them even offended her.

At first I experienced the interaction with her as "I + the minority woman." Years later, I learned that she experienced the interaction as "these one hundred white people + me + the five who see me." It was shocking to me when she explained what it was like for her. I learned that her fierce pose was because she too was afraid of us white folks.

Now I have to ask myself, *Am I going to be part of a vast similar (white) group? Or am I going to step out, face my fears and get to know a person? Can I open my arms and heart? Can I invite people of color into relationship with me?*

Letting God Heal Your Fears

Ephesians calls this pain of broken relationships between cultural groups "the dividing wall, . . . the hostility between us," and says it is only through Christ that the wall can be knocked down (Eph 2:14-16). If there isn't a wall of pain or hostility, is the wall apathy? Christ's love destroys apathy too. Doug and I define racial reconciliation as *Jesus' power through the cross restoring relationships between the races—replacing relationships characterized by divisions, partiality and the unjust use of human power with a new community based on God's love, healing, justice and shalom.*

Crosscultural relationships are challenging at times, but they are built on the same things that same-culture friendships are built on: love, kindness, doing fun things together (joy), telling the truth, finding ways the other person likes to be appreciated (generosity), faithfulness. Sound familiar? Many of these characteristics are the fruit of the Spirit, gifts God gives us when the Holy Spirit lives in us (Gal 5:22-23). When the cross takes down the walls, the Holy Spirit can fill us with love and begin to build godly relationships on a foundation of justice and well-being for everyone.

One way to face your deepest fears is an exercise a racially experienced white man taught me. Neil used to live in New York. Every day he walked past ethnic minority people who were poor and needy. To conquer his fear, he learned a simple exercise. When he felt afraid to face people who were different than him, he simply prayed, *This is a child of God.* Over and over again: *This one too, this person Jesus died for. This is a child of God. How can I hate this person? God loves him. How can I fear this person? God treasures her.* Now Neil is a deeply compassionate person.

I can relate to this. My church is in the urban center of the city where I live. We have several ministries to the poor. We run a homeless shelter and a food pantry. Women and children come and go from the food pantry, but often there is a group of black and white men hanging around the church in the morning when they leave the shelter. They may call out everything from loud pickup lines to obscenities. When I first started attending the church,

I was really afraid to walk with my kids past this crowd of men. I needed Neil's exercise, but I had no idea.

My little family usually sat in the back of the sanctuary because my children were young, wiggly and noisy. In our church, every week after the sermon we confess our sins to the Lord, receive absolution from the pastor and turn to speak peace to one another. After repenting, we say, "The peace of the Lord be with you." Then we can join together in Communion.

One Sunday two of the homeless men came inside the church. Soon I found myself speaking peace to them. In the following weeks I often found myself reflecting: *Am I at peace with them? How I can I speak God's peace to them inside the church if I act scared when I walk past them outside?*

Because of their initiative to enter my church, God convicted me of my fearful heart. Gradually, over a period of several years, I was able to listen to God's urging and begin to let God change me. First, I lifted my head as I walked past the crowd of men. I began to look them in the eyes. I began to see each person. I began to greet them. These days, sometimes we will stop and chat. Some days a person will ask me for lunch money or for a prayer. I find it a privilege to give these small gifts. Since God changed my heart, I have never again been cursed by these men. None are friends yet, but I am no longer their enemy.

As I allow God to minister to my heart, to open my arms and wait, I learn the path of friendly love with people who are not like me. I can take steps toward friendship. I can look around myself, asking, *Who is inviting me? Who has entered my context? Am I a member of a white crowd in certain places?* When I can identify those places, I can choose to act differently. I can start becoming a friend to people of color.

There are more difficult questions, though: *Where are the places where I am an enemy to people of color? What are the fears and hatreds that cause me to be an enemy? How can I allow God to transform my fears and hatred into love?*

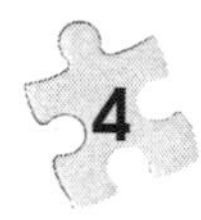

4

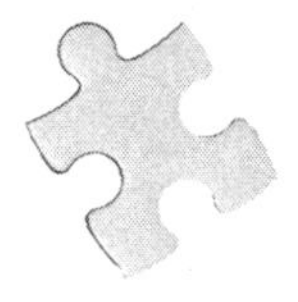

Going Deeper in Crosscultural Friendships

CONFLICT RESOLUTION STRENGTHENS THE BOND

Doug Schaupp

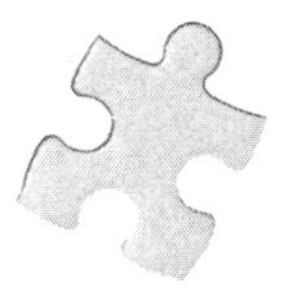

When I was in elementary school, my parents tried to teach my siblings and me how to express our feelings and work through our problems with each other. They created the "I don't like it" rule. When my brother or sister did something that made me angry, I was not allowed to yell or hit them. Instead I had to say, "I don't like it." And they magically had to stop.

I used this rule to my advantage, creating a personal force field that allowed me to walk through the house free from all sibling harassment. But despite my mastering this rule, I actually grew up lacking real skills in interpersonal conflict resolution. I subconsciously created a list of rules about conflict that shaped my friendships and interactions.

- ***True friends don't make waves.*** I wrongly believed that the best friendships are the ones where you just get along and there aren't any fights.
- ***Conflict is a sign that your friendship is flawed.*** I thought that avoiding conflict is a sign of relational strength. If there is a problem, the right thing to do is to just overlook it.
- ***Conflict weakens the bonds of trust in a friendship, so don't engage in it.*** You'll be sorry if you raise an issue with a friend and they never forgive you for it.

- ***Friendships naturally grow apart.*** I wanted friendships to stay close, but I did not know what to do when I drifted away from people.

As you can imagine, when I entered into discussions about race, these false assumptions about conflict multiplied the problems. I wanted calm waters, and when there were awkward issues and disagreements in my cross-ethnic friendships, I emotionally retreated.

How about for you? What were the rules for resolving conflict in your home?

In college I joined a Bible study group in InterVarsity Christian Fellowship. As we dug into passages of Scripture, I slowly realized that a number of my habits and values were out of sync with God's—including my fear of conflict.

Both Paula and I have been profoundly shaped by God through the book of Ruth. The story of Ruth begins with a struggling family who find themselves forced into a cross-ethnic situation. They are Jews, but because of a famine in their country they live in Moab, strangers in a strange land. To make matters worse, the father of the family dies. Now it is just Naomi and her two sons. These two Jewish men decide to marry Moabite women, Orpah and Ruth. Thus Naomi becomes the head of an international, cross-cultural household.

The five of them make the best of the situation for the next ten years, but then yet another crisis strikes: the two sons also die. All this in the first five verses of the book of Ruth!

What would you do if you were Naomi? She is alone with her two daughters-in-law who don't share her nationality, her culture or her religion. She decides to try her luck back in Israel, but she believes that Israel will not hold anything for her Moabite daughters-in-law. So she insists that they stay with their Moabite people and allow her to journey to Israel alone.

At first Ruth and Orpah resist her and declare their allegiance to her: "No, we will return with you to your people" (Ruth 1:10). But Naomi will have none of it. She repeats her command for them to stay with their people.

They are at an impasse, a moment of crisis. Orpah does the expected thing when she kisses her mother-in-law goodbye and returns to her people (1:14).

I have come to realize that such moments of crisis are an inherent part of cross-ethnic friendships. I don't like them, but I have come to terms with the fact that they are just part of the journey. In fact, I would even go so far as to say that you can't measure the strength of a cross-ethnic friendship BI, Before Impasse, only PI, Post Impasse. In a cross-ethnic friendship it is hard to know what you are both made of until you hit a serious difference or conflict. An impasse becomes a relational "gut check," exposing who you really are.

When Ruth and Naomi hit their impasse, Ruth's character is revealed. Instead of going along with the will of her mother-in-law, she gathers the strength to disagree and stand her ground. "But Ruth said, 'Do not press me to leave you or to turn back from following you! Where you go, I will go; where you lodge, I will lodge; your people shall be my people, and your God my God. Where you die, I will die—there will I be buried'" (1:16-17).

The stalemate is an opportunity for Ruth to show her deep loyalty and devotion across ethnic lines. As Ruth chooses to do good conflict with her mother-in-law, she in essence chooses to preserve the relationship. If she backs off, she loses Naomi.

How does Naomi receive the challenge? She is very impressed by Ruth's determination and has a change of heart, agreeing to bring her to Israel. The rest of the book of Ruth is about the amazing fruit that this decision bears for Ruth and Naomi. Because of how Ruth handles the conflict, their relationship Post Impasse is much more beautiful than Before Impasse.[1]

If Ruth had been afraid of pressing through her mother-in-law's intensity, we would probably have no reason to remember her. It is because Ruth chose well and entered into deeper commitment that she is honored in the Bible as a role model for us.

In chapter one I mentioned that my first year in college I had a roommate named Khalil. Things were going along well for the two of us as roommates until one day he shocked me. I came home from class and he was packing his stuff. He explained, "I'm moving in with my buddy down the hall. Don't worry, this doesn't have anything to do with you, Doug."

Though I was confused, I responded as Orpah did: I just resigned myself, taking him at his word and letting him go. Instead I should have gathered courage and used the crisis to probe and go deeper with Khalil and see if there were problems to resolve.

Jesus picks up this theme with surprising intensity in Matthew 18:15-20. To avoid any confusion about the centrality of working through relational impasses, Jesus gives us a blunt, step-by-step approach to right relationships. What do we do when we first realize there is a rift in a relationship? Do we talk to other friends and complain about how we were hurt? No, Jesus calls us to first go directly to the person who offended us. He does not allow us the option of merely letting the relationship drift (which was my natural mode while growing up). "If another member of the church sins against you, go and point out the fault when the two of you are alone" (Mt 18:15). Can you find any loopholes in this command?

When was the last time you were hurt by someone? Jesus' call is for you to get up the courage to go and talk it through with that person. I find that scary.[2]

As you probably know, some conflicts do not resolve nicely, and we need outside help to finish working it out. Never fear, Jesus has thought about that too. "But if you are not listened to, take one or two others along with you, so that every word may be confirmed by the evidence of two or three witnesses" (Mt 18:16). In our individualistic Western culture it seldom occurs to us to make this second step of reconciliation a priority. But mediating conflict is not only a good idea, it is commanded by Jesus.

As you and I extend ourselves in love across ethnic lines, we should expect to need to invite in a mediator to help straighten out tensions. During my years of working at cross-ethnic friendships, I have both needed the help of a mediator and played the role of mediator to repair relationships. Not only is the use of a mediator biblical, but in some cultures the use of a mediator to facilitate reconciliation is a mainstream practice. We need to understand, accept and adopt this practice whenever it's appropriate.

How do these passages speak to us as white people? As followers of Jesus, we must allow God to replace our subconscious rules about conflict resolution with his kingdom guidelines. Paula and I could write an entire book on white people and conflict resolution, but here we will merely touch on a few key points.

- ***Conflict resolution is not optional for Christians.*** Working through conflict is a normal part of life and healthy friendships in the kingdom of God.
- ***Conflict is about suffering with others and enduring in love, not about winning the argument.*** The goal is to "win back" our brother or sister as the end of Matthew 18:15 says, not to "be right." Beware of the natural tendency to become defensive. Instead we must trust God to defend us and heal our relationship.
- ***Each person in a conflict has a paradigm for how conflict is supposed to work, and we need to be aware of our biases.*** Each must identify both what we learned about conflict growing up and what our current mental model is for how disagreements should be resolved.
- ***Good conflict shows that you care enough to hang in there through glitches and more serious obstacles.*** While it is easier to just give up on a person, working through conflict can be a powerful expression of love and commitment. You and I have a choice each time we hit an impasse.
- ***There is a key difference between constructive conflict and harmful conflict.*** Harmful conflict tears people down with hurtful comments. In the name of honesty, it is tempting to unload: "You drive me crazy when you do that. Stop it!" A question is wiser than an accusation: "What was going on for you?" Then we can listen carefully to the other person and discern the issues that are under the surface for both of us.

Each culture has its own expectations of and approaches to the healthy resolving of interpersonal conflict. In fact, this may be one of the areas where the world's various cultures differ the most. Each of us is responsible to identify how we saw conflict handled in our family, in our community and in the media, because what we have seen is often what we will reproduce in our friendships.

So how do we white Americans handle conflict resolution? While there are some white people I know who are conflict-oriented, most white folks I have met are not very good at resolving interpersonal conflict. I am differentiating between the very specific act of resolving interpersonal conflict versus the more general white American trait of being direct, honest and sometimes blunt. Let me use my family as an illustration.

My parents encouraged quality conversation around the dinner table by creating a rule: during dinner each member of the family had to share one thing she or he had learned during the day. As I would go through the day, I would try to find something at school or in the newspaper to bring up during dinner to stimulate a discussion. Most days some disagreement would arise, and there would be a bit of banter around the table, bordering on a good-natured argument. In our family, intimacy often took the form of sharing our ideas, opinions and convictions. During dinner we almost never talked on a more personal level about how we were feeling. Because my family was rather direct in discussing ideas and convictions, I developed the misperception that we were good at resolving interpersonal conflict. The truth of the matter is that it wasn't until college that I learned what the Bible has to say about relational conflict. In the context of Christian community I began to focus on listening, sharing, forgiving and asking forgiveness.

In 1988 seven of us spent the summer in England studying, learning and extending ourselves in love to international students who had come to study in Oxford. This was my second summer mission experience, so I viewed myself as already knowing how to be a team player. But one person on our team started to drive me crazy. Sometimes during meals Susan would reach over to my plate, grab one of my french fries ("chips" in England) and proceed with dinner as if nothing had just transpired. Where was "May I have one?" or "Do you mind?"

One morning I was in the kitchen preparing food at the counter. Susan needed something on the other side of me. Without saying a word, she reached across me to get it. That was the last straw! I blurted, "Susan, you can't keep violating my personal space any time you feel like it."

There in the kitchen we listened to each other and talked things through. She explained that in Korean culture, a sign of comfort and friendship is to treat one another like family, and family members understand each other and look out for one another. There's no need for such formalities as "Excuse me" or "May I try some of your food?" In her Korean way, Susan was treating me like family and paying me the compliment of being relaxed in my presence, eating off my plate and reaching around me.

As she explained, I learned about my own subconscious set of rules. It dawned on me, *Wow, we white people are very dependent on verbal cues for interactions.*

That summer Susan and I resolved that conflict and others like it, and our friendship was the deeper for it. In fact, recently Susan wrote me a fabulous thirty-fifth birthday card, listing thirty-five things she appreciates about me. I am deeply grateful that instead of being offended by Susan and pulling back in my heart, we pressed through the conflict and pressed deeper into one another's lives. Today we reap the reward of real friendship based on truth and reconciliation.

Here are four key lessons I've learned from friends like Susan.

Listening to understand. When you sense misunderstanding or pain in a friendship, ask Jesus to give you the strength to apply his word in Matthew 18. Go to your friend, hoping not only to be understood but to understand him. When I enter into reconciliation conversations with a mindset of listening, I put my defensiveness aside and focus on "gaining back the brother or sister." After I have listened, I will sometimes summarize what he shared: "This is what I heard you saying. Did I hear you accurately?"

The hard work of listening helps us really connect, versus being offended by misunderstandings. This kind of listening is a form of suffering, because I am not in control when I put myself at my friend's feet in this way.

Sharing my perspective. It is not enough to listen. I need to also share how I was feeling and what I was trying to communicate. Because this is a natural weak area for me, I often take time to reflect beforehand in my journal. I write down what I value about this friendship and why it is worth entering into a reconciliation conversation. I write a list of my fears and pain, and I make note of ways I would be tempted to just unload on my friend.

I need to share my feelings honestly with my friend, without unloading. After I share, I need to be open to hearing that my perspective on him or my perspective on the problem is not accurate. Part of humility is to let my friend shape how I view him instead of just making up my mind about him on my own.

Asking forgiveness. In addition to clearing up misperceptions about one another, reconciliation includes both asking for and offering forgiveness.

When I hear that I have hurt someone else, I throw up a quick silent prayer, "God, please show me where I sinned in this. Help me to listen and repent."

There is an important difference between apologizing and asking forgiveness. To apologize is to say, "I am sorry that you got hurt," whereas asking forgiveness is saying, "I sinned against you. Please forgive me." Wherever possible, I choose to go the extra distance to ask forgiveness and not merely apologize. This is a concrete way that God teaches me humility. To ask forgiveness means I have to swallow my pride once again.

Offering forgiveness. When someone else asks for my forgiveness or apologizes to me, my natural response is to say, "That's okay." I have to resist this phrase because sin is not okay. Therefore I try to say, "I do forgive you, and I let it go in the name of Jesus."

Sometimes forgiving is easy, and sometimes it is very difficult. When it is tough, I ask to pray first. In prayer I can ask Jesus to give me the strength to do that which I cannot do in my own strength. In prayer I can ask God to show me a picture of my brother or sister in the Father's arms, and then it is easier to forgive.

To work through reconciliation effectively is to significantly strengthen the bond of your friendship. In fact, while resolving conflict may feel very scary to you, it may ironically be the first time that your nonwhite friend actually feels free to be real with you. The more you bond and connect, the more you care about things she cares about.

Friendship is the door to love and to giving our heart away. Once we give our heart, we are compelled to take action on things that otherwise don't move us. When a nonwhite friend shares her pain with us, it is no longer a conceptual issue to debate with her, but rather a friend to suffer with.

Making Friendship Real

Close friendships are one of the best vehicles for personal transformation that God offers us. As we give our heart to our friends and open our life fully to them, we are influenced and changed by them. For the rest of our life, we will be transformed inasmuch as we are giving our heart in love to others. Friendships are the refining fire of life, and we never "graduate" beyond needing them.

There are many excellent books you can read on forming friendships across ethnic lines. I (Doug) have been indelibly shaped by *More Than Equals* and *Breaking Down Walls.* I (Paula) have been shaped by *My First White Friend* and the crosscultural novels of Gish Jen, Amy Tan, Barbara Kingsolver, Sandra Cisneros and Ursula Hegi. Because of the vast resources available, we have chosen to offer only a few nudges for your journey.

If you have followed the flow of this book so far, you have had encounter experiences. You have hopefully responded with an eager and persistent learner's posture. Now it is fitting to go deeper with a few friends. Who are some people God has put in your life in whom you could invest more deeply? Ask God to increase your awareness of the ethnic minority acquaintances you could reach out to. Ask him for courage to go deeper with them.

1. Paula shared about being intimidated by the mother at the bus stop. Could you relate to what she was feeling? Are there ethnic minority people in your workplace or school who intimidate you? The normal response is to freeze up and pull away from people who arouse those feelings. What could it look like for you to persist in taking initiative with an intimidating person?
2. How do you feel about making a Ruth-like commitment to another person and their people? "Your people will be my people." What would it take for God to get you to this place of commitment and loyalty?
3. How do you feel about resolving conflict in your relationships? Do you avoid conflict? How did your family express hurt and come to reconciliation? What are the positive things your family taught you about reconciliation? What are the liabilities that you have to unlearn? What list of rules about conflict guides your behavior?
4. Have you ever asked a trusted friend or leader to help mediate a conflict you were having with another person? How did it go? How do you feel about trying a mediator the next time there is pain or damage in a friendship?

5

What Does the Bible Say About Displacement?

Doug Schaupp

How do we understand the process of growing from people who stumble into encounter moments into people who choose intentionally to enter displacement? Let's pick up where we left off with our overview of the book of Acts, because in Acts God leads his people into a similar growth transition.

All along God has intended to lead his people into crosscultural displacement for the sake of the gospel. In fact, this displacement component of the kingdom is such an indispensable part of Jesus' agenda that he puts the call front and center in several of his most pivotal vision statements: "Go therefore and make disciples of all nations" (Mt 28:19), and "You will be my witnesses in Jerusalem, in all Judea and Samaria, and to the ends of the earth" (Acts 1:8). Jesus makes it clear that to be his follower is to follow him into crosscultural displacement and love.

God's Shove

God creates his Jerusalem community to be an international community, which sets the stage for the irony I mentioned in chapter one. For the Hebrew followers of Jesus, the presence of their Hellenist sisters and brothers forces them into encounter, and God stretches them. On the flip side, the Hellenists are in an unavoidable displacement experience, which intensifies the pain when their widows are repeatedly neglected. Yet God had brought both the Hebrews and the Hellenists into this crosscultural community through an ambush of his Spirit (Acts 2), not through any carefully considered game plan of theirs. God was the overtly active agent to ensure that this international gathering bonded and forged a successful community so that through them he could demonstrate his amazing international heart for all to see.

While God was pleased to launch his church with a shove in the right direction, he soon switches modes by insisting that his people live up to the vision he has laid out for them, where we become Spirit-filled, proactive, crosscultural agents. God's intention is that stepping out in crosscultural love becomes a normal part of life for us Jesus followers, instead of a surprise phenomenon in Acts 2 moments. Therefore as Acts unfolds, God becomes increasingly blunt in calling us to displace ourselves. He guides his people through a paradigm shift, from being stumblers to becoming proactive seekers of godly displacement. What might have initially seemed optional becomes increasingly mandatory and mainstream in the community of obedient people who bear Jesus' name.

Most scholars agree that chapter 10 marks a profound turning point in the book of Acts. God does not merely remind Peter of the big picture he had laid out nine chapters earlier in Acts 1:8. Instead he makes it personal. Through a vision, God rebukes Peter three times, reopening a wound from when Peter denied Jesus three times, which effectively catches Peter's attention in the most poignant way imaginable. Why does God take such extreme steps in Acts 10? If Peter and his team in Jerusalem were basically on the right path of obedience, such a sharp rebuke would not be necessary. But time has run out for Peter and the Jerusalem leaders to make room in their busy schedules to extend themselves in love to the Gentiles. God is determined to get the church's attention, so he targets the "top dog" and shakes him to the core.

Though Jesus had clearly told Peter of his agenda to lead his disciples to the ends of the earth, Peter had not intentionally displaced himself for the sake of the gospel. Though Peter had repeatedly been exposed to and was aware of

God's heart for Gentiles, his lifestyle and leadership did not reflect that conviction.[1] To Peter's credit, in the events of chapters 10 and 11 he embraces God's rebuke and submits to discipleship and repentance on the way to becoming friends with a Gentile, Cornelius the centurion. As Peter puts on his 3-D glasses, he becomes proactive about taking the lead back in Jerusalem to help his community also embrace God's work among Gentiles (Acts 11:1-18). From this we can take hope that even though we, like Peter, will shrink back from stretching across ethnic lines, God will continue to nudge us along.

The Pivotal Transition: Becoming Proactive

After the Jerusalem leaders embrace this theological paradigm shift (Acts 11:18), Luke leaves us wondering who will be the ones to live out this vision and displace themselves for the sake of Jesus' gospel. Will it be Peter? Other apostles?

Luke proceeds with his narrative in a most unexpected way. He gives us a macro view of what was happening to those God had scattered from the Jerusalem church through persecution, forcing them out of their comfort zones. This is where we pick up the story in 11:19: "Now those who were scattered because of the persecution that took place over Stephen traveled as far as Phoenicia, Cyprus, and Antioch." How would these members of the Jerusalem church behave now that they were traveling to new cities? Would they recall the Acts 1:8 vision and displace themselves across ethnic and cultural lines? Or would they prefer to stick to their own, clinging to what was known and comfortable? Luke answers that question: "They spoke the word to no one except Jews" (11:19). Unfortunately, these followers of Jesus emulate what they had seen back in the Jerusalem community. They keep the gospel to themselves, avoiding displacement.

But these cautious disciples don't have the final word. God has a grassroots revolution planned among some daring followers of Jesus. "But among them were some men of Cyprus and Cyrene who, on coming to Antioch, spoke to the Greeks[2] also, proclaiming the Lord Jesus" (11:20). In stark contrast to those who avoid crossing cultural lines in their evangelism, these nameless heroes from Cyprus and Cyrene try something they have never seen done before.[3]

Is this daring evangelism a flash in the pan or something more? Let's look at God's response: "The hand of the Lord was with them, and a great number became believers and turned to the Lord" (11:21). God loves the courage of these disciples who follow his original Acts 1:8 plan and intentionally displace themselves by embracing Gentiles.

It is not the Jerusalem leaders who have the courage to pioneer a new model of church life but rather some anonymous rookies. Sometimes it is up to people who don't know better to take Jesus at his word and live out his priorities. All along Jesus intended for intentional displacement to be a mainstream priority for his disciples, but we have to wait until Acts 11:20 for the dam to break.

Word gets back to Jerusalem that Jews and Gentiles are worshiping together in Antioch. Who has ever heard of such a thing? "News of this came to the ears of the church in Jerusalem, and they sent Barnabas to Antioch" (11:22). What will Barnabas find in Antioch? Could this crosscultural church be of God?

Barnabas is a superb selection for various reasons. First, he is an insider in Jerusalem, fully trusted by the apostles; his birth name is Joseph, but the church leaders have given him the honorific title Barnabas, meaning "son of encouragement" (Acts 4:36). Second, since he was originally from Cyprus (4:36), he knows how to cross cultural barriers and is familiar with Gentiles. Third, he is a man of grace who holds out hope for people who break the mold, as we see in his embracing of Saul when no one else will (9:27). Thus when Barnabas arrives in Antioch to witness this cross-ethnic church, "he came and saw the grace of God, he rejoiced, and he exhorted them all to remain faithful to the Lord" (11:23).

Luke baits us by using an intriguing phrase: Barnabas "saw the grace of God." What exactly does he see? He sees the power of God to bring two "enemy" groups together in worship of Jesus. Only God can bring love between Jews and Gentiles. Seeing two distinct people groups worshiping together in Christian community authenticates the power and supremacy of Jesus' gospel.

Barnabas stays on to become the head pastor of this amazing church and works hard to strengthen this innovative model of cross-ethnic Christian community, which has displacement built into its very fabric.[4] Do the Antioch disciples also know that they are involved in forging a new model for church life? "It was in Antioch that the disciples were first called 'Christians'" (11:26). They embrace this new crosscultural name because they are aware that they are living in a crosscultural church.

God knows that growth into displacement will be difficult. Fortunately, he will bring along unconventional and courageous people to help open new doors. I am very grateful to God for friends like Andrea (chapter one), who showed me what displacement is all about long before I could hear God's call to it myself. Are you open to unconventional thinkers who challenge you to follow God's lead into displacement?

Embracing Partners for the Journey

Is this cross-ethnic breakthrough at Antioch God's plan for the future of his church? What would you do next if you were Barnabas, the leader of this unusual church? Barnabas thinks of someone who shares his love for both Jews and Gentiles: Saul. Immediately he recruits Saul to join him in developing the Antioch model of church life. "Then Barnabas went to Tarsus to look for Saul, and when he had found him, he brought him to Antioch" (11:25-26). Barnabas remembers God's special calling on Saul's life: "[Saul] is an instrument whom I have chosen to bring my name before Gentiles and kings and before the people of Israel" (Acts 9:15). Saul has a calling to both Gentiles and Jews, the mix found in this Antioch church.

Barnabas takes Saul under his wing, and together they learn about displacement dynamics as they lead Antioch. Together they integrate Jewish evangelism and Gentile evangelism, creating new categories for church life. Chapter 11 is a turning point in Acts: God's people cease to be passive about displacement and become proactive. The theological change happens in chapter 10, but the people who embrace the displacement inherent in the gospel are here in chapter 11.

On a sabbatical in 1999 I spent six months studying the book of Acts. One of my breakthroughs was a clearer view of Barnabas. I had pictured Barnabas as a model of generosity (he sold his property, 4:37) and of holding out hope for "long shots" (with Saul in 9:27). I still appreciate both those things about Barnabas, but I had missed what a pivotal trendsetter he is for developing models of ministry. Luke woke me up through his picture of

Barnabas as a daring and courageous leader in Antioch. Barnabas helps integrate Acts 1:8 into church life. He makes intentional displacement a mainstream Christian practice. God will no longer have to use waves of persecution (Acts 8) or sharply rebuke the leaders of the church (Acts 10) to propel them into displacement for the sake of the gospel. Luke honors Barnabas for being the leader who transformed how we think about both church life and missions. Thank God for leaders like Barnabas and Saul, who help guide us into changes God has for us!

Forging the Ultimate "Both/And" Ministry Model

What will Paul do with the Antioch model? Will it become one of many models he will use from time to time in his ministry? In Acts 13 Barnabas and Saul begin to plant churches around the Mediterranean, which becomes a life passion for Saul (his name changes to Paul in Acts 13). Paul goes from city to city, introducing people to Jesus and then gathering them into congregations. We see the influence of the Antioch model in all of his evangelism and church-planting ministry from Acts 13 until he dies.

Paul is a genius at contextualizing the gospel in each ethnic and cultural context. He is able to speak to the hearts and minds of very different types of people. The goodness of God and the attractiveness of Jesus are put into accessible terms that are easier for each group to grasp. The fruit of this approach is seen as scores of both Jews and Gentiles become disciples in each city he visits.

How does this flavor how Paul guides church life in the congregations he establishes? Will he take the easier route and have new converts worship and practice community in "separate but equal" congregations within each city? While there is some ambiguity about just how many of Paul's Jew/Gentile church plants actually practiced regular crosscultural table fellowship,[5] it is very clear that Paul's letters in the New Testament seek to preserve the fragile crosscultural communities he has founded.[6] Whereas Paul was very determined to make the first steps of Christian life attractive and uncomplicated for Jews and Gentiles alike, he switched approaches dramatically when it came to discipleship and church life. Paul became a master at leading his churches through this counterintuitive part of the kingdom of God: Jesus wants to meet us and win us over in our own cultural setting, but then, since he wants us to grow to become like him, he lovingly moves us out of our ethnic comfort zone. Paul guided a coalition of churches in the Roman Empire for whom navigating crosscultural complexities was a normal part of following Jesus on the path of Christian maturity. First Barnabas in Antioch and then Paul around the Mediterranean wove displacement into the fabric of discipleship, making it a normal part of Christian life.

How could this possibly work? Weren't there all kinds of difficult, nitty-gritty details of daily life that would derail such a complex community effort? Luke knew we might ask this question, so he kindly included a fascinating glimpse into crosscultural church leadership.

Navigating the Cross-Ethnic Crunch

A controversy arose in the church over how Jewish you have to be in order to make it into heaven. "Then certain individuals came down [to Antioch] from Judea and were teaching the brothers, 'Unless you are circumcised according to the custom of Moses, you cannot be saved'" (15:1). This group lobbied hard to tilt the table in favor of the Jews, asking all Gentile disciples to embrace the Jewish culture within the church. Remember, even though the Jews were a small minority of the population throughout the wider Roman Empire,[7] in the Christian movement the Jews were the majority and clearly held the power positions.

How do you think our friends Paul and Barnabas felt about this? The next verse tells us: "Paul and Barnabas had no small dissension and debate with them." They would not stand by and watch Christian Gentiles be forced into a new displacement experience while the Jews set up church dynamics to revolve around their culture. A heated debate ensued, and in the end God honored Paul and Barnabas's position. A council of church leaders agreed that Gentiles did not need to give up their ethnic identity and become Jewish in order to join the church and participate in the community. They could be saved in their own ethnic context.

As a result of this discernment, the council agreed to write a letter to the churches that had been agitated by the divisive and confusing teaching of the "Judaizers." Yet though the letter was written to help Gentiles be themselves in Christ, a curve ball is thrown at them at the end. "We should not trouble those Gentiles who are turning to God, but we should write to them to abstain only from things polluted by idols and from fornication and from whatever has been strangled and from blood" (15:19-20). On the one hand, the Gentiles avoided the circumcision knife, but on the other they were asked to abide by certain other rules. When I read the things that were required of them, I want to sing an old *Sesame Street* song, "One of these things is not like the others." Staying away from fornication makes perfect sense to me. But here are some Jewish dietary restrictions being added to the Gentile eating practices. Why were the Gentiles commanded to live like Jews? Was Jewish culture trumping Gentile culture after all?

The council was wading into the tricky waters of preserving table fellowship between two cultures whose dietary practices were incompatible. If Christians of both cultures continued to eat according to their own rules, there would be a breakdown of practical Christian community. That was utterly unacceptable. Therefore the council asked the Gentiles to accommodate the Jews' dietary concerns. Preserving intimate crosscultural community was essential and meant asking one ethnic group to accommodate the other's eating style. Because of the council's daring commands to the Gentiles, cross-ethnic Christian community was maintained, and the believers rejoiced at the news (Acts 15:31).

Implications for Our Lives from Antioch

An invitation to transformation is found throughout Scripture. Romans 12:2 puts it this way: "Do not be conformed to this world, but be transformed by the renewing of your minds." An ongoing part of following Jesus is handing him old ways of thinking and allowing him to transform our thinking along the lines of his kingdom.

Jesus invites us to get outside of ourselves by going to "make disciples of all nations." If we follow this call, we will step into displacement. This can happen in a variety of contexts: on campus, in the city, in church or in another country. What is one area of your life where you can allow yourself to be displaced for the sake of Jesus' gospel?

You and I will struggle with this call, just as the Jerusalem church did. God will nudge us along to help us move in the right direction. What are one or two current nudges from God in your life?

As we heed the call, God will continue to build communities like the one in Antioch, where displacement is woven into the fabric and where people of different ethnicities worship God together. God will raise up wise and daring leaders like Barnabas and Saul to lead these communities.

As God calls us to extend ourselves in love to other people groups, he will show us how to do it within their distinct culture and worldview. He will give us wisdom for how to engage them in a way that serves them.

Cross-ethnic communities will get snagged on nitty-gritty aspects of table fellowship. All members of the community will need to contribute to the strengthening of crosscultural fellowship. Everyone should find ways that their particular needs can be addressed and honored, and everyone should also stretch to get outside of their comfort zone.

We embrace the biblical call to displace ourselves precisely because this is God's pattern for helping us trust him and live out his love. We are not committed to displacement because we find it personally enriching and intriguing to explore other cultures (though it may well be), because we dislike our own culture, or because we hope to fix other people's cultures. We are committed to leaving our comfort zone because this is an important way that Christ is formed in us, and it is the pattern of life in the kingdom of God.

Wrap Up

Displacement is God's gift to us. It is his invitation to transformation. As we enter a new context, we cling to God profoundly. We can choose to walk into displacement, but if we don't we may find it happening to us anyway.

Many have gone before us. Let's remember Abraham. God invited Abraham into the journey of displacement and transformation: "Go from your country and your kindred and your father's house" (Gen 12:1). Remember Moses. He spent his life in one form of displacement after another. Daniel learned to thrive in God amidst displacement. And God built these lessons into the life of the Antioch church, creating a practicing community of mutual displacement as a model for the church. This is the biblical story of displacement.

But what does it look like in our lives today? The next chapter will offer a modern-day case study.

Can White Boys Hoop?*

Doug Schaupp

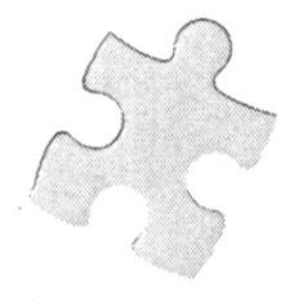

In February 1994 I stood terrified in front of an African American congregation. I had been assigned by the head pastor to lead the church into a celebration of Black History Month. There was a sinking feeling in my gut as I stepped into the large, authoritative wood pulpit. The audacity of my presence in this moment was overwhelming. I was being asked to explain to the church what it means to be African American, except they were the ones who had lived it and I was just beginning to learn about it. I had tried hard to avoid this assignment, but I lost. So I submitted and decided to give it my best shot.

As I gave my introductory comments, I noticed two new African American women sitting in the back pew. They caught my eye as they slapped each other on the back and pointed at me. They doubled over laughing and shaking. This white guy introducing them to Black History Month was the funniest thing they had ever seen. My heart sank into my stomach.

After the service I confronted the head pastor: "Why did you make me do that? Did you see those two women falling over themselves in the back pew?"

He listened, then calmly responded, "In this church each minister can lead the congregation. We don't practice partiality. The gospel of Jesus breaks down the walls between us, and we need to demonstrate that from

---

**Hooping* (whooping) is a style of preaching in some African American church traditions in which the preacher sings portions of the sermon.

up front. Some folks won't like it, but that is the gospel of Jesus that they are stumbling over."

Thus ended my protests. I was in over my head, right where Jesus had called me to be. Now there was no turning back.

Comfort Zones

I have a confession to make. I prefer to feel comfortable. I like social situations where I can be myself, where I am at ease and where I can relax. I like to know what is expected of me. On the flip side, I do not like situations where there are hidden expectations and I get blind-sided. I hate feeling stupid after discovering that I have insulted someone without meaning to at all. In a nutshell, I do not like being displaced.

So how did a comfort-loving white guy like me get to the place where I would join an African American church? Far and away the most important factor was soaking in the biblical mandate to move across ethnic lines (see chapter five). Second, God had led me into some helpful first steps while I was in college: I pursued some cross-ethnic friendships, participated in several crosscultural summer mission projects and took classes on Latino and African American history. After college Sandy and I got married, and in the process I began to cherish Sandy's Korean American heritage.

Displacement is choosing to place ourselves in an unfamiliar crosscultural situation. It is uncomfortable to be a minority. Crosscultural displacement is most successful when we commit ourselves to remain in this difficult setting and allow the learning experience to have its full impact.

Embracing Displacement

My whole attitude toward displacement changed in the summer of 1993. Before that I had felt confident that I could hang out with members of a variety of ethnic groups. I knew how to be sensitive and not say stupid or racist things. I felt that I was a good white person, not like those insensitive bad white people.

Then I had a light bulb moment, a wake-up call from God. Some light bulb moments are enjoyable, but this was not one of the enjoyable kinds.

In the wake of the L.A. riots, the ethnic and racial divides in our country and world were slowly eating away at me. Reading *More Than Equals* by Spencer Perkins and Chris Rice, I found that I could no longer avoid their troubling proposition: if I was not part of the ethnic solution, then I was inherently part of the ethnic divide. Which way would I choose? Would I stay in the comfortable world I had created, trying to feel good about myself, or would I set aside my comfort?

Stepping fully into another culture would let Jesus hold a mirror up to my face and show me who I really was. Once I saw things in that light, I submitted to God's prodding. I embraced the searing truth that until I fully displaced myself, I was indeed a part of the status quo ethnic divide.

By that point I had enough self-awareness to realize that unless the displacement was binding, I would do anything to return to something more comfortable when things got hard. So I said to Sandy, "For six years you have been fully committed to living out our racial reconciliation values. It is time for me to get on board with you. Can we take a concrete step together that I can't back out of?"

During that same season of life, we had been asking student leaders in InterVarsity to extend themselves across ethnic lines in their outreach on campus. They embraced the request, and as we prayed with them, we all received a conviction from God that we should extend ourselves in love to African American students on campus. Despite some initial enthusiasm about the idea, however, our efforts to build trust across ethnic lines were mostly unfruitful.

Sandy and I struggled with which direction to go in our personal displacement. We realized that if we were going to ask our student leaders to extend themselves in love to African Americans, we should be willing to do it first.

Sandy and I prayed, "Jesus, please lead us to an African American church where we can join the community and be transformed by you in the process." This was our Acts 10 moment. As with Peter, God nudged us to "go to Cornelius's house." We did not know where we were going, but we knew we needed to step out in faith.

A friend told us about a National Baptist church three miles from where we lived. The next Sunday we visited Calvary Baptist Church of Santa Monica. During the service there was a time for greeting the guests. No handshaking at this church, only warm, generous hugs. We were moved by the worship and energized by the preacher's message. Noticing that there was only one other white person there among nearly two hundred worshipers, though, we did feel a little out of context.

After returning a few more times, we made an appointment with Pastor Joseph Metoyer to ask about church membership.[1] As we sat in his living room asking questions about the church, he turned the conversation around to us and asked about our ministry. After a few minutes of sharing about our ministry with college students, he inquired, "Doug, are you licensed to preach?" I wondered, *What on earth is he talking about?*

My blank stare must have revealed my confusion. He repeated the question: "Has InterVarsity licensed you to preach?"

I responded tentatively, "Well—they like the fact that I preach, but I don't have a license per se."

He smiled. "It is my job to recognize the gifts that are in the church, no matter who has them. When I see the gift of preaching and the Lord's anointing, I have to license that person."

Part of me was very excited by his vision, but another part of me was intimidated and overwhelmed. Not sure what else to do, I just nodded and smiled awkwardly.

When we returned home, Sandy and I decided to join the church the next week. But we would hold on the licensing idea. First I would ask Pastor Metoyer to be my mentor.

Looking back, I see Pastor Metoyer walking in Barnabas's footsteps from Acts 11. Just as Barnabas had eyes of faith to see the grace of God in Antioch, Pastor Metoyer saw the way God was at work in our lives. He had no blueprint for partnering with a white leader, but he trusted that God had put us in his church for a reason. He was open to investing in partnership for the journey.

Over time we grew into the church family at Calvary Baptist. Each week church members were surprised to see us back again: "It is so great to have you back. I didn't think you would be back." At first I was bothered by their surprise, but I soon observed firsthand what caused their skepticism. Almost every week white folks visited, but few would ever return. They came for a taste of "the black experience" and returned to their own world again. Displacement for them was merely an enriching moment that didn't challenge or transform them.

After six months under the wing of my new mentor, I sensed a bond of trust with Pastor Metoyer. Our hearts were being knit together, which was a sign to me of God's grace on us. Now was the time to build on that grace. God was inviting me to another level of displacement. To be licensed in Calvary Baptist was to join the team of ministers who helped lead worship each Sunday. They sat up front in a row and faced the congregation together.

Taking this step would bring many new challenges my way. But in the end, to become the first white leader in Calvary Baptist's seventy-five-year history was to communicate to the church's people how committed we were to them. We heard the voice of Jesus in this decision. It was an opportunity to do what I had asked the student leaders to do: to intentionally displace ourselves and let Jesus change us in the process.

Displacement as a Path to Transformation

My first formal teaching opportunity at Calvary Baptist came one year after our decision to walk with Jesus into displacement. I can't remember the topic of the Wednesday night Bible study. What I do remember vividly is a panic attack in the middle of the Bible study as I looked out at a room of thirty to forty black faces focused back on me. I was committed to these people who were so different from me. What did I have in common with them? What was I doing here? A voice rang in my mind, *Doug, you don't belong here. Get out now!* Racked with fear, I barely made it through the Bible study.

When I got home, I was embarrassed for the way I was freaking out. Yet I was strangely happy, because I could feel the spiritual importance of this moment. I knew that displacement would bring out the worst of my fears and sin. Though I hated to see what had emerged from inside me, I sensed God was working to deliver a major blow to my ego, my independence and my white self-determination. These parts of me were on the ropes. My sinful self did not want to be exposed in the light of Jesus. So my sinful self was throwing a tantrum, trying to get me to bail out of this naive little experiment. *Doug, get out now! Back to your comfort zone.*

I decided to get tough with my sin and fears: *Shut up! I put my fears on the cross of Jesus. In the name of Jesus, I die to my old self.* I was experiencing the truth of the Scripture, "I have been crucified with Christ; it is no longer I who live, but Christ who lives in me" (Gal 2:20 RSV).

That night, the nails of the cross sank deeper into my soul, like a stake through the heart of my independence. My old self died a little bit more, and Jesus became more alive in me. Our old self can effectively avoid dying on the cross of Jesus until the day the press of concrete discipleship turns the tables on our sin.

The Joy of Bonding

After I joined the pulpit team and Sandy joined the choir, no one ever again expressed surprise that we kept showing up to church. The other six ministers received me warmly. Their affection for me and for each other showed in their humor. They started calling us "the Oreo Cookie Team." They joked, "We are black on one side, black on the other, and Doug in the middle," the cream filling. Or they would jest, "Doug, you are looking more like a black preacher every Sunday. I saw you take out the handkerchief and wipe your face as you preached."

In Acts 15 the leaders honor and protect table fellowship between Jews and Gentiles because that is where real Christian community is experienced. For me, the pulpit team was a place of "table fellowship" where the rubber hit the road in racial reconciliation.

Almost every Sunday afternoon my head would be spinning. Pastor Metoyer and I would talk on the phone, and he patiently answered my questions about what I had witnessed in church that day. He taught me about black church and where the traditions came from. These conversations were profound opportunities to understand what I was going through. Each Sunday I was slowly changing.

God was able to get my attention and expose a deeper layer of racism and racial fear in my heart and life. One day I was driving down the freeway. I wasn't thinking about anything in particular. A car passed on my left. As I looked over, I noticed that the car was old and beat up and that an African American man in his twenties was driving. The first thought that whispered in my ear was, *Watch out. He must have a gun.*

As soon as the thought registered, I was revolted. The thought tried to slip away from my consciousness just as quickly as it had arrived. But it was too late. *Hah! I caught you, my sinful wretched self! Why are you scared of that guy? If he came to Calvary on Sunday, you would embrace him during the welcome of visitors, and you would extend your heart in love to him. He might even become your friend. How dare you judge him! Repent, you stinking racist sinner.*

How many times in my life prior to that day had similar racist thoughts flashed across the computer screen of my mind without my noticing them? Displacement from my comfortable world helped me face my fears and biases. Bonding to the Calvary family gave me new positive images to replace my old warped pictures of African Americans. Jesus used this two-prong fork of displacement and bonding to deepen his work of sanctification in my life. Currently I still struggle against the partiality of my "old self," but during those Calvary Baptist years God brought me face to face with this element of myself for the first time.

I also began to notice and observe my core cultural beliefs. Before Calvary Baptist, I would not have had much of an answer to the question "Doug, what does it mean to be white?" The more I invested in another culture, the more opportunities arose to reflect on my own cultural values. I was learning to wear 3-D glasses, and I could simultaneously enjoy the amazing panorama of the African American culture and explore the texture and beauty of my white culture for the first time. (See chapter twelve.)

My first year on the pulpit team was like learning how to downhill ski amidst a team of experts. Everyone knew I was learning the basics, and they were patient with me. But there were many falls. All I could do was get up and try again. By the second year, I was beginning to understand the cultural signposts. I could increasingly catch what was happening in interactions. I saw how people operated by a subtle set of cultural rules. I slowly gained confidence in operating in that set of rules. Little did I know that God was preparing me for a showdown with the church mothers.

Playing on Their Turf

The showdown came in the spring of 1995. Pastor Metoyer and I had concocted a plan for a summer mission project: six Calvary Baptist high school students and a multiethnic team of six InterVarsity college students would partner for a five-week summer mission in Santa Monica. We formed discipleship pairs, with one InterVarsity student mentoring one Calvary Baptist high schooler throughout the mission. On paper the plan looked like a wonderful win/win scenario, good for the high schoolers and good for the InterVarsity students.

A few weeks before the project launched, I got a call from the chairman of the church board. He said, "The church mothers [the women of respect in the church over age fifty] are against your summer mission idea. I just have to warn you, they are furious. You need to meet with them at their next meeting."

My blood pressure doubled. I thought, *What could I have possibly done wrong?* I asked Pastor Metoyer what I should do. He said, "You don't have to face them if you don't want to. I will go to bat for you if you need it." I appreciated his supportive posture, but I realized that the Calvary Baptist way to handle this conflict would be for me to step up, have courage and talk with the mothers face to face.

When I walked into the Missionary Society meeting, I greeted the twenty church mothers, who were always friendly to me on Sundays. Today their tone was serious. "Minister Schaupp, why did you create your own missionary team here at Calvary Baptist and not consult the Missionary Society? This Missionary Society has been here for seventy-five years, and don't you dare think you can overlook us." They did not leave space for me to respond.

As I listened, I kept track of the issues they were raising so I could respond to each concern. They took turns expressing their frustration at being overlooked. As I stood in front of them in silence, I began to feel terrible about myself. Then I snapped out of it and told myself, *Doug, quit acting so white! Pull yourself together. They are engaging with you in their own way. Get on their turf and engage back with them.*

What should I say? I could see that the rules in this meeting did not fit my white grid. The women did not want a point-by-point response. They needed to know that their voice mattered and they were being listened to by a member of the pulpit team.

The last woman to stand was the most revered matriarch of the church, Mother Sanders. As she stood, she was so full of passion that she couldn't speak for about a minute. Instead she just swayed back and forth, gathering steam. Then she declared, "I try to love people in this church."

I interjected boldly, "Mother Sanders, you have loved me and my wife since the day we joined Calvary."

She looked me in the eye and shouted, "Yes, I have. I have loved you and your wife."

I jumped right back in: "And you have loved every UCLA student we have brought with us to visit."

She shouted back, "Yes, I have. I have loved each of them."

I continued, "These students need your prayer. They need more of God in their lives. And you have prayed for them."

She declared, "Yes, yes, I have prayed for them each week they come by."

She then swung her attention to the women around her: "Mothers, these students need our prayer this summer. Let's gather together to pray for these youth."

As if on cue, the mothers gathered around me to close in prayer, and Mother Sanders led us in praying for the Calvary high schoolers and the UCLA students.

Just like that, our hearts were knit together again. We had interacted in such a way that they felt listened to and taken seriously. According to their cultural rules, they now had participated in the decision. As a result, they were tremendously supportive of our mixed team all summer long. You better believe that they prayed us through that whole summer. And a wonderful summer it was.

That experience with the church mothers was a taste of heaven for me. God had transformed our disunity into community.[2]

LOOKING BACK

In hindsight, I see this process of displacement and healing as being like a baseball game. We step up to the plate of the Scripture and interact with

God. He pitches us some great passages, and we swing away. First base is our step of intentional displacement. Second base follows quickly thereafter, with bonding in the new cultural context. At third base we then step back, reflect and let the Holy Spirit bring to the surface the submerged things in our soul. Home plate, the goal of it all, is the joy of growing in sanctification, growing in ethnic self-awareness and experiencing the power of the cross to bring wholeness to broken relationships.

Calvary Baptist was my first effort at not merely stumbling into displacement but actually seeking it out in Jesus' name.

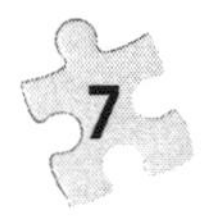

7

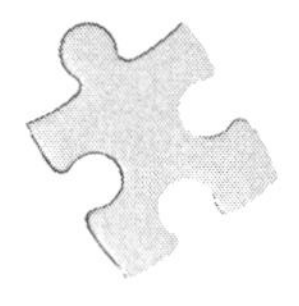

The Point of No Return

Doug Schaupp

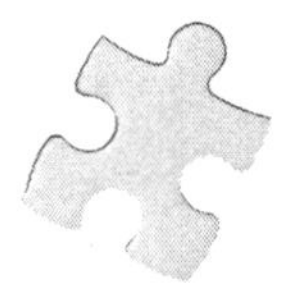

Growing up, I loved amusement parks, especially the roller coasters. I loved the whole experience: the anticipation, the thrill of defying gravity and then talking about it with friends afterward. Standing in line, I would watch those in front of me climb into the car, lower the safety bar over their shoulders and prepare for a wild ride. Some faces were full of excitement, but others were afraid and tentative. Then it would be my turn. The first leg of the coaster was always a long, slow ascent. Up, up, up. Clunk, clunk, clunk.

This long, slow ascent was pivotal for the roller-coaster experience, yet completely different from what would lie ahead. The way up was slow and jerky. The rest was speedy and smooth.

The moment of transition from the long, slow climb to racing through loops and turns was the apex, the point of no return. As we neared the top, I longed to hear the loud "click" of the car's disengagement, because then we were free to explode down the hill. After the apex, the motor was no longer needed. Our momentum would now be enough to take us all the way to the end.

Though I found the ascent tedious at times, as soon as we passed the point of no return, I immediately realized it was all worth it.

The life of following Jesus into displacement is like this roller-coaster experience. Phase one is being an observer. You stand in line, watching those who go before you as they enter into experiences of displacement. You know friends and have read books about people who have gone on summer missions projects or have moved overseas. You see the expressions of faith and fear on their faces and wonder whether someday you will similarly put yourself into out-of-control situations.

Then comes your turn. Phase two of displacement is when God gives you the courage to climb into the roller coaster. You jump into your first intentional displacement experience of being the minority. The rules are different, and you are the learner. The journey up the initial mountain might be a summer missions project in another country or in an urban setting. Or your slow ascent of displacement might begin when you sign up for a class on the African American experience.

As you ride up the hill, God expends a great amount of effort to help you climb against gravity. The ascent may be tedious and frustrating for you, or it may be thrilling. But the majority of white people in society are not on this roller coaster of displacement, and you rub against the grain. As you are changed along the upward slope of displacement, you have a very important decision to make: will you cross the point of no return and decide to remain on the journey of displacement for the rest of your life?

This is where my roller-coaster analogy breaks down. I have never been on a roller-coaster ride that includes a choice to disembark during the great ascent. Roller coasters are built so that if you lock in, you stay in. But on the spiritual roller coaster of intentional displacement, you and I have the strange ability to lift the safety bar and jump off the ride at any point.

Many white folks who begin the displacement journey jump off the ride before the apex, before the good part. Why? There are a million reasons to bail out before the point of no return.[1] The point is this: trying out the roller coaster of intentional displacement is very different from staying on past the point of no return.

Let's tackle the issue of control. When Sandy and I joined Calvary Baptist, we gave up the sense of controlling where the ride would take us. We committed ourselves and trusted Jesus for the best. That was a very different experience for me from the six-week summer mission in Mexico City I joined after my sophomore year in college. Halfway through the summer mission, I began to face parts of my personality I had never seen before. I was tossed back and forth by this chaos inside of me, and I hated it. What should I do? I could courageously face myself in the name of Jesus, or I could merely cope for a few more weeks, fixated on the promise of a quick return home.

The fact that we would soon get on a plane and stop feeling displaced gave me a false sense of control. I effectively avoided being changed by the displacement experience because soon the bar would lift and I would be "free."

In hindsight, that summer project was a pivotal part of my long, slow ascent. God used it to help me grow accustomed to being the minority, being a learner, being confused and not being in power. In fact, God led me through various powerful displacement experiences like this before I was willing to take the leap beyond the point of no return. My blindness lay in not seeing that I was avoiding the point of no return. I thought there was only the long, slow ascent, one summer mission after another.

The point of no return has everything to do with momentum. Both before and after the point of no return, the journey of following Jesus into displacement is marked by successes and failures, progress and setbacks, joy and heartbreak. But during the ascent, gravity is against us, and a few bad experiences can quickly grind us to a halt. We have no momentum on our side to keep us going when we feel inept and empty.

Yet once you have made the lifelong decision to be a white person who intentionally chooses to be in the minority, the suffering will hold less power over you. You will be able to stay in the game despite bumps and bruises. You have made it past the hard ascent, and you know you are in for the long haul.

Why is it necessary to make a lifelong commitment to following Jesus into displacement? Some kingdom values are reinforced in every church in the world; these values have considerable momentum. For example, jumping off the roller coaster of prayer would be really hard for me. Any church I have ever visited has encouraged prayer. God has put voices all around us inviting us to encounter God in prayer. I don't have to make a special lifelong commitment to prayer, because I already know that prayer is basic to life with God, and that message is reinforced on many sides.

But much of the church has lost the biblical value of displacement as a normal part of God's plan for his people. The message of Acts 11—17, the model of Antioch as a cross-ethnic community, and the clear leadership priorities of Barnabas and Paul are seldom preached. Displacement is a lonely message. In fact, some Christian leaders have written books saying that it is natural to live among your own people and it is fine to avoid displacement. No wonder we jump off before the point of no return.

What exactly is the decision we are making at this nebulous "point of no return"? The commitment to submit to Jesus and follow him into displacement all our days is a lordship commitment. It means a lifetime of allowing Jesus to call us out of comfort and ease and into places and communities where we are awkward and weak. Those of us who have made this commitment know that displacement will always be a part of what we do. Our worldview leads us to regularly ask, "Where in my life am I the minority, the learner, the one who is displaced?"

Sociologists Michael Emerson and Christian Smith, authors of *Divided by Faith,* interviewed hundreds of white Christians to discover which of them had been profoundly shaped by ethnic minority friends. They discovered the same thing we have discovered: while one-on-one friendships across ethnic lines are important, only by displacing ourselves into an ethnic minority community network does our worldview expand to see the world more as they do and our hearts expand in love to them. Unfortunately, few of their white interviewees had taken this pivotal step.[2]

Being committed to displacement does not mean that every single decision for the rest of your life is based solely on this one value. We do not become displacement addicts who pursue only the most bizarre displacement experiences. But following Jesus into displacement does become an indispensable part of our daily worldview, our value system and our lifestyle. If not at church, then in our neighborhood. If not where we live, then where we spend our summers or where we work or who is in our friendship circle. You and I have many decisions that can be influenced by a commitment to displacement.

Walking to the Altar

The roller-coaster analogy has a major weakness: it is not a relational image. Instead let's switch now to my favorite picture of making a "point of no return" decision: the wedding day. Hollywood likes to depict the inherent tensions in this particular point of no return. How many movies have you seen where there is a groom or bride sweating it out on their wedding day, debating one last time whether to take the plunge? The groom watches the bride walk down the aisle, glances nervously at his best man, then looks at the door and considers making a run for it. Or the bride refuses to leave her changing room as she ponders the fateful journey down the aisle to lifelong commitment to this one man.

What do they fear? As they commit themselves to one person for a lifetime, they say goodbye to all other options. They put to death all secret fantasies about who could be their perfect husband or wife. Commitment is the choice to focus. Focus is both a form of suffering and a form of liberation. Focus requires me to yield my independence, my autonomy and my sense of control over my future. It is no longer "my" future but "our" future. We hate to relinquish our sense of control. But focus is also a door to liberation, because I need to renounce all others in order to really give my heart to one. It is precisely by limiting my choices that I choose real, lasting love. It removes ambivalence. Prior to the altar, doubts can float through my mind when I come into any suffering: *Am I truly called to love this person?* After the point of no return, the doubts may resurface, but they no longer control me.

How does the marriage illustration shed light on our decision to become lifelong people of displacement? First, we need to fall in love with the groom before we come to the altar. It is Jesus who walks down the aisle, takes us by the hand and leads us across ethnic and cultural lines. It is his idea, not ours. He is our guide and our constant companion in the journey. If it were not for him, there would be no purpose in displacing ourselves for a lifetime.

As we fall in love with Jesus, we enjoy the process of courtship. Courting is an essential part of making a lifelong commitment. We begin with small steps of displacement to see if Jesus will indeed meet us in the process. We might have a delightful first go at displacement, or we might be miserable during the first summer displacement experience. More important than finding success in our first steps of displacement is that we encounter Jesus in the process. As we experience his presence and his leadership as the Good Shepherd, we grow in desire to trust him for a lifetime of obedient displacements.

If the idea of making a lifelong decision to be a person of displacement makes you anxious, turn to Jesus and ask him to give you small experiences of displacement to build your trust in him.

Once the trust is there, we must count the cost. *What kind of white person am I becoming in Christ?* Just as we renounce other romantic options when we get married, we need to renounce love of our own comfort when we give our life to Jesus. He tells us, "If you love your own life and cling to it, you will be lost. To become my follower, you must renounce your love of yourself and your comfort."[3] After counting the cost, we gather our friends, share our joy with them and take the plunge.

At the altar, we take vows to walk with each other through sickness, poverty and the hardships of life. This is the power of a strong marriage. Similarly, the decision to become a person of displacement is the decision to not walk away when things get difficult. Encounter is an experience we can leave behind when we want to. Displacement is entering fully into the community and relationships for the long haul.

Making the decision to stay committed is important precisely because we *do not want* to make this decision. Suffering is difficult even with those closest to us. How much more will we tend to run from suffering with people we cannot understand.

Displacement is not an abstract commitment. The power of displacement is found as we commit ourselves to people with all our heart.

> The word *compassion* is derived from the Latin words *pati* and *cum,* which together mean "to suffer with." Compassion asks us to go where it hurts, to enter into places of pain, to share in brokenness, fear, confusion, and anguish. Compassion challenges us to cry out with those in misery, to mourn with those who are lonely, to weep with those in tears. Compassion requires us to be weak with the weak, vulnerable with the vulnerable, and powerless with the powerless.[4]

The choice to "suffer with" is indeed a daily choice, but it is made easier once we have made the macro decision to give up control through displacement.

The Joy of the Plunge

Back in the 1970s there was a commercial that captivated my imagination. The shot began with a blistering hot day, and the actor was dripping with sweat. He was parched. Then someone poured a tall glass of delicious iced tea. As the actor picked up the glass, suddenly he was standing at the edge of a refreshing pool. On such a scorching day, there was only one smart thing to do: stretching out his arms, he began a free fall backwards. He splashed into the water, utter refreshment on his face.

Richard Foster put a kingdom spin on this image.[5] There are pivotal moments in a believer's life when we stand beside the pool of God's love and debate whether or not to do the back-flop. Will we do things in our own comfortable way, or will we take the risk to fall into God's arms? Falling backwards is counterintuitive. It is an ultimate act of relinquishing control and trusting what lies behind us. We wonder if God will step aside and watch us fall. Is God to be trusted so utterly? Foster calls this the prayer of relinquishment, the prayer of total surrender. Yet the image portrays a moment of complete freedom and bliss. Where else would you rather be on a hot day? Where else would you rather be than in the will of your good Father? It is utterly delightful to fall back into the safe and sure arms of our Heavenly Father.

Joining Calvary Baptist was both awkward and delightful. Because we took the plunge, God brought wave upon wave of spiritual vitality and renewal to our souls. We were refreshed and restored by God week after week.

The Way Up Is Down

Jesus surprises us when he says that the way to find life is giving our life away (Mk 8:35-37). The way to find strength is walking in our weakness. In Jesus' kingdom the way to greatness is servanthood and putting yourself at the bottom. True happiness is found as we pour ourselves out in God's power. Those who are lowly will be exalted. In this way Jesus' kingdom is counterintuitive.

For some, the invitation to displacement is unattractive and foreign. For some, Scripture has nothing to say about displacement. Because displacement is counterintuitive, they think that it cannot be of God. Displacement is viewed with suspicion.

Maybe simple pragmatic thinking would help. Would it help to be reminded that white people will become a minority in the United States before I die?[6] In that light, learning displacement is a wise way to prepare yourself and your children for the inevitable future.

For others, the call to the cross of Jesus is the call to find life by denying ourselves. The kingdom of God is naturally counterintuitive. The way up is via the downward path. That makes the call to displacement attractive and convincing.

When Peter sees Jesus walking on water, he has a compelling reaction. He has never seen his best friend do this before, but that does not bother him; in fact, it generally fits what he knows of Jesus. He calls out, "Jesus, if you are into walking on water, then I'm into it too. Call me to come to you, and I am there immediately" (Mt 14:28, my paraphrase). Peter's unbridled enthusiasm is because he knows Jesus. He knows Jesus offers joy and transformation. Where Jesus is, there we find true life.

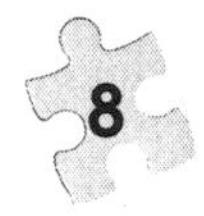

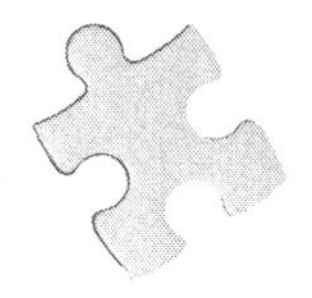

Being Colorblind

KINDERGARTEN OR COLLEGE?

Doug Schaupp

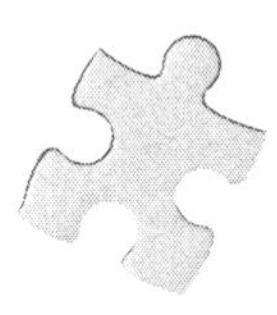

I hurried into the large parking lot of my grandmother-in-law's sprawling apartment complex in Korea Town. I was at least fifteen minutes late picking her up for church. As I turned the corner, my fears were realized. She was no longer standing on the curb where she waited patiently and dutifully every Sunday morning, dressed in her beautiful *hambok* dress.

This Sunday was different because my wife, Sandy, was out of town for the weekend, and I was picking up Halmonim all by myself.* Fortunately, Halmonim and I had a very friendly relationship. Each Sunday I would hug her and kiss her on the cheek, and she would inevitably blush, laugh a little and tell Sandy in Korean that I am a good husband. I knew that in Korean culture you don't kiss your elders on the cheek, but because I'm not Korean, the family cuts me some slack.

Apart from these wonderful smiles, bows, hugs and kisses, there is no other way for me to communicate with Halmonim. She doesn't speak a word of English, and I manage only a handful of Korean words.

I had forgotten to get the key to Halmonim's building from Sandy. Without the key I was powerless to get up to her third-floor apartment and bring her

---

**Halmonim* is the Korean word for grandmother, pronounced hal′-mo-neem. In Korean culture you don't use names, as in "Grandmother Lee"; the title is enough.

down to go to church. I got out of the car and looked up at her window. Gathering my strength, I yelled several times "Halmonim!" as loud as I could.

I forgot to mention that this apartment complex is mostly a Korean retirement community. It seemed like dozens of curtains immediately flew apart, and multiple grandmothers looked to see who was calling for them. You might imagine the surprise on their faces when they saw a white guy in a suit yelling for his Halmonim.

I continued to alternate between yelling and throwing pebbles at her window, and she eventually peered out and was delighted to see that her grandson-in-law had not forgotten her.

If we had not joined Sandy's family's church in 1997, I would not have had the opportunity to give my heart to Halmonim in particular and to Korean culture in general. The story of how God moved Sandy and me from Calvary Baptist to Wilshire Korean Presbyterian Church marks a milestone in our lives. I first heard about the ministry opening at Sandy's family's church from my friend Pastor Soon. He knew that the Korean church needed a minister for the twenty-something congregation, which they call the EM or English Ministry. When Pastor Soon first introduced the idea to me of our leaving our current church to take this other ministry position, I was baffled. I thought, *Why on earth is he recruiting me for this other church position? Doesn't he know how happily committed we are to Calvary Baptist?*

Later my thoughts went a little deeper: *If we were to move away from L.A. in five years, is there anything about our years here that I would regret?* This was a probing question. I had to admit, *Yes, I would regret not having invested more in Sandy's family and the Korean community.* I wondered if God might be in this invitation, but I honestly could not see how it would work to leave our church, which we loved.

I told Sandy about the idea of our taking this part-time position at her grandparents' church, ten miles away in Korea Town. Sandy was nervous about it. She had felt rejected by the people in that church when she was in high school because she didn't speak enough Korean, because she "wasn't Korean enough."

Sandy and I agreed to "put a fleece" out to the Lord. We would get together with Pastor Metoyer of Calvary Baptist, share the idea with him and see what he said. We had made a resolute commitment to be submitted to Pastor Metoyer, and we would not leave Calvary Baptist without his blessing. At our appointment with him, we told him the story of how we had been invited to serve at Sandy's family church.

Pastor Joe shocked us by saying, "That is the Lord! You need to go over there and invest in Sandy's family. You have already invested here in the black community, and our church will take great joy in commissioning you and sending you as missionaries to the Koreans." He laughed with delight at the idea.[1]

Back home, Sandy was still reluctant due to the lingering pain of repeated judgment by her own community. We prayed together, though, and I felt God was giving us the courage to take this new step. Sandy began warming up to it, despite the risk of being rejected again by her own ethnic group.

We did accept the invitation and served for two years as part-time pastors at her family's church. Reflecting on that time, Sandy said recently,

> This was probably the most significant step in my life for growing in my ethnic identity. I hadn't realized how much I had been negatively affected by my past experiences until this opportunity came up. I felt very vulnerable being there at first, but as time went on, the congregation was very open to us and was very honoring of us as their pastors. They very generously and warmly received us and learned from us and respected us. God used their kindness to replace my negative experiences.
>
> Because of our two years there, I no longer feel on the outside with Korean Americans. And I feel at peace with myself as a Korean American. Though I might not be considered "as Korean" as some other Korean Americans, I know inside that I'm Korean, and I don't feel like I have to prove myself to anyone, even if I may be judged by some.
>
> Doug played a pivotal role in this whole experience. He was the one who felt far more convicted about our taking the leadership position, in order to bless my family and thus bless me. Doug took the lead in displacing ourselves for the sake of joining that Korean community as the only white person in the wider congregation of about two hundred.

Without Doug's partnership, I doubt I would have faced my sense of alienation from the Korean community at that point in my life.

It is clear to me that Sandy is fearfully and wonderfully made (Ps 139:14). I admire the beautiful kingdom values God placed in her innermost being through her Korean heritage. But because of past rejection experiences, and since Sandy grew up in a primarily white context, these kingdom strengths were hazy for her early in our marriage. I am grateful to God that he worked through me to nudge Sandy along in her ethnic identity journey.

White people can be helpful to our ethnic minority friends as they explore how God has made them, if we learn to listen well and encourage them in a nonpatronizing way. Think about a few of your ethnic minority friends. How do they feel about their ethnic heritage? How connected are they to their ethnic community? What are some things you and I should know as we seek to be a blessing to our ethnic minority friends?

Kingdom Gems in Acts 17

In Acts 17 Paul preaches in Athens, which had a distinct worldview and culture. According to Athenian mythology, the Athenians had sprung directly from the gods themselves. This view of creation enhanced the Athenian sense of self-importance and the belief that they were the center of the world. How does Paul address this worldview?

> From one ancestor [God] made all nations *[ethnos]* to inhabit the whole earth, and he allotted the times of their existence and the boundaries of the places where they would live, so that they would search for God and perhaps grope for him and find him—though indeed he is not far from each one of us. For "In him we live and move and have our being"; as even some of your own poets have said,
>
> "For we too are his offspring." (vv. 26-28)

First, Paul says that all human beings and nations came from the same ancestor. As Paul traces the origin of all nations back to Adam, he is emphasizing our interconnectedness and our similarities. This declaration that we are all related would fly in the face of Athenian arrogance. It is an essential piece of biblical theology that we are children of the same God. In fact, a Christian attitude that is common today rests on our common origins. It is expressed something like this: "We are all one in Christ. What's the big deal about your culture and my culture?"

According to Paul, this attitude holds half the truth. As we grow up in our multiethnic world, accepting everyone as interconnected is an essential truth. But while being colorblind is an important starting place, it is a very poor ending place, especially for those of us who are interested in evangelism and missions.

Paul is not colorblind in Athens. He looks deeply into the soul of the Athenian people to see how God is at work in them. He assumes God is stirring them to grope after God in unique ways, since this is the sovereign purpose of all nations and ethnic groups.

Paul also has the humility to know that the way he searches for God is related to his Jewishness. He expects that the Athenians are being stirred to grope after God in completely different ways from what he is used to.

If Paul had been colorblind, he would have said to the Athenians, "We are all pretty much the same deep down inside, so I will preach to you from the Hebrew Scriptures." Actually he never quotes the Bible to them, for he knows that would not connect with them. Rather, he sees that God has embedded in the Athenian culture gems of truth and a distinctive openness to the gospel. Having come as a learner and observer of their heart yearnings and deepest needs, Paul learns from their poets and affirms the path of growth toward the kingdom that the Athenians are already on.

To be "colorblind" would have been a dual insult. First, it would have been an insult to the sovereign God; it would have meant ignoring how God was at work in the Athenians long before Paul showed up on the scene. Paul would have been arrogantly disregarding how the Holy Spirit was doing a unique work in them. And he would have been insulting the Athenians by ignoring their needs and assuming that they were basically Jewish just like him.

As you and I make friends across ethnic lines, we need an Acts 17:26-28 mindset. We need to open our eyes to God's unique work in their culture. What are the kingdom gems God has placed in their culture? How are they being led to grope after God? What strengths in their culture reflect the priorities of God and should lead us to praise God?

Like Sandy, many ethnic minority people bear some scars from their own community or carry the weight of some unresolved intraethnic issues. We should not assume that our ethnic minority friends have gotten their ethnic identity all nailed down. We cannot assume they know the particular kingdom strengths of their own culture. As we learn from them and alongside them about their ethnic heritage, we communicate to them that we value the fullness of who they are.

Why Can't We All Just Get Along?

How do you answer that perennial question? Sometimes our ethnic minority friends seem to be doing just fine, and we feel good about everyone just getting along. For me, Stanley Inouye has shed much light on this question through his exploration of the differences between how people of ethnic minority cultures experience life versus how white people tend to experience the world.

Inouye builds on research conducted on two different mission philosophies in Africa, one based on use of the general trade language and the other based on use of the tribal language of each group.[2] The first missionaries, who targeted a wider audience and communicated the power of Jesus through the trade language, saw initial results, but those converts struggled later in life. The second group of missionaries, who communicated the gospel in tribal languages, were able to tap into the "heart language" of each group.

> Those becoming Christians through their heart language were far more apt to find their way into local churches and become active members than those who committed their lives to Christ through trade languages. This seems to indicate that the heart language was attached to the values and beliefs that are more integrated and internalized, and the trade language was less attached. The gospel was able to touch and transform something deeper within when communicated through the language of home versus the language of commerce.[3]

Inouye diagrams this difference with two concentric circles, with the heart language as the smaller, internal circle and the larger circle representing the trade language.

Some ethnic minority folks are very aware that their set of internal cultural values is distinct from the set of values they operate by in public settings. They are consciously bicultural, moving from one style of communication in their "home" culture to an entirely different mode of relating in their "business" culture. Other ethnic minority folks switch subconsciously from their "trade" culture to their "heart" culture without knowing that their mode has changed.

The size of the internal heart language circle varies from person to person too. For some it is dominant, for others it is hardly noteworthy. Sandy's heart language played a larger role in her life than she initially knew.

In countries where white people are in the majority, our heart language blends nicely with the external trade language. Those who are in the majority culture feel integration between their heart language and their trade language. We don't have to intentionally switch modes from heart language to trade language when we go to work or go to the mall. Because the transition from heart to trade language is smooth for us, we often assume that others must similarly feel comfortable in mainstream culture.

But many ethnic minority folks have had to intentionally learn our mainstream culture, and it is not their heart language. In fact, they are greatly rewarded for assimilating as much as possible, using the trade language as much as possible. The more fluent they become in white values and white modes of interaction, the more "normal" and acceptable they become to the majority culture. There is a powerful pressure for them to focus entirely on their trade language, leaving them blind to the ways they are actually guided by their heart language.

Assimilation pressure can even cause our ethnic minority friends to forget that they are made in the image of God—or to wish that God had made them differently. As we learn to observe both the trade language and the heart language of our friends, we can become much more useful to them, serving them and understanding them more deeply.

Why We Couldn't Get Along

In 1997 I had a breakthrough experience regarding this paradigm of heart language versus trade language. I was coaching a multiethnic student leadership team that year, made up of five students, each with a different ethnic mix:

- Vikki, a Chinese American woman
- Sueann, a Korean American woman
- Stephanie, a biracial woman (half Japanese American, half white)
- April, a multiracial woman (one-quarter Filipina, one-quarter Chinese, half white)
- Marc, a white American guy

Marc worked it out with his parents for us to have a three-day leadership training retreat at their home. When we arrived, we faced a subtle dilemma: there were six of us, but there was bed space for only five. I offered to sleep on the floor in the office/den. For the first two days this sleeping configuration was acceptable to everyone. But not on the third.

A few hours before bedtime on our last night, Sueann began to inquire about people's sleeping situations. "Which bed are you sleeping on, Stephanie? How about you, April? Vikki?"

Each person wondered what on earth she was getting at. Why was she asking about this forty-eight hours into the retreat? Finally Sueann blurted out, "Stephanie, don't you care that Doug is sleeping on the floor?"

Stephanie was shocked, "Why are you picking on me? What are you talking about?"

I jumped in, "Sueann, I am perfectly happy sleeping on my air mattress."

The next day we were debriefing the retreat on the way home. The question came up, "Why did Sueann have that bizarre outburst about the beds?"

Sueann could not articulate why, out of the blue, she had become preoccupied with sleeping arrangements, and she felt embarrassed. She knew she had put Stephanie on the spot, but she could not explain where this came from.

Thinking back to Inouye's helpful categories, I said, "Is this what happened?" I offered that Sueann might have been operating in her trade language for two days with the rest of us. "Sueann, did something subtly switch inside of you yesterday, and all of a sudden your heart language took over and said to you, 'Wait a second, *Mok-sah-nim* [Korean word for "pastor"] is sleeping on the floor? How shameful!'? And you looked for a way to quickly resolve this shameful situation."

Sueann's eyes lit up. "That is exactly what happened! And I assumed that since I saw the sleeping situation in this new light, all the rest of you would see it this way also. I was surprised when you didn't see things through my shame/honor lens."

Stephanie felt relieved to understand Sueann's sudden urgency, and so did Sueann herself!

Without an understanding of trade language versus heart language, experiences like this would merely baffle me. I would be tempted to say, "Sueann, get over it! Let's just all get along." Instead I now can see that deep inside we operate out of different worldviews even when we share the same trade language. In multiethnic settings I even sometimes have the honor of helping to figure out the strange disconnects that come about because of this.

Being able to communicate through a shared trade language is a good starting point, but our ethnic minority friends are much deeper than our trade language can express.

Why Being Colorblind Is an Inadequate Goal

In the 1960s, the goal of becoming colorblind was a marked improvement for a society that had accepted overt racism as normal. But while becoming colorblind was an excellent corrective then, it is not a wise place to stay. To remain colorblind means I never look below the surface to understand the issues of heart language.

Here are a few reasons we need to graduate beyond colorblindness.

1. ***Colorblindness ignores the heart language of our ethnic minority friends.*** We ignore their deeper needs that they may or may not be aware of. Even if my ethnic minority friend is not aware of his heart language, that does not mean he isn't operating out of one at a subconscious level. If I want to be a good friend, I will not only see how he functions in majority culture but also look for signs of how his heart culture operates.
2. ***Colorblindness misses kingdom riches God intended for our blessing.*** Being colorblind means we don't look for the poets God has placed in each ethnic group and we miss the kingdom gems each group has to offer us. We are the poorer for not identifying and enjoying the riches our eth-

nic minority friends can offer us. We miss important gifts God intended to give us through them.

3. ***Colorblindness misses who people really are at their core.*** Being colorblind means you do not see the amazing details of God's craftsmanship in those of other cultures and ethnicities. It means you do not look insightfully into the people of color around you. Being colorblind is indeed better than burning crosses on people's lawns, but it is not living with open eyes.
4. ***Colorblindness assumes that everyone is "white like me."*** Since we feel reasonably comfortable in our majority trade language, we think everyone must feel as comfortable as we do. Without meaning any harm, we wrongly assume that their experience is just like ours.
5. ***Colorblindness makes us vulnerable to stumbling into an Acts 6 rift.*** If we overlook color, race, ethnic and cultural issues, we are setting ourselves up for the surprise moment when a schism emerges in our church, campus, neighborhood or business along the fault lines of ethnic communities. Our trade language in the majority culture may serve to keep relationships in a period of peaceful coexistence. But in the end our God-given differences will reemerge in inconvenient and potentially volatile ways.
6. ***Colorblindness numbs our hearts to the suffering of our friends.*** Other ethnic groups have suffered wave after wave of racism that I have not. Being colorblind ignores the ways our neighborhoods are built, our banks operate and our society runs. Being colorblind says that everyone has equal access to equal resources, which is not true, but it sure feels good to say it.

What If?

What if Moses' father-in-law had been colorblind? After living for years in the desert, Moses went to Jethro and said, "Please let me go back to my kindred in Egypt and see whether they are still living" (Ex 4:18). If Jethro were colorblind, he would have said something like "Moses, we are all one big happy family. You don't need to go and explore your ethnic heritage and stir up bad feelings. We don't see you as Jewish. We see you as being a Midianite just like us. Moses, can't we just all get along?"

What if Paul had tried to be colorblind? He would have said to his Gentile friends, "I don't see you as Gentile but just as people. I will treat you just like

I would treat my own people. As a sign of my fairness to you, please come and be circumcised, because that is how we Jews operate. What? You don't want to be circumcised like me? Why do you have to be so divisive? I am trying to prove to you how much I accept you by encouraging you to do things the way the rest of us Jews do them. I am so glad we can all be one in Christ."

If I had tried to be colorblind with Sandy, our marriage would have subtly come to be dominated by my majority culture rules. Sandy knows how to operate in the U.S. majority culture, so she could have played along with me for a few years. But over time, her core values and heart culture would have reemerged. I have seen other cross-ethnic marriages fall apart at just this point, when the ethnic minority spouse finally realizes that she or he has ignored something essential about herself or himself. It has been crucial that I "graduate" from the goal of being colorblind to the textured and complex world as God created it.

Sandy and I have worked hard to incorporate Korean values in our family. It is not just Sandy's job to bring in the ethnic flavor; I need to honor and inculcate Korean strengths into our boys just as much as she does. If the responsibility were only on her shoulders, that would not be a partnership. When I married Sandy, I also married into Korean culture. Part of my heart became Korean, because not only did I take Sandy to be mine but I also took her family and her culture to be mine.

I love telling Mark and David about their Korean strengths and the wonderful things about their ethnic heritage. Though Mark is only five when I write this, he knows that being Korean American is just how God intended for him to be and that he carries unique, God-given strengths. Thank God for the gift of 3-D glasses!

Making Displacement Real

You have been working on going deeper in one or two friendships. What have you learned about yourself in the process? You have probably been learning about commitment and about working through differences. That is wonderful progress.

It would be easy but naive to assume that friendship is the end. As we said earlier, friendships are pivotal for transformation. However, our own cross-ethnic friendships did not fundamentally transform our worldview. It took profound displacement to mold our worldview and take us beyond the point of no return. Only through displacement did we begin to see what it means that God has made us who we are in Christ.

It may be that for you section three has been the most exciting section of the book. Or perhaps this has been the most irritating or troublesome. We believe that the biblical call to displacement is God's word to us white people. This call to follow him into weakness and vulnerability is the door to the spiritual revolution that God wants to bring to us, his white people. But will we walk through it?

Here are a few discussion questions:

1. What did you find motivating in the Acts material in chapter five? Do you believe in the Antioch model of life and ministry? Consider doing an in-depth study of Acts 10—17. Name one person with whom you could study Acts.
2. What did you like about the Calvary Baptist story? Could you envision yourself in a situation like that in the future? What would God have to do to get you to take a step like that?
3. Which analogy do you find the most helpful for your personal life: the roller coaster, the wedding or the back-flop? How does that imagery help you think about your life?

You may have never been in a long-term setting where you were in the minority. For you, a step of application is to allow yourself to be displaced in some concrete way. What are some options for steps of displacement that you could take? What are your questions, your fears or your blocks?

If you live in an all-white neighborhood, this material will be more complicated for you to apply and integrate into your life. I know of churches that intentionally spend one week a year serving in ministries among the urban poor so that their members can experience the joy of kingdom displacement. You will similarly have to be proactive about finding a few things you can commit yourself to.

Some white folks resist displacement experiences because they fear feeling misunderstood, offending people and being ignorant or awkward. But stepping into displacement means that we *will* feel, do and be these things. We will discover that there are no "right" questions to ask. This is why we need Jesus to lead us into displacement. Our job is not to try to control the risk but to be willing to be uncomfortable in the name of Jesus. You and I need to become comfortable with being uncomfortable, to face our limitations and not run away.

One important way for us to displace ourselves is to submit to ethnic minority leaders in various contexts. Have you ever had an ethnic minority mentor? What would it be like for you to put yourself under the leadership and influence of an ethnic minority Christian? Can you name a few potential mentors in your city, your workplace, your campus or your church? Mentoring relationships tend to be more successful if they are focused on a concrete and realistic goal.[4] It would probably be more fruitful, then, for you to ask your potential mentor to recommend a book and discuss it with you than to just say, "Please teach me about the Latino experience."

Perhaps you have already had one or more clear displacement experiences of being in the minority; you decided to climb into that roller coaster and begin the long, slow ascent.

1. Briefly describe a displacement experience you have had. What was good about it, and what was hard? What is the "taste in your mouth" left from this and other displacement experiences?
2. Do you see displacement as a normal part of the Christian life?
3. Did you jump off the roller coaster at any point? If so, when and why?

You may be ready to cross the point of no return. God has been preparing you for this level of commitment in a number of ways.

1. Are you currently in the minority in your family, your neighborhood, your job or your church? Pick one of these areas and consider how you could grow in displacement there.
2. Ask God to speak to you about each of the areas of your life. Ask him to open doors of kingdom displacement.
3. If you decide to commit yourself to being a person of kingdom displacement for the rest of your life, be sure to share this with your family and friends. You will need help to keep this commitment.

If you are at this place of commitment, it is important to wisely differentiate places of *encounter* from your places of actual *displacement*. It is easy to mistake uncomfortable encounter experiences for displacement. Displacement involves being in the minority, being out of control, having given up power.

STAGE FOUR: **WHITE IDENTITY**

Living in the Truth About White History and Racism

Paula Harris

When whites choose to become the minority in numbers and in power, people of color start to tell us more stories about what whites have done. When they see our commitment to keep coming back to their church or stay in their neighborhood, they trust us a bit more. This is an invitation to us to learn the other side of the story. In order to become a godly white person in a multiethnic community, we have to learn the whole truth about interracial encounters.

Racism divides us. But what is it? Whites and people of color often don't agree. Whites have to learn to see and confront racial sin. We have to learn the truth about white history.

Perhaps my learning begins when I see pain on my nonwhite friend's faces and ask why. The Holy Spirit convicts me of my sin and strengthens me to confess it. Gradually I learn to see and understand racial dynamics around me, in my personal networks, in my church, my workplace and my city. God helps us understand our community more deeply and to confess and work to change our group's sins.

When I buy my first house, the black friends I've known since college are still renting. Why? I get promoted, several times over the years, but my Latino friends struggle to make ends meet. Why? I pray for them, but I also begin to wonder: *Do I have more opportunity than my nonwhite friends? Is it just? Is it right?* When I hear answers to my "whys," I begin to wonder, *is the explanation true?*

We white people have only part of the multiracial story. We only see in part. To see racial dynamics, I must learn to ask questions, to observe and talk about race.

Racism is a somewhat taboo subject in the dominant American culture. Most white people are not very comfortable talking about it. For the most part, mixed-race groups aren't comfortable talking about racial sin either. But if we are to achieve a godly multiracial community, we must break this taboo, put the subject out on the table and look at our different ways of understanding.

Racism has been defined as "a system of advantage based on race" or "prejudice plus power."[1] Neil Rendall, a white leader in InterVarsity's multiethnic ministry, says racism is "our denial that all people are made in the image of God." Doug and I think of racism as functioning both on the individual level (my racial partiality for my group) and on the group level (our racial partiality plus power). Sometimes we whites think of racism as individual acts of racial violence (lynching African Americans, for example, or the times some white soldiers intentionally killed Native Americans by giving them smallpox-infected blankets). It does include those sins, but it also includes community-wide acts of violence—acts of violence that are so familiar that they are hidden to well-meaning white people.

Here are some of the ways I learned to see racism. A few years ago, I moved into a multiracial neighborhood. My family lives on a mixed-race, mixed-income street. On the upper end of my street is a row of medium-sized houses. One day I realized that white people own most of the houses. Every white family is a combination of adults and young children, or simply one generation—an older couple. There are two black families who own houses; in one home there are two adult generations, the other has three generations of working adults. One older Asian couple lives here; I don't know them yet, but I think they are Chinese.

In the middle of my street there is a section of older duplexes. Rent for these duplexes is higher than mortgage payments on the houses (I wondered how much the rent was, so I called the landlord). The duplexes are filled with single white adults. The lower half of my street is apartments. Rent for the apartments is about two-thirds of a current mortgage payment, probably higher than the payments of those who bought houses here years ago. The apartments house a great assortment of single people and families; about half are black families, the other half a mix of Latino, Southeast Asian and a handful of whites. How did this happen? Is it okay?

At my kids' school, there is a similar mix of children. Before I moved here, I went to city hall to figure out what schools and neighborhoods were racially diverse and academically challenging. What schools would be a good environment for my biracial kids? The city publishes school performance reports for taxpayers. The reports are not mailed out, however, to the renters on my street, who are disproportionately people of color. Every year when academic performance standards are published, I read the racial comparisons. Every single year, black and Hispanic children in my city and state do worse in school than white children. High school kids around here say, "In West High the basement is full of minority kids"—that's where special ed is. "The top floor is white"—that's where college prep and advanced placement courses are taught.

The studies ask questions about the data. Reading the test score and grade comparisons, I can see them looking for the tangible cause of the racial inequity in academic performance. They compare financial situations: do white kids have better books and educational supplies at home? Maybe, but even when you compare minority and white families with equal income, white kids achieve more in school. They compare parents' education level: do kids whose parents are more educated do better in school? Well, yes, but if these factors are equalized (comparing parents with Ph.D.s to other Ph.D.s and high school grads with each other), white kids still do better in school. Is it that ethnic minority kids move more often and it's hard to learn that way? Well, sometimes, but comparing white and minority "lived-here-one-year" kids with each other and "lived-here-forever" kids with each other, the white kids still get better grades.

Under all the circumstances, white kids do better in school. No matter how researchers control the studies, comparing only children from similar households, white kids are achieving more. The unasked question is, Is there some kind of systemic bias? Do white kids benefit from subtle academic partiality? This question goes unasked because our culture considers this inequity a part of "normal" society. There must be a "normal" answer for the differing achievement. Racism can't possibly be that deep in our society. Can it?

This is one way I learned to see racism. The home ownership patterns and the school achievement patterns are both examples of systemic racism. Systemic racism is just what it sounds like: a racist system that operates broadly through a society or group, giving partiality to one racial group over another. Professor Beverly Daniel Tatum writes,

> I sometimes visualize the ongoing cycle of racism as a moving walkway at the airport. Active racist behavior is equivalent to walking fast on the conveyer belt. The person engaged in active racist behavior has identified with the ideology of white supremacy and is moving with it. Passive racist behavior is equivalent to standing still on the walkway. No overt effort is being made, but the conveyer belt moves the bystanders along to the same destination as those who are actively walking. Some of the bystanders may feel the motion of the conveyer belt, see the active racists ahead of them, and choose to turn around, unwilling to go to the same destination as the white supremacists. But unless they are walking actively in the opposite direction at a speed faster than the conveyor belt—unless they are actively antiracist—they will find themselves carried along with the others.[2]

Perhaps this is not how you have always understood racism. Racism has many faces.

Aware/Overt Racism

Most of us whites find it relatively easy to name the KKK as racist.[3] Lynching is racist. Genocide is racist. Hitler was racist. The Serbian genocide of Muslims was racist. If an ethnic minority person is dying and being raped because of his or her race, a racist was involved. That's obvious. This is racism we are aware of; it's blatant.[4] The solution seems obvious too: we must stop it. If the action was done by a racist person, we stop him or her. If it's a racist group or broad pattern like apartheid and genocide, society—whether local, national or international—must stop it. We have to corporately improve laws. We have to enforce good laws that have been ignored. Murderers must be forced to stop. Killers who profess to follow God must confess their sin and stop killing. Perhaps there should be attempts to reach out to the victim's family in reconciliation.

Racism operates on a physical level (killing), a spiritual level (immediate, and then eternal, separation from God), and an emotional and social level (hate). We must identify and repent from racism on all these levels.

More Subtle Racism

There are other types of racism than the aware/overt one. What I described on my street and in my kids' school, what I could describe in my church and at my workplace—these are also contexts where people of color are experiencing loss. They are losing the chance for a good education. They are losing the economic and emotional stability of owning their own home and land. Paul Kivel writes, "It's also an act of violence to be denied access to a job, housing, educational program, pay raise, or promotion *that one deserves.*"[5]

Let's look more deeply at the question of housing and land ownership. A few decades ago, when some of the older couples bought houses on my street, banks in the city practiced redlining. Not many black people got mortgage loans, and when they did it was only to buy in particular neighborhoods. A few generations ago, these same African American families' ancestors were forced to work as slaves without any income. Whites stole their labor, among other things. A few hundred years ago, the land where my house, my street and my whole city are built all belonged to the Ho Chunk tribe.

In the 1700s the Ho Chunk owned one-fourth of my state's land. In 1836 they were subjected to a forced relocation, and one in four died. In 1962 they owned only about five hundred acres. Today they do not even have a reservation.[6]

This might be less obvious, but if a person of color is experiencing systemic loss, probably someone stole something from them. It didn't "just happen" that white people own the land that used to belong to Native Americans.[7] It's not "normal" that most black people in America still don't own homes. The system is still based on earlier white violence.

Two dynamics are operating to maintain a racially stratified system. As a white person I am very privileged. Not all white people are better money managers; we don't necessarily deserve more loans. When I bought my second home, I had a bankruptcy and a foreclosure on my credit report. I got a chance anyway—other whites were partial to me. We don't inherently deserve higher-paying jobs. We don't inherently deserve better access to mortgages. At the three banks and mortgage companies where I compared rates and options, the employees I met were all white. White people decided if I would get a loan. The white mortgage officer I worked with knew the white guy who has been writing my paycheck for twelve years. Everyone who has ever given me a job was white. Everyone who has ever given me a raise or promotion was white. All my landlords and realtors have been white. These white people trust me more because I am white. Racial partiality has operated in my favor. They ask fewer questions. I look educated to them. I look reliable. I look predictable.

This partiality operates for me when I buy a house or a car, and it operates for me when I go to the neighborhood convenience store. It's interesting: as a white woman alone, I incite no interest. My checks are cashed without ID. I can wander around picking things up in a store. When I bring my black children along, though, suddenly I look slightly less reliable. My ID is checked. My kids and I are watched, and sometimes we are followed around the store to make sure we're not shoplifting.

The first time this happened, I brushed it off. The second and third, ninth and tenth times I thought, *Oh no, it's not possible.* But it does happen. Consistently.

Aware/Covert Racism

The other dynamic operating is that people of color are victims of racist discrimination. In World War II we put Japanese Americans in internment camps, but not Germans. Japanese American homes and businesses were confiscated, but not German ones.

Some white people actively steal opportunities from ethnic minorities. A few decades ago the banks in my city worked with a red line defining the areas on the city map where black people could or could not get mortgages. Then and now, there are all-white neighborhoods in my city. Today the areas that used to be inside the red line are still almost half African American, and the areas outside are still predominantly white.

Government studies show that there are still more than two million race-based housing discrimination crimes every year.[8] Most people of color eventually face housing discrimination. For this to happen, for all-white neighborhoods to be maintained, some white people say to minority people, whether with words or actions, "I don't like the look of you; I don't want to live with you." It's illegal, but it is happening.

This is called *aware/covert racism*. It's not hard. The partiality doesn't have to be publicly visible. A white person can just say to ethnic minority applicants, "That apartment's been rented" or "I need three months' rent as a deposit." For a system with racial privilege to operate once it is set up, all we whites have to do is ignore it. To deconstruct it, first we have to work hard to see it. Then we have to join forces with the people of color around us to rebuild a new, more just and godly system.

These days, thank God, there is an active fair-housing group in my city. Anybody can ask for an undercover investigation of a racist, or possibly racist, landlord. This is an attempt to break the cycle of aware/covert racism. Some white and nonwhite people concerned about justice came together to create this group.

Unaware/Covert Racism

Racism can operate even if you don't see it and don't intend it. My sister Holly is a teacher. Every year the state sends an educational tester to her classroom. The first year, almost all of the kids in Holly's class failed the basic academic test for kindergarten. They could not follow sequences. Their vocabulary was inadequate. The report came back concluding that the kids all needed special ed.

Holly's observation was, "This is a fairly average class. Maybe one or two could use some special tutoring, but most of the kids are normal. Some are very smart." So she asked the tester to return. As the test was repeated, Holly learned that to measure sequencing the white evaluator had asked each kid to explain the stages of making a peanut butter and jelly sandwich. This should be fairly simple for a five-year-old, but they all failed. Why? What was happening?

Holly realized, *None of these kids eat PBJ; they eat burritos and tamales for lunch. They're all Latino.* "Why don't you ask them what are the stages of making a burrito?" she suggested. All the kids but one passed this test. They passed easily, explaining clearly and sequentially how to make a burrito. That year they stayed out of special ed.

Now maybe it would be good for those kids to learn about making peanut butter sandwiches, but why? The point of the test was to measure the kids' capacity to give instructions in stages, with a defined sequence.

This situation reveals a racism that is more subtle. The white tester was unaware of racism at work. She would have been horrified to be called a racist. The tester didn't intend to hurt the kids. She didn't hate them. She didn't dislike them. She didn't consciously prefer white kids. She wasn't aware of her own partiality. She didn't have to *do* anything for unaware/covert racism to be at work.

The way this type of racism operated was hidden to both the tester and my sister the teacher, until Holly started actively thinking about it. Holly's reflection, *These kids don't need special ed,* caused her to try again, to ask hard questions. Only then was she able to uncover the unaware/covert racism that was at work and to explore the real abilities of the Latino children.

If Holly had not uncovered the racism at work, the kids and their parents would have been left to struggle with a reality gap. *The test says my kid needs special ed, but I think he is smart. What is true? Maybe I don't understand as much as I think I do.* (See the self-doubt beginning to take root?) Eventually, if this happens regularly, the white teachers and testers might have been left believing a lie, "Latino kids are not as smart as white kids." This test could affect the rest of these kids' lives, their education, future job possibilities and income.

The solution to the unaware/covert racism operating in this situation was a little more complex. Holly needed to submit the professional assessment to the "test" of the children. Do the kids understand sequencing or not? Do their parents think they need special ed? Does the teacher? What is the truth about the situation? Does the conclusion hold if I measure differently? What is the history? What is the wider cultural context? Holly even had to ask, what do the children eat? Uncovering this sort of racism required that Holly learn to see in a totally different way, with 3-D glasses.

Unaware/covert racism can operate despite our commitment to racial reconciliation, because we cannot see it very well. We whites are not aware of our own partiality; we don't know how to look for it, so it is hidden from us. People of color feel something is not right, but it's hard to name and describe. We white people want to excuse ourselves from it when it's pointed out to us. It makes us appropriately uncomfortable to think about racism operating in our hearts and around us. Kivel rightly observes, "People of color do not protest discrimination lightly. They know that when they do, white people routinely deny or minimize it, blame them for causing trouble, and then counterattack."[9] We create other explanations for the inequity.

If we are going to uncover racism, we cannot be satisfied with easy answers. Scripture says, "The wrath of God is revealed from heaven against all ungodliness and wickedness of those who by their wickedness suppress the truth" (Rom 1:18). The word that is translated "wickedness" can also be translated "injustice." If we continue to live in injustice or wickedness, what happens is that our thinking becomes cloudy, and "claiming to be wise, we become fools." Eventually, we exchange the eternal glory of God by putting something else in God's place (Rom 1:20-25). When we white people do not confront our own racism, we begin to put *ourselves* in God's place. We don't want to commit ourselves to learning to be simply human equals with people of color.

Underneath it all, we white people don't want to do the hard work of uncovering the racism in our systems. The abolitionist movement took decades to change slavery, and still it left us with a racially stratified economic system. How much easier it is to allow our partiality to go unacknowledged. We can just let the system work for us. We don't have to discriminate. The sad truth is, once a type of racism gets started, we don't need to do much for it to keep working. All we have to do is ignore it.

I can recognize unaware/covert racism when a white person (including me) objectifies a person of color, either individually or as a group. If an explanation for apparent inequity seems to demean a minority person, or assumes he is less intelligent or she is less diligent than the whites around, I must keep asking questions.

If whites and minorities have different analyses of the situation, I must keep seeking both perspectives in order to determine the truth. How did this happen? I need to put the situation in a broader context. Where are the roots? What is the history? What is the result? What fruit does the analysis produce in my own soul? (Does it allow me to self-justify, to perpetuate my own partiality? Am I caught up in pride?) What is the fruit in the soul of the ethnic minority person? (Does it cause inappropriate self-doubt? Does it cause self-protective anger? Does it cause self-blaming depression?) Asking these kinds of questions has taught me to see some of the racial dynamics that are operating in my world.

Unaware/Self-Righteous Racism

There is a final type of racism that I must include, because it is the type that most tempts me. Sadly, just as Romans says, "all have sinned and fall short of the glory of God" (Rom 3:23), it is also possible to say that all white people are tempted to be racists and imagine ourselves gods over others.

When we are deeply committed to being allies of people of color in the struggle against racial injustice, when we begin to think of ourselves as "antiracist whites," a different type of racism tempts us. Jenny Yamato describes it this way:

> The newest form of racism I'm hip to is unaware/self-righteous racism. The "good white" racist attempts to shame Blacks into being blacker, scorns Japanese-Americans who don't speak Japanese, and knows more about the Chicano/a community than the folks who make up the community. They assign themselves as the "good whites" as opposed to the "bad whites," and are often so busy telling people of color what the issues in the Black, Asian, Indian, Latino(a) communities should be that they don't have time to deal with their errant sisters and brothers in the white community. Which means that people of color are still left to deal with what the "good whites" don't want to . . . racism.[10]

This type of racism shames people of color. While I am shaming them, this type of racism lets me continue in pride and self-partiality, thinking, *I'm a good white. I'm not a racist.* My sin is left unacknowledged. Not only that, I am alienating myself from other whites and not actively dealing with the sin in my own community.

When I think and act as an unaware, self-righteous racist, Scripture says to me, "You have no excuse, whoever you are, when you judge others; for in passing judgment on another you condemn yourself, because you, the judge, are doing the very same things" (Rom 2:1). Am I thinking that I can escape the judgment of God? Can I judge other white people for doing what I do? Paul asks, shouldn't God's patience, God's kindness, lead me to repentance?

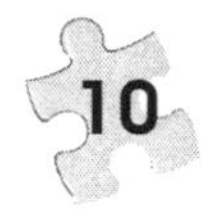

10

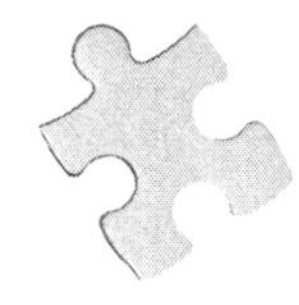

Open the Parachute

Doug Schaupp

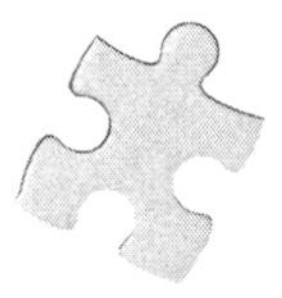

All my life I have consciously or subconsciously ordered the world into two groups of people: those who are similar to me and those who are different. In high school I loved to order the world between groups of people, and I eagerly celebrated with my friends how we were different from and better than others. First, there were "we" athletes versus "those" uncoordinated people. I felt better about myself because I was on the varsity wrestling team and a committed athlete. Then there were "we" cool partyers versus "those" nerds. We knew how to have a good time. And there were "we" nonconformists—my little group of friends versus "those" conformists. If the mainstream did things one way, we would intentionally do them another way. For example, we dyed our jeans purple and pink so that we would be distinct from the rest of "them" who wore blue jeans. I enjoyed being around people like me, and I generally avoided people who were different.

When I was a freshman in college, God threw my life into a spiritual revolution. One of the catalysts of transformation was my experience of being loved by the Christians in InterVarsity Christian Fellowship. As a new student, I was shocked to discover such love. Christians listened with rapt attention as I talked about my life, and they asked me insightful questions to help draw me out.

At first I misunderstood what the attention was all about. Being a self-absorbed person, I concluded that these Christians were amazed at how cool

I was. Just the opposite was true. Later I found out that they asked excellent questions and listened with loving patience not because of who I was but *despite* who I was. They treated everyone with this type of care and even extended themselves in love for an obnoxious freshman who thought he was the king of cool.

I noticed that my Bible study leader would hang out with everyone on the dorm floor, not just the cool people. He was indiscriminate in his love. As someone who put people into categories, I couldn't believe it. Following the example of these Christians, I started learning to listen, to ask good questions and to become captivated by those around me—even putting my book down when someone would walk into my dorm room, so that I could focus my attention on them.

Where did this practice of treasuring people originate? Looking back now, it is obvious. The practice of being captivated by people sprang out of the life and heart of Jesus. Jesus could always see the unique beauty and the image of God in everyone he interacted with. He let all manner of image-bearing individuals interrupt his schedule and occupy his attention. When a filthy leper came groveling to him, Jesus didn't see a beggar and an outcast. He saw a person made in God's image, starved for love and attention. He knew his pain and rejection. He was moved from his heart to hold him and heal him. Jesus was captivated by the leper. Jesus' life was marked by the kind of love that looks beneath the surface, and people flourished in his presence.

God knows how we are wired. He knows that you and I thrive when we are invested in and cared for. He wants us not only to be the joyful recipients of such love but also to have the honor of extending that love to others. Our Lord places this lavish love at the center of the Christian life. "Those who say, 'I love God,' and hate their brothers or sisters, are liars; for those who do not love a brother or sister whom they have seen, cannot love God whom they have not seen" (1 Jn 4:20).

Our problem is that you and I are not lavish in our love for all the people made in the image of God. Being captivated by others is hard work, and we tend to generalize about others as a way of conserving energy. As we interact with God's people of all *ethnos* (nations), our reaction should be fascination, appreciation, enjoyment and a near reverence for others. C. S. Lewis captures this eloquently:

> It is a serious thing to live in a society of possible gods and goddesses, to remember that the dullest and most uninteresting person you can talk to may one day be a creature which, if you saw it now, you would be strongly tempted to worship, or else a horror and a corruption such as you now meet, if at all, in a nightmare. . . . It is in the light of these overwhelming possibilities, it is with the awe and circumspection proper to them, that we should conduct all our dealings with one another, all friendships, all loves, all play, all politics. There are no ordinary people. You have never talked to a mere mortal. Nations, cultures, arts, civilizations—these are mortal and their life to ours is as the life of a gnat. But it is immortals whom we joke with, work with, marry, snub, and exploit. . . . Next to the Blessed Sacrament itself, your neighbour is the holiest object presented to your senses.[1]

Life is meant to be lived one person at a time. Our heart needs to become large enough to make room for each person we come across in our daily activity. All of us need to have our heart stretched. Therefore we should regularly find ourselves praying, "Father, show me how you see them. Help me feel for them how you feel for them."

Our hearts are like parachutes, built to expand to their fullness in the power of God's Spirit, enlarged for the journey. Unfortunately, most of us live with our parachute still collapsed, folded tightly in its chute pack. Jesus lived with his heart wide open and full of love, showing us what is possible as we open ourselves to God. His heart is on display on page after page of the Gospels, trying to inspire us to yearn for more from our own heart. He dares us to open our heart all the way, to be the open, beautiful parachute of love that is possible in God.

How do we step into this life of open-hearted love? In addition to praying daily for God to pour his love through us into everyone we come in contact with, we need to become aware of the straps and snags that hold our heart down. When I am feeling competitive or insecure around someone, it is virtually impossible for me to feel proper godly compassion for them. The same is true when I fear someone. Fear, anxiety, pride, confusion, indifference all snag and inhibit our hearts from expanding in love for those around us. What tends to hold your heart back from loving others?

How about race? What part does race play in whether our heart soars in love for each person we meet?

I have a confession to make. I am a recovering racist. I am a racist not because I burn crosses but because my heart snags when I am given an opportunity to love those different from me. My apathetic heart is ugly and indifferent. I am numb instead of compassionate.

I long to have a wide-open heart for all of God's people. I desperately want to be like Jesus as he fearlessly walked in compassion, unfazed by any differences. Though I have already dealt with a lot of my biases and blocks, I am always seeing more. The process of healing and transformation will last all my life. But the process of growth and healing has an explosive beginning point—the hardest step of all: real honesty with myself, with others and with God about my struggles.

You know how I said that in high school I divided the world between "us" and "them"? Well, I think we all do that. To be human is to play favorites. The biblical authors call this "favoritism" or "partiality." Without knowing it, we are always doing it. We subtly extend love and favor to those more like us, while we are tempted to withhold love from those different from ourselves. You and I are guilty of practicing partiality.

Everyone has secret fears and assumptions about others. The question is whether we will look deep inside and face ourselves in Jesus' grace. *Racism* is an ugly little word, and these days there are more reasons than ever to keep us from honestly facing our racism. In fact, in some circles we can get sued for admitting we are racist; no wonder we flee from this word like the plague. Yet avoidance only makes the problem worse.

The good news is that God is an expert in dealing with all forms of our partiality, including our racism. Once you are willing to admit your biases, fears and racism, you can make so much more progress in love. As you admit the truth about the straps and snags, God can break them and your heart can become much more like Jesus'.

The book of James provides us with a theological lens for understanding partiality, and chapter 2 is largely devoted to this theme of playing favorites. "My brothers and sisters, do you with your acts of favoritism really believe in our glorious Lord Jesus Christ?" (2:1). Playing favorites is so completely opposed to the priorities and way of Jesus that James wonders how Christians can be committed to Jesus and maintain this practice. He proceeds to use the illustration of how people in the church "take notice" of the rich and ignore the poor, "making distinctions" between one group and the other. Then he brings it home in verse 9: "If you show partiality, you commit sin and are convicted by the law as transgressors."[2] This is strong language for our common practice of playing favorites.

Though James is addressing a situation of partiality between rich and poor, Peter turns this same theological lens onto ethnic and cultural partiality. The book of Acts paints a powerful picture of God's trying to open the hearts of his people like a beautiful parachute, while they are reluctant. As we saw earlier in the book (see chapters one and five), God began Acts with this vision of his people extending themselves to all *ethnos,* including the Gentiles, but it took life-threatening crises to prod the people of God to open up. What held the church of God back from its calling? The straps and snags of partiality were never directly identified and broken.

God patiently waits for his church to become proactive in facing their snags of partiality, but by Acts 10 he has decided that it is time for overt sovereign intervention to get his point across. Acts 10 is the description of God bringing Peter to see his partiality and move through it. Later in Acts 10, Peter gives his first-ever sermon in a Gentile's house, and it is as much a confession for Peter as it is a sermon for them. He begins with a lesson he has just learned that very day, "I truly understand that God shows no partiality."

Daring to Ask the Question

God has a tricky job in helping Peter to face his partiality. Helping people face their partiality is difficult across the board, but I think it is particularly touchy for us white people.

I went to a national conference on racial reconciliation about five years ago, and at one point we were divided into ethnic-specific communities for group discussion. In our white group, one person decided that this was her opportunity to explain to the rest of us what is wrong with white people. She probably thought it would work well to exhort us about our racism. But her exhortation sounded an awful lot like a lecture.

I looked around the circle, and no one was listening. We just sat there, resentful, silent, waiting for her to shut up. Exhortation and lecturing were not the way to help us face our partiality and be energized for new steps of obedience.

God's way of getting Peter to change is ingenious. Instead of lecturing or exhorting him, God gives him a vision and gets Peter to start thinking about it (see Acts 10:9-17). The vision is not directly about racism but about food customs. Peter knows there is more to it, so he has to ponder it.

Asking questions and pondering are essential to seeing something new about yourself and God. Asking questions helps us lower our defenses and become more teachable. We begin to really want to see the truth about ourselves, instead of having someone else impose it on us. A truth discovered will tend to burrow far deeper into our heart and soul than a truth imposed from outside. Jesus often taught this way, using parables to ignite the curiosity of his hearers, enticing them to search for meaning.

God's goal is to get Peter to examine his thinking about Gentiles, his assumptions, his fears and his lifestyle. He is trying to engage his brain, his heart and all parts of his life in an elaborate paradigm shift. God is not imposing the "Theologically Correct" agenda on Peter, merely seeking to change Peter's vocabulary. God is going for full-life transformation.

Similarly, you and I will face ourselves only when we start asking good questions. *Why am I afraid of black people? Why do I ignore the Latino worker who does the gardening? Why do I eat lunch with people who look like me and not at that other table? Why do we go to this church and live in this neighborhood?* These are probing, unsettling questions without easy answers.

Take a moment right now and ask yourself one such honest question. If Paula and I can nudge you to ask yourself one disturbingly honest, probing question, we have accomplished our goal with this book. What do you need to begin pondering? Answers are much more comforting than good questions, but answers don't bring transformation. Are you ready to walk with the Holy Spirit into some rigorous soul-searching and pondering?

First, *listen to the tapes.* All of us have tapes that play in our head when we see people. Often the volume is turned down low so that we hardly notice. When you walk past a group of loud black people, what do you think or feel? Next time, pay very close attention so that your partiality will be exposed.

Now *embrace the conviction.* As God points out partiality in your life, welcome it. You don't need to be afraid of the Holy Spirit's conviction. Conviction is not his way of saying, "Shame on you." Rather, the Spirit brings conviction when he is ready to bring transformation. Feeling convicted is a great sign of a healthy conscience. The thing we *should* fear is numbness of soul and indifference.

Identify the origin of the stereotypes. Reflect back on formative racial lightbulb moments in your life. What did you learn from your family about ethnic minorities? What negative terms or assumptions did you hear in the home, in school or in church? When did you first become aware of being white? Did you think whiteness was better or worse than other ethnicities?

You could draw a timeline and make note of key racial experiences that have both shaped your own racial self-perception and shaped your view of various other groups. One of my friends, Lisa, decided to do personal interviews of our Greater Los Angeles InterVarsity staff team, asking these types of questions.[3] When she interviewed me, it was the first time I had ever told someone about certain formative childhood experiences. Why did I wait my whole life to examine and articulate the events that shaped my feelings about race and ethnicity? We white people have had the luxury of not having to ask those probing questions unless we want to.

In addition to the voices of fear and superiority, *listen for any lack of love and lack of interest.* Where do you have the opportunity to extend yourself in love, but hold back? Where are you numb and indifferent? Where is your heart snagged instead of enlarged like an open parachute?

How have your perceptions of others affected how you make decisions and live your life? Where do you live, go to church, study, shop, vacation?

Last year my wife and I led a group in a racial discussion called Race Matters.[4] As we facilitated the dialogue, one ethnic minority student, Charles,[5] shared about a dual wound he had experienced that very day: first, he was the recipient of a blast of direct racism; and second, when he shared the experience with his teammates, they rationalized it away.

We asked his white friend Kevin, "Why didn't you listen better or respond with compassion?"

Kevin confessed, "I have never personally experienced anything like that, so I figured it couldn't really have happened like he said."

I was momentarily stunned by his shameless honesty. It was the first time his eyes had been opened to the fact that he operated by a set of racist rules that subconsciously told him, *My view of life is the most reliable guide, and my experience will trump and invalidate any accounts that differ from mine. This racial thing isn't my problem, because there is no such problem.*

Because of the honesty of these two friends within a community of love and truth, a new layer of reconciliation was possible between them. Racism had been grasped, exposed and understood in a new way.

The process of repentance and liberation turned a corner in Kevin's life that day. Our white brother was able to have the parachute of his heart opened only because he was lovingly confronted with the snags of his racism. He would not have faced this part of himself alone. The internal tapes of racism were too subtle for him to notice.

The hard work of facing ourselves and our brokenness can seldom be done alone. Christian community is the best place to come into the light and find new life.

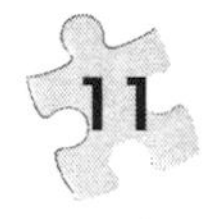

11

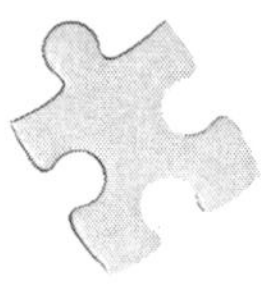

Who Are We? Who Do They Say We Are?

Paula Harris

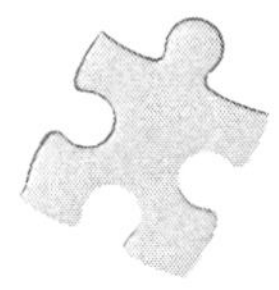

Do you trust God with the fact that you're white? Can you trust that God created you white on purpose and that God intends good to come of it?

The psalmist writes in wonder, "I praise you, for I am fearfully and wonderfully made. . . . My frame was not hidden from you, when I was being made" (Ps 139:14-15). "Frame" is not just about our dress or shirt size; it's our race, our body, everything that makes up our physical being, which God created. God carefully crafted us as an artist does a major artwork.

The same psalm closes, "Search me, O God, and know my heart; test me and know my thoughts. See if there is any wicked way in me, and lead me in the way everlasting" (Ps 139:23-24). To begin to see myself clearly and truthfully as a white person, I need to be willing to face whatever truth comes out. White people have perpetuated a lot of evil, and only a few of us made choices against it. It may help to learn the Jesus prayer: "Lord Jesus Christ, Son of God, have mercy on me, a sinner." There are some days I feel the need to repeat that prayer, as I face the truth about white history and white culture.

At the same time, we must have faith. White people must trust in God's goodness and God's faithfulness, in spite of human evil. The psalmist praises God for how God made us—in other words, your works are good, God! We need to acknowledge that however sinful we have been together, however sinful I have been (perhaps unwittingly), God created us. We whites need to submit to God's shaping power over our life and be willing to seek out God's ways. This paradox of human choice and God's sovereign goodness and power to redeem is the spiritual context for our challenging and often painful journey into understanding racial identity.

The Pain of Whiteness

In the Gospels, John the Baptist sends his disciples to Jesus, to discern who Jesus really is. The men come and ask him, who are you? Jesus answers them very simply: "Go and tell John what you have seen and heard . . ." (see Lk 7:18-23 or Mt 11:1-6). I am struck by Jesus' confidence, letting John and his disciples make up their mind about him based on their own observations. Do we also have courage to let our names and character be tested so simply by people's testimony to our actions and words?

Let's just admit it. It's not fun be pointed out as a white person. When we displace ourselves, we can be bombarded by our culture and by people of color with messages about whiteness, about white history, about racism, about our cultural dominance in multiethnic situations. A few years ago *Salon,* an online literary magazine, published an article called "The Unbearable Whiteness of Being." The author interviewed some white-power skinheads and wrote that for them,

> being white meant being rootless, causeless, no flag to wave, no people to feel loyal to, no one feeling loyalty to them. . . . For all their talk of racial pride, they didn't seem to like white people much. White meant weak. Greedy. Complacent. Most of all, lonely. They complained bitterly about how materialistic and bloodless white families had become.[1]

That is the skinheads, supposedly the "white pride" people.

When I read this article before the flag-waving that followed 9/11, I found myself relating to their description of white people. It shocked me to see white identity—even for a moment—the same way white supremacists see it. But how many of us who are antiracist[2] whites, deeply invested in racial reconciliation, can relate to these feelings?

My youngest sister, Holly, loves Latino people and culture. She's fair and freckled, like me, but if you closed your eyes and listened to her speak Spanish, you'd think she was Mexican. One day I asked her, "Why do you love them so much? How did this start for you?"

She told me, "Because they are alive. They have passion for life and they really love each other. They know what family and community really mean."

All of that is true, and Holly is right. But it left me wondering, *What does family mean to white people then? Where is our passion?* Most of the time the cultural and personal messages we hear about what it means to be white leave us feeling guilty, defensive or ashamed. Unfortunately, we are given very few spiritual or cultural resources to process these messages. Very few of us are reading Scripture in ways that speak into the interracial encounter from a white perspective.

Getting Whiter

As we go through the process of displacement, as we journey more and more deeply into another culture, we grow in many ways. We can feel our cross-cultural skills developing. We become more patient, more generous, more self-controlled, more kind as God grows the fruit of the Holy Spirit in our life. We know we are different people from what we were.

We might also experience some dissonance in relation to white friends and family as we grow to feel awkward in situations where previously we would have been oblivious. If we ignored racial jokes before, they bother us now. We have more awareness of the hidden messages whites convey about nonwhite people. Sometimes we feel tempted to think of ourselves as a "good white" and the others as "bad white people."

But oddly enough, even though we are growing, we begin to feel not less white but *more* white. Sooner or later, displacement will raise questions for us about white identity.

When I first enter an ethnic minority group, I always enjoy getting out of myself. I feel joyful, a fruit of the Holy Spirit. I love to learn about the other place, the other people, and celebrate the godly aspects of their culture. It's fun and stretching.

Then inevitably, as in the conflict between Doug and the church mothers, something happens that points out to me how very white I am. For white people this is a weird experience, because in an all-white group we don't notice our culture; it just operates.[3] It's in a mixed-culture group, and particularly in situations where we are in the minority, that we may be forced to notice ourselves. Anyone who is in a crosscultural situation starts to feel more aware of themselves. This is part of the social power of being in a context where we cannot fully predict what might happen and have to work hard at figuring out cultural cues and expectations.

Most of us white Americans can go a long time without the experiences that would hold up social mirrors to us. My biracial children, however, began to identify racial differences when they were toddlers. By the time they were in kindergarten, they began observing discrepancies in how often different races appeared on TV and how different people were treated according to their race. I heard questions like "Is that because he is black?" and had to wrestle with the answer. It was a shock to me as a white mother. As I sought counsel, I learned that this is very common for children of color. It had been totally unexpected for me, even though I had interacted with people of other races virtually from birth.

My family had many nonwhite friends, often in our home. At the age of two I had a black nanny. But I do not recall distinctly wrestling with the fact that I was white until I was in high school and began to observe that there were invisible racial lines drawn to indicate which guys a white girl could date.

When was the first time you realized you were white? How old were you? What were the circumstances? It probably depends somewhat on your circumstances, but many of us do not start our racial identity journey until we are truly immersed in a multiracial context. Sociologists who analyze group dynamics describe race names as a social construct, a cultural idea, not a biological one.[4] When we interact with other people who are racially different from us, they hold up social mirrors to us by naming and responding to us as individuals and as a group. What can we learn from looking in those mirrors?

Names We Are Given

When I was a teenager in Texas, black people called us "honky," which is offensive slang for a white person. It has an older meaning too. *Honky* is from the word *honq* in the West African Wolof language, and *honq* also means "red person" or "pink person."[5]

When I was a girl, my family lived in Papua New Guinea. The local people there are black; they called us "red" people because our skin turned bright red in the sun. If the white person was male, they'd call him "red boss" or "masta." That was the late 1960s; Papua New Guinea's political independence was in 1964, and colonial habits die slowly if they are not rooted out. Blacks called us a color before they learned to call us "the man" (oppressor).

There are other names for us too. I still remember the first time I was called "Slavemaster" by a black leader. My heart just ached with complaining inside that I'm a good person, that it's not fair to call me such horrible names. After he had left and I finished crying, I realized that he was making an observation about the way I was using my power: to exclude loud black people from access to the resources I controlled but allow cooperative, submissive black people access to the same resources. *Ouch.*

Now I should point out that I'd had no intention of doing that; I was simply applying values and policies that had been previously developed. It was my role that was functioning, not my values or motives. I was being "fair" about the rules. But he was correctly observing the result of my actions and calling me to account beyond my personal motives.

Once a Lakota man asked me, "Are you going to be my 'Great White Mother?'"

"Um—no . . ." I said. *I hope not,* I thought. I wanted to defend myself. *That wasn't me,* I thought. *I've treated you well, and respectfully. That was just history.* I realized long afterward that actually my friend was accurately using a power name for me as a white person. "White father" is what Native people were taught to call white leaders—both government officials and church leaders—in the 1800s, when we were systematically removing the Indian nations from America.[6]

Unfortunately, this is the history of Christian mission here in America, so it is *our* history. In his book *Missionary Conquest,* historian George Tinker documents the ways "the Christian missionaries—of all denominations working among American Indian nations—were partners in genocide."[7] Several Native American tribes, including the Hopi, have traditional cultural stories about looking for a white brother who will bring them news about God. Tragically, their experience with whites has led them to describe us as "white fathers" rather than white brothers and sisters. Today there are very, very few Christians among the Hopi.

My new friend was testing me, asking, Do you know the history? Are you also going to perpetuate that power structure, with me beneath you?

My interaction with the African American leader and with my Lakota friend is a very common experience in white-nonwhite relationships. Jane Lazarre writes of a similar interaction with her students. Her black husband, Douglas Hughes White, explains to her, "It doesn't matter what you meant." Finally she realizes:

> *It doesn't matter what you meant* when you are moving against a tide of history and social reality far more important than one white person's mistake. A white American either accepts the weight of this history or relinquishes the respect and possibility of authentic connection to Black Americans. . . . I encounter the same kinds of mistakes in my white friends, students and colleagues, and even at times in myself, all of the time. The mistake is followed quickly by a denial of its importance, as if language itself, individual words and sounds, did not have a history thick with hidden meanings not to be casually undone.[8]

Naming is not simply a current event, a choice in the moment. Naming, like all communication, exists in the context of a long history and in the wider context of white cultural practices in multiethnic interaction. We can learn a lot from it.

There are other names for us that we can learn from. We can learn from the names for a white stranger. "Stranger" could be a neutral idea or a positive one. Along the U.S.-Mexico border, though, I get called *gringa.*[9] *Gringa* literally means simply "white girl," but in Mexico it conveys the sense of an outsider—a person who is not trying to fit into the community, an ugly

American. *Güera* is a Spanish word for a white person that Mexicans use to describe only her skin color, without carrying the same ugly crosscultural connotation. *Güera* could describe my white, bicultural, bilingual sister Holly, *güero* her fair Latino husband. Interacting with Latinos, we have a choice: will I be a *gringa* or a *güera?* And this choice expresses itself in my life at every level. Will I taste the mango-pepper lollipop I'm offered? Will I submit to the teaching and correction of a Latino leader?

When I was in China as a missionary teacher, we whites were mostly called *wai guo ren,* which means "outside person." I looked very strange in China, with a high nose, light-colored hair and eyes, spots and hair on my skin. I was the only blond in the mid-sized city where I lived. One day as I was walking to the teacher's college where I worked, a little girl saw me. "Ghost demon!" she screamed (in Chinese). Her face registered total terror, and she turned and fled to her grandma, who said (in Chinese), "Yes, they are dangerous, but you can call her an 'outside person.' "

Afterward I went about trying to figure out what was being said and why, discovering both the surface and hidden meanings of the names being used about me and my people. In Chinese stories, demons are white. It was a good experience for me to be called "ghost demon" and "outside person," because it caused me to reflect more deeply on how we use names.

If you look at paintings from the European Middle Ages, of course, demons are black. One could argue that in contemporary American discourse—our papers, our TV news, most of the media—demons are still black and Latino. After 9/11 we demonized Arabs. We exclude each other by our racial categories. This is what the Bible calls partiality. When it's combined with power, it's far more dangerous.

Generally there is something to be learned from names we are called and the names we call others. It's important to address the internal response they evoke, as well as reflect on what truth lies behind the name they are using. Finally, we can bring that truth to God and pray for God's redemption. "Jesus have mercy" is, on its deepest level, a confession and a prayer for a new beginning.

Sometimes there is also confession I need to make to the other person, in order to receive their forgiveness and a chance for a new beginning in the relationship. Sometimes the sin involved is not my personal wrongdoing but a corporate sin that other whites have perpetuated. Then I have another choice. Will I have the humility to admit that I may benefit from other white people's racial sin? Will I take spiritual responsibility for my community, even if I don't see how I bear personal responsibility?

If I get to choose a name for myself, I prefer to be called "white" rather than "European American." Part of this has to do with looking unflinchingly at who we whites are as a group. Ruth Frankenburg, a white sociologist, writes in her *White Women, Race Matters: The Social Construction of Whiteness* that the term *European American* "deracializes." Using the ethnic term *European American* instead of the racial term *white* allows us to ignore the fact that we have been and still are in a position of power over people of other races. It lets us avoid the current racial hegemonic reality of white people in the United States and much of North and South America.

Frankenburg goes on to observe that whiteness or white cultural practice is—historically and currently—linked to dominance. "It is by and large the cultural practices of *white* people (though not all white people, and certainly to varying degrees) by means of which individuals in societies structured in racial dominance are asked to engage with the institutions of those societies."[10]

The White Power Club

What she is saying is critically important for us to understand. The point is not the name we choose for ourselves. The point is to recognize that it is through our race that we individual whites connect with the institutions and organizations that perpetuate whites' racial dominance.

Earlier I said that most sociologists and race studies scholars describe "race" as a social construct. That is true. But race is not a neutral social construct. It's a power club.[11] It's an idea other whites created that historically has been used to dominate and control people of color. We need to understand our racial dominance and confess it, individually and corporately. The names we get called are simply responses to our community's actions. They come from people of color standing outside the white club, looking in at us and telling us how it affects them.

I may hate the names we whites get called. They may be true or false about me as an individual. They usually cause me pain. But after wrestling with them on a deep level, I have to admit there is truth in the names. *Honky* went from meaning "red man" in precolonial independent Africa to meaning "oppressive man" in the post-Civil War South, because of many encounters between blacks and whites through the grueling years of kidnapping, sale and slavery. Likewise, *gringo* changed meanings and added its negative connotations over generations of encounters, as Mexico was forced geographically south and Mexican people were forced by the conquistadors and missionaries into working-class labor. The Hopi and other tribes, expecting a loving white brother who would introduce them more deeply to God, received a brutal and condescending "white father." Lord Jesus Christ, Son of God, have mercy on us sinners.

Along the way, white people had choices. Some of us were abolitionists; more were slave owners, and most simply ignored slavery. Sociologist Frankenburg writes about the way white racial identity is mostly claimed by white supremacists, leaving antiracist whites apparently without much of a racial genealogy.[12] There are moments of historical possibility we can remember. *How the Irish Became White* recounts one. Slavery had been illegal in Ireland since the twelfth century, when the Irish decided it was immoral to take white British prisoners of war and enslave them. Later when Irish people arrived in America, they observed the class and race structure. In the nineteenth century, sixty thousand Christians from Ireland signed a petition addressed to Irish Americans:

> The object of this address is to call your attention to the subject of SLAVERY IN AMERICA—that foul blot upon the noble institution and fair name of your adopted country. . . . America is cursed by slavery! . . . JOIN WITH THE ABOLITIONISTS EVERYWHERE! *They are the only consistent advocates of liberty.* Tell every man that you do not understand liberty for the white man, *and slavery for the black man;* that you are for LIBERTY FOR ALL, of every color, creed and country. Irishmen and Irishwomen! *Treat the colored people as your equals, as brethren.* By your memories of Ireland, continue to love liberty—hate slavery—CLING BY THE ABOLITIONISTS—and *in America you will do honor to the name of Ireland.*[13]

Most Irish Americans, however, chose not to join the abolitionists and freed slaves. They chose racism and economic opportunity over justice. It was 1842, decades before emancipation. Still, it is possible to observe that moment of choice, to look at the Christian appeal to moral values and godly cultural tradition, and wonder what would have happened if Irish immigrants to America had chosen differently.

We still have that choice today.

White and Free

Doug and I have enjoyed talking together about our experiences as white people. We both see our own racism. It's no secret; we've told you stories of how God has addressed our own racism and begun healing our racist hearts. We are learning to see the ways we join in racist structures and benefit from the choices of other whites. When we feel defensive about racism, thinking, *It wasn't me,* or *It's not that bad,* we look again. We ask ourselves, *Are there ways we benefit from what other whites have done?*

But we are free of white shame and guilt. We are free because when we are guilty, we admit it. We confess racial sin before God, and God forgives us. This sin grieves us and we mourn. We confess it before the people we personally have sinned against or those our group has sinned against. People of color are often willing to forgive us also. They almost always appreciate our telling the truth. It is very freeing to be forgiven.

If we feel ashamed about being white or about white racism, we ask God to give us a new vision of ourselves and others who are godly whites. What was God's intent in creating white people? It does not honor God or restore relationships for us to live in defensiveness, shame or guilt. We look for ways to join God in replacing the "moving sidewalk" of our racist culture with our own intentional antiracist choices. We look for ways to begin restoring what our people have broken, to make active, specific commitments to racial reconciliation and racial justice.

One day as Doug and I were sitting in Starbucks, we realized that we both have nonwhite friends and family who call us "white with a [colored] heart." Perhaps it seems unusual. We think it's simply an acknowledgment of commitment.

Recently I was at a birthday party for a friend and heard a black woman there call a white woman "sister" in front of the interracial group. It wasn't in passing: she went on to talk about their commitment to each other. The white woman beamed. She was clearly thrilled. It is wonderful to be received in this way.

As you commit yourself to allowing God to heal you from your personal racism and to loving people of color, as you commit yourself to allowing God to heal you from our communal racism and as you learn to do justice, God will go before you, and there will be great rewards.

MAKING ANTIRACISM REAL

Because racism is so complex and subtle, it's important that you ask God to show you the truth about your heart and broader racial patterns in society. Start with your heart, and move on to your understanding of history and the racial groups around you. Being confronted with our racism can produce different reactions in our heart.

1. We can defend ourselves, either personally or as a group. Ask God, "Is any of it true?" Examine your heart. Do you have *any* racial sin in your heart? Have you ever been hardhearted toward people of color? "You do well if you really fulfill the royal law according to the scripture, 'You shall love your neighbor as yourself.' But if you show partiality, you commit sin and are convicted by the law as transgressors. For whoever keeps the whole law but fails in one point has become accountable for all of it" (Jas 2:8-10).

   Is there any wrong we whites as a group have perpetuated? Start there, with any racial sin the Holy Spirit brings to your mind. Scripture says, " 'Because of the oppression of the weak and the groaning of the needy, I will now arise,' says the LORD. 'I will protect them from those who malign them' " (Ps 12:5 NIV). Ask God to give you a soft heart for everything that grieves God. Ask God to show you what is true about racism in America.
2. We can see our guilt. Once we are able to face what we have done personally and corporately, how do we get racism out of our life? Paul talks about guilt in 2 Corinthians 7:10: "For godly grief produces a repentance that leads to salvation and brings no regret, but worldly grief produces death." Godly grief is a heart that mourns, and the person who experi-

ences it is willing to repent. When you start to feel guilty, ask God to show you what the sin is. What do you need to repent for? Confess your sin to God. When you identify the specific sin, ask God to show you what godly habit to put in its place. Ask God to make you racially holy again. Ask God to show you what acts of righteousness and justice you should practice in place of your sin.

3. We can get caught in shame or "white guilt." White guilt isn't the true spiritual guilt that leads to repentance and freedom. It is a passive feeling of shame about being white. If we feel ashamed of being white, we are not confessing specific sin, replacing it with good choices and letting God restore us. Because we don't know how to transform those feelings of shame into life-giving repentance, we avoid the truth of our past and our present. We cannot handle the truth until we learn to repent. Feeling bad about ourselves doesn't help us, and it doesn't help our ethnic minority sisters and brothers. If you feel being white is bad, generally, ask God to show you the truth about white people and about yourself. There is some sin: what is it? It needs to be confessed and replaced with righteousness and justice. There are also some godly characteristics: what are they?

After you are honest before God and repent for what racism is in your heart, you are more ready to let God show you what is true about racism in our society. We can address aware/overt racism and aware/covert racism. If we are aware of it, we can more clearly replace the wrong with right. We replace greed with generosity. We replace intentional exclusion with intentional inclusion.

Most of us well-intentioned whites engage in more subtle types of racism that are hard for us to see. But God sends questions to our conscience, and we can learn to act on them instead of squelching them. If we don't see injustice, we can ask God to restore our racial conscience, to help us "see" racism.

Remember the special ed tester asking the first-generation Mexican American kids to make PBJs? Holly, the teacher, had to listen to other voices than the white expert's. She had to listen to her experience with the Latino kids and their parents. Remember Kevin, the white guy who couldn't quite believe Charles's experience of racism was real, because it had never happened to Kevin? Start looking for those kinds of situations, where white people and people of color are having two different experiences. Put on 3-D glasses; ask more questions of the situation.

Systemic racism, Beverly Tatum's "moving sidewalk," is found in a racist system that was set up a long time ago and works on our behalf. In order to start seeing how it works, you'll have to learn more about the history of various racial groups in America. Choose any people group and read the history of their interaction with whites—for example, *Bury My Heart at Wounded Knee: An Indian History of the American West,* or a history of slave owning like *Slaves in the Family.* Don't simply read it quickly for information; read it slowly before God. Ask God, "Please show me what we have done that offends you." Grieve the wrongs you read about, and repent of them in your daily prayers.

People get hurt easily in the multiethnic journey, and we white people are quick to give up. We call it "racial fatigue," but that is just a fancy label for unresolved pain. The cross of Jesus is enough for all our pain. We just keep coming to Jesus and let him heal our wounds.

The world is full of guilt-ridden, deflated white people who stop with false guilt and don't replace wrong choices with right ones. We need a generation of empowered, humble white people. But there is only one path to such freedom in Christ, and that is ongoing repentance, humility, self-awareness and a learner's posture.

Please learn to enjoy the process of repentance and transformation, because the only way to gain life is to lose life for Jesus' sake.

We pray, Jesus,
that truth about white people will be spoken
and truth will be received.
Keep us from the temptation of denial.
Give us the grace to look in the mirrors that are held up to us.
Give us the strength to fully listen to who people say we are,
as you were willing to do.
Teach us whites to see ourselves and to see our culture.
Teach us to discern where there is sin that we need to confess.
Give us daily the strength to repent.
Give us daily the faith to trust you to cleanse us from sin.
Give us daily the spiritual power to act in new ways.

Teach us to discern where there are seeds of godly choices in ourselves
and godly choices in our culture.
Give us the gratitude to praise you for the godliness that is within us.
Teach us to celebrate and build on the good you have put in us.
Lord, we pray with faith in your power
that you would mold us,
as white people, into the image of Jesus. Amen.

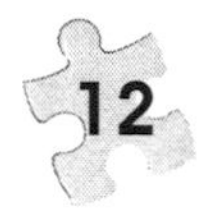

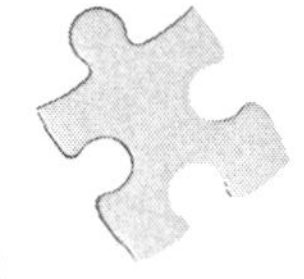

Can God Redeem White Culture?

Doug Schaupp

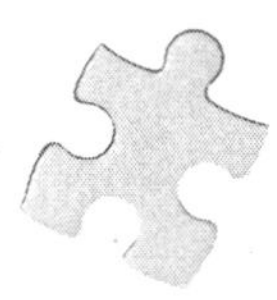

In the independent movie *My Big Fat Greek Wedding,* the bride is from a large extended family that had moved from Greece a few decades earlier. Her family is funny, loud, opinionated, vibrant, up-in-each-other's-business and generally winsome. They are quirky, but that is what makes them flavorful, compelling and attractive. You want to be around them, even though they are a bit of a handful.

On the groom's side, his parents are weak at conversation, awkward, private and bland. They are passive and boring. Who wants to be like them? Going to their house for dinner looks like cruel and unusual punishment. It seems the single best thing that has ever happened to these sheltered country-club members is to be loosened up by being forced to relate to the dynamic Greek family.

How do you feel as a white person seeing that movie? The ethnic Greek family, albeit flawed, was a hundred times more intriguing than the WASP parents. Do you ever feel like a bland white person in the midst of a truly flavorful multiethnic world?

Sometimes people at the local coffee shop ask me what I am writing as I bang away at my laptop. When they find out I am working on a book, they inevitably ask, "What is it about?"

Hmmm. How do I answer that question concisely? I usually answer by saying, "This book is for white people who have extended ourselves across ethnic lines and discover that everyone else seems to have a strong, well-defined set of cultural values. But when we look at ourselves, we ask, 'What culture do I have? What are my ethnic values anyway?'"

This description of the book often triggers a curious, pensive expression. One guy confessed, "I ask those questions every day of my life." Another woman declared, "I need to read that book."

Because many of us have that hunger, Paula and I thought about putting this chapter at the beginning of the book. Instead we place it here because we think this part of the discussion makes most sense once you have committed yourself to regularly cross racial lines. As we love other ethnic groups, understanding our cultural values and thus growing in self-awareness becomes a crucial act of love. *After* you have displaced yourself, it is fitting and natural to ask, "Who then am I as a white person? What do we bring to the table?" These are pivotal questions.

Many voices are telling us conflicting things about being white. Some say, "As long as you are white, you don't bring anything except problems." On the other hand, there are still some white supremacist voices that say being white is God's best gift. What do you say? Where do you fall on the spectrum between racial self-hatred on the one extreme and the KKK on the other? We come to this discussion from different places in the journey of white identity development.

After my sophomore year in college, I spent my first summer in another country. Although I had good intentions, I'm sure I was a pain in the neck for the teammates who had to put up with me for those six weeks in Mexico City. One of them finally had enough of my anti-U.S. complaints and confronted me: "Doug, do you think there is anything good about the United States?"

I paused to reflect. My teammates and I were all aware of the slowness of mail delivery in Mexico. In all seriousness, I said, "Why, yes. I like it that the United States delivers mail on time."

Since that time I have come to identify thousands of things that I appreciate about my country. You will see some of them later in this chapter.

Why was I able to find only one thing that I liked about my home country when I was a sophomore? I was pursuing a political science major, and I had spent a lot of time reading about mistakes our country had made both domestically and internationally. I was embarrassed about the downsides of our history. My coping mechanism was to emotionally distance myself from my country of origin and take on a jaded, critical mindset.

Similarly, in the years since I have found it far easier to pinpoint the downsides of being a white American than to have a balanced assessment of our culture and heritage. I thus began this journey unknowingly making my home in the self-hatred camp.

Why is this important for you to know? As I write about the wonderful things of God in our culture, I am being stretched in a whole new direction. Maybe for you it is easy to identify the things that make you confident about being white or being American. But if you're like me, this topic is a bit awkward.

THE WAY GOD WORKS

Paula has delved into the systems of white racism. What do we do with awareness of these things? In the Bible I've found a significant point of hope for our white identity.

In Genesis when God made humans, he placed us in a garden, his idea of perfection and utopia for us. Despite God's lavish provision, we decided to try life on our own terms. The moment Adam and Eve turned their backs on God, a horrible tearing happened: between us and God, between us and creation, and between one another. An awareness of human frailty crushed Adam and Eve. What would they do now that they had told God that they could handle life on their own? They would have to protect themselves. Their first act of self-protection was to sew fig leaves together as clothes, so that their shame would not be utterly overwhelming.

In Genesis 4 the line of Cain and the line of Abel reflect two ways of living in a post-Fall reality. Abel is snuffed out, and we see what comes of Cain's descendants. Scrambling to make a life for themselves, Cain's family built the first city (4:17), became ranchers (4:20), created music (4:21) and forged tools (4:22). In case we are not sure what to make of the industriousness of Cain's lineage, the next verse removes any ambiguity. We see in Lamech the ruthless and self-protective spirit of the Cain family line. "I have killed a man for wounding me, a young man for striking me. If Cain is avenged sevenfold, truly Lamech seventy-sevenfold" (4:23-24). Lamech and his family do not have a God who will protect them, so he protects them by using his own strength and by the crafting of civilization.

If I had only the first five chapters of the Bible and had to guess how the rest of it would unfold, I might guess that God would abolish the city—center of civilization—as a symbol of rebellion, and heaven would be an idyllic scene of Eden revisited. But that isn't the way God works. God's glory is multiplied precisely because he can redeem that which was produced for human self-justification and infuse it with heaven. God's ability to enter into our depravity and brokenness is seen in that the new utopia is our rebellion redeemed. Heaven is not Eden revisited; it is the city perfected (see Rev 3:12; 21:2; 22:14). Without a doubt, God can be trusted to redeem the fruits of human pride and rebellion.[1]

Our God who can redeem the city can also redeem brutal suffering and evil. That gives me great cause for hope and joy. As I, a white man, submit to God and walk in the path of repentance, God can take something that my ancestors meant for oppression and transform it into something good. As I learn humility and servanthood, God can redeem the best parts of my white heritage and use them for kingdom blessing. The sin of my ancestors does not have to be the final word regarding my identity and my life. As I walk with Jesus, he can transform my depravity into something beautiful. Being white can be beautiful too.

How can we identify and affirm the kingdom values that are sovereignly embedded in white *ethnos*?[2] Every culture, including ours, has a God-given upside that echoes biblical values. We must not be ashamed of the positive values embedded in our ethnic DNA. On the flip side, every culture, including ours, has a warped downside that we have used for evil and that God sorely needs to redeem. As we look at white values, we must be aware that any cultural strength can be (and has been) warped, abused and taken to an unhealthy extreme.

What then are the kingdom gems God has placed in white culture?[3] In what ways is God bringing good out of our culture? What are the strengths in our culture which reflect the priorities of God and for which we should praise God?[4] Since many white Americans today are generally not accustomed to celebrating the distinctive values and customs of our culture, and since we come from many different ethnic heritages (from Greek to WASP, Swedish to South African), there is no consensus about which values are particularly *white*. Where then are we to turn?

In my experience, the most successful approach for discovering our cultural strengths is storytelling about our families. In several InterVarsity conferences for white American students, we have divided into small groups and discussed the question, "What are the positive values that have been passed on to you from your parents or grandparents?" This question creates a great discussion, and a surprising sense of commonality emerges through stories and illustrations.

Try it now! Get out a pen or pencil and jot down a quick phrase or memory in response to each of the following questions.

1. What kinds of positive values did your parents imprint on you while you were growing up? What did they emphasize repeatedly?
2. How did your family handle money? What did your family teach you about finances when you were growing up?
3. What has your family taught you about hard work? How do (or did) your parents approach work?
4. What did you learn about your ability to choose a direction in life? What happened when you disagreed with your parents about your career plans, your lifestyle choices or your relationships?
5. What did you learn in your family about education? What did your parents or grandparents say about that while you were growing up?
6. What is your family's style of taking risks or being innovative? How does your family approach problem solving?
7. How did your family feel about the need to be fair and equitable? If you had siblings, how was each of you treated?
8. How does your family feel about cheering for the underdog?

As we have discussed questions like these with other white people, we have often found agreement in values by telling positive family stories. Let me quickly add that many of our families have also been places of pain and shame, not just good values. For those of us who have high levels of brokenness in our families, this exercise may not be very helpful. Also, if you are like me, you can think of white people who don't fit these general trends, or you can think of socioeconomic variables that limit the accuracy of generalizations. I can quickly think of ways that all these cultural traits have been abused and turned into tools of evil too. This chapter will be helpful only if you put on a "sociologist hat" and allow yourself to observe general trends in your family and beyond. Of course at many times white people have not lived up to these values. And there are certainly other cultures that share these values. We do not have a corner on the market.[5] In the exploration that follows, I will rely heavily on anecdotes from my family, since it has been my main source of cultural values.

1. The Importance of Self-Determination

All my life, my parents have told me that I can be whatever I want to be. They have played the role of cheerleaders, encouraging me to dream big dreams and then to pursue them. Their role as they saw it was not to tell me what path to walk on but rather to gently encourage me to walk on whatever good path I might desire.

As a sophomore and junior in college, I came to believe I should follow Jesus' model of a life of generosity, of sharing all I had. My parents had kindly loaned me a family car because I was 350 miles away at school. I let them know that I was loaning out the car to my college friends as an act of generosity. My family did not make a practice of loaning out our cars. After several intense phone conversations, I expected they would take the car away from me. But my dad did the opposite. Though he did not agree with my practices, he graciously upgraded our auto insurance so that I could continue to pursue my conviction about generosity without exposing my parents to risky liability. This was a very supportive move by my parents, as they accommodated my strange lifestyle decision instead of controlling it. All my life they have played this role: "We support you in what you think is best for your life and future."

Throughout my youth and my formal education, my parents encouraged me to try all kinds of sports, music, drama and leadership activities. They made it clear that a good education for life goes beyond academics. School was never merely for training my mind; it was for opening doors of exploration so that I would become a well-rounded "Renaissance person." By exposing me to many opportunities, they helped me discern what I like and who God has created me to be.

Our parents do not want to play the role of tyrant or monarch in our lives. Since the Revolutionary War, we Americans carry a sense deep in our collective psyche that this is to be avoided at all costs. "Modern individualism emerged out of the struggle against monarchical and aristocratic authority that seemed arbitrary and oppressive to citizens prepared to assert the right to govern themselves."[6]

In God's hands, our self-determination is a gift, but on our own, it becomes a form of arrogance and self-deception. In Luke 15 Jesus tells the story of the "prodigal son." How does the father respond when his youngest son wants to throw his life away? Instead of trying to control his son and force him down a particular life path, the father allows the son to choose his own path, though surely his poor decisions would cost him dearly in due time. God graciously allows us to walk our own path. Self-determination is worth the risk of bad decision making.

2. The Significance of the Individual

White Americans believe that each person, if they put their mind to it, has the potential to be a catalyst for great change. Ours is a very low "power distance" culture in which any individual can challenge or offer an opinion to any person in a power position.[7] We uphold the ideal that everyone has the right to speak their mind and thereby shape society. We honor individuals who go against the grain and stand up for their convictions, even though they may stand alone.

Something deep in me has always hoped to amount to something. From time to time a voice in me says, *Doug, it's time to step up, to trust God and believe him for the impossible. It is okay if you are the only one with this vision, because it is more important to do the right thing than to fit in with everyone else.* You and I are built to believe that God can work in and through an individual.

The LORD saw that the wickedness of humankind was great in the

> earth, and that every inclination of the thoughts of their hearts was only evil continually. And the LORD was sorry that he had made humankind on the earth, and it grieved him to his heart. So the LORD said, "I will blot out from the earth the human beings I have created—people together with animals and creeping things and birds of the air, for I am sorry that I have made them." But Noah found favor in the sight of the LORD. (Gen 6:5-8)

One person, Noah, made an impact on God as he pondered how to deal with the earth, and Noah shaped human history.

3. The Entrepreneurial Spirit and Problem Solving

Growing up, when I ran into an impasse or a seemingly impossible situation, I would go to my dad for help. Each time Dad would hook me with the same response: "That would be a difficult problem for the average person, but not for someone exceptional like you. You will be able to solve that problem in a snap." Although this answer was infuriating at the time, I did begin to believe it was true.

My parents themselves lived by this type of life philosophy. When they were first married, they read a book called *How to Turn $1,000 into $1,000,000 in Your Spare Time*. Its premise was that someone who invests $1,000 in rental income property at age twenty will be worth $10,000 at age thirty, $100,000 at age forty and $1 million by age fifty. My parents followed the book's advice carefully, and through hard work and entrepreneurial risk taking, they gained the results that the book promised. This success forged a sense of optimism in them about problem solving and risk taking, which they in turn have passed to us, the next generation of problem solvers. Some people call this the "can-do" attitude.

Our focus on problem solving and innovative solutions leads to an uncommon level of freedom to fail. Thomas Friedman sees this on a wider scale, quoting a Silicon Valley venture capitalist: "The view here is that you are always better and wiser for having failed. . . . People say, 'Oh, he went bankrupt on that first venture? I bet he learned something from that, so I'll bankroll him again.'"[8] We want people to try new ways to solve problems.[9]

Proverbs 31:10-32 describes an amazingly resourceful woman. She does not wait for anyone to give her permission to create a side business and break into the garment industry. As she works hard day and night, she translates her initial successes into the opportunity to buy land. "She considers a field and buys it; with the fruit of her hands she plants a vineyard" (Prov 31:16).

4. The Belief That Hard Work Is Important

My parents have a strong work ethic. They don't complain about long hours or the rigors of work. My siblings and I all had assigned chores each week; we didn't like them, but we knew it was just part of being family. Our parents didn't have to beat the value of work into my head, they just modeled it.

When I was in junior high, I got my first job, selling door to door. When I was in high school, my dad said to us kids, "How would you like to have the experience of starting your own business? We could start a wholesale sunglasses business." We didn't know any better, so we agreed to the plan. The first year was grueling as we went from store to store, trying to convince each owner to put our plastic rack of $3.99 sunglasses on his or her counter. We were rejected ten times for every one time we got a customer. But by the second year we had a strong base of stores that carried our product, and I could see how the hard work had paid off. I am very grateful that appreciation for work is a basic part of my life, passed down from generations before me.

In their seminal book *Habits of the Heart,* Robert Bellah and colleagues look into the soul of America past and present and identify the basic motivation to "'make something of yourself' through work."[10] Richard Brookhiser also observes this trend in our past. "One of Herbert Hoover's cousins once asked their grandmother if it was true that they were related to John Wesley, and got the following response: 'What matter if we descended from the highest unless we are something ourselves? Get busy.'"[11] Hoover's grandmother, like my grandmother, would not let anyone rest on status or reputation.

"In all toil there is profit, but mere talk leads only to poverty" (Prov

14:23). In God's kingdom there is a high regard for all work, and we pursue it with joy.

5. Deferred Gratification and Fiscal Integrity

When my friend Nate was growing up, his parents put three jars on his shelf: one for God, one for savings and one for spending. Every time he got money, he had to divide it equally between the three jars. Sandy and I have adopted this three-jar policy and do the same thing with our five-year-old son.

When I was growing up, my parents encouraged me to put any money I was given into my savings account. Instead of buying a candy bar, I learned to postpone gratification and save up for the stereo, the scooter or the new pair of skis. I got my first credit card in junior high, but I seldom used it.[12]

Throughout my youth, my parents owned rental property, but they had me convinced that our family was barely above the poverty line. We literally bought all our clothes at Goodwill and secondhand stores. Kmart was too expensive for us. When we went to McDonald's®, we were permitted to order only two hamburgers and a milk; fries and soda were entirely out of our price range.

Looking back, I don't remember being upset about this. I honestly thought we were just scraping by. Recently my dad was mistaken for a homeless man at the coffee shop he frequents. He is certainly not homeless, but he cares so little about how he looks that he could pass for it. This part of my ethnic heritage has been a tremendous gift to me.

Scripture says, "Go to the ant, you lazybones; consider its ways, and be wise. Without having any chief or officer or ruler, it prepares its food in summer, and gathers its sustenance in harvest" (Prov 6:6-8). Why do ants save their food instead of consuming it on the spot? God has somehow implanted in them an instinct to defer gratification and save up their food for when they will need it most.

6. A Strong Conscience for Fairness

Being fair is one of my mom and dad's highest parenting values. If they do something for one of us children, they are adamant about doing the same for the rest of us. Having any bias toward one child is anathema to them. Playing favorites is seen as extremely unfair and even hurtful.

I went to a small private college, and they paid my tuition. My brother and sister attended state schools, and their (lower) tuition was paid as well. When we had all finished college, my parents wrote them checks making up the difference. Mom and Dad were determined to be absolutely fair by us. To this day they are careful to count how much money they spend on each of us and even how much time they spend with us.

One of my heroes of fairness is our first president, George Washington. Garry Wills in *Certain Trumpets* highlights attributes of Washington's character that are worth emulating. Wills argues that it would have been easy for Washington to become a dictator rather than to bow out of office after two terms.

> Washington's refusal to bring about a strong central government by seizing power is his greatest legacy to the nation. . . . He wielded power by yielding it. . . . His accomplishment was so great and unusual that it is hard to estimate at its true worth. . . . During the early struggles of the nation, Washington was himself the unifying icon, the symbol of the whole process. He had to replace his own glamour with the more impersonal symbols of power—the Constitution, the flag, the offices of government, the courts.[13]

Washington was a man of discipline, conscience and convictions that drove him to value fairness to his country over personal gain and prominence. Brookhiser uses the terms *conscience* and *civic-mindedness* to describe these white traits. "In societies ruled by conscience, people stop for red lights at three o'clock in the morning. In societies with less alert monitors, people drive on the sidewalk."[14]

Scripture puts it, "A false balance is an abomination to the LORD, but an accurate weight is his delight" (Prov 11:1). Buying and trading in biblical times was done with a system of scales and balances. It was tempting to rig the balances so that you could get more money out of a transaction, and no one would know if the scales were a bit biased. God, who sees all things, calls us to exercise self-control and integrity, to be the same people in private that we are when everyone is looking.

Cultural Gifts

You may relate to all or some of these values. In my experience these are key elements of our white *ethnos,* and I believe God has woven these values into our culture because they echo some biblical values. As we explore these and other values in our ethnic heritage, we must recognize that God's gracious hand has given us these good gifts. All cultures reflect God in important ways and also reflect the fallenness of our humanity. White culture is like any other in this.

We need to praise God for how he has placed kingdom gems in every culture, including our own. As you and I allow God to humble us and redeem our ethnic "junk," these kingdom gems become brighter and more able to serve the whole body of Christ. We have a tendency to misuse, spoil and at times hurt people with God's gifts. But this is not God's intention. He is working to redeem our culture and thereby teach us to serve humbly with what he has given us.

13

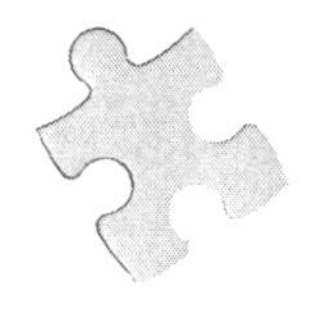

Finding Our White Identity in Christ

Doug Schaupp

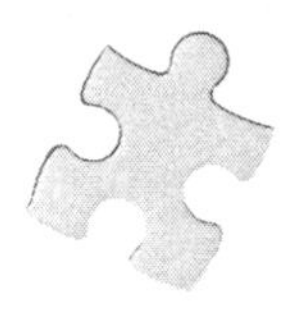

I was a speaker at a conference for white college students called "Rooting Our White Identity in Jesus." I began my session by asking the group of seventy students, "How many of you struggle with feeling bad about yourselves for being white?" Without hesitation, the majority of hands shot into the air.

I then asked, "Would a few of you please share a story with us?"

One woman said, "I was taking a Latino Studies class. The TA approached me and told me, 'Since you are white, you cannot speak in class.'"

I probed: "How did that make you feel? How did you respond?"

She confessed, "I felt terrible about myself. I felt condemned. I just sat through the class hating it."

A handful of others told of similar experiences of feeling guilty for the color of their skin. They talked about being frozen in shame, anger, resentment and confusion. They were unsure how to be themselves as white people.

What has happened to us white people? Would you have raised your hand?

Foundations of White Identity

I went on to ask the students, "What has been pivotal for you in the foundation of your white identity?" This was a much harder question for them to answer. Many had never been conscious of any process of forming their ethnic identity.

Turning to the Scripture, we discussed Romans 12:1-2, which commands us to not be conformed to the voices around us but rather to let God transform our minds and hearts according to the kingdom of God. Since there are many strong opinions today about how we are supposed to feel about being white, it is easy to be conformed to the wrong things. We must not conform to and base our identity on criticism of our ethnicity. Instead we need (and long) to be transformed by God and rooted in his kingdom perspective on us.

God infused our gathering with a new passion to become proactive and discern how to build a healthy identity as white people.

What complicates the process of developing our ethnic identity in Jesus is that we are surrounded by clamoring voices. If we are not thoughtful and intentional about which voices we listen to, we will by default conform our white identity to the loudest voices.

We are faced with two challenges. The first challenge to live well as white people is discerning what Jesus has in mind for us within his kingdom. The second challenge is "abiding in the vine" (see Jn 15:4) and abiding in biblical passages; this is the one antidote to being conformed to the world. Lest we be lulled into thinking that this process is automatic, the author of Hebrews urges us to gear up for a tough battle. "Take care, brothers and sisters, that none of you may have an evil, unbelieving heart that turns away from the living God. But exhort one another every day, as long as it is called 'today,' so that none of you may be hardened by the deceitfulness of sin" (Heb 3:12-13).

The Pressure of Partial Truths

Most of the students at the conference struggled with feeling bad about themselves. Using the language of Hebrews, we could say that they were struggling with unbelieving hearts, hearts that were locked onto partial truths instead of abiding in the truth of Scripture. Partial truths had made their hearts and minds discouraged and hazy.

Picture a pool table with pockets on the sides and in the corners. Except this pool table is not flat; it is bowed up in the middle, so that the pool balls all naturally roll away from the center toward the pockets.

In the center of this picture is life in the kingdom of God. This is where we white followers of Jesus want to abide, find joy and root our identity in the truth about ourselves in Christ. We are the pool balls, and though we try to hold to the truths about ourselves in Christ, we easily roll to the sides of the table. The pockets are partial truths that sound true and appear believable: cluelessness, defensiveness, cheap grace, pride, passivity, the language of awareness, and shame and condemnation. These traps keep our minds deceived so we fail to see the truth about God and ourselves.

There is no particular order to which hole we find ourselves in on a given day. Pick your poison. We struggle with different things at various seasons of life. It could be any or all of the following seven partial truths.

1. Cluelessness. The partial truth of this corner says, "We need to overlook race and ethnicity and just get along with each other. We already make too big of a deal about this ethnic stuff. Can't we all just get along?" Some of us live in the clueless partial truth because we have never been in a crosscultural situation or relationship. But the rest of us have chosen to live under this half-truth because we prefer it.

Remember Kevin in chapter ten, who couldn't accept his friend Charles's experience of racism? Kevin is a classic example of the way we choose to put on white blinders when we are confronted with facts that do not jive with our rosy worldview. We say, "Because I have not seen this type of thing, it cannot exist."

That is not the way of the kingdom. As Jesus tells his good Samaritan story, he makes it clear that a pivotal difference between the religious leaders who avoid the suffering man and the Samaritan who is a neighbor is the word *saw:* "When he saw him, he was moved with pity" (Lk 10:33). If Kevin had not taken off his blinders, he would not have been able to see and have pity.[1] If we are going to be a neighbor, we must open our eyes and let God change our heart.

2. Defensiveness. This partial truth whispers in our ear, "Don't listen to them. They don't know you. They don't know what you have been through. You are more committed than they think." Defensiveness quickly parades before our mind's eye the ways we have already grown. We resent people who question this or make us feel bad about being white. Defensiveness makes us resentful and bitter.

3. ***Cheap grace.*** This partial truth sounds so legitimate. We know there are problems with the world. We know we are not perfect. As soon as we feel pangs of guilt, we quickly cast ourselves on the mercy of Jesus. "There is no condemnation in Christ Jesus. So any feelings of guilt or condemnation are not of God. I'm forgiven by the blood of Jesus. I don't need to look at sin in my life. I just need to accept forgiveness by faith." With cheap grace, "no contrition is required, still less any real desire to be delivered from the sin."[2] This kind of self-talk aborts the work of the Spirit in our life. God wants to do something profound in us, but we keep him at arm's length with this mentality.

4. ***Pride.*** This voice says, "No one gave you a hand up in life. Your family made it this far by hard work and determination. Anyone who really applies himself or herself can do just as well as you have."

Obviously, a strong work ethic and resourcefulness are very desirable, and they are honored in Scripture (see Prov 31:10-31). But this partial truth is slippery, because it blinds us to all the ways we have indeed been helped to get where we are. "What do you have that you did not receive? And if you received it, why do you boast as if it were not a gift?" (1 Cor 4:7). The truth is that God and people have poured gifts into our lives since the day we were born. We are not self-made people. We are the result of a massive investment by our families and many people.

5. ***Passivity.*** This is one of the most lethal voices for us white people. It says, "What difference can you make? You know how hopeless this whole racial mess is. Don't bother with it. If you talk about it, people will only get their feelings hurt once again. Just let it slide." Or else it masks itself behind the politically correct movement: "It is important for you to be sensitive to others. Don't say offensive things. Watch your language. If you just avoid saying racist things, the whole thing will go away." We become discouraged, frozen, fearful and defeated, yet we may not even know it.

6. ***The language of awareness.*** There is one more insidious area, which borders on the kingdom of God. We are told by wise friends to read books, watch documentaries and gain knowledge about the past and today. There are tremendous things to be gained from reading a book. Obviously Paula and I hope that *our* book proves helpful! However, my reading a book and then employing new words does not guarantee that I am more loving, more courageous, more humble or more free to follow Jesus wherever he leads.

As you become more educated in crosscultural dynamics, please be properly apprehensive of making awareness your goal. It is not an end in itself but a step on the way. Our goal is courageous obedience to Jesus in all the fullness of his kingdom. The right words without obedience are cheap.

7. Shame and condemnation. This partial truth says, "White people have done so many bad things in history and even today that you should just feel terrible about yourself. That is the only fitting state for you." When we think of ourselves as white people, we are ashamed and paralyzed. This is a particularly difficult struggle for us. It sometimes leads to ethnic self-hatred, wishing we were another ethnic group.

The apostle Paul says that we have two choices when we feel guilty: "For godly grief produces a repentance that leads to salvation and brings no regret, but worldly grief produces death" (2 Cor 7:10). In my experience, the easiest emotional reaction to seeing my mistakes and shortcomings is to plunge into worldly grief and regret. Sliding into the pit of worldly guilt can be very subtle. The next thing I know I feel terrible about myself.

In chapter ten I recounted taking part in a group that was lectured at by a white participant about our weaknesses as white people. What was our reaction to her words? To quietly stew in white resentment. We were offended by being put once again in the pit of worldly regret. That pit does not open out to life, and we are tired of living there.

Unfortunately, once we get sick of the pit of white shame, it is tempting to set our defensiveness up against it "so you can't send me there again."

An Integrated Kingdom Identity

Partial truths, though powerful, do not have the final word. Jesus is stronger than any partial truth. Jesus gives us his Spirit so we can choose for his kingdom over and over again. We do not need to settle for bouncing between those traps.

You and I are learning to find our place in our multiethnic world. If we are to live with joy, courage, compassion and conviction in multiethnic settings, it is essential that we discern God's voice amidst the cacophony of other voices. We know the voice of our Good Shepherd. He calls us by name, and we are determined to heed him alone. His is the only voice that gives us life and sets us free.

Here is an attempt at picturing an integrated identity in Jesus amidst multiethnic realities. Five kingdom values will particularly aid us in our ethnic identity development.[3] On the pool table, these five values would be clustered together on the raised center, where we long to reside. Our home is found in humility, long-suffering love, community, empowerment for engagement and freedom in Christ.

1. Humility. Jesus gives us a very helpful tool for our growth in humility in Luke 14:7-11, in the form of instructions on seating at a wedding reception. As is common in such events, the guests take mental note of who gets to sit closest to the people being honored. Jesus' analogy taps into one of the most visceral parts of being human. *Am I being honored, or am I being shamed? How do I compare to the others around me in this situation? I wish I were getting recognized too.*

Fortunately, Jesus has an excellent remedy for people who struggle with comparison. "Do not sit down at the place of honor. . . . But when you are invited, go and sit down at the lowest place, so that when your host comes, he may say to you, 'Friend, move up higher' " (Lk 14:8, 10).

As white people, we have inherited the seat of honor in our world. (This will be explored at length in chapter sixteen.) It is tempting to stay put in our place of privilege, but Jesus says that's not a very good idea. Jesus promises that it will go well for those who go out of their way to choose a position of humility. "For all who exalt themselves will be humbled, and those who humble themselves will be exalted" (Lk 14:11). We have our Lord's reliable promise that if we step into humility, we will be exalted by him in due time.

In my experience, humility is not much fun. It is not the natural instinct of my heart. One day I was stirred, though, as I read about a monk from St. Francis of Assisi's community who was falsely accused of rebellion against the government. As people brought accusations against him, he would merely respond, "I am worse than you think." Fortunately, St. Francis himself happened upon the scene just as the authorities were about to execute this humble prisoner, and was able to save him.

Humility does not stand up for itself. Humility is not defensive. Humility agrees with Jesus as he uncovers the evil and racism inside each one of us. "It is from within, from the human heart, that evil intentions come. . . . All these evil things come from within, and they defile a person" (Mk 7:21-23). Humility welcomes the conviction of the Holy Spirit. Once we embrace the truth that we are inherently broken and fearful beings, we can drop our defenses and give Jesus permission to transform any areas of our lives that he wants to address.

Last year I was talking with Angela,[4] an African American friend. At one point she said, "There is something I need to clear up with you. I really should have talked to you about this two years ago, so let me begin this conversation by apologizing for not being prompt in resolving issues with you."

My heart stopped for a moment. *What on earth is she going to bring up with me? What did I do?*

Angela continued, "Do you remember several years ago when I was eating Thai food with you and Sandy? Well, you told me that the kind of ministry I do is really worthless, a basic waste of time. Your comment really hurt me. Why did you say that?"

I was shocked. My mind raced through my recollections of that dinner, what the restaurant looked like, what we talked about. Though parts of the conversation were vivid in my memory, I had no memory of saying anything like that.

Defensiveness jumped up into my throat. My options ran through my head: *Why would I be so insulting to someone I respect? I don't think I said anything like that.* But I bit my tongue. I remembered St. Francis's friend. I remembered Jesus calling me to the lowly seat of humility. I chose to submit to Angela's memory of the interaction instead of mine, because I know I can have a selective memory that thinks only the best of me.

I responded, "I am so sorry I said that to you. I have no idea why I said that. But I do know that I struggle with self-justification. And I sometimes put other people down in order to try and feel better about myself. I am so embarrassed that I made you feel small so that I could make myself feel big. That was terrible. I honestly do not have any firsthand experiences with the kind of ministry that you do. How dare I pass judgment on something I have never seen! Thank you for having the courage to bring it to my attention. I respect you more for that. Please forgive me for sinning against you." She was very gracious, and she forgave me.

Did I do the right thing? What would you have said?

Humility does need to go hand in hand with empowerment and freedom, which we will explore later in this chapter. But I believe that in this conversation Jesus was offering me an opportunity to take the lowly seat, to embrace humility and to reiterate to my friend what I already know to be true about myself: I am a sinner, I am self-deceived. She didn't have to convince me of any of these things, because I already knew them about myself. Once I saw Jesus inviting me to humility, it was no longer a battle of who could remember the conversation better. Because of the presence of Jesus, my repentance was sincere and honest.

White people need to become comfortable with giving up power in relationships, with having people call us on our sin and with assuming the posture of a learner. Humility is a wonderful kingdom safeguard.

2. Long-suffering love. Breaking down the walls between people is hard work. We need the power of God's love to sustain us over the long haul. Setbacks, conflicts and failures are inevitable in cross-ethnic relationships. We should not be surprised if miscommunication and misunderstandings derail our best efforts. But we must not give up. We must endure in love.

White people can tend toward problem solving in relationships. Sometimes our most sincere problem-solving efforts are received as acts of love, and sometimes they are not. When your ethnic minority friend shares pain or frustration, ask yourself, "Is now the time to problem solve, or is the loving thing to patiently listen?" As kingdom white people, we want all we do to be rooted in love, since only love lasts forever (1 Cor 13:1-8).

You and I regularly run out of love for those around us. We get hurt, and our hearts close off from others. We hate failure, and when we see our weaknesses, we pull back. The call to be people of love is not a call to stir up feelings of love on our own. Instead we come just as we are to Jesus and ask him again and again to give us his eyes to see this person or these people rightly. "Jesus, show me how you feel about this person. Fill me with your compassion for her. Take my fears and racism. Transform my small heart with your huge, passionate heart. Let your love for her flow through me."

3. Community. A major way that Jesus works his transformation in us is through experiences of community. As we walk with him into community situations, he shows us what we need to learn and gain from other people and shows us what we bring as gifts. We are not created to go through life as autonomous, independent individuals. Rather, as people of the kingdom of God we are knit together in Jesus' body. We do not protect ourselves from the other parts of the body. We embrace all the parts of the body.

For many white people, embracing our need for community is not easy. Many of us have been raised to believe that at age eighteen we are on our own in the world. It is accepted as healthy and normal to individuate quickly from our parents. We have been taught that it is a noble goal to be self-sufficient, to not need other people. We each need to pull our own weight, to work hard and pull ourselves up by our own bootstraps. While there are some wonderful things about these values, they can keep us from acknowledging our need for community. If we are going to become the kind of kingdom white people Jesus is seeking, we need to have a more communitarian outlook on life.

4. Empowerment for engagement. We white people can be strangely passive at times. If we try to become sensitive in cross-ethnic situations, we can end up being wallflowers. Jesus commands us to be servants in our speech and actions, so we must learn to be sensitive and honor people of other ethnicities in what we say. However, if we focus *only* on becoming sensitive, our courage will wither and die. Just being sensitive is not enough.

I met Molly at our first "5-in-1" InterVarsity conference, at which we divided into five different ethnic-specific tracks. She was a white senior who had friends from various ethnic minority groups. She told me how her friends would confide to her all the things white people do that irritate them. She tried to rid herself of any trace of these offensive behaviors. She knew how to use all the right words around her friends, but inside she was crushed. She was not a woman of courage and truth; instead she lived under a shadow of self-hatred and self-condemnation. That weekend God broke her free from that bondage. God empowered her to be herself in those relationships, to bring who she is to the table.

My wife, who is Korean American, has a number of white friends. Many of them, she laments, are stuck under a cloud of "white guilt." When we white people are afraid of saying the wrong thing, we just keep our mouths shut. Sandy wants friends who can enter into give-and-take with her on key issues and be honest about what is happening in the friendship. This is her response to white friends whose courage has been sapped: "Please reengage with me. Find your voice again. What good are you to me if you just sit there feeling bad about yourself?"

Jesus has something far better for us than merely struggling to be "the good white person." He wants to fill us with his Spirit and make us courageous, fearless and proactive advocates—empowered white people with a voice.

5. Freedom in Christ. In the kingdom of God, Jesus wants us free to be fully ourselves, just as he has made us. God did not make a mistake in making you and me white. Being white is beautiful in God's eyes. We too are created in the image of God.

There are some white folks who are committed to cross-ethnic relationships but struggle with self-hatred. They wish they were not white. Yet Jesus died for white people just as for every other group of people he created. The ultimate proof that someone is beloved by God is Jesus' death.

When I live under a sense of self-hatred and condemnation, I declare through my actions that the power of the cross is not enough to liberate a sinner like me. My situation is *not* more powerful than the blood of Jesus. As I open up my whole life to the blood of Jesus, he promises to work in me and through me. No shame allowed! Freedom is found as we embrace a Psalm 139 spirituality on the one hand ("I am fearfully and wonderfully made") and a Psalm 51 spirituality on the other ("Create in me a clean heart, O God, and put a new and right spirit within me"). To live in both is to find freedom.

I do not want to pretend that embracing these kingdom truths is easy. There are all kinds of voices competing to tell us who we are. Which ones should I internalize and which ones should I not? How am I supposed to feel about our history? How am I supposed to feel about people who hate me because of the color of my skin? This is very emotionally complex. But

Jesus is large enough to handle the complexities. He can still teach me to live well in his kingdom in the midst of many voices and judgments. Jesus is a very good Shepherd, and that means we have great hope as we continue in this journey.

Making White Identity Real

This section on racism and identity was the hardest of the five sections for us to write. In five chapters we tried to touch on the most important issues in sorting out who we are as white people. We placed the identity section here because a preoccupation with white ethnic identity prior to a commitment to displacement and love, and an understanding of racism, could become narcissistic and warped. Once we are firmly planted in Jesus' call to lay down our lives for his sake, then we can more safely explore questions of our identity in Christ. Questions that are normal and healthy at a later point in the journey could have been destructive and confusing at an earlier point. Truth about who we are apart from love is nothing but a clanging cymbal.

This section contains both the bad news and the good news, the downside and the upside. How do you make sense of the different themes? Sometimes in the kingdom of God and in life in general, there are tensions that never go away. We don't like these tensions, but trying to explain them away would mean plugging our ears to part of the truth.

On the one hand, we need to open our ears and listen to who we are from the perspective of our ethnic minority brothers and sisters. We need to listen carefully to how they see us and what they call us. We need to study history humbly and not run away. We look at the past and say, "Yes, and we white people probably did even worse than that." We enter into mourning and weakness. We let our hearts be broken. We search our hearts and let the pain shape us. This is grueling, but as we follow Jesus on this path of lowliness, he will exalt us and bring us new life.

On the other hand, we need to filter the voices of others. Ultimately we need to let God and no one else define us. His is the only voice that can shape and guide us. We will submit only to our heavenly Father. We resolutely hide our identity in Christ, our fortress from the winds of popular opinion.

This tension is not easy, but it is good. It reflects the complexity of reality. There will be times when we get confused and make mistakes—when we confuse the voice of others with the voice of God. But the only true failure would be to lose hope and give up. The call for us is to embrace the complexity and surrender it to God, who is generous to give us wisdom when we ask for it (Jas 1:5). God will be faithful to us for the entire journey.

1. What are some painful things you have heard others say about white people? How did you feel when you heard them? What is the thing you need to pay attention to from each voice?
2. Psalm 139 says that you are beautifully and wonderfully made. What positive things have you heard others say about white people?
3. Do you ever experience white shame or condemnation? How do you move from that feeling into an empowered attitude?
4. Which of the partial truths do you sometimes listen to or fall into?
5. How did you feel as you read the positive descriptions of white values? Which of those do you relate to?

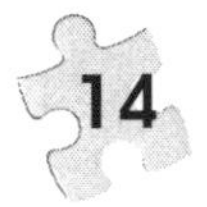

I Want a Friend, She Wants Justice

Paula Harris

Shortly after I finished college, God led me into a series of displacement experiences. I was working hard to learn about race and to recognize racial injustice. God grew my capacity to repent and be free of racial sin.

My friends who were people of color taught me a lot, from practical crosscultural lessons to a deeper understanding of their experiences in America. Now we would think, and I certainly thought at the time, that I was able to be a great friend back to them. And I was, to some of them, as well as I knew how. I was deeply aware of them as people. I had learned to judge people individually, by their character and not by their race. The white value of fairness was deeply ingrained in me, and instinctively I wanted to make sure that all my friends had a fair chance.

But interracial friendship was not enough. Seeing racism was not enough. I had to start doing something about it.

After leaving China, I joined InterVarsity's missions department in order to bring together what I had learned about race in America and missions internationally. When I first started leading short-term missions trips, I believed strongly that they should be interracial teams, based on the missionary model found in Acts. I could envision a community based on justice and was trying to use my power as a leader to build it. So I sought to recruit students of color and mixed-race teams of staff who could work together to lead and pastor them. I would give the vision for missions, my vision for a mixed-race team and why it is important that people of all cultures be involved in mission—and invite students to come along.

Some responded enthusiastically. Some said no thanks. Some were hostile, probably because of experiences with other whites. Some had practical obstacles we needed to work through, like finances or family concerns. But students of color often responded beyond this with what I came to interpret as "tests" for me: "I believe you, but . . ." "What if . . . ?" "Are you going to . . . ?"

I was shocked that they didn't trust me. I knew how to fit in to their culture. They were obviously interested. We worked through all the usual obstacles. But still, they asked directly and indirectly, "Can I trust you?"

Honestly, I felt betrayed. I had gone not only the extra mile but ten miles, or twenty. I felt so strongly, *I'm different from other whites. I deserve your trust. How dare you not believe me?*

Being Tested for Justice

Maybe you can relate to the experience of being tested in positive or negative ways by a person of color. Maybe you weathered it better than I did. The truth is, I realized later, these students did see my heart. What they were testing was my commitment to justice. They were testing me because they saw what I was doing and thought, *Perhaps this white person is worthy of my trust.* They responded, naturally from their perspective, by testing me. They had not met white people who deserved their trust. They were cautiously moving forward, testing me and waiting to see how I responded.

The first time I was tested, I confess I just got mad and dismissed the person. Eventually I realized that being tested is an opportunity to respond appropriately, to take further action, to develop trust and work together to build a just community. Scripture says, "Whenever you face trials of any kind, consider it nothing but joy, because you know that the testing of your faith produces endurance; and let endurance have its full effect, so that you may be mature and complete, lacking in nothing" (Jas 1:2-4).

In "Letter from Birmingham Jail" Dr. Martin Luther King Jr. offers insight into why the students might have tested me. He was writing in response to eight white clergymen who had actively denounced the civil rights movement, but he also addresses people like me, white people of goodwill toward African Americans, white people trying to build good relationships:

> I must confess that over the past few years I have been gravely disappointed with the white moderate. I have almost reached the regrettable conclusion that the Negro's great stumbling block in his stride toward freedom is not the white Citizen's Counciler or the Ku Klux Klanner, but the white moderate . . . who paternalistically believes he can set the timetable for another man's freedom. . . . Shallow understanding from people of good will is more frustrating than absolute misunderstanding from people of ill will. Lukewarm acceptance is much more bewildering than outright rejection. . . .
>
> Perhaps I was too optimistic; perhaps I expected too much. I suppose I should have realized that few members of the oppressor race can understand the deep groans and passionate yearnings of the oppressed race, and still fewer have the vision to see that injustice must be rooted out by strong, persistent and determined action.[1]

As King articulates, the second reason the black students tested me is that they suspected we had different hopes. I did not truly understand their concerns. I wanted to include them in the multicultural community. I wanted to reflect the gospel in many cultures. I wanted to have good individual relationships with the staff and students. I wanted them to be involved in missions. These were all great desires, rooted in Scripture. I had hopes and dreams that honored God. But I wanted to do this on a personal, individual level, while acting as if there were no injustice between my people and their people.

So the students tested me, first to see if I could understand the "groans and yearnings" of oppression, and second to see if I understood that there was injustice between us and we must take action together to root it out. The students could receive me in relationship, but they could not join a "just community" on unequal footing. I needed to commit myself to working actively for justice. They wanted a commitment to justice that they could see.

God gradually used the students' questions, and their leaders' wisdom, to help me grow in a practical commitment to justice. Were there economic inequities? I found scholarships for the students of color and worked with leaders from their communities to identify fundraising goals that were challenging but possible. Were there power divisions and all-white leadership on our team? I recruited ethnic minority staff to come with us. For each ethnic minority group, I studied their heritage in missions and told them how important it was, how important they were.

We whites, valuing fairness, want to think our achievements have been based on a fair system. Not everybody sees it this way. My friend Terry told me the story of a man who had a visitor. The man offered his visitor a meal, and they had a pleasant conversation. Then when it came time to go home, the visitor stayed on the couch. His host felt fine about that.

The next night, the visitor insisted on taking a bedroom. The man was gracious; the couch might not have been comfortable. The visitor soon invited his friends over, and they too needed places to sleep. The man let them in also. Soon there were so many visitors that they took over the house, pushing the man and his whole family into a back closet.

My friend Terry is from the Micmac nation of Canada. My own family is German and Irish. His story is a parable of the ways that generations of our peoples have interacted. Can I truly call myself his friend and ignore the fact that I'm sitting in his living room, acting as if it's mine?

Terry led me, telling me a parable that gently corrected my perception if I had ears to hear it. A younger Native person might have tested me to see if I could perceive the inequity in the system clearly enough for him to trust me to do justice as a leader.

What is it like in your context? Are the leaders all white, or is there some diversity? Do the people of color who lead have real power—money to spend, decisions to make for themselves and others, opportunities to shape the community's values and activities? If you are a leader yourself, in what ways are you inviting people of color to share your power? When you invite them, have you been tested? How did you respond?

Responding to Injustice

God also longs for justice. You might go so far as to say God finds individual relationships without justice inadequate. In Isaiah 1 God confronts injustice, saying to his people, in effect, "I can't stand being with you! Stop worshiping me. My soul hates it. Clean yourself up! Stop doing evil! Do justice! Rescue the oppressed!" (Is 1:11-17). Jesus honors justice and setting things straight in society. When his mom prays over him, thanking God for bringing the Messiah, she says God has brought the powerful down, will lift the lowly up, will feed the hungry and send the rich away empty (Lk 1:51-53). In Jesus' first sermon he says that he is calling out good news to the poor, setting prisoners free, healing the blind and freeing the oppressed (Lk 4:18-19).

Let's take one of the categories Jesus used in his sermon. Who are the prisoners in our country? What are the facts? Over half of those on death row are people of color. Black men alone make up over 42 percent of all death row prisoners, though they account for only 6 percent of people living in the United States.[2] So when you read your paper, if it says the local district attorney (D.A.) has decided to pursue a death sentence, remember that 98 percent of the D.A.s in death-penalty states are white, while 74 percent of the defendants are people of color.

What can you do? You could take a stand against the death penalty, or if you believe the death penalty is appropriate, you could work with an advocacy group to make sure that it is implemented fairly. You could get involved with a ministry to prisoners like Prison Fellowship, or take a Christian prayer partner and start visiting people in prison. You could pay a legal bill for a group that addresses issues of legal justice like the Southern Poverty Law Center. You could make a donation for the human rights of prisoners in America through a group like Amnesty International. You can keep yourself informed about local cases and pray for the people who appear in the news.

Let's take another of Jesus' categories. Who are the poor in our country? What are the facts? According to the U.S. Census Bureau, in 2002 the average Native American household income was $32,000, Latino household income $33,000 and black household income $29,000. White family income was $47,000. Asian household income was $55,000, reflecting both higher education level and families with multiple working generations living together.[3] Jesus says he came to turn this upside down. Why don't we?

When I learned the income gap, I asked myself, *What can I personally do about the national household income gap? Okay, I have responsibility to hire people for my department. I can't change the national income figures, but I can make sure my own hiring is fair.* As a supervisor, I don't practice affirmative action, I practice "affirmative recruitment." I work hard to make sure that I recruit as many qualified candidates who are people of color as I have white applicants. To correct for bias in the process, I appoint a mixed-race, mixed gender interview team. Then we screen rigorously and choose the best person.

Learning facts about injustice helps me understand what is happening in the broader context of my relationships with people of color. Sure, they want me as a friend. Sure, when I displace myself I am working hard at learning about their culture. But when I am an unseeing friend, when I pretend that everything is okay, it is deeply painful to them. If I truly love them the way Jesus loved us, then I will also be committed to justice. I will see the racist system of partiality that gives me more opportunity, and I will take practical steps in the opposite direction.

Sometimes I wonder how much Zacchaeus the tax collector actually stole money from the Jews and how much he just took advantage of a system set up in his favor.[4] After he came to Jesus, Zacchaeus promised to give away half his wealth and repay fourfold anything he had stolen (Lk 19).

Likewise, the rich ruler came to ask Jesus, "How can I be saved?" Jesus' reply was "Sell everything you own and give the money to the poor; then you can follow me" (see Lk 18). The text doesn't tell us anything about how the man got his wealth, whether legally or illegally. He just had it. In any case, the rich guy couldn't obey; it was too hard. He walked away from Jesus instead.

I know a white professor who earns his salary legitimately yet lives on a fraction of his income so he can give the rest to the poor. I deeply admire him. His heart is soft toward God, and he quickly obeys God's Word. If we want to come to God with a clean heart and clean hands, we will be committed to economic and systemic justice.

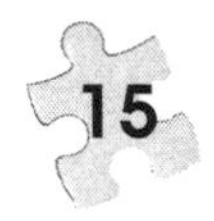
15

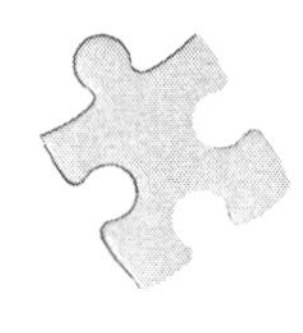

Responsibility Is Not a Four-Letter Word

Doug Schaupp

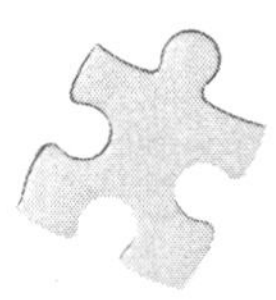

I sat down to watch *Spider-Man* expecting nothing more than an action movie with big special effects. Instead I was moved by the film's insight into human nature and the way life works.

The lead character, Peter Parker, first unveils his amazing strength by defeating the local wrestling champion for a three-thousand-dollar prize. When Parker goes to collect, the owner breaks his word and gives Parker a mere one hundred dollars. When he protests that he needs the money, the boss zips him with a potent one-liner: "I missed the part where that's my problem."

A minute later, a thief holds up the same boss at gunpoint and makes off with the heap of cash from that evening. The thief makes his getaway, running right past Peter Parker. Parker has a critical choice to make: to step in and get involved or to numb his conscience, telling himself that it's okay to let injustice go unnoticed. Wounded by the snub he has just experienced, he chooses to let the thief go.

Later when the owner confronts Parker for letting the criminal go by, he turns his one-liner right back on him. "I missed the part where that's my problem," he says cynically. A few hours before, Parker's uncle had warned him, "Be careful who you become." That advice turns out to be prophetic, because Parker is now well on the path to becoming just like that owner, jaded and frozen in heart.

How did this happen? In the first part of the movie, Peter Parker is a nice guy, the kind of person who will go out of his way for someone else. The turning point is when Parker gets infected by the owner, who is a carrier of a lethal and very contagious disease: viewing one's responsibility in the narrowest possible terms.

When we spend time with someone who reduces his role in life to merely the very few things that he cannot possibly avoid doing, we are in danger of emulating him. Everything else falls into the category of "not my responsibility, *and I resent the very fact that you think it is my problem.*" This attitude rubs off on Parker in just one bad interaction. Is that realistic or unrealistic? I say realistic.

This scene could well be titled "The Temptation of Peter Parker." Parker is tempted to become reductionistic, and he plays right into the hands of the tempter, becoming like him.

The poignancy of the scene is in its universality. You and I have each faced this same temptation many times over. *Why should I care?* Before we even know what is happening, a voice in our head lets us off the hook with some version of *I missed the part where that is my problem.* The voice is probably not that cynical. It is probably more of an overwhelmed voice: *I wouldn't even know where to begin with that problem.* Or a sympathetic *I feel so sorry for them.* It is ironic that I can use my feelings of sympathy to let myself off the hook just as easily as I can use cynicism or fear.

We daily have opportunities to step in the way of small injustices and try to do the right thing, but we freeze, silently echoing the sentiment, *I missed the part where that is my problem.* These sins of omission can easily sneak under the radar of our conscious mind and usually go unnoticed by others.[1]

Who suffers because of our sins of omission? Seldom do I pay the price for my own sins of omission, and that is why they are so dangerous and slippery. In *Spider-Man* Peter Parker does pay for his sin of omission. The criminal proceeds to shoot and kill his uncle on the way out of the arena. Parker's sin of omission translates directly into a sin of commission against his family. The exact impact of his choice to limit his responsibility stares him in the face.

What does he do with this unavoidable link between his inaction and his uncle's death? With courage, he steps up to the plate of reality and changes his definition of *responsibility.* His life changes because he embraces the world around him with its potential for beauty and its cycles of evil.

I once asked a group of college guys, "Is *responsibility* a good word or a bad word?" They all agreed: *responsibility* is a bad word. They told me that the word *responsibility* is unappealing because it speaks of being tied down, of being boring.

How do you feel about the word *responsibility*? Personally, I have come to love the word. Responsibility gets things done, makes a difference and creates room for courage. Responsibility opens the door to freedom and liberation. Once I embrace my God-given responsibility, I can become the person of courage and truth God has meant for me to be.

We live in a world where most white people look at racism and say, "I missed the part where that is my problem." How then do you and I avoid this temptation to shirk our responsibility? How do we begin to respond to the racism of our world, without being crushed in the process?

Generational Sin, Generational Responsibility

One of the most common ways white people avoid responsibility is by not understanding that past sins of racism continue to damage and cripple our country, our churches, our campuses and ourselves. How do we wrap our mind around the fact that sins from the past still influence the state of affairs today?

After I graduated from college, I had dinner with Bob, an old family friend. About halfway through dinner, Bob tried to pay me a compliment: "Doug, you are just like your parents. You have gotten so much from them."

Inside my gut, something rose up in protest. I wanted to shout, "No, I am the product of my own decisions. I've chosen my own goals and values. They haven't been handed down to me."

In hindsight, I have come to see that Bob is right. I am the product of generations who have invested in me and shaped who I am—most directly my parents, but also countless others, both living and dead. But honestly, I much prefer to view myself as an island, an autonomous agent. Americans are some of the most independent people in the world, and I am a product of that rampant individualism.

What does Scripture have to say about how we are influenced by those who came before us? Exodus 34:6-7 describes God as "abounding in steadfast love and faithfulness, keeping steadfast love for the thousandth generation, forgiving iniquity and transgression and sin, yet by no means clearing the guilty, but visiting the iniquity of the parents upon the children and the children's children, to the third and the fourth generation." In contrast to how I want to see myself, God says that I am the recipient of blessings from those who came generations before me and also of curses from those who came generations before.

Intellectually, I can see this through the lens of modern psychology when it tells me that children of divorce, abuse or addiction are more likely than their peers to grow up and choose similar patterns of divorce, abuse and addictions. Yet when it comes to racism, I would far prefer to think that the racial sins of our forefathers and foremothers have magically evaporated into thin air during the past century. Somehow Dr. Martin Luther King Jr. and the civil rights leaders waved their wand and leveled the playing field, and thus ended the generational sin cycle.

But that is not the way Exodus describes the sin problem. God says that I am not cleared of the sin that was done in this country three or four generations ago. My white ancestors repeatedly and systematically mistreated Native Americans, African Americans, Latin Americans, Asian Americans. Though I never met them, I am still the recipient of their spiritual heritage. I have inherited the lie that I can love people like me and not care about those different from me, and everything will be fine between God and me. That is a wicked falsehood. The bad news is that you and I live under the influence of generational sin, and we don't even know it.

Nehemiah: Stepping into the Gap

As we begin to see clearly the problem of sin and racism both in us and around us, what are we supposed to do about it? Nehemiah is a superb example of a leader who grasps the complexity of generational sin, responds directly and actually sees the cycle of generational sin broken in his day. If we all embrace the path that Nehemiah walked before us, we too may see the cycle of white generational sin broken in our day.

God promised that he would walk with his people and protect them as long as they trusted him and abided in his commands. But if his people turned their hearts away and walked in their own path, God would give them over to their rebellion and let them be scattered by another nation. "If you are unfaithful, I will scatter you among the peoples; but if you return to me and keep my commandments and do them . . . I will gather [my people]" (Neh 1:8-9). Unfortunately Israel did rebel, and therefore it was taken over by the Persian Empire. The educated Jews were taken from their homeland and had to live in exile in the land of their oppressors.

Nehemiah had various reasons to limit his sense of responsibility for Jerusalem and the plight of his people. First, he was born in exile and had never visited his homeland. He did not know what Jerusalem looked like. There was no firsthand experience to help him care. Second, Nehemiah had done well for himself and was respected enough to win a power position in the Persian government. He had much to lose if his cause backfired. Third, Nehemiah had done nothing to cause this problem. Those who rebelled against God had lived several generations before him, and he did not walk in their wicked ways. God was not angry with Nehemiah, and Nehemiah was not "responsible" for the situation.

Here are the steps that God leads Nehemiah through in transforming him and giving him a sense of responsibility to become part of the solution. What if we let God transform us into white servants with a godly sense of responsibility?

1. Nehemiah investigates. He approaches those who have seen Jerusalem firsthand. He wants to learn and have his eyes opened. "I asked them about the Jews that survived, those who had escaped the captivity, and about Jerusalem" (1:2). The fact that he doesn't know firsthand does not keep him from learning.

We fear learning because of what that will do to the safe little world we have created. Like Nehemiah, we need to gather our courage to ask hard questions about the suffering of our ethnic minority friends. An honest question allows the experience of another to shape our worldview. It is a step of vulnerability to ask someone what their experience of racism has been.

2. He listens and lets their experience move him. "When I heard these words I sat down and wept" (1:4). Instead of using his own experience to trump their story of suffering and shame, he allows his heart to care about their experience.

This is the most pivotal step in dealing with racism. To let our heart be moved is to open the door of our life to the rest of the world. To be moved as your ethnic minority friend tells you her story of suffering is to free your heart from the cage of self-protection and defensiveness.

But this is a scary step of profound vulnerability and humility. It can be frightening to learn that the way I view myself and the world is sorely incomplete. To open my heart to the stories of others is to release control and accept suffering, facing the fact that we cannot solve the problem in a neat, efficient way. Will you let yourself become vulnerable to your friends?

3. He enters into mourning. Nehemiah is able to look directly at the evil that has befallen his people because he has a spirituality of mourning. "[I] mourned for days, fasting and praying before the God of heaven" (1:4). He does not begin by trying to solve the problem, though he is a superb problem solver. He does not craft a plan of action with a team of committed friends. In fact, it seems he's initially unsure if he is even supposed to be a part of the solution. Instead he allows himself to sit powerless in the presence of God.

To mourn is to tell God, "This is not the way it is supposed to be." To mourn is to let God reshape what we care about. We prefer to fix things—but the world is far too broken; we can't fix it all. We must intentionally develop a deeper spirituality of mourning that can handle the messiness of our world. We miss the part where racism is our problem because we miss the part where we take it to God and interact with God over it.

4. Nehemiah puts his trust back in God. He affirms that God is the trustworthy One and that the best way to live is by walking with God in his good advice. "God . . . keeps covenant and steadfast love with those who love him and keep his commandments" (1:5). This is a crucial step, because without it mourning can lead to despair and cynicism. Mourning in and of itself does not lead us to God. Godly mourning must be linked to worship and to recommitting our lives to our good God.

5. He steps up to take responsibility. Nehemiah can now safely enter into ownership of the problem. "I now pray . . . confessing the sins of the people of Israel, which we have sinned against you. Both I and my family have sinned. We have offended you deeply, failing to keep the commandments" (1:6-7). He squarely faces the blame and says, "We brought this oppression on ourselves. We sinned. We were warned not to turn our backs on God, but we didn't listen. Forgive us." Then he torques it up a notch by making it personal. Nehemiah does not just point to his people who have offended God; he also points to himself and his family. This is daring! As far as we can tell, Nehemiah himself did not break the Ten Commandments. But part of stepping up to the plate of responsibility is saying, "This is my problem. I own it. Have mercy on me, Lord." This is not a step of self-hatred or shame. When we own a problem in a healthy way, it is actually a great step of liberation.

Nehemiah's ability to embrace his people and the wrong they have done before God is a profound mystery to white people. Extending our heart and our sense of responsibility to all white people in America seems completely out of the question. We say defensive things such as "My family never owned slaves" or "My parents started out poor too."

Let us instead swallow our pride and, like Nehemiah, confess the sins of our white people, past and present. "Lord, we white people have sinned against you. We set up our country's economy and social system so that we would get the best at the expense of nonwhite people. We trusted in this prowhite system for our good and happy future, instead of trusting the Lord of the universe to provide for us. I and my family have sinned against you. We have subtly and not so subtly benefited from this prowhite world every day of our lives. Have mercy on a sinner like me." For those of you who are familiar with this type of vicarious praying or identificational repentance in other areas of life, please lead the way in racial reconciliation too.

6. He does not sugarcoat the problem. "We have offended you deeply, failing to keep the commandments, the statutes, and the ordinances that you commanded your servant Moses" (1:7). Nehemiah does not make excuses for his people or try to convince God to lighten up on them. He affirms that God is justified in bringing punishment and scattering his people for their disobedience. Nehemiah does not play the victim card. Nor does he try to sweep the sin under the carpet and just pray for God's blessing in an undiscerning way.

7. He takes God at his word. "If you return to me and keep my commandments and do them, though your outcasts are under the farthest skies, I will gather them from there and bring them to the place at which I have chosen to establish my name" (1:9). Nehemiah sits in the presence of God both as an individual and as a representative of God's people. He reminds God of his promise to break the curse and gather his people when repentance has happened. In effect he is saying, "We are coming back to you right now. Please honor your promise to us."

8. Nehemiah gets involved in the solution. During this season of mourning and repentance, God has won over Nehemiah's heart completely. He now cares so much about the problem that he asks God to let him become part of the solution. In essence he says, "Give me success today as I approach the king to foot the bill for this venture" (see 1:11). Nehemiah is open to being a key part of the solution only because he has gone deep with God. May the same be true of us.

9. He becomes aware of his access to resources. Nehemiah is not a rich man, but he knows someone with great resources. It might have been tempting to think, *I would get involved in helping Jerusalem if only I had more money.* Instead he looks around and realizes that he has access to the king, if he can muster the courage to ask. He has been put in this position "for such a time as this," and he makes the most of his access to power. King Artaxerxes opens up the checkbook and gives Nehemiah a forest of timber and the position of governor with all its privileges. When Nehemiah travels to Jerusalem, he has excellent resources at his disposal.

It has been hard for me to see and admit, but you and I have incredible access to white privilege. Even if you want to bury your head and refuse to acknowledge your access to power, you and I will never change the color of our skin and our access. If you do nothing about your access to resources, you will continue to benefit personally—directly or indirectly—from how our country is set up. Let us instead follow in Nehemiah's footsteps and become aware of our access to King Artaxerxes. Each of us should create a game plan for how we will intentionally use and share the resources to which we have access.

A Good Word

In 1993 a Latina woman, Maria,[2] stood up to speak in front of one hundred of her UCLA peers at the end of our InterVarsity fall conference. She was angry: "Does any one else here care that I am just about the only Latina person here?"

I was leading the sharing time, and I had no idea what to say. *How do I respond to her anger?* In typical white fashion, I decided to just move on. I spotted someone in the room who I knew would have something more positive to share, and I called on them to "lift" the sharing toward a more encouraging note.

Fast-forward to 1998. We were in a Race Matters community discussion, and Alex said to a room full of seventy-five UCLA peers, "Does any one else care that I'm the only Latino here?"

It was another intense moment, as we could all see his sadness and anger. This time I said to the group, "Alex has just raised an issue with us. What are we going to say to him?"

Students shared their hearts with Alex, and soon we gathered around him to pray for him. I prayed, "God, put it on the hearts of some in this room to spearhead a new outreach to Latino students here on campus."

Within a year God brought thirty Latino students to our Latino family night, and the InterVarsity ministry at UCLA has never been the same since.

What happened to me between 1993 and 1998? God had transformed me from a white person who said, "I missed the part where that is my problem," to a white person who said, "We together open our hearts to that problem in the name of Jesus." Thank God that *responsibility* is a good word in the kingdom of God.

Nearly ten years ago, a handful of InterVarsity alumni relocated into an urban poor neighborhood in South Central Los Angeles. During their college years they had studied the Scriptures and heard God's call into displacement and compassion. They formed an intentional Christian community and looked for opportunities to minister to their neighbors.

A block from their house there was a liquor store that had become a drug distribution and prostitution hub. Because they had made this neighborhood their home, the household of Christians could not ignore the call to take a step of responsibility. After praying and talking together, they petitioned the city government to revoke the liquor store license. God honored their stand, and the liquor store soon closed.

Today that community of relocaters has become the core of a new church. Ministry is thriving, and the good news is being lived out.

Consider the following questions to help you become a white person who says, "I can open my heart and own that problem."

1. How are you feeling about the word *responsibility?* What do you like about it, and what makes you resistant toward it?
2. Have you ever said, "Racism is not my problem. My family never did those things"? How do you feel about Nehemiah and his ability to embrace all the foolish and sinful things his people did in their rebellion against God?
3. When was the last time your heart was moved by the story of one of your ethnic minority friends? What would it look like for you to allow your heart to be increasingly shaped by the experiences of ethnic minority folks around you?
4. How do you feel about mourning? When was the last time you sat before God in prayer and mourned for fifteen minutes about a situation of injustice? What will it take for you to be willing to let God lead you into more messy mourning situations?
5. Are you open to repenting on behalf of our people? Are you open to letting God break your heart for us white people? Please try that in prayer this week.
6. You and I have direct and indirect access to white privilege. Is that hard or easy for you to see and acknowledge? A few weeks ago I took a risk with our staff team. I said, "Who here has parents or family members who are worth more than $500,000? If you do, please know that you have access to wealth. Please form a proactive game plan about how you will share that wealth over your lifetime. Don't just hoard it."

How about you? Are your parents worth more than $500,000? Let God lead you into becoming part of the solution. Form a proactive game plan for how to use those resources for the good of the poor and oppressed, for the good of all of God's people.[3] If you don't form a game plan, you will still use those resources, but in the way that most white people do: for yourself.

I love Nehemiah. He is one of my top heroes of the faith, and he particularly speaks to my identity as a white person. I pray that God makes me like Nehemiah and raises up among us a new generation of Nehemiahs. I hope you will join me in this prayer and journey to embrace this responsibility.

16

Betraying White Privilege, Plundering White Power

Paula Harris

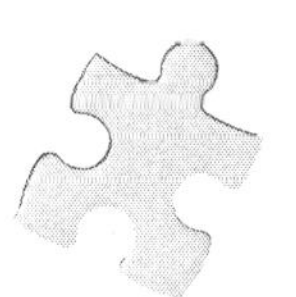

Clearly, white people are not the first people in history to have power over another group. We are not the first to abuse our power. What are we supposed to do about it? What does Scripture say to majority culture people who have power over other ethnic groups? What is God's intent?

Intercultural power differences are everywhere in Scripture—from the Jews relating to the Egyptians, Babylonians or Assyrians in the Old Testament, to the Jewish-Roman conflict in New Testament-era politics or the Jewish-Gentile conflict in the church. In these broader cultural conflicts, the character of a person's heart is magnified, reflected first in his or her deeds and also in the community's corporate action.

Take the Egyptians and the Hebrews, two ethnic groups. The land belongs to the Egyptians, but the Israelites are hard workers and prolific childbearers; soon they are everywhere. When a new Egyptian king comes into power, he sees this and says to his people: "Look, the Israelite people are more numerous and more powerful than we. Come, let us deal shrewdly with them, or they will increase and, in the event of war, join our enemies and fight against us and escape from the land" (Ex 1:9-10). In Pharaoh's statement we can discern the seeds of *personal racism:* he clearly is showing partiality to the Egyptian people over the Hebrews. He is fearful of the Hebrews and is speaking and acting in such a way as to divide the Egyptians from the Israelite people.

As a group, the Egyptians respond to their king's message and set up *a racially stratified system:* "Therefore [the Egyptians] set taskmasters over [the Israelites] to oppress them with forced labor. . . . But the more they were oppressed, the more they multiplied and spread, so that the Egyptians came to dread the Israelites" (Ex 1:11-12).

You can see here how the racism of one person (the king) comes to infect relations between two nations. His partiality spreads because of his power and the actions he has called his people to take. Out of their dread, the Egyptians "became ruthless" against the Israelites and "made their lives bitter" (1:13-14). You can see the Egyptians' racism spreading and deepening in their relations with the Israelites. What did it take for the Egyptians to ignore the bitterness of the Israelites' lives?

As the Egyptian people ignore their neighbors' lives, the king is free to step further into his Egyptian supremacy, and he commands the murder of Hebrew boy babies. First he commands the Hebrew midwives, then "all his people," to drown the babies (1:15-16, 22).

Can you imagine being an Egyptian at this moment? What would you do? When do you stop and say no? Is it at murder? Or earlier, at forced labor? Or at the level of partiality, preferring Egyptian people over Israelites?

In retrospect it's easy enough to see how the system of racism and then slavery developed. Scripture helps us see it, by conflating hundreds of years of history into a few short verses in Exodus 1. We could easily document the same sort of development in North America: European immigration, Native American slavery, the devastation caused by the accidental spreading of European disease among Native peoples, the *intentional* exposure of Native people to European disease, the exploitation of intertribal warfare and then finally the genocide.

Three Choices in a Racist System

Alongside the development of racist systems in Egypt, there is also an antiracist development—again because of individual choices. Moses' parents choose not to drown him but float him in a basket, creatively both obeying the law to "throw them into the Nile" and saving their boy when they can no longer hide him. This is an act of civil disobedience, like Rosa Parks's deciding to sit down where it was illegal.

What's significant to our questions about majority culture people is that Pharaoh's own daughter, an upper-class Egyptian, also conspires to save the baby. Seeing the basket, she sends her maid for it (she could have ignored it), she opens it (she could have had the maid "deal with" it), and "she took pity on him," saying, "This must be one of the Hebrews' children" (2:5-6). She lets herself feel what his own family must feel. His sister bravely offers to find a Hebrew wet nurse, and Pharaoh's daughter agrees.

There's no secret. Each group knows that Hebrew boys are being murdered, that this baby legally ought to be murdered, and the Egyptian princess stands against it. Not only does she save the baby, she pays his mother to nurse him, and after he is weaned she adopts him, giving him the bicultural name Mosheh.[1] We may think this is a relatively safe choice for her. Actually it is quite risky. "There is no reason to assume that this daughter of Pharaoh would have been in a position of power or influence. Harem children by the score existed in every court, and daughters were considered less highly than sons."[2]

So the story already poses a choice to us white people: are we going to be like Pharaoh or like Pharaoh's daughter? At this point in the text there is no sense that either of them is following God. Their choices are purely on the human level. Later, while Moses is being reformed in the Midian desert, back in Egypt the Israelites go from being victims of forced labor (1:13-14) to being slaves (2:23). Our choices about race and ethnicity have an enormous cost for ethnic minority people.

As we follow the story of Exodus, God says, "The cry of the Israelites has now come to me; I have also seen how the Egyptians oppress them" (3:9). It's no secret who the bad guys are in the story. Now, we would think, the Egyptians are about to be judged, to receive the wrath of God. Don't they deserve it? Don't *we* deserve it? Indeed there are a few promises to the Israelites that could be read as threats against Egypt. God will compel their freedom with "a mighty hand" (3:19).[3] God will "strike Egypt" (3:20). The Israelites will "plunder" Egypt (3:22).

Not only that, but the Egyptians' story begins to be told on an explicitly religious level as well as the human and political one. When the Israelites hear that God has remembered them, they fall down and worship (4:31). Moses and Aaron ask first that Pharaoh free them for a three-day festival to celebrate God, and Pharaoh's response is to deny God: "Who is the LORD, that I should heed him and let Israel go?" (5:1-2).

We know the story: backlash. To punish the slaves for asking, Pharaoh commands the (Egyptian) taskmasters and (Israelite) supervisors to make their labor harsher (chap. 5). God does threaten to judge Egypt, in 6:6 and 7:4.

What is striking in the context is that God threatens to judge Egypt not only to free the Israelites, the people of the covenant, but also so that *the Egyptians* "shall know that I am the LORD" (7:5, 17; 8:10, 22; 9:14; 14:4, 18). The Egyptians have choices during the plagues. Some Egyptians imitate Pharaoh, who chooses to harden his heart against God and human suffering. Even as he's rejecting God, Pharaoh is using religious language and promising to be righteous, but his actions prove he's a liar. First he asks Moses to "pray to the LORD" to take away the plague (8:8-10, 28; 9:28; 10:17). Then he admits, "I have sinned; the LORD is in the right, and I and my people are in the wrong" (9:27, also 10:16-17). Each time he promises to do right and release the Israelites. Yet over and over again he ignores Moses, ignores God and ignores those of his own leaders who plead on the Israelites' behalf (8:19; 10:7). Pharaoh uses words of repentance about the racist system he leads, but his actions are the opposite, because his heart is hard.

On a very basic level, the few Egyptians who make good choices are being driven by fear: they are figuring out who's in power. At first the Egyptian magicians are able to duplicate the acts of God. But by about the third plague, they—the Egyptian court magicians—are giving testimony to God. "This is the finger of God!" they say (8:19). (Ironic that it's not the whole hand, just the finger.)

After a few more plagues, God says to Pharaoh, "Look, I'm sending the plagues so that you and your officials and your people know there is no one like me. I could have wiped you Egyptians off the earth, but instead I've let you live, to show my power and extend my name among all nations." But "you are still exalting yourself against my people"—a fairly explicit description of racism (see 9:13-17).

The ten plagues, each one of which confronts a deity and power of Egypt, are an incredible act of God's mercy to the Egyptian people. By the seventh plague, God gives warning instructions to the Egyptians: "I'm sending a massive hailstorm; get the humans and animals into shelter" (see 9:18-19). There begins to be a division: "Those officials of Pharaoh who feared the word of the LORD hurried their slaves and livestock off to a secure place. Those who did not regard the word of the LORD left their slaves and livestock in the open field" (9:20-21).

After the next threat, Pharaoh's officials even urge him, "Let these people go, get rid of Moses, Egypt is ruined!" (see 10:7). After the final plague, the Egyptians are all in mourning; they urge the Israelites to leave quickly, and they let themselves be plundered (12:33-36.) The Egyptians have finally chosen to do something right, out of fear. It doesn't last. When the immediate difficulty is resolved, Pharaoh's army follows his choice, pursues the Israelites and dies in the Red Sea.

Thus there are three paths: (1) Pharaoh's hard heart, lying promises and evil deeds; (2) the Egyptian people's fearful hearts, going along with whoever seems most powerful; and (3) Pharaoh's daughter's merciful heart, which causes her to reach across racial and economic lines and adopt Moses, whom God uses to save his people.

None of the Egyptians are shown worshiping the Lord; none are shown leaving home along with the people of Israel. But we have to wonder if there was this ultimate path available to them: to join the Israelites in following God.

Choosing for the Just Community

Exodus shows us clearly how a racist system was set up, how it was maintained and how it was undermined. We get a picture of dominant-culture individuals and the paths available to us. Most encouragingly, we get a picture of God's intent for the Egyptians: to worship the Lord and release their neighbors. While the Israelites *are* set free, the Egyptians never tap into what is available to them.

As members of the ruling class of North America, we will have to choose a path, a way to relate to people of color. Pharaoh's path is a great temptation. Even if we have begun to confront our own racism, it is easy to have a racist heart and to build or participate in a racist system to protect ourselves and our people. Even if we have let God uproot the racism in our heart, on this path the next temptation to us is to *change only our words.* It's not possible to betray white privilege with words alone.

What groups are you a part of? Where can your groups make choices to live out justice, choices expressed in what you do, not only what you say? Are you—as an individual or a member of a group—involved in any situations where you make decisions about whites and people of color? Can you find ways to practice "affirmative recruitment" and restore what has gone wrong?

The second path that tempts us is the path of expediency. The Egyptian people had it pretty good. Hebrews were doing the worst labor, for free. It was a great country, a fruitful land. There is a profound temptation for us to follow the easy way and say yes to the most powerful. When Pharaoh was most powerful, the Egyptians said okay to Hebrew slavery. "It's the way things work, it must be okay." When God was shown to be more powerful, they let the Hebrews go.

It is not meaningful to plunder white power out of fearful expediency. To follow this path, the Egyptians did not have to do anything. This is the default. Are there any interracial situations in which you are acting out of expediency—where the system is set up and it's working okay for you? Dr. King said, "We will have to repent . . . not merely for the hateful words and actions of the bad people, but also for the appalling silence of the good people."[4] Are you just doing what is expedient?

The third path is that of Pharaoh's daughter. She started on a good path with her act of mercy. Like her, we may not have enough power to protect ourselves within the human system (as a daughter she would have been subject to Pharaoh's command). But her courageous deed was used by God to empower Moses and thus eventually to free the entire people. Where is God moving your heart for the suffering of people of color? What courageous deeds might God call you to? Have you asked God? Have you looked around?

The path we want to be on is following and worshiping God. This is the path of Moses, obeying God. It is available to us, and I believe it may have been available to the Egyptians, because after the account of the Israelites' flight Exodus goes on immediately to describe the commandments and laws by which the Israelites are to live, including treating resident aliens with compassion.

On this path God takes sides. Clearly God is on the side of the oppressed. Clearly the role of God's people is to call out for deliverance, to obey, to have faith. Sometimes God calls them to do weird things, as when Moses had to strike his sister with leprosy. Sometimes God shows power. Sometimes God seems absent, such as when the bricks had to be made without resources. Changing racist systems doesn't happen overnight and doesn't happen without cost and patience. Changing the system takes prayer and intervention by God. Changing the system takes interracial partnerships and obedient action by people.

This story is very meaningful to me. I can relate to Pharaoh's daughter's risk. I long to be on the path following God, preparing for worship.

In order to prepare for worship, Pharaoh's daughter would have had to lay down all of her privilege. In order to join the people following God, she would have had to leave her wealth, her people and her place.

On this path, my privilege as a white person is nothing to me. Sometimes, as for the rich ruler, white privilege is an obstacle—something that would call me back into the palace and away from God. It is not something to be guarded. Sometimes my privilege is something God has given me to spend on behalf of those who do not have it.

When I'm spending my privilege for others, speaking up for them or confronting an evil that everybody has been ignoring, I am often terrified. Sometimes I think I'll be fired; sometimes I fear that I'll lose my white friends. I struggle with all sorts of real or imagined fears—the heritage and call of white racism. But God's call is clear: to follow, into the desert.

Making the Just Community Real

Part of God's transformation in our lives is to mobilize us into action on behalf of others. Some of us are easily stirred to actions of justice. Others of us will be propelled into a cause only if we have been personally affected by the injustice.

Sympathy is the first level of caring about others. It is a fine starting place but a poor ending place. Jesus' call is to *compassion.* If we invite Jesus into our sympathy, he will teach us the way of compassion. Compassion is much more dangerous, because we don't know where it will lead us. In compassion we give our heart away like Nehemiah and Pharoah's daughter, and we must follow our heart. In Scripture, compassion leads to advocacy. Love without action is empty. Love in action on behalf of others is central to Jesus' kingdom.

Advocacy is the process of walking in the shoes of others and then letting their experiences of injustice move us to action on their behalf. Advocacy is not self-righteous; it is our courageous alignment with those who are oppressed or in need. You don't need to have the right answers or even know what course of action to take. Sometimes our mere presence as white people who are aligned with the oppressed can bring attention to the problem. Once you are aligned, God will meet you there, and together the group will receive the wisdom you need for the next steps.

As people of the kingdom, we should expect that Jesus will lead us into compassion and advocacy. Keep your eyes open to these opportunities, and do not be surprised when the door opens.

Questions for Reflection

1. Have you ever benefited from someone's advocacy? When did someone go to bat for you? How did that feel?
2. What does it feel like to be sympathetic with someone who is being wronged? How do you know when your sympathy has turned into compassion?
3. Think of a time when your compassion led you to become an advocate for someone. What did it take to mobilize you as an advocate?
4. Do you see yourself as someone who has access to resources or power? Give an example.

Next Steps

1. Make a habit of reading articles once a month about the issues facing your

ethnic minority friends. What are the people of color around you up against on your campus? in your city? What is their story? What do they pray about? Pray for them, and ask God to show you what he is doing in their midst.

2. As you read and pray, ask your friends of color what they think about these issues. Learn from them and with them. Pay particular attention to how different ethnic minority communities view and respond to national events in which race is an issue.
3. Focus is important for making an impact. Ask God to give you an area of injustice or oppression to care about and advocate against.
4. Read books on justice and injustice. Randy White's *Journey to the Center of the City,* for example, will inspire and help equip you for being a person of God's justice.

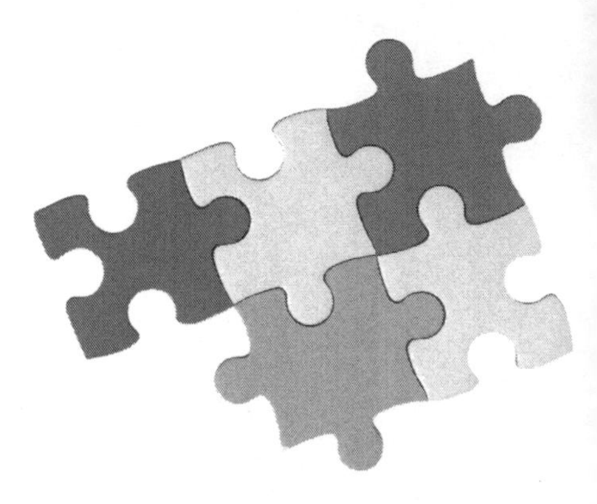

Conclusion

THE WAY, THE TRUTH AND THE LIFE

Paula Harris

Our racism is simultaneously the worst we have ever done and the pointer to the best we could do. We can never undo it, never fully restore it, never heal the people we have wounded. This is why Scripture teaches us that true religion is to "do justice . . . love kindness, and . . . walk humbly with your God" (Mic 6:8). It can also be stated as "Be peace and do justice."

Doug and I have told you many stories, some of suffering and some of love. Richard Rohr writes: "The path of prayer/love and the path of suffering seem to be the two Great Paths of transformation. Suffering seems to get our attention; love and prayer seem to get our heart and our passion."[1] I believe these two paths are really two faces of the one path Jesus leads us on. The face of prayer and love, or love and prayer, will finally lead us into suffering and self-denial. There is no love that does not lay itself down for the other.

In my priest's last sermon before retiring, he said, "Love is the ability to feel passion about the good of another, to prefer the other before yourself, to feel alive and feel joyful in the presence of the other. Love is characterized by passion, commitment and involvement; these are the three great characteristics of love."[2]

Likewise, and in the opposite direction, the path of suffering, if accepted in and through prayer, if redeemed by God, leads ultimately to love. When we suffer and obey God, we encounter the call to forgive. To be forgiven, to follow Christ into the presence of God, we must also forgive. To be loved, we must also learn to love.

Human reality has a cruciform shape. The direction of our souls and spirits, the only path to God, is the shape of the cross, the path of Christ.

> God is to be found in *all things,* even and most especially in the painful, tragic, and sinful things, exactly where we do not want to look for God. The crucifixion of the God-Man is at the same moment the worst thing in human history and the best thing in human history.[3]

As the apostle Paul puts it in Philippians, after describing the fruit of enduring hardship (1:12-26) and the hope set before us (1:27-30), the path of Christ is to serve like Christ (2:1-11), to be "poured out" in love like Paul, Timothy and Epaphroditus (2:17-30).[4] Here is true righteousness, Paul teaches, not in works, not in the law—in other words, not in human religion (3:1-9). True righteousness is not in blood, not in race, not in tribal community (3:1-7). Whatever good these offer, Paul says, he counts as loss. He sees these things as garbage, compared to knowing Christ. "I want to know Christ and the power of his resurrection and the sharing of his sufferings by becoming like him in his death" (3:10).

What is Christ's model? Where is the place we will find joy? Where will we find true love? Where can we experience godly multiracial community? The way is to "in humility regard others as better than yourselves. Let each of you look not to your own interests, but to the interests of others" (Phil 2:3-4).

Like Christ Jesus, white people have certain equality and power. Like Christ, let us also not regard equality or power or glory as things to grasp for, but let us empty ourselves, and take on the form of *slaves* (2:5-7). Can we do that truly, in our communities that bear his name? Let us white people, if we are his followers, humble ourselves and be obedient to God, even unto death (2:8). This is the only path for Christ-followers. Human reality, spiritual reality, has this cruciform shape.

We can choose it. We can enter the path by following Jesus into suffering, by following Jesus into prayer, into love. They all take us the same place: to the cross.

Or we can wait for it to come to us. Especially as Americans, and as whites, we want things to turn out easy. We medicate our smallest pains. But any pain, any suffering, may teach us to seek God. It can teach us to pray, to forgive, to love. It may not even be our own suffering. We may be so moved by the suffering of those nearby or far away that it leads us to prayer and love. However, suffering may not come to us in this life. God may not give us suffering. We may choose to ignore others' suffering and experience mostly the goodness of human life. We have that choice. But even then, the path of the cross will come to us on the last day, when we face Jesus in the new kingdom. We can seek it, we can stumble on it, or we can deny it, but this is the way.

Jesus said, "I am *the way,* and the truth, and the life. No one comes to the Father except through me" (Jn 14:6, emphasis mine). It is through this path of love, prayer and the suffering of Jesus that we are restored. Through Christ, we are released from our sin into the presence of God. By modeling our life on Jesus and walking obediently on Jesus' path, we are released from our racism into the life of the multiethnic church of God.

"In Christ," Paul writes in Ephesians, we become "holy and blameless before [God] in love" (Eph 1:4). Because of Christ, people of color are often able to forgive us and receive us as brothers and sisters. In Christ Jesus, and by following Jesus' way, we whites who have been estranged from others, and estranged from God, have been brought near.

> He is our peace; in his flesh he has made both groups into one and has broken down the dividing wall, that is, the hostility between us. He has abolished the law with its commandments and ordinances, that he might create in himself one new humanity in place of the two, . . . and might reconcile both groups to God in one body through the cross. (Eph 2:14-16)

The place of truth and unity at the beginning of the world, in Eden's garden, was relating to God, worshiping God and receiving God's words as true so that we might obey them (Gen 2—3). The Fall irrevocably changed that. Divisions, injustice, personal racism and systemic racism exist, and God longs to transform them. The power of the cross is sufficient to restore us and give us strength to respond like Zacchaeus, giving our money away, or like the community leaders in Acts 6, constructing a new distribution system. The place of truth and unity at the end is the same—relating to God, worshiping God together, receiving and confessing God's words as true (Rev 15:3-4)—but it is radically transformed. Every race is there. Every ethnic group worships God.

This is what we are waiting for. This must be what we are building together in the church. The path to it is the path of believing in Jesus as truth, following Jesus as the way and living like Jesus as true life.

Notes

Why This Book?

[1]Martin Luther King Jr., "I Have a Dream," speech delivered on the steps of the Lincoln Memorial in Washington, D.C., on August 28, 1963, available at <http://www.stanford.edu/group/King/publications/speeches/address_at_march_on_washington.pdf>.

[2]InterVarsity Christian Fellowship/USA was founded in 1941 and serves students on about six hundred college and university campuses around the United States. For more information, please visit the website at <www.intervarsity.org>.

[3]Feel free to contact us: Doug_Schaupp@ivstaff.org and PHarris@ivcf.org.

[4]Paula Rothenberg, "How It Happened: Race and Gender Issues in U.S. Law," in *Race, Class and Gender in the United States: An Integrated Study,* ed. Paula S. Rothenberg, 2nd ed. (New York: St. Martin's, 1992), pp. 239, 264.

[5]See, for example, Benjamin DeMott, *The Trouble with Friendship: Why Americans Can't Think Straight About Race* (New York: Atlantic Monthly Press, 1995).

[6]The Urbana Student Mission Convention is a triennial conference sponsored by InterVarsity Christian Fellowship for the purpose of helping students understand God's mission to the world and consider how they could contribute in missions. For more information, see <www.urbana.org>.

Chapter 1: Stumbling into Encounter

[1]I first heard this "seeker" and "stumbler" language from Alex Van Riesen in 1990 as he taught on this passage.

Chapter 2: Giving Your Heart Away

[1]In Kenya people speak Swahili and English, among other languages—not Portuguese.

[2]E. Thomas Brewster and Elizabeth S. Brewster, *Bonding and the Missionary Task: Establishing a Sense of Belonging* (Pasadena, Calif.: Lingua House, 1982), pp. 4-5.

Chapter 3: Making and Keeping Friendships with People of Color

[1]Miroslav Volf, *Exclusion and Embrace: A Theological Exploration of Identity, Otherness and Reconciliation* (Nashville: Abingdon, 1996), p. 141.

[2]Ibid., p. 142.

[3]Ibid., pp. 143-44.

Chapter 4: Going Deeper in Crosscultural Friendships

[1]Read Ruth 2—4 for yourself to see what great things come out of Ruth's clinging to Naomi.

[2]Jesus also addresses the flip side of conflict resolution. Sometimes I am the one who has been offended (Mt 18), but sometimes I am the one who has offended someone else (Mt 5:23-24).

It doesn't matter if I have been on the giving or receiving end of the impasse. I am called to heal the relationship, period.

Chapter 5: What Does the Bible Say About Displacement?

[1]It had taken a crisis to stir the disciples in Jerusalem to advance the vision by extending themselves to the Samaritans. "Now those who were scattered went from place to place, proclaiming the word" (Acts 8:4). Amazing ministry broke forth in Acts 8, but it was only because God used a wave of persecution to mobilize his people.

[2]This word can be translated either "Greeks" or "Hellenists." (Hellenists are international Jews, which means they are ethnically Jewish but were born in Gentile countries. Greeks are entirely different.) Later in the chapter we see that this development in Antioch is shocking enough to require an investigation from the Jerusalem leaders. What kind of ethnic crisis in Antioch would stir the Jerusalem leaders to the point of wondering if this movement was of God or not? Since Hellenists had already been reached in Jerusalem, merely reaching Hellenists in Antioch would not require a Jerusalem investigation. But reaching Greeks would challenge the Jerusalem worldview.

[3]These Hellenists had been born in an international context and thus had prior crosscultural experiences. The gospel broke forth from an all-Jewish context through the lives of bicultural Jews. Likewise, Paula and I are deeply indebted to courageous bicultural white people who have paved the way before us on this journey of displacement. We need bicultural role models to take us out of our comfort zone and show us what love can look like across ethnic lines.

[4]Church growth thinkers cannot fathom God's ability to build a cross-ethnic church like this one, where relational displacement is normal. Peter Wagner, a major church growth theorist, concedes in his commentary on Acts that his theory cannot allow for a cross-ethnic church in Antioch, so he is forced to impose his worldview onto the text. "What meaningful social interaction the Gentile and the Jewish churches in Antioch might have had is unknown. But if what we know about intercultural communication applied then as it does now, whatever social interaction they might have had with each other would have been a secondary social relationship. Their primary relationships would have been with fellow Jews or fellow Gentiles" (C. Peter Wagner, *Acts of the Holy Spirit* [Ventura, Calif.: Regal, 2000], pp. 249-50).

[5]"Table fellowship" is the term used to describe intimate community between friends. It is the type of reclining around a meal that Jesus practiced with his disciples (see Jn 13:23-25).

[6]For example, in Galatians 2:11-14, Peter is pulling back from practicing table fellowship with Gentile Christians. His aloofness from the Gentiles stokes the flames of an ethnic rift in the church. When Paul sees this, he demands that Peter change his ways and renew his commitment to displacing himself for the sake of the Gentiles. And in Ephesians 2:11-22 Jews and Gentiles are exhorted toward unity, called to see how Jesus "has made both groups into one" (v. 14).

[7]Records indicate that the Jewish community represented 10 percent of the entire Roman Empire.

Chapter 6: Can White Boys Hoop?

[1]Dr. Metoyer now is head pastor of ACTS, A Church That Studies, in Santa Monica, California.

[2]This story has a nice ending, but often it is messier than this. And the ethnic minority communities that receive us as learners can pay a high price for "educating" us. We should be sensitive to their experience of us in the midst of our displacement.

Chapter 7: The Point of No Return

[1]The safety bar releases only for white people on the roller coaster of displacement. Often our ethnic minority friends don't have a choice about displacing themselves. They are a minority in a world that is not their own.

[2]Michael Emerson and Christian Smith, *Divided by Faith: Evangelical Religion and the Problem of Race in America* (New York: Oxford University Press, 2000), p. 132.

[3]My rough paraphrase of Mark 8:34.

[4]Henri J. M. Nouwen, Donald P. McNeill and Douglas A. Morrison, *Compassion: A Reflection on the Christian Life* (New York: Doubleday, 1982), p. 4.

[5]Richard J. Foster, *Prayer* (San Francisco: HarperCollins, 1992), p. 48.

[6]"The magic year, say our national number crunchers, appears to be 2056, when European Americans will be less than 50 percent of the population" (Paul Tokunaga, *Invitation to Lead: Guidance for Emerging Asian American Leaders* [Downers Grove, Ill.: InterVarsity Press, 2003], p. 173).

Chapter 8: Being Colorblind

[1]This was six years after the L.A. riots, and there was still a well-known rift between these two ethnic communities.

[2]Stanley K. Inouye, *Foundations for Asian American Ministry* (Monrovia, Calif.: Iwa, 2001), p. 19.

[3]Ibid., p. 21.

[4]J. Robert Clinton and Paul D. Stanley, *Connecting* (Colorado Springs: NavPress, 1992), p. 197.

Chapter 9: Living in the Truth About White History and Racism

[1]Beverly Daniel Tatum, *Why Are All the Black Kids Sitting Together in the Cafeteria? And Other Conversations About Race* (New York: BasicBooks, 1997), p. 7.

[2]Ibid., pp. 11-12.

[3]The Ku Klux Klan is a terrorist white supremacy group. It is infamous for being a secret society of white men who violently terrorize people of color by burning crosses, threatening families, beating and lynching leaders, and holding parades to demonstrate their power, all the while dressed in white sheets and hidden under white masks. The usual targets of the Klan are African Americans, but Mexicans, Jews, Catholics, women and "traitors to the white race" have also been victims. The KKK was founded in 1865, shortly after the slaves were freed in the United States, and had a resurgence beginning in 1965 in reaction to the achievements of the civil rights movement.

[4]The "aware/overt" category and the other categories of racism come from Jenny Yamato, "Something About the Subject Makes It Hard to Name," in *Race, Class and Gender in the United States: An Integrated Study*, ed. Paula S. Rothenberg, 2nd ed. (New York: St. Martin's, 1992), p. 59.

[5]Paul Kivel, *Uprooting Racism: How White People Can Work for Racial Justice* (Gabriola Island, B.C., Canada: New Society, 2002), p. 101, emphasis added.

[6]Patty Loew, *Indian Nations in Wisconsin: Histories of Endurance and Renewal* (Madison: Wisconsin Historical Society Press, 2001), pp. 40, 46, 41.

[7]Ho Chunk negotiator Little Elk said, "Do you want *our* country? Yours is much larger than ours. . . . Do you want *our* wigwams? You live in palaces. My fathers, what can be your motive?" Quoted in ibid., pp. 44-45.

[8]Kivel, *Uprooting Racism*, p. 101.

[9]Ibid.

[10]Yamato, "Something About the Subject," p. 59.

Chapter 10: Open the Parachute

[1]C. S. Lewis, *The Weight of Glory and Other Essays* (San Francisco: HarperSanFrancisco, 2001), pp. 45-46.

[2]The NRSV translates the same Greek word, *prosopolepsia,* as "favoritism" in verse 1 and as "partiality" in verse 9 (James Strong, *Strong's Exhaustive Concordance, Greek Dictionary* [Grand Rapids: Baker, 1991], pp. 4382, 4380).

[3]Lisa Harper, "The Colors of Us," 2001, <http://www.intervarsity.org/socal/assets/multiethnic/beingwhite.htm>.

[4]Race Matters is an InterVarsity community-healing event in which we bring to the surface the hidden pain and biases in multiethnic communities and work toward reconciliation and advocacy. See our Race Matters Handbook at <http://www.intervarsity.org/socal/assets/multiethnic/beingwhite.htm>.

[5]The names in this story have been changed.

Chapter 11: Who Are We? Who Do They Say We Are?

[1]Kathy Dobie, "The Unbearable Whiteness of Being," *Salon*, July 19, 1999, <www.salon.com/news/feature/1999/07/19/white>.

[2]I use the term *antiracist* for a person who is clearly committed to understanding and confessing his or her own racism as well as understanding and deconstructing the racist systems he or she participates in. To learn more, see Joseph Barndt, *Dismantling Racism: The Continuing Challenge to White America* (Minneapolis: Augsburg Fortress, 1991), or Paul Kivel, *Uprooting Racism: How White People Can Work for Racial Justice* (Gabriola Island, B.C., Canada: New Society, 2002).

[3]Of course in an all-white mixed-ethnicity group, such as European and American whites, I would experience the culture clash and increased self-awareness that Doug calls 3-D glasses.

[4]Birgit Brander et al., eds., *The Making and Unmaking of Whiteness* (Durham, N.C.: Duke University Press, 2001).

[5]"From a blend of Wolof *honq,* 'red, pink, of light complexion' and *hunky,*" *The American Heritage Dictionary of the English Language,* 4th ed. (Boston: Houghton Mifflin, 2000), s.v. "honky."

[6]For more information on how this name functioned, and the history itself, see Dee Brown, *Bury My Heart at Wounded Knee: An Indian History of the American West* (New York: Henry Holt, 1970).

[7]George Tinker, *Missionary Conquest: The Gospel and Native American Cultural Genocide* (Minneapolis: Fortress, 1993), p. 4.

[8]Jane Lazarre, *Beyond the Whiteness of Whiteness: Memoir of a White Mother of Black Sons* (Durham, N.C.: Duke University Press, 1996), p. 32, italics in the original.

[9]"A disparaging term for a foreign woman in Latin America, especially an American or English woman. From Spanish, feminine of *gringo,*" *American Heritage Dictionary,* s.v. "gringa."

[10]Ruth Frankenburg, *White Women, Race Matters: The Social Construction of Whiteness* (Minneapolis: University of Minnesota Press, 1993), p. 632, italics in the original.

[11]For example, see Noel Ignatiev, "The Point Is Not to Interpret Whiteness but to Abolish It," *Race Traitor,* 1997, p. 1, <www.postfun.com/racetraitor/features/thepoint.html>, or George Lipsitz, *The Possessive Investment in Whiteness: How White People Benefit from Identity Politics* (Philadelphia: Temple University Press, 1998).

[12]Frankenburg, *White Women, Race Matters,* p. 632.
[13]Noel Ignatiev, *How the Irish Became White* (New York: Routledge, 1995), p. 10.

Chapter 12: Can God Redeem White Culture?

[1]I am indebted to Ray Bakke for his insights into God's redemption of the city. I heard him lecture on this topic at Occidental College in 1987.
[2]The topic of the fall and redemption of cultures is a complicated subject, worthy of an entire book. For our purposes here, it is sufficient to say that we agree with the orthodox Christian position that every culture is warped and fallen, none better or worse than the next, all in need of the redemption of Christ.
[3]While there are some international commonalities among white people on various continents, here I will focus on white values in the United States.
[4]There are many variables that make it difficult to nail down the strengths of our Anglo-American heritage. In an era of globalization, white culture has been exported, blended and morphed so that it is present in many continents and in many forms. See Thomas Friedman, *The Lexus and the Olive Tree* (New York: Anchor, 1999), pp. 367-78, for a summary of some of these variables.
[5]Another way to understand our cultural values is to look at ourselves through the eyes of another culture. For a helpful chart comparing American and Puerto Rican values, see Orlando Crespo, *Being Latino in Christ* (Downers Grove, Ill.: InterVarsity Press, 2003), p. 89.
[6]Robert Bellah et al., *Habits of the Heart* (Berkeley: University of California Press, 1985), p. 142.
[7]Eric H. F. Law, *The Wolf Shall Lie Down with the Lamb: A Spirituality for Multicultural Leadership* (St. Louis, Mo.: Chalice, 1993), p. 21.
[8]Harry Saal, quoted in Friedman, *Lexus and the Olive Tree,* p. 370.
[9]Bellah et al., *Habits of the Heart,* pp. 41-44.
[10]Ibid., p. 65.
[11]Richard Brookhiser, *The Way of the WASP: How It Made America and How It Can Save It . . . So to Speak* (New York: Free Press, 1991), p. 31.
[12]The rise of rampant materialism and credit card debt in the United States over the past several decades has undermined much of this good value. However, we still see enough of it in us to include it here.
[13]Garry Wills, *Certain Trumpets: The Nature of Leadership* (New York: Simon & Schuster, 1994), pp. 152-54.
[14]Brookhiser, *Way of the WASP,* p. 31. For an account of the limitations of this commitment to fairness, see Bellah et al., *Habits of the Heart,* pp. 25-26.

Chapter 13: Finding Our White Identity in Christ

[1]A philosophical rationale for remaining clueless is the traditional American self-concept that we are supposed to be a "melting pot" for immigrants. As long as the melting pot is our vision, there is no need for any of us to try to understand the journeys that others have walked. We assume the suffering of our neighbors will melt away.
[2]See Dietrich Bonhoeffer, *The Cost of Discipleship* (New York: Macmillan, 1956), chap. 1, for an excellent description of the problem of cheap grace. The quote here is from p. 37.
[3]It is crucial that we not become reductionistic in our understanding of the kingdom of God. But while we recognize that Jesus' kingdom is much more than living out these five values, these identity values have special importance for white people as we live as Jesus' followers

in this multiethnic world.

[4]Her name has been changed, though I did receive my friend's permission to tell this story.

Chapter 14: I Want a Friend, She Wants Justice

[1]Martin Luther King Jr., "Letter from Birmingham Jail," p. 1, at <http://www.stanford.edu/group/King/popular_requests/frequentdocs/birmingham.pdf>.

[2]Equal Justice USA, "How Racism Riddles the U.S. Death Penalty," quoted at <http://www.quixote.org/ej/moratorium_now/broch_race.html>.

[3]Statistics from <http://www.census.gov/hhes/income/income02/3yr_avg_race.html>.

[4]Craig Keener says, "Zacchaeus could have become rich without cheating, but it seems that he had cheated anyway" (Keener, *The IVP Bible Background Commentary: New Testament* [Downers Grove, Ill.: InterVarsity Press, 1993], p. 240).

Chapter 15: Responsibility Is Not a Four-Letter Word

[1]Sins of *omission* happen in the moments when we could extend ourselves in love but instead hold back. We neglect to obey God and do the right thing. Sins of *commission* are the more obvious ones, negative behaviors that are visible to all.

[2]Her name has been changed.

[3]For another perspective on this process of growing in godly responsibility, please see Orlando Crespo's seven point process in *Being Latino in Christ* (Downers Grove, Ill.: InterVarsity Press, 2003), pp. 96-99.

Chapter 16: Betraying White Privilege, Plundering White Power

[1]In Hebrew the word means "drawn out"; literally he is drawn out of the water, but figuratively it forecasts his drawing his people out of Egypt. In Egyptian the word means "is born," possibly giving him a dynastic identity as a prince of Egypt. Elaine Phillips, "Exodus," in *The IVP Women's Bible Commentary*, ed. Catherine Clark Kroeger and Mary Evans (Downers Grove, Ill.: InterVarsity Press, 2002), p. 30.

[2]John H. Walton, Victor H. Matthews and Mark W. Chavalas, *The IVP Bible Background Commentary: Old Testament* (Downers Grove, Ill.: InterVarsity Press, 2000), p. 78.

[3]This image, the outstretched arm, was one usually reserved for Pharaoh, to show his power accomplishing mighty acts. See ibid., p. 81.

[4]Martin Luther King Jr., "Letter from Birmingham Jail," p. 1, at <http://www.stanford.edu/group/King/popular_requests/frequentdocs/birmingham.pdf>.

Conclusion: The Way, the Truth and the Life

[1]Richard Rohr, *Everything Belongs: The Gift of Contemplative Prayer* (New York: Crossroad, 1999), pp. 16-17.

[2]John Fetterman, sermon delivered at Grace Episcopal Church, Madison, Wis., June 30, 2002.

[3]Rohr, *Everything Belongs*, p. 151.

[4]Craig Keener, *The IVP Bible Background Commentary: New Testament* (Downers Grove, Ill.: InterVarsity Press, 1993), pp. 558-62.

Bibliography

Appiah, K. Anthony, and Amy Gutmann. *Color Conscious: The Political Morality of Race*. Princeton, N.J.: Princeton University Press, 1996.

Ball, Edward. *Slaves in the Family*. New York: Farrar, Straus and Giroux, 1998.

Barndt, Joseph. *Dismantling Racism: The Continuing Challenge to White America*. Minneapolis: Augsburg Fortress, 1991.

Bellah, Robert, et al. *Habits of the Heart*. Berkeley: University of California Press, 1985.

Bonhoeffer, Dietrich. *The Cost of Discipleship*. New York: Macmillan, 1956.

Brander, Birgit, et al., eds. *The Making and Unmaking of Whiteness*. Durham, N.C.: Duke University Press, 2001.

Brewster, E. Thomas, and Elizabeth S. Brewster. *Bonding and the Missionary Task: Establishing a Sense of Belonging*. Pasadena, Calif.: Lingua House, 1982.

Brookhiser, Richard. *The Way of the WASP: How It Made America and How It Can Save It . . . So to Speak*. New York: Free Press, 1991.

Brown, Dee. *Bury My Heart at Wounded Knee: An Indian History of the American West*. New York: Henry Holt, 1970.

Carmichael, Alexander. *Carmina Gadelica: Hymns and Incantations*. Edinburgh: Floris, 2001.

Clinton, J. Robert, and Paul D. Stanley. *Connecting*. Colorado Springs: NavPress, 1992.

Crespo, Orlando. *Being Latino in Christ*. Downers Grove, Ill.: InterVarsity Press, 2003.

Delgado, Richard, and Jean Stafancic. *Critical White Studies: Looking Behind the Mirror*. Philadelphia: Temple University Press, 1997.

DeMott, Benjamin. *The Trouble with Friendship: Why Americans Can't Think Straight About Race*. New York: Atlantic Monthly Press, 1995.

Dobie, Kathy. "The Unbearable Whiteness of Being." *Salon*, July 19, 1999. <www.salon.com/news/feature/1999/07/19/white>.

Ellis, Carl, Jr. *Free at Last*. Rev. ed. Downers Grove, Ill.: InterVarsity Press, 1996.

Emerson, Michael O., and Christian Smith. *Divided by Faith: Evangelical Religion and the Problem of Race in America*. New York: Oxford University Press, 2000.

Foster, Richard J. *Prayer*. San Francisco: HarperCollins, 1992.

Frankenburg, Ruth. *White Women, Race Matters: The Social Construction of Whiteness.* Minneapolis: University of Minnesota Press, 1993.

Friedman, Thomas. *The Lexus and the Olive Tree: Understanding Globalization.* New York: Anchor, 1999.

Gen, Jish. *Typical American.* New York: Plume Contemporary Fiction, 1992.

Golden, Marita, and Susan Richards Shreve, eds. *Skin Deep: Black Women and White Women Write About Race.* New York: Anchor, 1995.

Harper, Lisa. "The Colors of Us." 2001. <http://www.intervarsity.org/socal/assets/multiethnic/beingwhite.htm>.

Hegi, Ursula. *Tearing the Silence: Being German in America.* New York: Simon & Schuster, 1997.

———. *The Vision of Emma Blau.* New York: Simon & Schuster, 2002.

Ignatiev, Noel. *How the Irish Became White.* New York: Routledge, 1995.

———. "The Point Is Not to Interpret Whiteness But to Abolish It." *Race Traitor,* 1997. <http://www.postfun.com/racetraitor/features/thepoint.html>.

Inouye, Stanley K. "Core Values/Survival Values Diagram." In *Foundations for Asian American Ministry.* Monrovia, Calif.: Iwa, 2001.

Keener, Craig. *The IVP Bible Background Commentary: New Testament.* Downers Grove, Ill.: InterVarsity Press, 1993.

King, Martin Luther, Jr. "I Have a Dream." Text available at <http://www.stanford.edu/group/King/publications/speeches/address_at_march_on_washington.pdf>.

———. "Letter from Birmingham Jail." Text available at <http://www.stanford.edu/group/King/popular_requests/frequentdocs/birmingham.pdf>.

———. *The Peaceful Warrior.* New York: Pocket Books, 1968.

Kivel, Paul. *Uprooting Racism: How White People Can Work for Racial Justice.* Gabriola Island, B.C., Canada: New Society, 2002.

Kochman, Thomas. *Black and White Styles in Conflict.* Chicago: University of Chicago Press, 1981.

Kroeger, Catherine Clark, and Mary Evans, eds. *The IVP Women's Bible Commentary.* Downers Grove, Ill.: InterVarsity Press, 2002.

Law, Eric H. F. *The Wolf Shall Lie Down with the Lamb: A Spirituality for Multicultural Leadership.* St. Louis, Mo.: Chalice, 1993.

Lazarre, Jane. *Beyond the Whiteness of Whiteness: Memoir of a White Mother of Black Sons.* Durham, N.C.: Duke University Press, 1996.

Lederach, John Paul. *The Journey Toward Reconciliation.* Scottdale, Penn.: Herald, 1999.

Lewis, C. S. *The Weight of Glory and Other Essays.* San Francisco: HarperSanFrancisco, 2001.

Lipsitz, George. *The Possessive Investment in Whiteness: How White People Benefit from Identity Politics.* Philadelphia: Temple University Press, 1998.

Loew, Patty. *Indian Nations in Wisconsin: Histories of Endurance and Renewal.* Madison: Wisconsin Historical Society Press, 2001.

Loewen, James. *Lies My Teacher Told Me: Everything Your American History Textbook Got Wrong.* New York: Touchstone, 1995.

Nouwen, Henri J. M., Donald P. McNeill and Douglas A. Morrison. *Compassion: A Reflection on the Christian Life.* New York: Doubleday, 1982.

Perkins, Spencer, and Chris Rice. *More Than Equals.* Downers Grove, Ill.: InterVarsity Press, 1993.

Raybon, Patricia. *My First White Friend: Confessions on Race, Love and Forgiveness.* New York: Penguin, 1996.

Roediger, David. *Colored White: Transcending the Racial Past.* Berkeley: University of California Press, 2002.

Rohr, Richard. *Everything Belongs: The Gift of Contemplative Prayer.* New York: Crossroad, 1999.

Rothenberg, Paula S., ed. *Race, Class and Gender in the United States: An Integrated Study.* 2nd ed. New York: St. Martin's, 1992.

Tatum, Beverly Daniel. *Why Are All the Black Kids Sitting Together in the Cafeteria? And Other Conversations About Race.* New York: BasicBooks, 1997.

Tinker, George. *Missionary Conquest: The Gospel and Native American Cultural Genocide.* Minneapolis: Fortress, 1993.

Tokunaga, Paul. *Invitation to Lead: Guidance for Emerging Asian American Leaders.* Downers Grove, Ill.: InterVarsity Press, 2003.

Volf, Miroslav. *Exclusion and Embrace: A Theological Exploration of Identity, Otherness and Reconciliation.* Nashville: Abingdon, 1996.

Wagner, C. Peter. *Acts of the Holy Spirit.* Ventura, Calif.: Regal, 2000.

Walton, John H., Victor H. Matthews and Mark W. Chavalas. *The IVP Bible Background Commentary: Old Testament.* Downers Grove, Ill.: InterVarsity Press, 2000.

White, Randy. *Journey to the Center of the City.* Downers Grove, Ill.: InterVarsity Press, 1996.

Wills, Garry. *Certain Trumpets: The Nature of Leadership.* New York: Simon & Schuster, 1994.

Washington, Raleigh, and Glen Kehrein. *Breaking Down Walls.* Chicago: Moody Press, 1993.